DM 120,—

D1735255

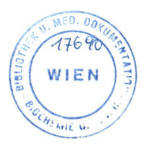

17690
WIEN
BIBLIOTHEK U. MED. DOKUMENTATIO.
BIOCHEMIE U.

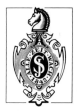

The Epstein-Barr Virus

Edited by M. A. Epstein and B. G. Achong

With 72 Figures and 29 Tables

Springer-Verlag
Berlin Heidelberg New York 1979

M.A. Epstein, M.A., M.D., Ph.D., D.Sc., F.R.C. Path., F.R.S.
B.G. Achong, M.B., B.Ch., B.A.O., M.D.

Department of Pathology, The Medical School, University of Bristol, University Walk, Bristol BS8 1TD (England)

ISBN 3-540-09272-2 Springer-Verlag Berlin Heidelberg New York
ISBN 0-387-09272-2 Springer-Verlag New York Heidelberg Berlin

Library of Congress Cataloging in Publication Data. Main entry under title: The Epstein-Barr virus. Bibliography: p. Includes index. 1. Epstein-Barr virus. 2. Lymphocyte transformation. 3. Viral genetics. 4. Viral carcinogenesis. I. Epstein, Michael Anthony. II. Achong, B.G., 1928–. QR400.2.E68E65 616.01'94 79-4370.

This work is subject to copyright. All rights are reserved, whether the whole or part of the material is concerned, specifically those of translation, reprinting, re-use of illustrations, broadcasting, reproduction by photocopying machine or similar means, and storage in data banks.
Under § 54 of the German Copyright Law where copies are made for other than private use, a fee is payable to the publisher, the amount of the fee to be determined by agreement with the publisher.

© by Springer-Verlag Berlin Heidelberg 1979
Printed in Germany.

The use of registered names, trademarks, etc. in this publication does not imply, even in the absence of a specific statement, than such names are exempt from the relevant protective laws and regulations and therefore free for general use.

Typesetting, printing and bookbinding: Oscar Brandstetter Druckerei KG, 62 Wiesbaden. 2123/3140-543210

Preface

The Epstein-Barr virus was discovered 15 years ago. Since that time an immense body of information has been accumulated on this agent which has come to assume great significance in many different fields of biological science. Thus, the virus has very special relevance in human medicine and oncology, in tumor virology, in immunology, and in molecular virology, since it is the cause of infectious mononucleosis and also the first human cancer virus, etiologically related to endemic Burkitt's lymphoma and probably to nasopharyngeal carcinoma. In addition, continuous human lymphoid cell lines initiated and maintained by the transforming function of the virus genome provide a laboratory tool with wide and ever-growing applications.

Innumerable papers on the Epstein-Barr virus have appeared over recent years and reports of work with this agent now constitute a veritable flood. The present book provides the first and only comprehensive, authoritative over-view of all aspects of the virus by authors who have been the original and major contributors in their particular disciplines.

A complete and up-to-date survey of this unique and important agent is thus provided which should be of great interest to experts, teachers, and students engaged in cancer research, virology, immunology, molecular biology, epidemiology, and cell culture. Where topics have been dealt with from more than one of these viewpoints, some inevitable overlap and duplication has resulted; although this has been kept to a minimum, it has been retained in some places because of positive usefulness.

M. A. Epstein
B. G. Achong

List of Contents

B. Hampar

G. Henle and W. Henle

M. A. Epstein and B. G. Achong

Key to Abbreviations

ADLC	antibody-dependent lymphocytotoxicity
B cell/lymphocyte	bone marrow-derived lymphocyte
BL	Burkitt's lymphoma
BUDR	5-bromodeoxyuridine
CF	complement fixing/fixation
CMV	cytomegalovirus
CPV	carp pox virus
DEAE	diethyl-aminoethyl-dextran
EA	early antigen
EA (D)	early antigen (diffuse)
EA (R)	early antigen (restricted)
EAV	equine abortion virus
EBNA	EBV nuclear antigen
EBV	Epstein-Barr virus
EMA	early membrane antigen
GPHV	guinea pig herpesvirus
HSV	herpes simplex virus
HVA	herpesvirus ateles
HVP	herpesvirus papio
HVS	herpesvirus saimiri
HVT	herpesvirus of turkeys
IBR	infectious bovine rhinotracheitis virus
IF	immunofluorescence
IM	infectious mononucleosis
IUDR	5-iododeoxyuridine
LA	late antigen
LCL	lymphoblastoid cell lines
LHV	Lucké's herpesvirus
LMA	late membrane antigen
LYDMA	lymphocyte-detected membrane antigen
MA	membrane antigen
MATSA	Marek's disease tumor-associated surface antigen
MDV	Marek's disease virus
MPMV	Mason-Pfizer virus
NPC	undifferentiated nasopharyngeal carcinoma
PFU	plaque forming units
p. i.	post inoculation

PRV   pseudorabies virus

T cell/lymphocyte   thymus-dependent lymphocyte
TD_{50} dose of virus transforming 50% of a series of
                            cultures

UV   ultraviolet

VCA   viral capsid antigen
VZV   varicella-zoster virus

List of Contributors

B. G. ACHONG
University of Bristol, Bristol (England)

A. ADAMS
University of Göteborg, Göteborg (Sweden)

Y. BECKER
The Hebrew University, Jerusalem (Israel)

F. DEINHARDT
Ludwig Maximilians-Universität, München (Federal Republic of Germany)

J. DEINHARDT
Ludwig Maximilians-Universität, München (Federal Republic of Germany)

M. A. EPSTEIN
University of Bristol, Bristol (England)

I. ERNBERG
Karolinska Institutet, Stockholm (Sweden)

B. HAMPAR
Frederick Cancer Research Center, Bethesda, MD (USA)

H. ZUR HAUSEN
University of Freiburg, Freiburg (Federal Republic of Germany)

G. HENLE
University of Pennsylvania, Philadelphia, PA (USA)

W. HENLE
University of Pennsylvania, Philadelphia, PA (USA)

G. KLEIN
Karolinska Institutet, Stockholm (Sweden)

G. MILLER
Yale University, New Haven, CT (USA)

K. NILSSON
University of Uppsala, Uppsala (Sweden)

J. S. PAGANO
University of North Carolina, Chapel Hill, NC (USA)

J. H. POPE
Queensland Institute, Brisbane (Australia)

J. E. SHAW
University of North Carolina, Chapel Hill, NC (USA)

J. L. STROMINGER
Harvard Medical School, Boston, MA (USA)

G. DE-THÉ
Faculty of medicine A. Carrel, Lyon and IRSC Villejuif (France)

D. THORLEY-LAWSON
Harvard Medical School, Boston, MA (USA)

1 Introduction: Discovery and General Biology of the Virus

M. A. Epstein and B. G. Achong

Department of Pathology, The Medical School, University of Bristol, University Walk, Bristol BS8 1TD (England)

A. INTRODUCTION

By the beginning of the 1960s viruses causing tumors in animals had been known for more than 50 years (Gross, 1961), but at that time there was no such agent with a convincing etiologic link to human cancer. Since then a remarkable association has been uncovered between a new herpesvirus and malignancy in man; the association has been established by work of many different kinds, but the original discoveries which provided the impetus for this work resulted from experiments undertaken because of clinical and epidemiologic observations on an unusual lymphoma of children in Africa.

The first account of this lymphoma (Burkitt, 1958) attracted little attention. However, in March 1961 Denis Burkitt, then an unknown surgeon working in Uganda, addressed a staff meeting at the Middlesex Hospital Medical School, London (Fig. 1), and presented for the first time outside Africa his pioneer studies which seemed to show that the distribution of the tumor was determined by geographic features affecting climate. That the incidence of what soon came to be known as Burkitt's lymphoma (BL) was influenced by temperature and rainfall suggested at once that some biologic factor was concerned, and of these a climate-dependent arthropod vector seemed the most likely. If an insect or other arthropod were indeed spreading the tumor the further important implication followed that a transmissible agent such as a virus must be involved in causation. It was this exciting hypothesis which was directly responsible for our immediate decision to seek for possible oncogenic viruses in BL material.

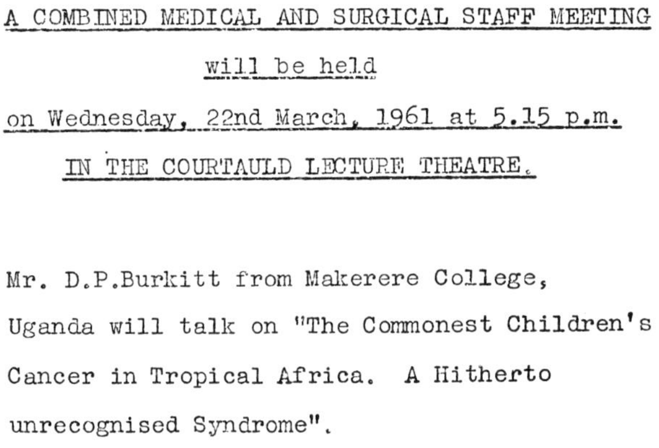

A COMBINED MEDICAL AND SURGICAL STAFF MEETING

will be held

on Wednesday, 22nd March, 1961 at 5.15 p.m.

IN THE COURTAULD LECTURE THEATRE.

Mr. D.P.Burkitt from Makerere College,

Uganda will talk on "The Commonest Children's

Cancer in Tropical Africa. A Hitherto

unrecognised Syndrome".

Fig. 1. Photograph of the original notice announcing a staff meeting at the Middlesex Hospital, London, at which Burkitt gave the first account outside Africa of the clinical and epidemiologic features of the lymphoma which now bears his name. From Epstein, M. A.: Long-term tissue culture of Burkitt's lymphoma cells. In: Burkitt's lymphoma. Burkitt, D. P., Wright, D. H. (eds.). Livingstone, 1970: Courtesy of the editors and publisher

Although the original concept of case-to-case infection mediated by a climate-dependent arthropod vector (Burkitt, 1962 a, b) required revision as epidemiologic information accumulated (Haddow, 1964), other explanations for the role of temperature and rainfall have emerged (Burkitt, 1969) and the idea of an infectious cause has remained constant (Chap. 14).

B. DISCOVERY OF EBV

I. PRELIMINARY INVESTIGATIONS

As part of the various investigations on BL undertaken in our laboratory at the Middlesex Hospital Medical School, virologic studies were of prime importance. BL biopsy samples were deep-frozen immediately after removal and were flown overnight from Uganda to London. On arrival the tumor material was thawed and prepared in many different ways for inoculation into newborn mice, embryonated hen eggs, and test tissue culture systems in order to isolate any viruses which might have been present. However, these early experiments proved uniformly negative and thin sections of tumor samples were therefore searched in the electron microscope in an effort to find unusual viruses which might not be demonstrable by standard biologic isolation procedures; such direct examinations were likewise negative.

It was then considered (Epstein et al., 1964a) that success might be achieved if BL cells from biopsy samples transported at room temperature could be grown in vitro away from host defences so that an otherwise inapparent oncogenic virus might be able to replicate, as happens with cultured cells from certain virus-induced animal tumors (Bonar et al., 1960). Because of this, it was decided that in the further search for virus in BL, high priority should be given to the establishment of lines of the tumor cells capable of growing in continuous long-term culture, even though the prospects for accomplishing this with a lymphoid tumor were unpromising. For, at that time, no member of the human lymphocytic series of cells had been grown as a permanent line in vitro despite repeated efforts ever since the earliest phases of the tissue culture technique (Woodliff, 1964).

II. CULTURE OF BURKITT'S LYMPHOMA CELLS AND FINDING OF THE VIRUS

After a long series of trial methods a successful procedure for culturing BL tumor cells was evolved in the latter part of 1963 and the EB1 line of continuously growing BL-derived lymphoblasts was established (Epstein and Barr, 1964); a full account of both the preliminary trials and the definitive culture technique was given the following year (Epstein and Barr, 1965).

As soon as sufficient material could be spared from the first EB1 cultures, electron microscopy was undertaken; pelleted cells were examined in thin sections, virus particles were observed in a cell within the very first grid square to be searched, and the virus was immediately recognized as a morphologically typical member of the herpes group (Epstein et al., 1964b). When first seen there was naturally no means of knowing which herpesvirus was involved, but it was thought unusual that a member of the herpes family was being carried as an inapparent infection in a continuous human cell line without causing destruction of the cultures. Preliminary biologic tests for herpesviruses were applied to the virus-bearing EB1 cells using embryonated hen eggs, HeLa cells, and young mice inoculated intracerebrally, but in each case the results were negative. When further extensive virologic investigations were also negative (Epstein et al., 1965) it became obvious that the agent was unlike any known herpesvirus since it showed a complete lack of biologic activity in any of the standard test systems. With such uncharacteristic negative attributes it is clear that the virus would not have been readily detected other than with the electron microscope and it is fortunate that the work was going forward in a laboratory where this type of examination was regularly undertaken even when more ordinary biologic tests had failed. Indeed, it would appear that this was the first viral agent to be discovered solely by electron microscopy.

III. CONFIRMATION OF THE VIRUS IN OTHER CELL LINES AND ORIGIN OF ITS DESIGNATION

Following these initial studies, a similar herpesvirus was demonstrated by electron microscopy in numerous further cell lines established from BL tumors occurring in patients from widely separate parts of the world; a similar virus was also found in lymphoblastoid lines established from blood both from normal donors and from patients with leukemia, other cancers, and infectious mononucleosis (IM).

Although the significance of herpesvirus-containing cell lines originating from all these many sources was not understood at the time (Sect. C.I.2 below), the virus itself showed in every case the same inertness in biologic tests as the original agent in the EB1 line of BL cells. As a result, it was recognized that a new and distinct virus was in question and this soon came to be designated as the Epstein-Barr virus (EBV) after the cell line in which it was first found. This early work has been documented and discussed previously (Epstein, 1970; Epstein and Achong, 1973a).

IV. CONFIRMATION OF THE UNIQUENESS OF EBV

In addition to the biologic singularity of EBV, evidence for its immunologic uniqueness was soon forthcoming. Antisera to known herpesviruses did not react in indirect immunofluorescence tests with cells carrying the virus (Henle and Henle, 1966a, b), while artificial antisera raised in rabbits against purified preparations of the virus showed that the herpes agents in several different lymphoid cell lines were identical, as well as quite distinct from other human herpesviruses (Epstein and Achong, 1968a, b). In view of this, it is only natural that later investigations have also firmly established the biochemical uniqueness of EBV (Chaps. 5, 6, 7, and 8).

C. GENERAL BIOLOGY

Despite the confusing presence of EBV in cell lines from healthy people and patients of many kinds (Sect. C.I.2 below), the association of EBV with BL steadily continued to strengthen (Chaps. 4 and 14) and a new and similar association emerged with one other human cancer, nasopharyngeal carcinoma (NPC) (Chaps. 4 and 15). Because of this, investigations on EBV have accelerated year by year and an immense body of information has been accumulated both on it and on its general biologic behavior.

I. INCIDENCE AND EFFECTS OF INFECTION

EBV is transmitted horizontally and infects all human populations (Henle and Henle, 1966 a, b; Moore et al., 1966; Henle and Henle, 1967; Gerber and Rosenblum, 1968; Goldman et al., 1968; Svedmyr and Demissie, 1968; Demissie and Svedmyr, 1969; Pereira et al., 1969; Chap. 4).

Natural primary infection usually takes place in childhood without disease manifestations (Henle and Henle, 1970; Chap. 4), but whatever the circumstances, it is always accompanied by permanent seroconversion and harboring of the virus for the rest of the individual's life. This harboring is manifested, first, as a nonproductive latent infection (Fig. 2) of a small number of circulating lymphocytes, and second, as a productive infection (Fig. 2) somewhere in the oro- or nasopharynx with liberation of infectious virus into the buccal fluid. It is, of course, the infectious virus shed in this way into buccal fluids which is responsible by horizontal transmission for all natural primary infections.

If primary infection is delayed until late adolescence or young adulthood, this event leads to IM in about 50% of cases (Niederman et al., 1970; University Health Physicians et al., 1971; Chap. 13). Delayed natural primary infection is more frequent in the privileged classes of developed societies than in lower socioeconomic groups, thus explaining why IM is commonest among the affluent (Henle and Henle, 1969; Henle and Henle, 1973). In developing countries primary infection affects almost all children before the age of 10 so that very few young adults are susceptible and IM is virtually unknown (Henle and Henle, 1969; Diehl et al., 1969; Chaps. 13 and 18). The size of viral dose and mode of infection, together probably with host physiologic and immunologic state, evidently determine the frequent occurrence of IM in primarily infected young adults in developed countries. The relationship of outbreaks of IM to

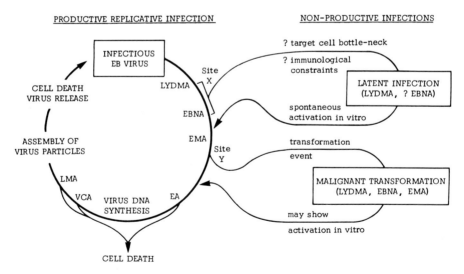

Fig. 2. Antigen expression in cells during various forms of infection by EB virus in vivo. *LYDMA*, lymphocyte-detected membrane antigen; *EBNA*, EBV nuclear antigen; *EMA*, early antigen; *VCA*, viral capsid antigen; *LMA*, late membrane antigen. From Epstein, M. A., Achong, B. G. (1977b): Courtesy of the editor and publisher

kissing among young people has long been recognized (Hoagland, 1955) and can now be understood as being due to the ingestion by previously uninfected individuals, when kissing, of large doses of EBV shed orally by seropositive healthy subjects who usually have never shown signs of their original primary infection. This mechanism forms a contrast to the situation in young children where more indirect methods of spread operate, probably being responsible for the smaller infecting doses which seem to play a part in determining inapparent infections without symptoms (Henle and Henle, 1970). In this context it should be noted that although most IM occurs in those aged 15 to 25 where EBV is usually transmitted by kissing, primary infection in children and in older adults can very occasionally also be accompanied by the fully developed disease (Horwitz et al., 1976; Ginsburg et al., 1977).

1. Virus in the Buccal Fluid

The incidence of people shedding EBV from the mouth varies in different populations and under different conditions. In Western communities $\sim 20\%$ of healthy seropositive individuals are shedders at any one time (Golden et al., 1973; Chang et al, 1973), but the rate rises significantly to 50% of seropositives among those subjected to immunosuppressive therapy (Strauch et al., 1974); similarly, a raised incidence of shedders has been observed in a developing country, probably because of the immunosuppressive effects of endemic malaria (Gerber et al., 1976). During IM 75%–92% of patients shed infectious EBV into the oropharynx (Miller et al., 1973; Golden et al., 1973; Gerber et al., 1976; Niederman et al., 1976). It has been assumed in the past that the productive infection in the oropharynx takes place exclusively in B lymphocytes (bone narrow-derived lymphocyte), probably in Waldeyer's ring, since only B cells are known to have demonstrable receptors for EBV (Pattengale et al., 1973; Jondal and Klein, 1973). However, the finding of EBV at the orifice of Stensen's duct has led to the suggestion that salivary gland epithelial cells may also be involved (Niederman et al., 1976), while the demonstration of EBV replication in the malignant epithelial cells of NPC (Trumper et al., 1976, 1977) has raised the possibility that some normal cells of the nasopharyngeal epithelium may likewise support virus production. A recent claim based on in situ nucleic-acid cytohybridization, that EBV replication takes place in oropharyngeal epithelial cells (Lemon et al., 1977), though attractive, requires considerable further experimental investigation.

2. Virus-Carrying Cells in the Circulation

The latent infection of lymphocytes (Fig. 2) certainly only involves B cells; for, quite apart from their possession of receptors for the virus, cells of this type have been shown actually to carry the viral genome in vivo (Crawford et al., 1978). It is the small number of these genome-containing B lymphocytes in the peripheral circulation which provides the starting point for the continuous EBV-carrying lymphoblastoid lines that can be established in vitro from blood or lymph-node biopsies of seropositive people (Diehl et al., 1968; Nilsson et al., 1971; Chap. 11). The phenomenon occurs irrespective of whether the seropositive individual is perfectly healthy or suffering from some coincidental clinical condition, and it was the bewildering ability to establish EBV-carrying cell lines from the blood of patients with a variety of tumors and other diseases which led to confusion before the significance of latent B cell infection in all seropositive people was understood. In this connection it should be noted that EBV genome-containing B cells are present in blood during IM in higher numbers than in seropositive healthy subjects (Henle and Henle, 1972) and cell lines can therefore be established more easily from the former than the latter (Diehl et al., 1968; Henle and Henle, 1972).

II. TYPES OF CELLULAR INFECTION

During the course of the various types of infection which may be established by EBV in susceptible cells, different expressions of virus-determined antigens are seen. Four of these antigens were discovered by the use of naturally occurring human antibodies, namely (1) EBV nuclear antigen (EBNA) (Reedman and Klein, 1973), which is a DNA-binding nonhistone protein probably acting as a gene regulator (Baron et al., 1975; Luka et al., 1977); (2) membrane antigen (MA) (Klein et al., 1966), which has been subtyped into early (EMA) and late (LMA) components (Ernberg et al., 1974; Silvestre et al., 1974); (3) early antigen (EA) (Henle et al., 1970), which likewise has two subtypes, diffuse (D) and restricted (R) (Henle et al., 1971); and (4) viral capsid antigen (VCA) first described by Henle and Henle (1966 b). In addition, there is a fifth antigen, lymphocyte-detected membrane antigen (LYDMA), discovered in the course of cytotoxicity tests using killer T cells (thymus dependent lymphocyte) specifically active in vitro against EBV genome-containing B cells (Svedmyr and Jondal, 1975; Klein, E. et al., 1976 a). A full account of these antigens is presented in Chap. 3.

1. Productive Infection

The sequence of events whereby EBV infection leads to a productive replicative cycle (Table 1 and Fig. 2) has been deduced from observations on the productively infected cells which form a small proportion of the population in "producer" cell lines (Sect. C. IV below). The first antigen expressed is EBNA, presumably preceded or accompanied by LYDMA. This is followed by EMA expression, by the making of EA which inhibits cellular RNA, DNA, and protein synthesis (Gergely et al., 1971), then by virus DNA synthesis, and finally by the production of VCA and LMA to provide components for the assembly and release of infectious virus particles (Fig. 2).

As with all herpesviruses the release of infectious particles inevitably leads to death of the infected cell (Roizman, 1972; Epstein and Achong, 1973 b) and this type of infection is therefore sometimes described as "lytic". In addition, it should be noted that even if the cycle is aborted before the assembly and release of virus, progress through it as far as the production of EA, VCA, or LMA, likewise commits the cell inevitably to death (Fig. 2).

2. Latent Infection

In addition to productive infection, EBV can also bring about two types of nonproductive infection (Table 1). The first of these, latent infection, occurs as has

Table 1. Various forms of infection by EBV in vivo in man[a]

---

1. *Productive replicative infection*
   virus replication leading to cell death
   (as in the oropharynx of infected individuals).
2. *Nonproductive infection* — can be activated to productive cycle.
   a) *Latent infection*
      virus genome expressed to give LYDMA and ? EBNA
      (as in some peripheral B cells of all infected individuals).
   b) *Malignant transformation*
      virus genome expressed to give only the earliest antigens and ? cell changes of malignancy
      (as in BL showing LYDMA, EBNA, EMA; and NPC showing EBNA).

   N. B.: In marmosets EB virus certainly induces malignant transformation with EBNA expression, to
   give malignant lymphomas.

---

[a] LYDMA, lymphocyte-detected membrane antigen;
   EBNA, EBV nuclear antigen;
   EMA, early membrane antigen;
   BL, Burkitt's lymphoma;
   NPC, nasopharyngeal carcinoma.

already been mentioned in the few virus genome-containing B cells of all seropositive individuals. The evidence that the infection in these cells is indeed of the latent type is of several different kinds. Thus, infectious virus cannot be detected when the cells are freshly removed and disrupted (Rickinson et al., 1975) but only becomes manifest if intact cells are cultured, when the latent infection is activated so that infectious virus is liberated into the medium where it infects and transforms (see Sect. C.IV.2 below) coresident, uninfected B cells (Rickinson et al., 1974, 1977 a, b).

This phenomenon of latency by EBV in lymphocytes with its ability to be activated corresponds with the state of latency shown by all herpesviruses. Thus, herpes simplex virus-1 (HSV-1) latent in the trigeminal ganglion is activated to a productive infection when the ganglion cells are cultured (Bastian et al., 1972; Plummer, 1973; Baringer and Swoveland, 1973; Baringer, 1975), and both HSV-2 in sacral ganglia (Baringer, 1974, and 1975) and varicella-zoster virus (VZV) in dorsal root ganglia (Bastian et al., 1974; Shibuta et al., 1974) behave in the same way. But of far more significance in relation to EBV, since it provides an even closer parallel, is the latency behavior of lymphotropic herpesviruses; human cytomegalovirus (CMV), mouse CMV, and herpesvirus saimiri (HVS) in its natural squirrel monkey host, all establish latent, nonproductive infections in lymphocytes from which infectious virus can only be recovered if the undisrupted cells are cocultivated with a susceptible monolayer (Lang, 1975; Olding et al., 1975, 1976; Oldstone et al., 1976; Falk et al., 1972).

Although, as already pointed out, EBV genome-containing B lymphocytes are present in the peripheral circulation of all seropositive individuals, since they are at least 5000 times more numerous during IM (Rocchi et al., 1977), most work on this type of cell has been carried out using blood from IM patients. It is evident that the latently infected genome-containing B cells must express LYDMA on the plasma-lemma since IM killer T cells are specifically activated to recognize this antigen (Svedmyr and Jondal, 1975; Hutt et al., 1975; Royston et al., 1975; Rickinson et al., 1977c). It has been reported that EBNA-expressing B lymphocytes are present in the peripheral blood during the very earliest stages of acute IM (Klein, G. et al., 1976), but it has not yet been established whether these are latently infected cells or lymphocytes at the beginning of a productive infection (Fig. 2) which have escaped into the circulation but have not yet been eliminated by specific immunologic responses (Epstein and Achong, 1977a). It is thus still not clear whether or not latently infected cells express EBNA (Crawford et al., 1978) as well as LYDMA.

What arrests and holds latently infected cells at this very early stage in the productive replicative cycle (Fig. 2, *site X*) is not known, but this might be a result of such factors as bottlenecks in metabolic pathways resulting from inherent characteristics of particular B target cells which become infected or the operation of immunologic constraints. In any event, as mentioned above, the arrest breaks down when the cells are placed in culture away from host responses, with activation of infectious virus production.

3. Malignant Transformation

The second type of nonproductive infection by EBV relates to malignant transformation (Table 1). EBV has been shown to cause fatal, malignant reticuloproliferative disease on experimental inoculation into cotton-top marmosets (Shope et al., 1973) and owl monkeys (Epstein et al., 1973a, b, 1975), and confirmation showing a dose response has been obtained with the first of these species (Deinhardt et al., 1975). Thus, it has been demonstrated unequivocally that EBV can be directly oncogenic in vivo (Chap. 16).

With the two human EBV-associated malignant tumors, African BL and NPC, the relationship of the virus to the tumor cells closely resembles the malignant transformation type of infection seen with known oncogenic animal DNA viruses in the cells of the tumors they cause. In African BL cells, EBV causes the expression only of the earliest antigens, namely EBNA (Lindahl et al., 1974) which seems to correspond to the nuclear T neoantigens of animal tumor viruses, and LYDMA (Jondal et al., 1975) and EMA (Klein et al., 1966; Silvestre et al., 1974; Ernberg et al., 1974) corresponding to the transplantation membrane neoantigens. The events of the replicative cycle are here likewise arrested, but by some factor associated with malignant change and at a different stage (Fig. 2, *site Y*) from that of latency. In the case of NPC, only EBNA has so far been found in the malignant epithelial tumor cells (Huang et al., 1974), but with so many T cells infiltrating NPC tumors (Jondal and Klein, 1975; Klein, E. et al., 1976b) and some evidence that these are activated against LYDMA (Klein, E. et al., 1976b) it seems possible that this latter antigen is also expressed.

III. HOST REACTIONS

1. Pathogenesis of Infectious Mononucleosis

Enough is now known about the general biology of EBV to permit a comprehensive understanding of the way in which the virus actually produces the clinical manifestations of IM in those undergoing natural primary infection accompanied by the disease. A full account of the pathogenesis of IM has recently appeared (Epstein and Achong, 1977a) and further aspects are dealt with at length in Chap. 13. Understanding of the changes underlying IM is of considerable importance in its own right, but it has also, by analogy, provided extensive insights into the events which take place as a result of clinically inapparent primary infection.

2. Clinically Inapparent Infection

As in IM, EBV probably gains access to susceptible, EBV antibody-negative individuals via the oropharynx and sets up a productive infection at this site. However, in contrast to IM and probably because of a small infecting dose and individual physiologic (including factors related to age) and genetically determined immunologic resistance, this process and its consequences are held in check.

Only relatively few B lymphocytes in the lymphoid tissue of the oropharynx become involved and the number releasing virus and virus-determined antigens during productive infection, or arrested in latent infection and expressing LYDMA (Fig. 2), remains limited. In consequence, the vigorous antibody response and huge T cell reaction seen in IM as a result of widespread B cell infection fail to develop and no symptoms are engendered (Epstein and Achong, 1977a). Instead, a situation exactly like the postconvalescent steady state of IM is established at an early stage; virus production continues at a low level in a pool of cells somewhere in the oropharynx with intermittent release of infectious virus into the mouth (Gerber et al., 1972; Golden et al., 1973; Chang et al., 1973), together with the escape of a few latently infected B cells, expressing LYDMA, into the peripheral circulation. The low-level oropharyngeal virus replication brings about a lifelong maintenance of moderate levels of antibodies to VCA, MA, and EBNA (Henle and Henle, 1970; Hewetson et al., 1973), while the presence of the few latently infected B cells in the circulation is responsible for the ability to establish EBV-carrying cell lines in culture from the peripheral blood (Moore et al., 1967; Gerber and Monroe, 1968). It would appear that a few residual, specific memory T cells also continue to be present (Gergely et al., 1977) and destroy latently infected LYDMA-positive B lymphocytes, which are then replaced by others arrested in this state (Fig. 2) from the pool of virus-producing cells.

The interactions of all the above phenomena seem to reach a particular level of balance in each individual and the effects of immunologic changes on such components as virus shedding have already been noted.

3. EBV-Associated Tumors

Full descriptions both of host responses in BL and NPC, and of all aspects of the striking relationship of EBV to these tumors are given in Chaps. 4, 6, 7, 8, 14, 15, and 18.

IV. RELATIONSHIP OF EBV-CARRYING CELL LINES TO TYPES OF INFECTION

1. Lines Established by Transformation in vitro

When EBV is added to human B lymphocytes in culture the infected cells are transformed so as to acquire the power of unlimited in vitro proliferation (Henle et al.,

1967; Pope et al., 1968; Chap. 10). This EBV-induced transformation satisfies many of the generally accepted criteria for malignant transformation in vitro by known oncogenic viruses (Rapp and Westmoreland, 1976). Thus, EBV-transformed lines show (1) changed morphology to a blastoid form, (2) permanent growth, (3) ability to grow in semisolid medium (Mizuno et al., 1976), (4) loss of contact inhibition (Glaser and Rapp, 1972), (5) altered surface properties, (6) addition of stable, inheritable, viral genetic material, (7) presence of virus-specific functions, and (8) stimulation of cellular DNA synthesis (Chaps. 3, 10, and 11). Nevertheless, the cell lines resulting from transformation by EBV in vitro are certainly different in important biologic respects from the cell lines that are formed by direct outgrowth when the malignant cells of BL are placed in culture (Sect. C.IV.3 below). These differences probably reflect qualitative differences between malignant transformation in vivo (Chaps. 14 and 15). Whether or not this explanation ultimately proves to be correct, a great deal of factual information is available on the events which accompany in vitro transformation by the virus.

It has been estimated that with EBV about ten physical particles per cell are required to cause transformation in unfractionated mononuclear leukocyte cultures (Robinson and Miller, 1975; Henderson et al., 1977; Sugden and Mark, 1977). However, these calculations do not take account of the fact that only the B cells in such populations are susceptible nor of the recent claim that among B cells only those bearing S-Ig (M) constitute the target for the virus (Katsuki et al., 1977). Thus, the transforming dose is likely to be closer to 1:1 as has sometimes been suggested (Sugden and Mark, 1977); but even with a ratio of 10:1, EBV is clearly the most efficient in vitro transforming DNA virus known (Pagano, 1975; Robinson and Miller, 1975; Rapp and Westmoreland, 1976). In any event, all susceptible B lymphocytes must carry EBV receptors and these have been shown to correspond with C3 receptors on the plasmalemma and may indeed be identical with them (Yefenof et al., 1976; Yefenof and Klein, 1977).

Fetal human B lymphocytes have been thought in the past to be more susceptible to transformation by EBV in vitro than those of adult origin (Dalens et al., 1975; Gerber et al., 1976; Henderson et al., 1977). This seeming refractoriness of adult B cells has now been shown to be spurious and due in reality to suppression of their proliferation by accompanying adult T cells in a manner which does not occur with fetal T cells (Thorley-Lawson et al., 1977).

After infection, the first-known antigen to be expressed is EBNA which is seen by ∼ 12 h (Menezes et al., 1978; Einhorn and Ernberg, 1978; Takada and Osato, 1978), and is presumably preceded or accompanied by LYDMA (Crawford et al., 1978). EBNA expression is independent of cellular DNA synthesis and is followed by blastogenesis at ∼ 24 h and cellular DNA synthesis at ∼ 36 h (Takada and Osato, 1978). At an as yet undetermined stage after EBNA expression the virus DNA is replicated to give up to 60 genome equivalents per cell; following this genome amplification, some viral DNA molecules are linearly integrated into host cell DNA, perhaps on one or more of chromosomes 3, 4, 5, 6, and 10 (Glaser et al., 1975), whereas the remainder stays free as circular molecules (Chap. 8). The transformation event takes place around this time, and it has been speculatively suggested that it may be related either to the amplification of the genome load or to the integration of some EBV DNA molecules (Thorley-Lawson and Strominger, 1976; Chap. 9). In any case, it should be noted that the transformation event and EBNA induction are two independent steps (Menezes et al., 1978; Takada and Osato, 1978); indeed the mere presence of EBNA certainly does not indicate that the cell is in a transformed state since this antigen is also expressed early in the productive replicative cycle (Fig. 2) (Ernberg et al., 1976 Chap. 3). It should also be noted that whereas the whole viral genome is necessary for transformation (Henderson et al., 1978), only about 5% is required to maintain the transformed state (Orellana and Kieff, 1977).

Cell lines arising as a result of in vitro transformation by EBV are not uniform in their expression of viral functions. Although all transformed cells display EBNA and LYDMA, there are, at one extreme, lines in which at any one time a small, variable minority of the cells passes spontaneously into the full productive replicative cycle with release of infectious virus; such producer lines tend to arise when adult B lymphocytes have been the target for the virus and tend to carry a large number of viral genome equivalents (Pritchett et al., 1976; Gerber et al., 1976). There are also lines in which some cells spontaneously start on the productive cycle, express late viral antigens, but die without producing virus particles. Yet other lines are found in which there are no cells which enter a productive cycle spontaneously, but where entry into the cycle can be induced by halogenated pyrimidines (Chap. 12); these inducible lines tend to carry a somewhat smaller viral genome load. Finally, at the other extreme there are lines in which all the cells remain stable in the transformed state expressing EBNA and LYDMA and are totally resistant to the inducing effect of halogenated pyrimidines; it is interesting that the noninducible lines tend to carry a small number of viral genome copies and to originate by the transformation of fetal B lymphocytes (Pritchett et al., 1976; Gerber et al., 1976; Pagano et al., 1976). Irrespective of the number of cell generations through which a line passes, it will maintain its own particular load of genome equivalents per cell at a constant level (Thorley-Lawson and Strominger, 1976) and there is some evidence that the intensity of EBNA staining is directly related to the size of this genome load (Ernberg et al., 1977).

Although no fully permissive cell type has yet been identified for EBV production either in vivo or in vitro, it is clear that the few cells replicating infectious virus in producer lines are permissive, even if the majority of the cells are not. It might be that in vivo many more B lymphocytes can be permissive and can thus take part in replicating the infectious virus which is shed in the buccal fluid. Why some cells in producer lines make virus, why some cells in other lines are inducible, and why in yet other lines all cells remain stably transformed and totally noninducible is not understood. However, it seems likely that the various differences are determined by the particular genome load interacting with a series of blocks or bottlenecks in metabolic pathways which operate at different points in the virus replicative cycle (Fig. 2) and which vary in different classes of B cells within the target population. The differences in behavior in lines arising after EBV transformation of fetal or adult lymphocytes (Miller and Lipman, 1973) certainly suggest that this is a likely explanation.

2. Lines from Seropositive Individuals

As pointed out above, all seropositive individuals (whether healthy or with IM, BL, NPC, or some irrelevant clinical condition) have in their peripheral blood a few latently infected cells that are activated to a productive infection when placed in culture. It is the infectious virus liberated in this way which infects coresident uninfected B cells and transforms them to give cell lines (Rickinson et al., 1974, 1975, 1977a, b; Rocchi et al.,

1977; Crawford et al., 1978) in exactly the same way as occurs when the virus is added in vitro to B lymphocytes from seronegative sources. This two-step mechanism bringing about in vitro transformation accounts for the fact that lines derived from blood of seropositive people are exactly similar in all respects to the lymphoblastoid lines obtained by experimental in vitro transformation by EBV (Chap. 11).

It is obvious from the foregoing that the two-step mechanism also provides an explanation for the origin of the lymphoblastoid lines that have been grown from NPC biopsies (de-Thé et al., 1969, 1970; Achong et al., 1971; Epstein et al., 1971). This squamous epithelial tumor always contains a considerable lymphocyte infiltration (Shanmugaratnam, 1971), of which a few must be latently infected B cells capable of starting lines in vitro in this way.

3. Lines from Burkitt's Lymphoma Biopsies

It has long been recognized that the EBV genome-containing lymphoid lines that arise when African BL biopsies are placed in culture, do so by the direct outgrowth of the malignant tumor cells. This has been clearly established by studies of cytogenetic, IgM specificity, and isoenzyme markers in the original tumors and the lines derived from them (Nadkarni et al., 1969; Gripenberg et al., 1969; Fialkow et al., 1970; Manolov and Manolova, 1972).

These BL lines have recently been shown to differ perceptibly from the lymphoblastoid lines, which arise either from the transformation of B lymphocytes by EBV in vitro or by the two-step mechanism when the latently infected B cells present in the blood of all seropositive individuals are cultured.

The BL lines have monoclonal derivation, aneuploidy with a no. 14 chromosome marker, morphologic uniformity within each line, characteristic surface glycoprotein patterns, and the ability to form tumors in nude mice; in contrast, lymphoblastoid lines have polyclonal derivation, diploidy without the chromosome marker, morphologic heterogeneity within each line, a different surface glycoprotein pattern, and no capacity for growth in nude mice (Chap. 11). The likelihood that these differences probably reflect qualitative differences between malignant transformation by EBV in vitro and in vivo has already been pointed out. Despite the biologic differences, BL lines resemble lymphoblastoid lines in showing a similar spectrum in the expression of virus functions, ranging from producer lines, through inducible lines, to totally noninducible lines.

4. Lines from Subhuman Primates

Just as with human lymphocytes, so too have EBV-carrying lymphoblastoid lines been established from the lymphocytes of a variety of subhuman primates (marmosets, owl monkeys, gibbons, squirrel and cebus monkeys) either by transformation with EBV in vitro or by culture from the blood of infected animals (Miller et al., 1972; Werner et al., 1972; Miller and Lipman, 1973; Falk et al., 1974; Chap. 16). Like human lines, all the monkey lines tested are of B cell origin (Falk et al., 1974; Rabin et al., 1975) and produce EBV-determined antigens and virus particles (Miller et al., 1972; Miller and Lipman, 1973; Falk et al., 1974). In this connection it has been noted that at least some

EBV-carrying lines established from subhuman primates have a rather high proportion of producer cells and liberate unusually large amounts of extracellular infectious virus into the culture medium (Miller and Lipman, 1973; Epstein et al., 1973b). In addition to this tendency to virus production, marmoset lymphocytes are said to be 1000 times less sensitive to transformation by EBV in vitro than human fetal lymphocytes (Henderson et al., 1977).

Marmoset cells transformed into continuous lines by EBV in vitro (Miller et al., 1972) grow to give malignant tumors when inoculated into autologous hosts (Shope et al., 1973). This clearly demonstrates that with marmoset cells EBV brings about malignant transformation in vitro and seems to indicate that the same change probably occurs when human cells are transformed in these circumstances, since the process appears to be exactly similar in the two cases; for obvious reasons, the decisive inoculation experiments cannot be performed with the human material. To complete the parallel with the various types of EBV infection in man, EBV genome-containing B cell lines can be obtained when samples of EBV-induced subhuman primate lymphomas are placed in culture (Epstein et al., 1973b; Miller et al., 1977) and these lines appear to have a monoclonal origin just like BL-derived lines (Rabin et al., 1977).

Finally, it is of interest that several species of old-world primates (chimpanzee, baboon, and orangutang) have recently been shown to have their own transforming lymphotropic herpesviruses, which are closely related to EBV (Chap. 17).

V. VIRUS ISOLATES AND THE SEARCH FOR STRAIN DIFFERENCES

The lack of a fully permissive cell system suitable for conventional virologic tests has hampered from the outset many aspects of work with EBV. Virus isolation has been particularly difficult and has had to rely in practice either on transformation procedures making use of B lymphocytes from uninfected donors (Henle et al., 1967; Pope et al., 1968; Moss and Pope, 1972; Chap. 10), or on the cultivation of EBV-containing cells to give lines carrying the virus, as was done with the BL cells in which the agent was first discovered.

Despite the difficulties, EBV isolates have been made over the years from a wide variety of different sources. The virus was available from the beginning in cultured BL cells and has been obtained recently from the actual malignant epithelial cells of NPC (Trumper et al., 1977). Virus has also been isolated from the buccal fluids of normal seropositive individuals, patients with IM, and patients with BL, as well as from the genome-containing lymphocytes in the blood of IM patients, normal seropositives, and seropositives with various coincidental diseases.

Every naturally occurring isolate has yielded virus capable both of transforming B lymphocytes in vitro and of effecting a productive replicative viral cycle (Fig. 2), since if appropriate target cells are used for the transformation, producer lines emerge which contain the usual small number of cells undergoing productive infection. The fact that the transforming function of all EBV isolates predominates over the virus replicative function in in vitro systems is clearly an attribute of currently available target test cells. It has already been pointed out that the same virus isolate has been shown to give nonproducer or producer lines depending on whether it was used to transform fetal or adult lymphocytes (Miller and Lipman, 1973), while the infectious virus in every isolate from buccal fluid for example, irrespective of the transforming ability it shows in vitro, must obviously have arisen through the expression of productive replicative functions in vivo even though the fully permissive cell for this has not yet been identified. The recent finding that disodium phosphonacetate blocks EBV production in nontoxic doses (Summers and Klein, 1976; Nyormoi et al., 1976; Yajima et al., 1976) has made it possible to investigate the transforming and replicative functions of EBV separately, since they show differing sensitivities to inhibition by the drug (Rickinson and Epstein, 1978; Chap. 9).

Only one strain of virus fails to conform to the standard biologic behavior pattern and this, the P_3HR-1 strain, was obtained by experimental selection during cloning procedures in the laboratory (Hinuma et al., 1967). For the past few years, P_3HR-1 virus has lacked transforming ability (Miller et al., 1974), but it originally had this (Gerber et al., 1969) like its fully transforming parent strain (Jijoye) (Henle et al., 1967); in view of the uniqueness of the P_3HR-1 strain, it is best regarded as a rare, defective laboratory mutant. One might expect that virus lacking a biologic function would also lack part of the complete viral genome, yet the P_3HR-1 strain contains 15% more DNA sequences than transforming strains (Pritchett et al., 1975; Menezes et al., 1976; Chap. 8). The P_3HR-1 strain is also peculiar in that it seems to consist of a heterogeneous population of EBV DNA molecules (Fresen et al., 1977) which could not be found in a transforming strain when appropriate comparisons were made (zur Hausen and Fresen, 1977).

With EBV playing such widely differing roles as harmless commensal in the great majority of normal human beings (Sect. C.I above), causative agent of IM (Chap. 13), transforming agent for primate lymphocytes in vitro (Chap. 10), oncogenic virus in subhuman primates (Chap. 16), and suspected tumor virus in African BL (Chap. 14) and NPC (Chap. 15), considerable efforts have been made to ascertain whether these different activities are associated with different strains of the virus. The results of these efforts so far agree that, apart from P_3HR-1, all EBV isolates from whatever source show such biologic, biochemical, and antigenic similarities as not to suggest major strain variations (Kawai et al., 1973; Nonoyama and Pagano, 1973; Kieff and Levine, 1974; Menezes et al., 1975; Miller et al., 1976; Pagano et al., 1976; Gerber et al., 1976; Fialkow, 1976; Kaschka-Dierich et al., 1977; Sugden, 1977). In the absence of evidence for strain differences, it would seem that the different roles played by EBV are related instead to the selective expression of different viral functions (virus production/latency/malignant transformation), depending on which of various subtypes of target cells become infected, together with the influence on this of varying host responses.

REFERENCES

Achong, B. G., Mansell, P. W. A., Epstein, M. A., Clifford, P.: An unusual virus in cultures from a human nasopharyngeal carcinoma. J. Natl. Cancer Inst. **46**, 299–307 (1971)

Baringer, J. R.: Recovery of herpes simplex virus from human sacral ganglions. N. Engl. J. Med. **291**, 828–830 (1974)

Baringer, J. R.: Herpes simplex virus in human sensory ganglia. In: Oncogenesis and herpesviruses II. de-Thé, G., Epstein, M. A., zur Hausen, H. (eds.), Part 2, pp. 73–77. Lyon: IARC 1975

Baringer, J. R., Swoveland, P.: Recovery of herpes-simplex virus from human trigeminal ganglions. N. Engl. J. Med. **288**, 648–650 (1973)

Baron, D., Benz, W. C., Carmichael, G., Yocum, R. R., Strominger, J. L.: Assay and partial purification of Epstein-Barr virus nuclear antigen. In: Epstein-Barr virus production, concentration and purification. Internal Technical Report 75/003, pp. 257–262. Lyon: IARC 1975

Bastian, F. O., Rabson, A. S., Yee, C. L., Tralka, T. S.: Herpesvirus hominis: isolation from human trigeminal ganglia. Science **178**, 306–307 (1972)

Bastian, F. O., Rabson, A. S., Yee, C. L., Tralka, T. S.: Herpesvirus varicellae isolated from human dorsal root ganglia. Arch. Pathol. **97**, 331–333 (1974)

Bonar, R. A., Weinstein, D., Sommer, J. R., Beard, D., Beard, J. W.: Virus of avian myeloblastosis. XVII. Morphology of progressive virus-myeloblast interactions *in vitro*. Natl. Cancer Inst. Monogr. **4**, 251–290 (1960)

Burkitt, D.: A sarcoma involving the jaws in African children. Br. J. Surg. **46**, 218–223 (1958)

Burkitt, D.: A children's cancer dependent on climatic factors. Nature **194**, 232–234 (1962a)

Burkitt, D.: Determining the climatic limitations of a children's cancer common in Africa. Br. Med. J. **1962 b II**, 1019–1023

Burkitt, D. P.: Etiology of Burkitt's lymphoma – an alternative hypothesis to a vectored virus. J. Natl. Cancer Inst. **42**, 19–28 (1969)

Chang, R. S., Lewis, J. P., Abildgaard, C. F.: Prevalence of oropharyngeal excretors of leukocyte-transforming agents among a human population. N. Engl. J. Med. **289**, 1325–1329 (1973)

Crawford, D. H., Rickinson, A. B., Finerty, S., Epstein, M. A.: Epstein-Barr (EB) virus genome-containing, EB nuclear antigen-negative B-lymphocyte populations in blood in acute infectious mononucleosis. J. Gen. Virol. **38**, 449–460 (1978)

Dalens, M., Zech, L., Klein, G.: Origin of lymphoid lines established from mixed cultures of cord-blood lymphocytes and explants from infectious mononucleosis, Burkitt lymphoma and healthy donors. Int. J. Cancer **16**, 1008–1014 (1975)

Deinhardt, F., Falk, L., Wolfe, L. G., Paciga, J., Johnson, D.: Response of marmosets to experimental infection with Epstein-Barr virus. In: Oncogenesis and herpesviruses II. de-Thé, G., Epstein, M. A., zur Hausen, H. (eds.), Part 2, pp. 161–168. Lyon: IARC 1975

Demissie, A., Svedmyr, A.: Age distribution of antibodies to EB virus in Swedish females as studied by indirect immunofluorescence on Burkitt cells. Acta Pathol. Microbiol. Scand. **75**, 457–465 (1969)

de-Thé, G., Ambrosioni, J. C., Ho, H. C., Kwan, H. C.: Lymphoblastoid transformation and presence of herpes-type viral particles in a Chinese nasopharyngeal tumour cultured *in vitro*. Nature **221**, 770–771 (1969)

de-Thé, G., Ho, H. C., Kwan, H. C., Desgranges, C., Favre, M. C.: Nasopharyngeal carcinoma. I. Types of cultures derived from tumour biopsies and nontumourous tissues of Chinese patients with special reference to lymphoblastoid transformation. Int. J. Cancer **6**, 189–206 (1970)

Diehl, V., Henle, G., Henle, W., Kohn, G.: Demonstration of a herpes group virus in cultures of peripheral leukocytes from patients with infectious mononucleosis. J. Virol. **2**, 663–669 (1968)

Diehl, V., Taylor, J. R., Parlin, J. A., Henle, G., Henle, W.: Infectious mononucleosis in East Africa. East Afr. Med. J. **46**, 407–413 (1969)

Einhorn, L., Ernberg, I.: Induction of EBNA precedes the first cellular S-phase after EBV-infection of human lymphocytes. Int. J. Cancer **21**, 157–160 (1978)

Epstein, M. A.: Aspects of the EB virus. Adv. Cancer Res. **13**, 383–411 (1970)

Epstein, M. A., Achong, B. G.: Specific immunofluorescence test for the herpes-type EB virus of Burkitt lymphoblasts, authenticated by electron microscopy. J. Natl. Cancer Inst. **40**, 593–607 (1968a)

Epstein, M. A., Achong, B. G.: Observations on the nature of the herpes-type EB virus in cultured Burkitt lymphoblasts, using a specific immunofluorescence test. J. Natl. Cancer Inst. **40**, 609–621 (1968b)

Epstein, M. A., Achong, B. G.: The EB virus. Annu. Rev. Microbiol. **27**, 413–436 (1973a)

Epstein, M. A., Achong, B. G.: Various forms of Epstein-Barr virus infection in man: established facts and a general concept. Lancet **1973b II**, 836–839

Epstein, M. A., Achong, B. G.: Pathogenesis of infectious mononucleosis. Lancet **1977a II**, 1270–1273

Epstein, M. A., Achong, B. G.: Recent progress in Epstein-Barr virus research. Annu. Rev. Microbiol. **31**, 421–445 (1977b)

Epstein, M. A., Barr, Y. M.: Cultivation *in vitro* of human lymphoblasts from Burkitt's malignant lymphoma. Lancet **1964 I**, 252–253

Epstein, M. A., Barr, Y. M.: Characteristics and mode of growth of a tissue culture strain (EB1) of human lymphoblasts from Burkitt's lymphoma. J. Natl. Cancer Inst. **34**, 231–240 (1965)

Epstein, M. A., Barr, Y. M., Achong, B. G.: Avian tumor virus behavior as a guide in the investigation of a human neoplasm. Natl. Cancer Inst. Monogr. **17**, 637–650 (1964a)

Epstein, M. A., Achong, B. G., Barr, Y. M.: Virus particles in cultured lymphoblasts from Burkitt's lymphoma. Lancet **1964 b I**, 702–703

Epstein, M. A., Henle, G., Achong, B. G., Barr, Y. M.: Morphological and biological studies on a virus in cultured lymphoblasts from Burkitt's lymphoma. J. Exp. Med. **121**, 761–770 (1965)

Epstein, M. A., Achong, B. G., Mansell, P. W. A.: A new virus in cultures of human nasopharyngeal carcinoma. In: Proceedings 1st International Symposium of the Princess Takamatsu Cancer Research Fund.: Recent advances in human tumor virology and immunology. Nakahara, W., Nishioka, K., Hirayama, T., Ito, Y. (eds.), pp. 163–171. Tokyo: University of Tokyo Press 1971

Epstein, M. A., Hunt, R. D., Rabin, H.: Pilot experiments with EB virus in owl monkeys *(Aotus trivirgatus)* I. Reticuloproliferative disease in an inoculated animal. Int. J. Cancer **12**, 309–318 (1973a)

Epstein, M. A., Rabin, H., Ball, G., Rickinson, A. B., Jarvis, J., Meléndez, L. V.: Pilot experiments with EB virus in owl monkeys *(Aotus trivirgatus)* II. EB virus in a cell line from an animal with reticuloproliferative disease. Int. J. Cancer **12**, 319–332 (1973b)

Epstein, M. A., zur Hausen, H., Ball, G., Rabin, H.: Pilot experiments with EB virus in owl monkeys *(Aotus trivirgatus)* III. Serological and biochemical findings in an animal with reticuloproliferative disease. Int. J. Cancer **15**, 17–22 (1975)

Ernberg, I., Klein, G., Kourilsky, F. M., Silvestre, D.: Differentiation between early and late membrane antigen on human lymphoblastoid cell lines infected with Epstein-Barr virus. I. Immunofluorescence. J. Natl. Cancer Inst. **53**, 61–65 (1974)

Ernberg, I., Andersson-Anvret, M., Klein, G., Lundin, L., Killander, D.: Relationship between amount of Epstein-Barr virus-determined nuclear antigen per cell and number of EBV-DNA copies per cell. Nature **266**, 269–271 (1977)

Ernberg, I., Masucci, G., Klein, G.: Persistence of Epstein-Barr viral nuclear antigen (EBNA) in cells entering the EB viral cycle. Int. J. Cancer, **17**, 197–203 (1976)

Falk, L., Wolfe, L. G., Deinhardt, F.: Isolation of *Herpesvirus saimiri* from blood of squirrel monkeys *(Saimiri sciureus)*. J. Natl. Cancer Inst. **48**, 1499–1505 (1972)

Falk, L., Wolfe, L., Deinhardt, F., Paciga, J., Dombos, L., Klein, G., Henle, W., Henle, G.: Epstein-Barr virus: transformation of non-human primate lymphocytes *in vitro*. Int. J. Cancer **13**, 363–376 (1974)

Fialkow, P. J.: Clonal origin of human tumors. Biochem. Biophys. Acta **458**, 283–321 (1976)

Fialkow, P. J., Klein, G., Gartler, S. M., Clifford, P.: Clonal origin for individual Burkitt tumours. Lancet **1970 I** 384–386

Fresen, K. O., Merkt, B., Bornkamm, G. W., zur Hausen, H.: Heterogeneity of Epstein-Barr virus originating from P3HR-1 cells. I. Studies on EBNA induction. Int. J. Cancer **19**, 317–323 (1977)

Gerber, P., Monroe, J. H.: Studies on leukocytes growing in continuous culture derived from normal human donors. J. Natl. Cancer Inst. **40**, 855–866 (1968)

Gerber, P., Rosenblum, E. N.: The incidence of complement-fixing antibodies to herpes simplex and herpes-like viruses in man and rhesus monkeys. Proc. Soc. Exp. Biol. Med. **128**, 541–546 (1968)

Gerber, P., Whang-Peng, J., Monroe, J. H.: Transformation and chromosome changes induced by Epstein-Barr virus in normal human leukocyte cultures. Proc. Natl. Acad. Sci. USA **63**, 740–747 (1969)

Gerber, P., Nonoyama, M., Lucas, S., Perlin, E., Goldstein, L. I.: Oral excretion of Epstein-Barr virus by healthy subjects and patients with infectious mononucleosis. Lancet **1972 II**, 988–989

Gerber, P., Nkrumah, F. K., Pritchett, R., Kieff, E.: Comparative studies of Epstein-Barr virus strains from Ghana and the United States. Int. J. Cancer **17**, 71–81 (1976)

Gergely, L., Klein, G., and Ernberg, I.: Host cell macromolecular synthesis in cells containing EBV-induced early antigens, studied by combined immunofluorescence and radioautography. Virology **45**, 22–29 (1971)

Gergely, P., Ernberg, I., Klein, G., Steinitz, M.: Blastogenic response of purified human T-lymphocyte populations to Epstein-Barr virus (EBV). Clin. Exp. Immunol. **30**, 347–353 (1977)

Ginsburg, C. M., Henle, W., Henle, G., Horwitz, C. A.: Infectious mononucleosis in children. Evaluation of Epstein-Barr virus-specific serological data. J. Am. Med. Assoc. **237**, 781–785 (1977)

Glaser, R., Rapp, F.: Rescue of Epstein-Barr virus from somatic cell hybrids of Burkitt lymphoblastoid cells. J. Virol. **10**, 288–296 (1972)

Glaser, R., Nonoyama, M., Shows, T. B., Henle, G., Henle, W.: Epstein-Barr virus: studies on the association of virus genome with human chromosomes in hybrid cells. In: Oncogenesis and herpesviruses II. de-Thé, G., Epstein, M. A., zur Hausen, H. (eds.), Part 1, pp. 457–466. Lyon: IARC 1975

Golden, H. D., Chang, R. S., Prescott, W., Simpson, E., Cooper, T. Y.: Leukocyte-transforming agent: prolonged excretion by patients with mononucleosis and excretion by normal individuals. J. Infect. Dis. **127,** 471–473 (1973)

Goldman, M., Reisher, J. I., Bushar, H. F.: Serum-antibodies to Burkitt cell virus. Lancet **1968 I,** 1156

Gripenberg, U., Levan, A., Clifford, P.: Chomosomes in Burkitt lymphomas. I. Serial studies in a case with bilateral tumors showing different chromosomal stemlines. Int. J. Cancer **4,** 334–349 (1969)

Gross, L.: Oncogenic viruses, 1st ed. Oxford, London, New York, Paris: Pergamon Press 1961

Haddow, A. J.: Age incidence in Burkitt's lymphoma syndrome. East. Afr. Med. J. **41,** 1–6 (1964)

Henderson, E., Miller, G., Robinson, J., Heston, L.: Efficiency of transformation of lymphocytes by Epstein-Barr virus. Virology **76,** 152–163 (1977)

Henderson, E., Heston, L., Grogan, E., Miller, G.: Radiobiological inactivation of Epstein-Barr virus. J. Virol. **25,** 51–59 (1978)

Henle, G., Henle, W.: Studies on cell lines derived from Burkitt's lymphoma. Trans. NY Acad. Sci. **29,** 71–79 (1966a)

Henle, G., Henle, W.: Immunofluorescence in cells derived from Burkitt's lymphoma. J. Bacteriol. **91,** 1248–1256 (1966b)

Henle, G., Henle, W.: Immunofluorescence, interference, and complement fixation technics in the detection of the herpes-type virus in Burkitt tumor cell lines. Cancer Res. **27,** 2442–2446 (1967)

Henle, W., Henle, G.: The relation between the Epstein-Barr virus and infectious mononucleosis, Burkitt's lymphoma and cancer of the postnasal space. East. Afr. Med. J. **46,** 402–406 (1969)

Henle, G., Henle, W.: Observations on childhood infections with the Epstein-Barr virus. J. Infect. Dis. **121,** 303–310 (1970)

Henle, W., Henle, G.: Epstein-Barr virus: the cause of infectious mononucleosis – a review. In: Oncogenesis and herpesviruses. Biggs, P. M., de Thé, G., Payne, L. N. (eds.), pp. 269–274. Lyon: IARC 1972

Henle, W., Henle, G.: Epstein-Barr virus and infectious mononucleosis. N. Engl. J. Med. **288,** 263–264 (1973)

Henle, W., Diehl, V., Kohn, G., zur Hausen, H., Henle, G.: Herpes-type virus and chromosome marker in normal leukocytes after growth with irradiated Burkitt cells. Science **157,** 1064–1065 (1967)

Henle, W., Henle, G., Zajac, B. A., Pearson, G., Waubke, R., Scriba, M.: Differential reactivity of human serums with early antigens induced by Epstein-Barr virus. Science **169,** 188–190 (1970)

Henle, G., Henle, W., Klein, G.: Demonstration of two distinct components in the early antigen complex of Epstein-Barr virus-infected cells. Int. J. Cancer **8,** 272–282 (1971)

Hewetson, J. F., Rocchi, G., Henle, W., Henle, G.: Neutralizing antibodies to Epstein-Barr virus in healthy populations and patients with infectious mononucleosis. J. Infect. Dis. **128,** 283–289 (1973)

Hinuma, Y., Konn, M., Yamaguchi, J., Wudarski, D. J., Blakeslee, J. R., Grace, J. T.: Immunofluorescence and herpes-type virus particles in the P_3HR-1 Burkitt lymphoma cell line. J. Virol. **1,** 1045–1051 (1967)

Hoagland, R. J.: The transmission of infectious mononucleosis. Am. J. Med. Sci. **229,** 262–272 (1955)

Horwitz, C. A., Henle, W., Henle, G., Segal, M., Arnold, T., Lewis, F. B., Zanick, D., Ward, P. C. J.: Clinical and laboratory evaluation of elderly patients with heterophil-antibody positive infectious mononucleosis. Am. J. Med. **61,** 333–339 (1976)

Huang, D. P., Ho, J. H., Henle, W., Henle, G.: Demonstration of Epstein-Barr virus-associated nuclear antigen in nasopharyngeal carcinoma cells from fresh biopsies. Int. J. Cancer **14,** 580–588 (1974)

Hutt, L. M., Huang, Y. T., Dascomb, H. E., Pagano, J. S.: Enhanced destruction of lymphoid cell lines by peripheral blood leukocytes taken from patients with acute infectious mononucleosis. J. Immunol. **115,** 243–248 (1975)

Jondal, M., Klein, G.: Surface markers on human B and T lymphocytes. II. Presence of Epstein-Barr virus receptors on B lymphocytes. J. Exp. Med. **138,** 1365–1378 (1973)

Jondal, M., Klein, G.: Classification of lymphocytes in nasopharyngeal carcinoma (NPC) biopsies. Biomedicine **23,** 163–165 (1975)

Jondal, M., Svedmyr, E., Klein, E., Singh, S.: Killer T cells in a Burkitt's lymphoma biopsy. Nature **255,** 405–407 (1975)

Kaschka-Dierich, C., Falk, L., Bjursell, G., Adams, A., Lindahl, T.: Human lymphoblastoid cell lines derived from individuals without lymphoproliferative disease contain the same latent forms of Epstein-Barr virus DNA as those found in tumor cells. Int. J. Cancer **20,** 173–180 (1977)

Katsuki, T., Hinuma, Y., Yamamoto, N., Abo, T., Kumagai, K.: Identification of the target cells in human B lymphocytes for transformation by Epstein-Barr virus. Virology **83,** 287–294 (1977)

Kawai, Y., Nonoyama, M., Pagano, J. S.: Reassociation kinetics for Epstein-Barr virus DNA: nonhomology to mammalian DNA and homology of viral DNA in various diseases. J. Virol. **12,** 1006–1012 (1973)

Kieff, E., Levine, J.: Homology between Burkitt herpes viral DNA and DNA in continuous lymphoblastoid cells from patients with infectious mononucleosis. Proc. Natl. Acad. Sci. USA **71,** 355–358 (1974)

Klein, E., Klein, G., Levine, P. H.: Immunological control of human lymphoma: discussion. Cancer Res. **36,** 724–727 (1976 a)

Klein, E., Becker, S., Svedmyr, E., Jondal, M., Vánky, F.: Tumor infiltrating lymphocytes. Ann. NY Acad. Sci. **276,** 207–216 (1976 b)

Klein, G., Clifford, P., Klein, E., Stjernswärd, J.: Search for tumor-specific immune reactions in Burkitt lymphoma patients by the membrane immunofluorescence reaction. Proc. Natl. Acad. Sci. USA **55,** 1628–1635 (1966)

Klein, G., Svedmyr, E., Jondal, M., Persson, P. O.: EBV-determined nuclear antigen (EBNA) positive cells in the peripheral blood of infectious mononucleosis patients. Int. J. Cancer **17,** 21–26 (1976)

Lang, D. J.: Transfusion and perfusion-associated cytomegalovirus and Epstein-Barr virus infections: current understanding and investigations. In: Transmissible disease and blood transfusion. Greenwalt, T. J., Jamieson, G. A. (eds.), pp. 153–169. New York, San Francisco, London: Grune & Stratton 1975

Lemon, S. M., Hutt, L. M., Shaw, J. E., Li, J-L. H., Pagano, J. S.: Replication of EBV in epithelial cells during infectious mononucleosis. Nature **268,** 268–270 (1977)

Lindahl, T., Klein, G., Reedman, B. M., Johansson, B., Singh, S.: Relationship between Epstein-Barr virus (EBV) DNA and the EBV-determined nuclear antigen (EBNA) in Burkitt lymphoma biopsies and other lymphoproliferative malignancies. Int. J. Cancer **13,** 764–772 (1974)

Luka, J., Siegert, W., Klein, G.: Solubilization of the Epstein-Barr virus-determined nuclear antigen and its characterization as a DNA-binding protein. J. Virol. **22,** 1–8 (1977)

Manolov, G., Manolova, Y.: Marker band in one chromosome 14 from Burkitt lymphomas. Nature **237,** 33–34 (1972)

Menezes, J., Leibold, W., Klein, G.: Biological differences between Epstein-Barr virus (EBV) strains with regard to lymphocyte transforming ability, superinfection and antigen induction. Exp. Cell Res. **92,** 478–484 (1975)

Menezes, J., Patel, P., Dussault, H., Bourkas, A. E.: Comparative studies on the induction of virus-associated nuclear antigen and early antigen by lymphocyte-transforming (B95-8) and non-transforming (P$_3$HR-1) strains of Epstein-Barr virus. Intervirology **9,** 86–94 (1978)

Menezes, J., Patel, P., Dussault, H., Joncas, J., Leibold, W.: Effect of interferon on lymphocyte transformation and nuclear antigen production by Epstein-Barr virus. Nature **260,** 430–432 (1976)

Miller, G., Lipman, M.: Release of infectious Epstein-Barr virus by transformed marmoset leukocytes. Proc. Natl. Acad. Sci. USA **70,** 190–194 (1973)

Miller, G., Shope, T., Lisco, H., Stitt, D., Lipman, M.: Epstein-Barr virus: transformation, cytopathic changes, and viral antigens in squirrel monkey and marmoset leukocytes. Proc. Natl. Acad. Sci. USA **69,** 383–387 (1972)

Miller, G., Niederman, J. C., Andrews, L-L.: Prolonged oropharyngeal excretion of Epstein-Barr virus after infectious mononucleosis. N. Engl. J. Med. **288,** 229–232 (1973)

Miller, G., Robinson, J., Heston, L., Lipman, M.: Differences between laboratory strains of Epstein-Barr virus based on immortalization, abortive infection, and interference. Proc. Natl. Acad. Sci. USA **71,** 4006–4010 (1974)

Miller, G., Coope, D., Niederman, J., Pagano, J.: Biological properties and viral surface antigens of Burkitt lymphoma- and mononucleosis-derived strains of Epstein-Barr virus released from transformed marmoset cells. J. Virol. **18,** 1071–1080 (1976)

Miller, G., Shope, T., Coope, D., Waters, L., Pagano, J., Bornkamm, G. W., Henle, W.: Lymphoma in cotton-top marmosets after inoculation with Epstein-Barr virus: tumor incidence, histologic spectrum, antibody responses, demonstration of viral DNA, and characterization of viruses. J. Exp. Med. **145,** 948–967 (1977)

Mizuno, F., Aya, T., Osato, T.: Growth in semisolid agar medium of human cord leukocytes freshly transformed by Epstein-Barr virus. J. Natl. Cancer Inst. **56,** 171–173 (1976)

Moore, G. E., Grace, J. T., Citron, P., Gerner, R., Burns, A.: Leukocyte cultures of patients with leukemia and lymphomas. NY State J. Med. **66,** 2757–2764 (1966)

Moore, G. E., Gerner, R. E., Franklin, H. A.: Culture of normal human leukocytes. J. Am. Med. Assoc. **199,** 519–524 (1967)

Moss, D. J., Pope, J. H.: Assay of the infectivity of Epstein-Barr virus by transformation of human leucocytes *in vitro*. J. Gen. Virol. **17**, 233–236 (1972)

Nadkarni, J. S., Nadkarni, J. J., Clifford, P., Manolov, G., Fenyö, E. M., Klein, E.: Characteristics of new cell lines derived from Burkitt lymphomas. Cancer **23**, 64–79 (1969)

Niederman, J. C., Evans, A. S., Subrahmanyan, L., McCollum, R. W.: Prevalence, incidence and persistence of EB virus antibody in young adults. N. Engl. J. Med. **282**, 361–365 (1970)

Niedermann, J. C., Miller, G., Pearson, H. A., Pagano, J. S., Dowaliby, J. M.: Infectious mononucleosis. Epstein-Barr virus shedding in saliva and the oropharynx. N. Engl. J. Med. **294**, 1355–1359 (1976)

Nilsson, K., Klein, G., Henle, W., Henle, G.: The establishment of lymphoblastoid lines from adult and fetal human lymphoid tissue and its dependence on EBV. Int. J. Cancer **8**, 443–450 (1971)

Nonoyama, M., Pagano, J. S.: Homology between Epstein-Barr virus DNA and viral DNA from Burkitt's lymphoma and nasopharyngeal carcinoma determined by DNA-DNA reassociation kinetics. Nature **242**, 44–47 (1973)

Nyormoi, O., Thorley-Lawson, D. A., Elkington, J., Strominger, J. L.: Differential effect of phosphonoacetic acid on the expression of Epstein-Barr viral antigens and virus production. Proc. Natl. Acad. Sci. USA **73**, 1745–1748 (1976)

Olding, L. B., Jensen, F. C., Oldstone, M. B. A.: Pathogenesis of cytomegalovirus infection. I. Activation of virus from bone marrow derived lymphocytes by *in vitro* allogenic reaction. J. Exp. Med. **141**, 561–572 (1975)

Olding, L. B., Kingsbury, D. T., Oldstone, M. B. A.: Pathogenesis of cytomegalovirus infection. Distribution of viral products, immune complexes and autoimmunity during latent murine infection. J. Gen. Virol. **33**, 267–280 (1976)

Oldstone, M. B. A., Haspel, M. V., Pellegrino, M. A., Kingsbury, D. T., Olding, L.: Histocompatability complex and virus infection latency and activation. Transplant. Rev. **31**, 225–239 (1976)

Orellana, T., Kieff, E.: Epstein-Barr virus-specific RNA. II. Analysis of polyadenylated viral RNA in restringent, abortive, and productive infections. J. Virol. **22**, 321–330 (1977)

Pagano, J. S.: Diseases and mechanisms of persistent DNA virus infection: latency and cellular transformation. J. Infect. Dis. **132**, 209–223 (1975)

Pagano, J. S., Huang, C-H., Huang, Y-T.: Epstein-Barr virus genome in infectious mononucleosis. Nature **263**, 787–789 (1976)

Pattengale, P. K., Smith, R. W., Gerber, P.: Selective transformation of B lymphocytes by EB virus. Lancet **1973 II**, 93

Pereira, M. S., Blake, J. M., Macrae, A. D.: EB virus antibody at different ages. Br. Med. J. **1969 IV**, 526–527

Plummer, G.: Isolation of herpesviruses from trigeminal ganglia of man, monkeys, and cats. J. Infect. Dis. **128**, 345–348 (1973)

Pope, J. H., Horne, M. K., Scott, W.: Transformation of foetal human leukocytes *in vitro* by filtrates of a human leukaemic cell line containing herpes-like virus. Int. J. Cancer **3**, 857–866 (1968)

Pritchett, R. F., Hayward, S. D., Kieff, E. D.: DNA of Epstein-Barr virus. I. Comparative studies of the DNA of EBV from HR-1 and B95-8 cells. Size, structure and relatedness. J. Virol. **15**, 556–584 (1975)

Pritchett, R., Pedersen, M., Kieff, E.: Complexity of EBV homologous DNA in continuous lymphoblastoid cell lines. Virology **74**, 227–231 (1976)

Rabin, H., Wallen, W. C., Neubauer, R. H., Epstein, M. A.: Comparisons of surface markers on herpesvirus-associated lymphoid cells of nonhuman primates and established human lymphoid cell lines. In: Comparative leukemia research 1973. Leukemogenesis. Ito, Y., Dutcher, R. M. (eds.), pp. 367–374. Tokyo, Basel: University of Tokyo Press/Karger 1975

Rabin, H., Neubauer, R. H., Hopkins III, R. F., Levy, B. M.: Characterization of lymphoid cell lines established from multiple Epstein-Barr virus (EBV-) induced lymphomas in a cotton-topped marmoset. Int. J. Cancer **20**, 44–50 (1977)

Rapp, F., Westmoreland, D.: Cell transformation by DNA-containing viruses. Biochem. Biophys. Acta **458**, 167–211 (1976)

Reedman, B. M., Klein, G.: Cellular localization of an Epstein-Barr virus (EBV)-associated complement-fixing antigen in producer and nonproducer lymphoblastoid cell lines. Int. J. Cancer **11**, 499–520 (1973)

Rickinson, A. B., Jarvis, J. E., Crawford, D. H., Epstein, M. A.: Observations on the type of infection by Epstein-Barr virus in peripheral lymphoid cells of patients with infectious mononucleosis. Int. J. Cancer **14**, 704–715 (1974)

Rickinson, A. B., Epstein, M. A., Crawford, D. H.: Absence of infectious Epstein-Barr virus in blood in acute infectious mononucleosis. Nature **258**, 236–238 (1975)

Rickinson, A. B., Finerty, S., Epstein, M. A.: Comparative studies on adult donor lymphocytes infected by EB virus *in vivo* or *in vitro:* origin of transformed cells arising in co-cultures with foetal lymphocytes. Int. J. Cancer **19,** 775–782 (1977a)

Rickinson, A. B., Finerty, S., Epstein, M. A.: Mechanism of the establishment of Epstein-Barr virus genome-containing lymphoid cell lines from infectious mononucleosis patients: studies with phosphonoacetate. Int. J. Cancer **20,** 861–868 (1977b)

Rickinson, A. B., Crawford, D., Epstein, M. A.: Inhibition of the *in vitro* outgrowth of Epstein-Barr virus-transformed lymphocytes by thymus-dependent lymphocytes from infectious mononucleosis patients. Clin. Exp. Immunol. **28,** 72–79 (1977c)

Rickinson, A. B., Epstein, M. A.: Sensitivity of the transforming and replicative functions of Epstein-Barr virus to inhibition by phosphonoacetate. J. Gen. Virol. **40,** 409–420 (1978)

Robinson, J., Miller, G.: Assay for Epstein-Barr virus based on stimulation of DNA synthesis in mixed leukocytes from human umbilical cord blood. J. Virol. **15,** 1065–1072 (1975)

Rocchi, G., de Felici, A., Ragona, G., Heinz, A.: Quantitative evaluation of Epstein-Barr-virus-infected mononuclear peripheral blood leukocytes in infectious mononucleosis. N. Engl. J. Med. **296,** 132–134 (1977)

Roizman, B.: The biochemical features of herpesvirus-infected cells, particularly as they relate to their possible oncogenicity, a review. In: Oncogenesis and herpesviruses. Biggs, P. M., de-Thé, G., Payne, L. N. (eds.), pp. 1–17. Lyon: IARC 1972

Royston, I., Sullivan, J. L., Periman, P. O., Perlin, E.: Cell-mediated immunity to Epstein-Barr virus-transformed lymphoblastoid cells in acute infectious mononucleosis. N. Engl. J. Med. **293,** 1159–1163 (1975)

Shanmugaratnam, K.: Studies on the etiology of nasopharyngeal carcinoma. In: Int. Rev. Exp. Pathol. **10,** 361–413 (1971)

Shibuta, H., Ishikawa, T., Hondo, R., Aoyama, Y., Kurata, K., Matumoto, M.: Varicella virus isolation from spinal ganglion. Arch. Virusforsch. **45,** 382–385 (1974)

Shope, T., Dechairo, D., Miller, G.: Malignant lymphoma in cottontop marmosets after inoculation with Epstein-Barr virus. Proc. Natl. Acad. Sci. USA **70,** 2487–2491 (1973)

Silvestre, D., Ernberg, I., Neauport-Sautes, C., Kourilsky, F. M., Klein, G.: Differentiation between early and late membrane antigen on human lymphoblastoid cell lines infected with Epstein-Barr virus. II. Immunoelectron microscopy. J. Natl. Cancer Inst. **53,** 67–74 (1974)

Strauch, B., Andrews, L-L., Siegel, N., Miller, G.: Oropharyngeal excretion of Epstein-Barr virus by renal transplant recipients and other patients treated with immunosuppressive drugs. Lancet **1974 I,** 234–237

Sugden, B.: Comparison of Epstein-Barr viral DNAs in Burkitt lymphoma biopsy cells and in cells clonally transformed *in vitro.* Proc. Natl. Acad. Sci. USA **74,** 4651–4655 (1977)

Sugden, B., Mark, W.: Clonal transformation of adult human leukocytes by Epstein-Barr virus. J. Virol. **23,** 503–508 (1977)

Summers, W. C., Klein, G.: Inhibition of Epstein-Barr virus DNA synthesis and late gene expression by phosphonoacetic acid. J. Virol. **18,** 151–155 (1976)

Svedmyr, A., Demissie, A.: Age distribution of antibodies to Burkitt cells. Acta Pathol. Microbiol. Scand. **73,** 653–654 (1968)

Svedmyr, E., Jondal, M.: Cytotoxic effector cells specific for B cell lines transformed by Epstein-Barr virus are present in patients with infectious mononucleosis. Proc. Natl. Acad. Sci. USA **72,** 1622–1626 (1975)

Takada, K., Ostato, T.: Analysis of the transformation of human lymphocytes by Epstein-Barr virus. I. Sequential occurrence from the virus-determined nuclear antigen synthesis, to blastogenesis, to DNA synthesis. Intervirology **11,** 30–39 (1978)

Thorley-Lawson, D. A., Chess, L., Strominger, J. L.: Suppression of in vitro Epstein-Barr virus infection. A new role for adult human T lymphocytes. J. Exp. Med. **146,** 495–508 (1977)

Thorley-Lawson, D., Strominger, J. L.: Transformation of human lymphocytes by Epstein-Barr virus is inhibited by phosphonoacetic acid. Nature **263,** 332–334 (1976)

Trumper, P. A., Epstein, M. A., Giovanella, B. C.: Activation *in vitro* by BUdR of a productive EB virus infection in the epithelial cells of nasopharyngeal carcinoma. Int. J. Cancer **17,** 578–587 (1976)

Trumper, P. A., Epstein, M. A., Giovanella, B. C., Finerty, S.: Isolation of infectious EB virus from the epithelial tumour cells of nasopharyngeal carcinoma. Int. J. Cancer **20,** 655–662 (1977)

University Health Physicians and PHLS Laboratories.: Infectious mononucleosis and its relationship to EB virus antibody. Br. Med. J. **1971 IV,** 643–646

Werner, J., Henle, G., Pinto, C. A., Haff, R. F., Henle, W.: Establishment of continuous lymphoblast cultures from leukocytes of gibbons (Hylobates lar). Int. J. Cancer **10,** 557–567 (1972)

Woodliff, H. J.: Blood and bone marrow cell culture. London: Eyre & Spottiswoode 1964

Yajima, Y., Tanaka, A., Nonoyama, M.: Inhibition of productive replication of Epstein-Barr virus DNA by phosphonoacetic acid. Virology **71**, 352–354 (1976)

Yefenof, E., Klein, G.: Membrane receptor stripping confirms the association between EBV receptors and complement receptors on the surface of human B lymphoma lines. Int. J. Cancer **20**, 347–352 (1977)

Yefenof, E., Klein, G., Jondal, M., Oldstone, M. B. A.: Surface markers on human B- and T-lymphocytes. IX. Two-color immunofluorescence studies on the association between EBV receptors and complement receptors on the surface of lymphoid cell lines. Int. J. Cancer **17**, 693–700 (1976)

zur Hausen, H., Fresen, K. O.: Heterogeneity of Epstein-Barr virus II. Induction of early antigens (EA) by complementation. Virology **81**, 138–143 (1977)

2 Morphology of the Virus and of Virus-Induced Cytopathologic Changes

M. A. Epstein and B. G. Achong

Department of Pathology, The Medical School, University of Bristol, University Walk, Bristol BS8 1TD (England)

A. INTRODUCTION

From the first moment of sighting, it was immediately recognized that the virus in cultured Burkitt's lymphoma (BL) lymphoid cells was morphologically typical of the herpes family (Fig. 1) (Epstein et al., 1964 a). This observation was never in doubt and led to the description of the agent in the early years as "herpes-like" or "herpes-type" (Stewart et al., 1965; Rabson et al., 1966; Hinuma et al., 1967; Henle et al., 1967).

By the time that the designation Epstein-Barr Virus (EBV) began to come into general use (Henle et al., 1968), the biologic, immunologic, and biochemical singularity of the virus was being firmly established (Epstein et al., 1965 a; Henle and Henle, 1966 a, b; Epstein and Achong, 1967, 1968 a, b; zur Hausen et al., 1970) and it was clear that this new and unusual member of the human herpesvirus group required extensive investigation.

B. VIRUS MORPHOLOGY

I. STRUCTURE OF THE VIRION

EBV particles from whatever source have proved structurally indistinguishable. It was thought at first that EBV might perhaps be slightly smaller than other herpesviruses, but this view probably arose as a result of the particular preparative techniques used; the influence of different dehydration and embedding procedures on virus size has long been recognized in thin-sectioned material (Epstein, 1962), as has the flattening effect of drying in whole mount, negatively stained preparations. Although comparative studies taking these factors into account have not been undertaken, it is not now considered that there are significant size differences between EBV and other members of the herpes group and in every other detail of morphology EBV is an absolutely typical herpesvirus.

1. The Immature Particle (Nucleocapsid)

In thin sections of productively infected cells, immature particles are present in both the nucleus and cytoplasm (Figs. 1, 2, 3, 9, and 10). Such particles show a hexagonal

Fig. 1.[1] Survey picture of the first EBV particles to be found in a cell of the earliest EB1 (BL-derived) culture ▶ examined by electron microscopy. The cell membrane crosses the *upper right corner* with the nucleus in the *lower right portion* of the field; the nucleoplasm shows greatly reduced electron opacity and the double nuclear envelope includes a short region of reduplication. The cytoplasm contains several mature EBV particles (*v*) within membrane-bounded spaces, some immature particles (*iv*), and sheaves of electron-dense altered microtubules cut in various planes. In addition, there is a large lipid body *(below left)*, some rough endoplasmic reticulum (*er*), and many scattered free ribosomes (× 51,000). From Epstein, M. A., Achong, B. G., Barr, Y. M. (1964a): Courtesy of the editor

---

[1] All the figures, except Figs. 4 and 5, show electron micrographs of thin sections of cells fixed in glutaraldehyde followed by osmium tetroxide, embedded in epoxy resin, and stained in the section with uranyl acetate.

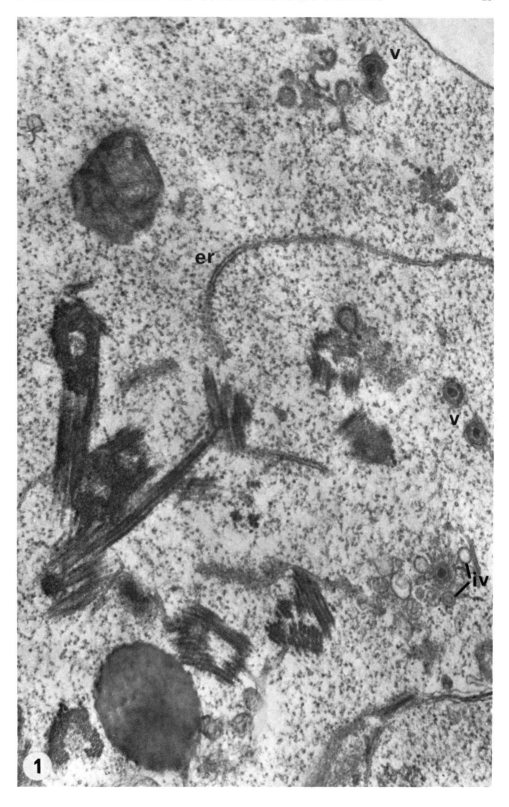

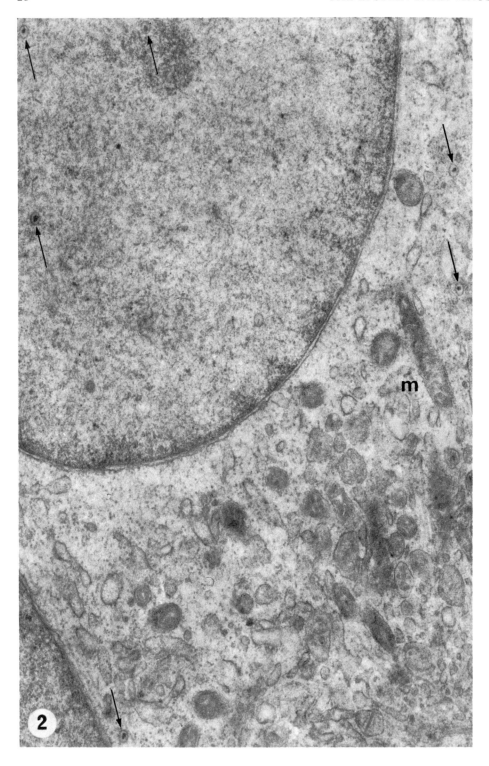

profile when appropriately oriented to the plane of section, measure about 80 mμ in diameter, and are either empty or contain a central dense or ring-shaped nucleoid or core (Figs. 1, 2, 3, 9, and 10) (Epstein et al., 1964a, b, c; 1965a).

With negative-contrast preparations, irrespective of whether the virus has been examined after purification procedures (Toplin and Schidlovsky, 1966) or directly within fragmented cells (Hummeler et al., 1966), the immature particles again appear hexagonal, but also exhibit triangular surface facets covered by hollow, tubular capsomeres (Figs. 4 and 5). The capsomeres measure 12 mμ in length, have a central hole 4 mμ in diameter, show center-to-center spacing of 12 mμ, and are regularly arranged in hexagonal array surrounded by six neighbors, except where corner capsomeres lie in fivefold symmetry. Negative staining studies have also shown that the immature particle is an icosahedron with 162 capsomeres and a diameter of 100 mμ (Toplin and Schidlovsky, 1966; Hummeler et al., 1966; Yamaguchi et al., 1967). This slightly larger size as compared to that found in thin sections results from the flattening effects occurring during negative staining added to the small amount of shrinkage which accompanies embedding for sectioning. Slightly damaged immature particles are penetrated by contrast medium when negatively stained and this has confirmed that they are either empty (Fig. 4) or contain central, dense or ring-shaped cores (Fig. 5).

2. The Mature Enveloped Particle

When sectioned, the mature EBV particle with its additional outer enveloping membrane measures about 120 mμ across and always contains a dense central nucleoid or core of around 45 mμ diameter (Fig. 6). The invariable presence of the dense core suggests that this structure must be developed in the immature particles before maturation and that therefore immature particles which are empty or have ring-shaped nucleoids are either defective and never destined to mature, or represent developmental stages on the way to the dense-cored form (Epstein et al., 1964a, b, c; 1965a).

Intact mature particles are not usually found in negatively stained material; the preparation procedure usually causes slight damage to the envelope which therefore appears collapsed and penetrated by negative stain, allowing the immature component within to be visualized (Toplin and Schidlovsky, 1966; Hummeler et al., 1966). Mature EBV particles are not therefore suitable for measuring in such material.

II. VIRUS MATURATION

1. Envelopment

As with all herpesviruses, the maturation of EBV virions takes place by immature particles budding through cellular membranes and becoming enveloped in a portion of

◀ **Fig. 2.** Part of the lobed nucleus, bounded by its intact double envelope, and the adjacent cytoplasm of a productively infected cultured human lymphoid cell. Immature EBV particles can be seen in both the nucleus and cytoplasm *(arrows);* the cell shows such characteristic virus-induced cytopathologic changes as marginated chromatin, low electron opacity in the nucleoplasm, and altered cristae in the mitochondrion *(m)*. (× 37,500)

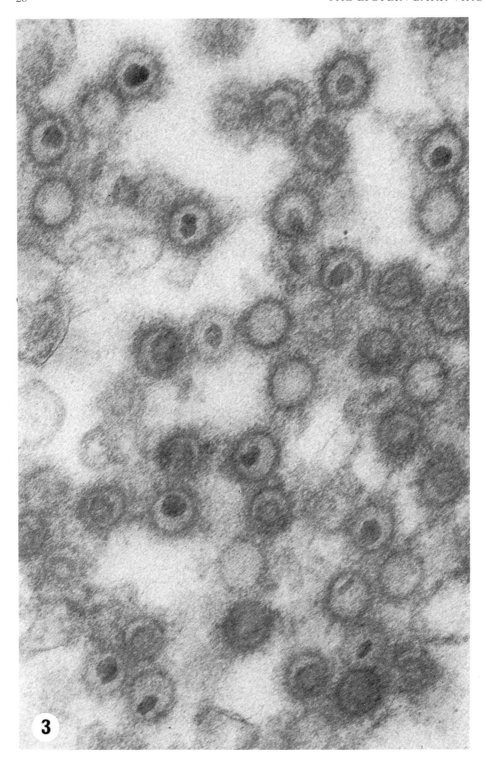

3

the membrane as they pass through (Figs. 7 and 8). Intranuclear immature particles bud at the inner nuclear membrane (Figs. 8 and 9) and cytoplasmic immature particles either at smooth membranes of the endoplasmic reticulum (Fig. 10) or at the plasmalemma (Fig. 7); in consequence, mature particles accumulate in the perinuclear space (Fig. 9), within membrane-bounded cytoplasmic spaces (Figs. 6 and 10), and just outside the cell membrane (Fig. 11).

2. Incorporation of Antigens in the Virion

The early observations on the structure of immature and mature EBV particles and on the mechanism of envelopment have been solidly confirmed (Stewart et al., 1965; Epstein et al., 1965b; O'Conor and Rabson, 1965; Rabson et al., 1966; Epstein et al., 1967; Dalton and Manaker, 1967; Grace, 1967; Pope et al., 1968). Furthermore, it is now clear that during the development and maturation of EBV only two virus-determined antigens are known to be incorporated in the virion. Thus, viral capsid antigen (VCA) (Chap. 3) occurs in the nucleus and cytoplasm of the infected cell (Henle and Henle, 1966b) where it takes part in the formation of the hollow tubular capsomeres of the immature particles which appear at these two sites. In addition, membrane antigen (MA) (Chap. 3) which is present in the membranes of infected cells, is acquired by the mature particle during envelopment by budding, thus becoming a structural component of the viral envelope (Silvestre et al., 1971). On the other hand, human leukocyte antigens (HL-A), which are of course unrelated to EBV, are not picked up in this way (Silvestre et al., 1974) despite being present on the cell membrane; this absence is particularly surprising since there is a 36-fold enhancement in the expression of HL-A in EBV-infected cells (McCune et al., 1975).

C. VIRUS-INDUCED CYTOPATHOLOGIC CHANGES

Although there is no fully permissive system for EBV replication, "producer" lymphoid lines, which include at any one time a small number of cells undergoing a virus replicative cycle (Chap. 1), show characteristic fine-structural cytopathologic changes in those cells assembling the virus particles. These changes, first described by Epstein et al. (1964a, c; 1965a, b), consist of some or all of the following:

1. A striking concentration of the chromatin into dense, marginated clumps with decreased electron opacity of the remaining nucleoplasm (Figs. 1, 2, 9, and 10). This rearrangement of the chromatin underlies the appearance at the light microscope level of the classical Cowdry type-A inclusion body of herpesvirus-infected cells.

2. Fragmentation and multilayered reduplication of the nuclear envelope (Fig. 1) with nucleocytoplasmic continuity between segments of the nuclear membrane.

◀ **Fig. 3.** Group of cytoplasmic immature EBV particles, either empty or with a central ring-shaped or dense nucleoid or core. A hexagonal profile can be seen in particles appropriately oriented to the plane of section. (× 150,000)

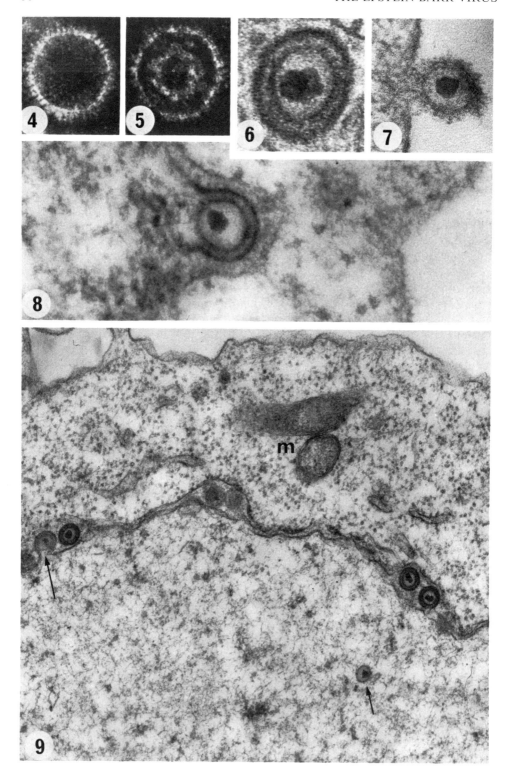

3. Mitochondrial changes in which the cristae and matrix are replaced by a beaded or clubbed electron-opaque material (Figs. 2, 10 and 11).

4. Sheaves of unusual electron-opaque, altered microtubules (Figs. 1 and 10).

5. Unusual, intranuclear ring-shaped structures of unknown nature, sometimes associated with immature EBV particles, accompanied occasionally by intranuclear filaments.

The association of these changes with EBV production was soon confirmed in numerous studies (Rabson et al., 1966; Epstein et al., 1967; Dalton and Manaker, 1967; Pope et al., 1968; Hampar et al., 1972) and it is of interest that similar sheaves of altered microtubules are known to occur in cells producing other tumor-associated herpesviruses (Fawcett, 1956; Epstein et al., 1968), while the nuclear ring-shaped structures and filaments have long been recognized in herpesvirus-infected cells in general (Morgan et al., 1959; Murphy et al., 1967; Epstein et al., 1968).

It is now clear that the above characteristic cytopathology induced in lymphoid cells by EBV replication is not restricted to this cell type. Recent experiments with the squamous epithelial cells of nude mouse-passaged nasopharyngeal carcinoma (NPC) have shown that activation of virus production can be induced in vitro by treatment with 5-bromodeoxyuridine (BUDR) (Trumper et al., 1976) or in some cases merely by the nude mouse environment (Trumper et al., 1977), and when this occurs, the epithelial cells involved show exactly the same changes (Fig. 12).

The naturally occurring cytopathologic changes discussed so far have obviously not been able to provide information on the earliest steps whereby EBV enters and infects cells, since recognizable changes do not arise until the end of the virus replicative cycle (Chap. 1). The early stages of the cycle can only be investigated under experimental conditions. Indeed, a recent study, although giving some useful information on these early stages, was based on a highly artificial system in which a nonproducer BL cell line (Raji), already carrying the EBV genome, was superinfected with the uniquely unusual

◀ **Figs. 4 and 5.** Details of immature EBV virions penetrated by negative stain; the hexagonal shape is evident and hollow tubular capsomeres can be well seen in side view at the surface of the profile. One particle is empty, while the other has a central ring-shaped nucleoid. Whole mount negative-contrast preparations made with phosphotungstic acid. (× 275,000)

Fig. 6. Mature EBV particle with its additional cell membrane-derived outer envelope. The particle lies in a cytoplasmic space the limiting membrane of which crosses the *upper right corner* of the field. (× 225,000)

Fig. 7. Small area of the surface of a productively infected lymphoid cell. An immature EBV particle is in the process of maturation by budding through the plasmalemma into the extracellular space and is almost enveloped by a portion of the cell membrane. (× 120,000)

Fig. 8. Detail of nucleus *(left)* and cytoplasm, with the plasmalemma on the *extreme right.* The double nuclear envelope crosses the center of the field with an immature EBV virion maturing by budding into the perinuclear space. (× 120,000)

Fig. 9. Nucleus *(below)* and cytoplasm of an EBV-producing lymphoid cell. Mature EBV has accumulated in the perinuclear space after budding from the nucleus through the inner nuclear envelope. This process of budding can be seen on the *left (long arrow);* there is also an immature particle in the nucleus *(short arrow).* Virus-induced cytopathologic change is evident in the altered mitochondria *(m)* and the extremely electron-lucent nucleoplasm. (× 46,250)

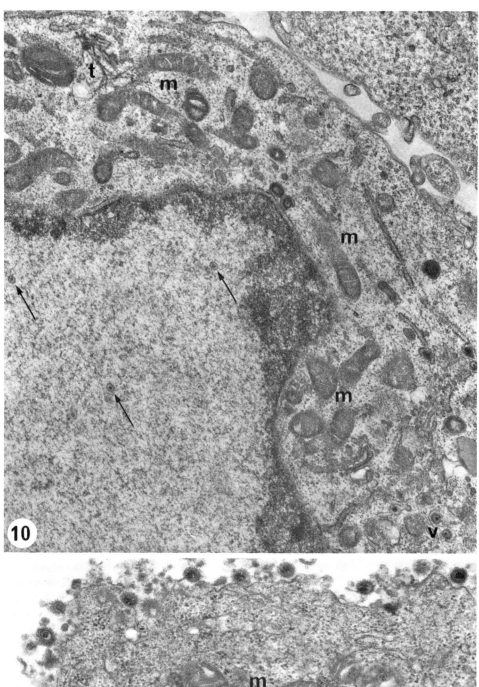

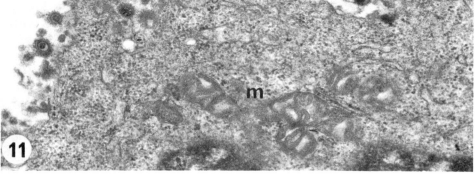

nontransforming mutant P₃HR-1 strain of EBV (Chap. 1). Nevertheless, it would seem that EBV enters the cell by fusion of the envelope membrane with the plasmalemma, after which the nucleocapsid migrates towards the nucleus where it disintegrates, presumably to liberate its DNA for infection of the cell (Seigneurin et al., 1977).

D. COMMENT

The crucial importance of fine structural studies in the discovery of EBV has already been stressed (Chap. 1). The recognition of the agent as a herpesvirus (Epstein et al., 1964 a) was of no particular significance at the time, since herpesviruses were not then known to be oncogenic. However, the subsequent demonstration of the natural etiologic role of herpesviruses in the malignant lymphoma of Marek's disease (Churchill and Biggs, 1967; Solomon et al., 1968; Epstein et al., 1968) and the Lucké frog carcinoma (Mizell et al., 1969; Naegele et al., 1974), and of the experimental carcinogenicity of subhuman primate herpesviruses in South American monkeys, marmosets, and laboratory rabbits (Meléndez et al., 1969; Morgan et al., 1970; Daniel et al., 1970; Meléndez et al., 1972), soon provided important implications for EBV in relation to the comparative aspects of herpesviruses and cancer (Chap. 17). Indeed, Marek's lymphoma and its causative herpesvirus, as the first naturally occurring malignant tumor to be controlled by a viral vaccine (Churchill et al., 1969; Okazaki et al., 1970), are of quite outstanding consequence for long-term goals with EBV (Chap. 19).

The finding by electron microscopy of immature EBV particles in the cytoplasm as well as in the nucleus, with maturation by budding at both sites (Epstein et al., 1965 a), is not in agreement with biochemical and morphologic data on some other herpesviruses, which stress the exclusively nuclear site of assembly of immature particles (Roizman, 1972). However, unequivocal morphologic evidence for both cytoplasmic and nuclear virus assembly has been obtained with the Lucké herpesvirus (Lunger et al., 1965), varicella-zoster virus (VZV) (Achong and Meurisse, 1968), Marek's disease virus (MDV) (Epstein et al., 1968) and, most tellingly, with herpesvirus saimiri (HVS) where the extremely slow replicative cycle has permitted the separation of an initial cytoplasmic phase of virus assembly from a subsequent nuclear phase (Morgan et al., 1976).

The further fine structural finding that MA is incorporated into the viral envelope during virus maturation by budding (Silvestre et al., 1971) provides a clear explanation for the fact that antibodies to MA are the virus-neutralizing antibodies (Pearson et al.,

◀ **Fig. 10.** Survey of a lymphoid cell producing EBV and showing characteristic virus-induced cytopathology. Mature particles lie in the cytoplasm (at *v*) within a membrane-bounded space, with immature particles in the nucleus *(arrows)*. The nucleus shows clumped, marginated chromatin with loss of nucleoplasmic electron-density, while the cytoplasm contains altered, electron-opaque microtubules (*t*) and mitochondria with clubbed cristae (at *m*). (× 28,000)

Fig. 11. Detail of the surface of an EBV-producing lymphoid cell showing mature particles accumulated outside the plasmalemma after budding at that site. Mitochondria with clubbed cristae are present in the cytoplasm (at *m*) and clumped chromatin lies in the nucleus at the *bottom of the field*. (× 32,000)

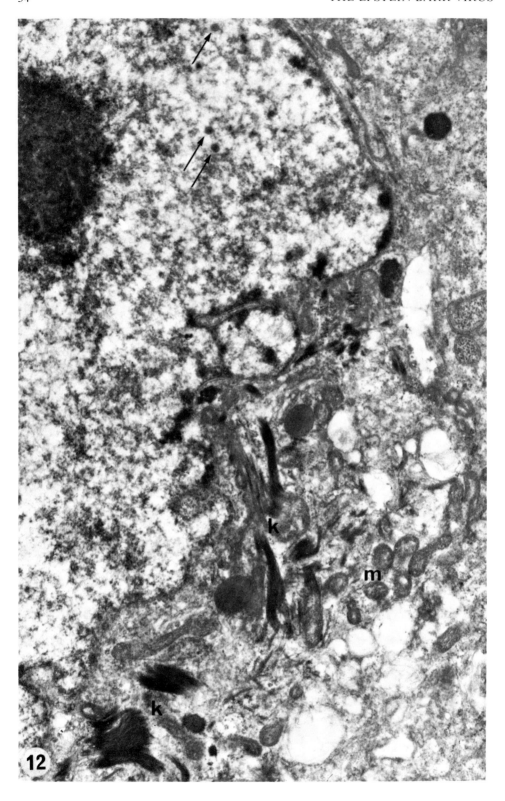

1970, 1971; de Schryver et al., 1974, 1976); the importance of viral DNA-free cell membrane preparations expressing MA as a possible vaccine for human use has already been pointed out (Epstein, 1976) and is discussed further in Chap. 19.

REFERENCES

Achong, B. G., Meurisse, E. V.: Observations on the fine structure and replication of varicella virus in cultivated human amnion cells. J. Gen. Virol. **3,** 305–308 (1968)

Churchill, A. E., Biggs, P. M.: Agent of Marek's disease in tissue culture. Nature **215,** 528–530 (1967)

Churchill, A. E., Payne, L. N., Chubb, R. C.: Immunization against Marek's disease using a live attenuated virus. Nature **221,** 744–747 (1969)

Dalton, A. J., Manaker, R. A.: The comparison of virus particles associated with Burkitt lymphoma with other herpes-like viruses. The University of Texas M. D. Anderson Hospital and Tumor Institute 20th Annual Symposium on Fundamental Cancer Research. Carcinogenesis: a broad critique. pp. 59–90. Baltimore: Williams and Wilkins 1967

Daniel, M. D., Meléndez, L. V., Hunt, R. D., King, N. W., Williamson, M. E.: Malignant lymphoma induced in rabbits by *Herpesvirus saimiri* strains. Bacteriol. Proc. 195 (1970)

De Schryver, A., Klein, G., Hewetson, J., Rocchi, G., Henle, W., Henle, G., Moss, D. J., Pope, J. H.: Comparison of EBV neutralization tests based on abortive infection or transformation of lymphoid cells and their relation to membrane reactive antibodies (anti MA). Int. J. Cancer **13,** 353–362 (1974)

De Schryver, A., Rosén, A., Gunvén, P., Klein, G.: Comparison between two antibody populations in the EBV system: anti-MA *versus* neutralizing antibody activity. Int. J. Cancer **17,** 8–13 (1976)

Epstein, M. A.: Observations on the fine structure of mature herpes simplex virus and on the composition of its nucleoid. J. Exp. Med. **115,** 1–12 (1962)

Epstein, M. A.: Epstein-Barr virus – is it time to develop a vaccine program? J. Natl. Cancer Inst. **56,** 697–700 (1976)

Epstein, M. A., Achong, B. G.: Immunologic relationship of the herpes-like EB virus of cultured Burkitt lymphoblasts. Cancer Res. **27,** 2489–2493 (1967)

Epstein, M. A., Achong, B. G.: Specific immunofluorescence test for the herpes-type EB virus of Burkitt lymphoblasts, authenticated by electron microscopy. J. Natl. Cancer Inst. **40,** 593–607 (1968 a)

Epstein, M. A., Achong, B. G.: Observations on the nature of the herpes-type EB virus in cultured Burkitt lymphoblasts, using a specific immunofluorescence test. J. Natl. Cancer Inst. **40,** 609–621 (1968 b)

Epstein, M. A., Achong, B. G., Barr, Y. M.: Virus particles in cultured lymphoblasts from Burkitt's lymphoma. Lancet **1964 a I,** 702–703

Epstein, M. A., Barr, Y. M., Achong, B. G.: A second virus-carrying tissue culture strain (EB2) of lymphoblasts from Burkitt's lymphoma. Pathol. Biol. (Paris) **12,** 1233–1234 (1964b)

Epstein, M. A., Barr, Y. M., Achong, B. G.: Avian tumor virus behavior as a guide in the investigation of a human neoplasm. Natl. Cancer Inst. Monogr. **17,** 637–650 (1964 c)

Epstein, M. A., Henle, G., Achong, B. G., Barr, Y. M.: Morphological and biological studies on a virus in cultured lymphoblasts from Burkitt's lymphoma. J. Exp. Med. **121,** 761–770 (1965 a)

Epstein, M. A., Barr, Y. M., Achong, B. G.: Studies with Burkitt's lymphoma. Wistar Inst. Symp. Monogr. **4,** 69–82 (1965 b)

Epstein, M. A., Achong, B. G., Pope, J. H.: Virus in cultured lymphoblasts from a New Guinea Burkitt lymphoma. Br. Med. J. **1967 I,** 290–291

Epstein, M. A., Achong, B. G., Churchill, A. E., Biggs, P. M.: Structure and development of the herpes-type virus of Marek's disease. J. Natl. Cancer Inst., **41,** 805–820 (1968)

◀ **Fig. 12.** Malignant epithelial cell from a nude mouse-passaged NPC in which EBV replication was activated in vitro by BUDR; the squamous nature of the cell is evident from the presence of dense cytoplasmic bundles of keratin fibrils (*k*). The nucleus lies on the *left;* it shows loss of electron density, small clumps of marginated chromatin, and immature EBV particles *(arrows)*. The cell is degenerating, with cytoplasmic vacuolation and changes in the mitochondrial cristae (at *m*). (× 20,000)

Fawcett, D. W.: Electron microscope observations on intracellular virus-like particles associated with the cells of the Lucké renal adenocarcinoma. J. Biophys. Biochem. Cytol. **2**, 725–747 (1956)

Grace, J. T.: Hematopoietic cell cultures and associated herpes-type viruses. Cancer Res. **27**, 2494–2499 (1967)

Hampar, B., Derge, J. G., Martos, L. M., Walker, J. L.: Synthesis of Epstein-Barr virus after activation of the viral genome in a "virus-negative" human lymphoblastoid cell (Raji) made resistant to 5-bromodeoxyuridine. Proc. Natl. Acad. Sci. USA **69**, 78–82 (1972)

Henle, G., Henle, W.: Studies on cell lines derived from Burkitt's lymphoma. Trans. NY Acad. Sci. **29**, 71–79 (1966a)

Henle, G., Henle, W.: Immunofluorescence in cells derived from Burkitt's lymphoma. J. Bacteriol. **91**, 1248–1256 (1966b)

Henle, W., Diehl, V., Kohn, G., zur Hausen, H., Henle, G.: Herpes-type virus and chromosome marker in normal leukocytes after growth with irradiated Burkitt cells. Science **157**, 1064–1065 (1967)

Henle, G., Henle, W., Diehl, V.: Relation of Burkitt's tumor-associated herpes-type virus to infectious mononucleosis. Proc. Natl. Acad. Sci. USA **59**, 94–101 (1968)

Hinuma, Y., Konn, M., Yamaguchi, J., Wudarski, D. J., Blakeslee, J. R., Grace, J. T.: Immunofluorescence and herpes-type virus particles in the P_3HR-1 Burkitt lymphoma cell line. J. Virol. **1**, 1045–1051 (1967)

Hummeler, K., Henle, G., Henle, W.: Fine structure of a virus in cultured lymphoblasts from Burkitt lymphoma. J. Bacteriol. **91**, 1366–1368 (1966)

Lunger, P. D., Darlington, R. W., Granoff, A.: Cell-virus relationships in the Lucké renal adenocarcinoma: an ultrastructure study. Ann. NY Acad. Sci. **126**, 289–314 (1965)

McCune, J. M., Humphreys, R. E., Yocum, R. R., Strominger, J. L.: Enhanced representation of HL-A antigens on human lymphocytes after mitogenesis induced by phytochemagglutin or Epstein-Barr virus. Proc. Natl. Acad. Sci. **72**, 3206–3209 (1975)

Meléndez, L. V., Hunt, R. D., Daniel, M. D., Garcia, F. G., Fraser, C. E. O.: Herpesvirus saimiri. II. An experimentally induced primate disease resembling reticulum cell sarcoma. Lab. Animal Care **19**, 378–386 (1969)

Meléndez, L. V., Hunt, R. D., King, N. W., Barahona, H. H., Daniel, M. D., Fraser, C. E. O., Garcia, F. G.: *Herpesvirus ateles,* a new lymphoma virus of monkeys. Nature New Biol. **235**, 182–184 (1972)

Mizell, M., Toplin, I., Isaacs, J. J.: Tumor induction in developing frog kidneys by a zonal centrifuge purified fraction of the frog herpes-type virus. Science **165**, 1134–1137 (1969)

Morgan, C., Rose, H. M., Holden, M., Jones, E. P.: Electron microscopic observations on the development of herpes simplex virus. J. Exp. Med. **110**, 643–656 (1959)

Morgan, D. G., Epstein, M. A., Achong, B. G., Meléndez, L. V.: Morphological confirmation of the herpes nature of a carcinogenic virus of primates *(Herpes saimiri)*. Nature **228**, 170–172 (1970)

Morgan, D. G., Achong, B. G., Epstein, M. A.: Morphological observations on the replication of herpesvirus saimiri in monkey kidney cell cultures. J. Gen. Virol. **32**, 461–470 (1976)

Murphy, F. A., Harrison, A. K., Whitfield, S. G.: Intranuclear formation of filaments in herpesvirus hominis infection of mice. Arch. Ges. Virusforsch. **21**, 463–468 (1967)

Naegele, R. F., Granoff, A., Darlington, R. W.: The presence of the Lucké herpesvirus genome in induced tadpole tumors and its oncogenicity: Koch-Henle postulates fulfilled. Proc. Natl. Acad. Sci. USA **71**, 830–834 (1974)

O'Conor, G. T., Rabson, A. S.: Herpes-like particles in an American lymphoma: preliminary note. J. Natl. Cancer Inst. **35**, 899–903 (1965)

Okazaki, W., Purchase, H. G., Burmester, B. R.: Protection against Marek's disease by vaccination with a herpesvirus of turkeys. Avian Dis. **14**, 413–429 (1970)

Pearson, G. Dewey, F., Klein, G., Henle, G., Henle, W.: Relation between neutralization of Epstein-Barr virus and antibodies to cell-membrane antigens induced by the virus. J. Natl. Cancer Inst. **45**, 989–995 (1970)

Pearson, G., Henle, G., Henle, W.: Production of antigens associated with Epstein-Barr virus in experimentally infected lymphoblastoid cell lines. J. Natl. Cancer Inst. **46**, 1243–1250 (1971)

Pope, J. H., Achong, B. G., Epstein, M. A.: Cultivation and fine structure of virus-bearing lymphoblasts from a second New Guinea Burkitt lymphoma: establishment of sublines with unusual cultural properties. Int. J. Cancer **3**, 171–182 (1968)

Rabson, A. S., O'Conor, G. T., Baron, S., Whang, J. J., Legallais, F. Y.: Morphologic, cytogenetic and virologic studies *in vitro* of a malignant lymphoma from an African child. Int. J. Cancer **1**, 89–106 (1966)

Roizman, B.: The biochemical features of herpesvirus-infected cells, particularly as they relate to their possible oncogenicity – a review. In: Oncogenesis and herpesviruses. Biggs, P. M., de-Thé, G., Payne, L. N. (eds.), pp. 1–17. Lyon: IARC 1972

Seigneurin, J-M., Vuillaume, M., Lenoir, G., de-Thé, G.: Replication of Epstein-Barr virus: ultrastructural and immunofluorescent studies of P₃HR1-superinfected Raji cells. J. Virol. **24**, 836–845 (1977)

Silvestre, D., Kourilsky, F. M., Klein, G., Yata, Y., Neauport-Sautes, C., Levy, J. P.: Relationship between the EBV-associated membrane antigen on Burkitt lymphoma cells and the viral envelope, demonstrated by immunoferritin labelling. Int. J. Cancer **8**, 222–233 (1971)

Silvestre, D., Ernberg, I., Neauport-Sautes, C., Kourilsky, F. M., Klein, G.: Differentiation between early and late membrane antigen on human lymphoblastoid cell lines infected with Epstein-Barr virus. II. Immunoelectron microscopy. J. Natl. Cancer Inst. **53**, 67–74 (1974)

Solomon, J. J., Witter, R. L., Nazerian, K., Burmester, B. R.: Studies on the etiology of Marek's disease. I. Propagation of the agent in cell culture. Proc. Soc. Exp. Biol. Med. **127**, 173–177 (1968)

Stewart, S. E., Lovelace, E., Whang, J. J., Ngu, V. A.: Burkitt tumor: tissue culture, cytogenetic and virus studies. J. Natl. Cancer Inst. **34**, 319–327 (1965)

Toplin, I., Schidlovsky, G.: Partial purification and electron microscopy of the virus in the EB-3 cell line derived from a Burkitt lymphoma. Science **152**, 1084–1085 (1966)

Trumper, P. A., Epstein, M. A., Giovanella, B. C.: Activation *in vitro* by BUdR of a productive EB virus infection in the epithelial cells of nasopharyngeal carcinoma. Int. J. Cancer **17**, 578–587 (1976)

Trumper, P. A., Epstein, M. A., Giovanella, B. C., Finerty, S.: Isolation of infectious EB virus from the epithelial tumour cells of nasopharyngeal carcinoma. Int. J. Cancer **20**, 655–662 (1977)

Yamaguchi, J., Hinuma, Y., Grace, J. T.: Structure of virus particles extracted from a Burkitt lymphoma cell line. J. Virol. **1**, 640–642 (1967)

zur Hausen, H., Schulte-Holthausen, H., Klein, G., Henle, W., Henle, G., Clifford, P., Santesson, L.: EBV DNA in biopsies of Burkitt tumours and anaplastic carcinomas of the nasopharynx. Nature **228**, 1056–1058 (1970)

3 EB Virus-Induced Antigens

I. Ernberg and G. Klein

Department of Tumor Biology, Karolinska Institutet, S-10401 Stockholm 60 (Sweden)

A. INTRODUCTION

The study of antigenic markers and antibodies directed against them has occupied a central position in all Epstein-Barr virus (EBV) research, ever since the discovery of the virus. Detailed seroepidemiologic studies on the distribution and pathogenic significance of virus infections, retrospective and prognostic studies on patients with EBV-related diseases, and tracing of early events during primary viral infection of normal cells in vitro are only some of the areas that were largely or entirely based on antigen-antibody tests. Serology played a primary role in establishing the relationship between the virus and the three EBV-related diseases: infectious mononucleosis (IM), Burkitt's lymphoma (BL), and nasopharyngeal carcinoma (NPC). Furthermore, the majority of viral infectivity assays are based on antigen induction in appropriate target cells.

This predominance of serology is due to the unusual properties of the virus-host cell interaction. The virus does not pass through a full replicative cycle upon infection of appropriate target cells. The spontaneous or induced virus cycle that occurs in some lymphoid cell lines and affects only a minority of the target cells, as a rule, is the only regularly available source of viral products. In a heterogeneous cell population, the detection of antigenic markers at the single cell level by methods like immunofluorescence plays a predominant role.

The central importance of EBV antigens for virtually all EBV work has led to numerous studies concerned with antigenic specificity, time of appearance, and role of the different antigens in relation to the virus cycle and virus-host cell relationships. Recently several investigators have started to characterize the antigens biochemically. However, with few exceptions (Zajac and Ogburn, 1975; Vestergaard et al., 1978), monospecific xenogeneic antisera against purified antigens have not yet been produced. Due to this fact and to the easy availability of high-titered human sera containing by now well-characterized combinations of antibodies against the various EBV-induced antigens, such sera are the generally accepted reagents for antigen detection. This also has some advantages. Human antibodies are specific for the different EBV antigens and there are as a rule no problems of background reactions (apart from sera of patients with autoimmune or rheumatoid diseases) when human target cells are used. With some antigens, like the EBV nuclear antigen (EBNA), it is important to exclude other anti-nuclear antibodies, particularly in tumor patient sera. This poses no major difficulty, however, as long as appropriate EBV-negative control cells are tested in parallel.

Table 1 summarizes the methods that have been used for the detection of different EBV-associated antigens. Among the serologic methods, immunofluorescence has been most widely used, ever since the initial development of the area and until today. However, important information was also obtained with other methods, particularly complement fixation (CF), immunodiffusion, and radiolabeled antibody studies. In addition to serologic assays, some EBV-determined antigens were detected by means of their reactivity with immunocompetent cells, but the relationship between serologically defined antigens and antigens detected by the cell mediated reactions is not well established.

Table 1. Methods for detection of EBV-associated antigens

Immunofluorescence	
Membrane antigen (MA)	Klein et al., 1966
Early antigen (EA)	Henle et al., 1970
Viral capsid antigen (VCA)	Henle and Henle, 1966
Nuclear antigen (EBNA)	Reedman and Klein, 1973
Immunodiffusion	Old et al., 1966; Konn et al., 1967
Heat-resistant soluble antigens (S)	Reedman et al., 1972
Heat-labile/heat-stable antigens	Demissie and Svedmyr, 1973
Complement fixation	Armstrong et al., 1966
Heat-resistant soluble antigens (S)	Gerber and Birch, 1967; Pope et al., 1969
Heat-resistant virion antigens	Vonka et al., 1970
Heat-labile sedimentable	Walters and Pope, 1971
^{125}I-*labeled antibodies*	Inoue and Klein, 1970
Extracted antigen	Lamon et al., 1974 a, b; Brown et al., 1975; Ernberg and Brown, 1975; Dölken and Klein, 1977 a, b
Autoradiography	Moar et al., 1977, 1978 a
Immunoferritin-labeled antibodies	Sugawara and Osato, 1970
Peroxidase-labeled antibodies	Bahr et al., 1976; Stephens et al., 1977
Passive hemagglutination	Ogburn and Zajac, 1977
Detection by immunocompetent cells	
Cytotoxic killer T cells	Svedmyr and Jondal, 1975

B. ANTIGEN DETECTION METHODS

Electron microscope evidence for the existence of EBV was first reported in 1964 (Epstein et al., 1964). Antigenic tests were first published in 1966. Three papers appeared that year, describing three different methods. Henle and Henle (1966) demonstrated a brilliant intracellular antigen in acetone-fixed cell smears of certain BL-derived lines, by indirect immunofluorescence with sera from BL patients and some normal human sera. This was the first detection of the viral capsid antigen (VCA) complex. Armstrong et al. (1966) showed that cells of certain BL lines reacted with similar sera in a CF assay. When the cells were disintegrated by freezing and thawing or by sonication the antigen titers increased. Subsequently, disrupted cell preparations were used, clarified by low-speed centrifugation. Antibodies to this crude antigen were detectable in nearly all BL patients and also in 60% of all healthy American adults tested.

Nearly all the CF-positive sera also reacted in the immunofluorescence assay developed in the same laboratory (Henle and Henle, 1966), but the reverse was not always true.

In 1966, Old et al. reported that about two-thirds of the BL and NPC patients tested had antibodies to a crude antigen extracted from the BL cell line, Jijoye (Pulvertaft, unpublished), as detected by immunodiffusion; up to five distinct, precipitating lines could be detected with some antisera.

In the course of subsequent development, a number of EBV-determined antigens were defined, mostly by direct and indirect immunofluorescence tests. There are four main groups of such antigens which differ in serologic specificity, cellular localization, and expression during the viral cycle. They are: VCA (Henle and Henle, 1966), the early antigen (EA) complex (Henle et al., 1970), the membrane antigen (MA) (Klein et al., 1966, 1967), and EBNA (Reedman and Klein, 1973). As a rule, the latter can only be detected by the highly sensitive anti-complement immunofluorescence (ACIF) method (Hinuma et al., 1962).

When properly performed, the fluorescence tests have the advantage of simplicity and specificity. Also they permit in situ studies on the distribution of antigen-positive cells and antigen localization. By combining two fluorescent dyes, two different antigens can be visualized in the same cell by two-color fluorescence (Klein et al., 1971).

EBV antigens have recently been detected in situ by alternative methods, such as radioiodinated antibodies combined with radioautography (Moar et al., 1977, 1978 a, b) and peroxidase-labeled antibodies (Stephens et al., 1977). The higher sensitivity of the two latter techniques is advantageous in a variety of studies.

For antigen isolation, purification, and characterization, it is important to have methods that permit the detection of soluble antigens. The original CF test described by Armstrong et al. (1966), has been developed further (Gerber and Birch, 1967; Gerber and Deal, 1970; Vonka et al., 1970). Pope et al. (1969) detected only one EBV-related CF antigen in EBV genome-carrying but virus-nonproducer Raji cells. This antigen was not sedimentable at 60,000 g for 2 h and was therefore designated as the soluble (S) antigen. Later it was shown (Walters and Pope, 1971) that virus-producing lines contain the S antigen that was relatively heat-resistant, and two other EBV-related components in addition, a heat-resistant virion component and a heat-labile sedimentable component.

Recently, a more sensitive CF test was developed for the detection of the S antigen, based on the labeling of the target erythrocytes with ^{51}Cr and measuring the isotope activity released (Baron et al., 1975).

Among the antigens detected by immunodiffusion, only a soluble, heat-resistant antigen could be found in all EBV-carrying cell lines (Stevens et al., 1970 a, b; Reedman et al., 1972; Demissie and Svedmyr, 1973) while two heat-stable and one heat-labile antigens were found in virus-producer lines (Demissie and Svedmyr, 1973; Demissie, 1973). Immunodiffusion is a relatively insensitive method and requires large amounts of material for antigen extraction. It would be interesting though if the immunoprecipitation in gels of EBV antigens could be developed. The potentialities of some semiquantitative high resolution method such as crossed immunoelectrophoresis (Weeke, 1973) have not yet been explored in the EBV field. Indirect single radial immunodiffusion (ISRD) as applied by Matsuo et al. (1976) would be another sensitive method.

Using ^{125}I-labeled antibodies against judiciously selected target cell combinations, exposed as particulate-bound or solubilized material, it has been possible to detect EA, MA, VCA, and EBNA (Lamon et al., 1974 a, b; Brown et al., 1974, 1975; Ernberg and Brown, 1975; Dölken and Klein, 1977 a, b).

Svedmyr and Jondal (1975) detected an EBV-related, previously unknown and so far serologically undefined cell surface antigen by exposing EBV-carrying lines and

EBV-negative controls to purified T cells (thymus-dependent lymphocytes) of acute IM patients. While certain non-T cells of normal and IM bloods are nonspecifically cytotoxic, purified T cells of IM patients killed only EBV-carrying but not EBV-negative lines. The specific killer T cells appear and disappear in relation to the acute phase of IM. The responsible antigen was designated as lymphocyte-detected membrane antigen (LYDMA).

Table 2 lists the antigens detected in virus-producer and EBV genome-carrying but nonproducer lines.

Since immunofluorescence has led to the clearest definition of the antigens, the following presentation will largely focus on the antigens defined by this method. Due consideration will be given to antigens detected by other methods, where feasible.

Table 2. EBV antigens detected by different methods in EBV-carrying virus-producer and nonproducer lines

Method	Antigen	Virus-producer lines	EBV genome-carrying nonproducer lines
T cell-mediated lymphocytotoxicity	LYDMA	+	+
Immunofluorescence[a]	MA	+	−
	EA	+	−
	VCA	+	−
	EBNA[b]	+	+
Immunodiffusion	S, heat-resistant[b]	+	+
	Heat-labile, soluble	+	−
Complement fixation	S, heat-resistant[b]	+	+
	Heat-resistant, virion	+	−
	Heat-labile, sedimentable	+	−

[a] Also detectable by other methods, such as ^{125}I-labeled antibodies, peroxidase-labeled antibodies, and passive hemagglutination (Inoue and Klein, 1970; Lamon et al., 1974a, b; Dölken and Klein, 1977a, b; Stephens et al., 1977; Ogburn and Zajac, 1977).

[b] There is suggestive evidence that these represent the same antigen (Reedman et al., 1972; Klein and Vonka, 1974; Ohno et al., 1977b).

C. MEMBRANE ANTIGEN

MA was first detected in 1966 (Klein et al., 1966) by indirect immunofluorescence staining of fresh biopsy cells with patients' sera. Only BL cells gave a positive reaction; lymph nodes or bone marrow of the BL patients and lymphoid cells of healthy donors were negative (Klein et al., 1966, 1967). In addition to the BL patients' sera, antibodies that reacted with the BL tumor cells were also found in a variety of other sera from healthy and diseased donors. The EBV specificity of the membrane reaction could be established by the blocking of direct membrane immunofluorescence (Klein et al., 1969). EBV-specific membrane fluorescence could also be demonstrated on some of the BL-derived cell lines. A variable number of cells showed positive membrane fluorescence in the different lines (Klein et al., 1968; Yata and Klein, 1969; Yata et al., 1970).

Pearson et al. (1970) found a good correlation between EBV-neutralizing and anti-MA titers but not between neutralizing and anti-VCA or anti-EA titers in a carefully selected spectrum of sera where sufficient discordance existed between anti-MA and -VCA titers to allow a separate evaluation. This suggested that anti-MA antibodies have neutralizing activity and it seemed likely that MA is present on the viral envelope. This was directly confirmed by immunoferritin labeling and electron microscopy (Sugawara and Osato, 1970; Silvestre et al., 1971). In addition to the MA specificity, shared with the cell membrane, the viral envelope also has some additional antigenic specificities of its own, as shown by a subsequent paper of De Schryver et al. (1974). These investigators compared the anti-MA titer, measured by the blocking of direct membrane fluorescence, with the virus-neutralizing titer, as measured in three different tests, in a collection of patients' and control sera.

Yata et al. (1970) showed that synthesis of MA was inhibited by protein and RNA synthesis inhibitors, but not by DNA synthesis inhibitors. Low doses of actinomycin D and mitomycin C actually increased the number of MA-positive cells, possibly due to the induction of the lytic cycle. Gergely et al. (1971 a) showed that P_3HR-1 virus superinfection induced MA synthesis in MA-negative Raji cells both in the presence and absence of DNA synthesis (inhibited by cytosine arabinoside). This further confirmed the independence of MA of DNA synthesis, whereas puromycin completely prevented MA induction.

One difficulty with P_3HR-1 virus superinfection experiments for the study of MA induction lies in the fact that superinfectable, EBV receptor-positive cells adsorb virus particles and the latter give a brilliant MA staining, due to the presence of MA on the viral envelope. This difficulty was avoided when it was found (Sairenji and Hinuma, 1975; Dölken and Klein, 1976) that adsorbed MA-positive material could be removed from the cell surface by proteolytic enzyme digestion, e. g., papain or trypsin. Following this "cleaning", MA synthesis "from within" could be followed in a more objective fashion. These experiments confirmed the conclusion that de novo MA synthesis depends on protein but not on DNA synthesis.

Blocking of direct anti-MA fluorescence has shown that MA is actually an antigen complex with three distinguishable binding sites for human antibodies. Anti-MA sera may contain antibodies against one, two, or three specificities (Svedmyr et al., 1970).

In addition to the "early" (i. e., viral DNA synthesis independent) MA, designated EMA, additional membrane antigen components were found that were only made after viral DNA synthesis and were designated late membrane antigen (LMA). LMA was made only in the cells that have passed into the late viral cycle and have synthesized viral DNA. LMA could be differentiated from EMA by absorption and blocking tests (Ernberg et al., 1974; Sairenji et al., 1977).

Cells that express EMA but not LMA still had the ability for continued growth and division. They were not yet committed to virus production and cell death (Ernberg and Killander, unpublished observations). This conclusion also agrees with the fact that in virus-producer lines MA is often present on a much larger number of cells than the intracellular, virus-cycle related antigens, EA and VCA, and the same is true of BL biopsy cells where no EA or VCA can be demonstrated.

Recently MA-reactive material was solubilized and attached to columns to serve as the target for radioiodinated antibody tests (Dölken and Klein, 1977 a) and both direct binding and blocking assays were successfully used to demonstrate the presence of the antigen. This method should be helpful in further detecting the various immunologic subspecificities and also as an aid to purification and characterization.

By coupling anti-MA sera to glass bead columns, antigen-positive cells could be retained selectively (Dalianis et al., 1977; Dalianis, Moar, Ernberg, unpublished observation).

Antibodies against cell surface antigens can also be demonstrated by the antibody-dependent cell mediated cytotoxicity (ADCC) test. EBV-carrying target cells were killed by Fc receptor-carrying effector cells of the K-type (Pearson and Orr, 1976). The sensitivity of this method was considerably higher than of the fluorescence test, as judged by the comparative antibody titrations. However, it has not yet been critically established which antigen is detected by this method (Pearson and Orr, 1976; Pearson et al., 1978)

The properties of the immunofluorescence-defined EMA and LMA are summarized in Table 3.

Table 3. Properties of the EBV-associated membrane antigens

	EMA	LMA
Detected by[a]	Immunofluorescence, ^{125}I-antibodies, peroxidase-labeled antibodies	
Function	Structural components of virus envelope	
Subcomponents	R, M, K	—
Relation to viral cycle	Dependent on protein and RNA synthesis, but not on DNA synthesis	Dependent on protein, RNA and DNA synthesis.
Relation to cell cycle	Compatible with cell growth and division	Incompatible with cell division
Biochemical characteristics	Not known	Not known

[a] Membrane antigens are also detected by antibody-dependent cellular cytotoxicity (ADCC) (Pearson and Orr, 1976) and by cytotoxic T cells from patients with acute IM (Svedmyr and Jondal, 1975; Sect. G). The antigen(s) detected by the latter method are not identical with the MA detected by immunofluorescence and their relationship to the ADCC-detected antigen is unclear.

D. THE EARLY ANTIGEN COMPLEX

The existence of what later became identified as the EA complex was first suspected when a certain discrepancy was found in the number of immunofluorescence-positive cells in a virus-producer line after staining with EBV-positive sera from healthy donors, compared to the staining obtained with the sera of certain tumor patients, particularly BL and NPC, or from patients with acute IM (Henle et al., 1970). A larger number of cells was stained by the latter sera than by the former. Even more importantly, the sera of normal EBV-positive donors often failed altogether to react with EBV (P_3HR-1 virus substrain) -superinfected Raji cells, whereas the sera of patients with ongoing EBV-associated diseases regularly reacted. This complex picture was understood when it was shown that P_3HR-1 virus infection of Raji cells induces predominantly EA, which differs from VCA in immunologic specificity. Also, while healthy seropositive donors rarely have antibodies to EA, patients with ongoing EBV-related diseases very frequently do.

EA could be subdivided into two components, different in serologic specificity and also in cellular distribution. One antigen, designated "restricted" (R) was confined to the cytoplasm. The other, "diffuse" (D) was more finely dispersed and could be found in both nuclei and cytoplasm (Henle et al., 1971). D appears before R during the early stage of the viral cycle (Henle et al., 1971).

A curious difference was found in the activity of sera from patients with EBV-related diseases against the two subcomponents. Anti-EA sera of acute IM patients contained anti-D antibody more frequently than anti-R. In contrast, BL patients' sera were more frequently anti-R or R + D than anti-D alone. NPC patients' sera often contained both antibodies, with anti-D being usually predominant (Chaps. 4, 13 and 14). While the reasons for these differences are not known they have a certain diagnostic (and also prognostic) significance (Chaps. 4, 13, 14, and 15).

The two EA subcomponents are also distinguishable on the basis of their resistance to certain fixatives. The R component is destroyed by 95% ethanol or methanol, but is preserved by acetone. The D antigen is not alcohol-sensitive, but it is somewhat more easily digested by proteolytic enzymes than R (Henle et al., 1971).

The appearance of EA is the first definite sign that the cell has entered into the lytic cycle (Gergely et al., 1971 b, c). Double immunofluorescence studies showed that all VCA-positive cells contained EA as well. EA-positive cells without detectable VCA are seen during the early stage of the superinfection experiment, as already mentioned and also in some producer lines where there is a block between EA and VCA (Gergely et al., 1971 a, c; Klein et al., 1976 c). Production of EA is not dependent on DNA synthesis: inhibition of detectable DNA synthesis by cytosine arabinoside does not decrease the number of EA-positive cells after P_3HR-1 viral superinfection, whereas the appearance of VCA is completely prevented by DNA inhibitors (Gergely et al., 1971 c). Parallel immunofluorescence and autoradiography have shown that EA-positive cells are already characterized by a progressive inhibition of cellular nucleic acid and protein synthesis. In contrast to MA and VCA, EA cannot be demonstrated in the virion and must therefore be classified as a nonstructural antigen complex (Silvestre et al., 1971).

In addition to immunofluorescence, EA has also been detected by a number of other methods, such as by ^{125}I-antibodies in solution and on autoradiograms (Ernberg and Brown, 1975; Moar et al., 1977, 1978 a), immunodiffusion (Demissie, 1973) and passive hemagglutination (Ogburn and Zajac, 1977).

There is no information about the chemical composition of the EA complex. It may be heat-labile, destroyed at 56 °C after 30 min (Demissie, 1973) (Table 4).

Table 4. Properties of the EA complex

Detected by	Immunofluorescence, complement fixation, immunodiffusion, ^{125}I-labeled antibodies, passive hemagglutination.
Distribution	Early after infection in the nucleus; later in both cytoplasm and nucleus.
Function	Not known; nonstructural "early" virus induced. Synthesized independently of viral DNA synthesis.
Subcomponents	Two identified: R = restricted and D = diffuse.
Molecular properties	R is removed by some alcohols (ethanol, methanol); D is not. D is more sensitive to proteolytic enzymes than R.
Molecular weight	Not known.

E. THE VIRAL CAPSID ANTIGEN

VCA is the first EBV antigen that was detected (Henle and Henle, 1966) by indirect immunofluorescence and in the early papers of the EBV literature it is often called "the EBV antigen". Early studies on the specificity of VCA or, more appropriately, the VCA complex were important in establishing that EBV was not a previously known member of the herpes group, since there was no serologic cross reactivity between it and any viral antigen determined by previously known herpesviruses. Antibodies against this antigen, and against MA as well, were subsequently detected in the sera of BL patients, and also in other human sera and pooled human gamma globulin (Chap. 4).

Already at an early stage of these studies it was established that the small number of VCA-positive cells corresponded to the virus producers. This was shown by the following evidence:

a) The frequency of VCA-positive cells, by immunofluorescence, corresponded closely to the fraction of virus particle-containing cells on electron microscope examination of the same lymphoid lines (Henle and Henle, 1966; Hinuma et al., 1967).

b) Immunofluorescence (VCA)-positive cells were picked individually, embedded, and thin-sectioned for electron microscopy. All VCA-positive cells examined contained a large number of virus particles, whereas similarly prepared VCA-negative cells of the same culture contained none (zur Hausen et al., 1967; Epstein and Achong, 1968).

c) VCA antibody-positive, but not negative sera, reacted with nonenveloped viral nucleocapsids derived from virus-producing cultures, inducing the formation of a thick immunoglobulin coat on the virus particles that were also partly agglutinated, as shown by negative-contrast electron microscopy (Henle et al., 1966; Mayyasi et al., 1967).

Subsequently it was also shown that anti-VCA antibodies only reacted with naked but not with enveloped virus particles (Silvestre et al., 1971). It is thus well established that VCA is a structural component of the virus capsid.

Becker and Weinberg (1972) demonstrated seven major proteins associated with the virus particles after separation on SDS-gels, which correlated with the major herpes simplex proteins. They have not been correlated to antigenic activity, however. Dolyniuk et al. (1976 a, b) have demonstrated 33 major proteins associated with EBV particles on SDS-polyacrylamide gel electrophoresis ranging in molecular weight from 28,000 to 290,000. Seven of these proteins could be localized to the nucleocapsid.

VCA has also been detected by ^{125}I-labeled antibodies (Lamon et al., 1974 a, b), immunoperoxidase (Stephens et al., 1977), and by an immune rabbit serum, absorbed with EBV-negative cells (Vestergaard et al., 1978).

The properties of VCA are summarized in Table 5.

Table 5. Properties of VCA

Detected by[a]	Immunofluorescence, immunoferritin-labeled antibodies, ^{125}I-antibodies, peroxidase-labeled antibodies.
Distribution	In nucleus and cytoplasm of cells containing virus particles.
Function	Structural component of virion capsid.
Biochemical characteristics	Not known[b].

[a] A heat-stable, soluble antigen detected by immunodiffusion (Demissie, 1973) or CF (Walters and Pope, 1971) may be related to the VCA complex.

[b] Dolyniuk et al. (1976b) found seven nucleocapsid proteins on SDS-polyacrylamide gel electrophoresis after purification of virus and enrichment of nucleocapsids, with molecular weights 28×10^3, 37×10^3, 47×10^3, 52×10^3, 144×10^3, 160×10^3 and 275×10^3. They have not been related to antigenic reactivity.

F. THE EBV NUCLEAR ANTIGEN

EBNA was originally detected in the nucleus of all EBV-genome-carrying in vitro cell lines and in BL biopsy cells (Reedman and Klein, 1973; Reedman et al., 1974). Subsequently EBNA has also been demonstrated in the epithelial cells of NPC (Huang et al., 1974; Klein et al., 1974). Furthermore, a small number of EBNA-positive B blasts was detected in the circulation of patients in the acute phase of IM (Klein et al., 1976a).

As a rule, EBNA cannot be demonstrated by direct or indirect fluorescence (although there are some exceptions). It was originally detected and is regularly demonstrated by a three-layer ACIF technique. This method, originally worked out by Hinuma et al. (1962) for other antigen-antibody systems amplifies antigen-antibody reactions, due to the large number of activated C3 molecules bound to each complement fixing antigen-antibody complex (Liabeuf et al., 1975). It is more readily visualized by an appropriate anti-C3 (anti-β_1 C/β_1 A) fluorescent conjugate than can be achieved by the direct or indirect tagging of immunoglobulins.

As already mentioned in the introduction, there is strong evidence that EBNA is identical with the complement-fixing, heat-stable, soluble (S) antigen and perhaps also the S antigen detected by immunodiffusion (Reedman et al., 1972; Klein and Vonka, 1974). Klein and Vonka (1974) showed a close correlation between anti-EBNA and anti-CF (S) titers, while there was no such correlation with the antibody titers against

EA or VCA. EBNA-reactivity during purification could be followed by the CF assay (Baron et al., 1975; Luka et al., 1977). Definite evidence for the identity of EBNA and the S antigen was found when the purified CF moiety could be bound to acid-fixed cell nuclei. Upon ACIF staining, a brilliant fluorescent EBNA reaction was obtained (Ohno et al., 1977 b). This technique is now designated as the acid fixed nuclear binding (AFNB) method. Acid extraction or, alternatively, proteolytic digestion on preexisting nuclear proteins is essential to achieve EBNA binding, with subsequent staining (Luka et al., 1978 a). The AFNB method is useful for the monitoring of antigen purification. Also it serves as an amplification method for DNA-binding nuclear antigens that are present in subliminal concentrations in nuclei to give in situ staining, as in the herpesvirus papio system (Ohno et al., 1977 a) or in BL tumor biopsy material (Luka et al., 1978 a).

In the original paper of Reedman and Klein (1973) it was demonstrated that EBNA binds to the chromosomes. In interphase nuclei, EBNA could be demonstrated on chromatin fibrils by horse-radish peroxidase labeled antibodies and electron microscopy (Bahr et al., 1975; Shamoto and Suzubi, 1976). Subsequently it was shown (Luka et al., 1977) that EBNA binds to double-stranded DNA, but less to single-stranded DNA. There is no apparent specificity of this DNA binding: EBNA binds to DNA of any source (Ohno et al., 1977b). It cannot be excluded that high affinity binding sites exist, as has been found with other DNA binding nuclear antigens determined by transforming viruses, e. g., SV40 (Reed et al., 1975; Jessel et al., 1975)

Lenoir et al. (1976) characterized EBNA by sucrose gradient centrifugation, gel filtration, and ion-exchange chromatography. They found a sediment coefficient of 8.5 S corresponding approximately to a molecular weight of 180,000 daltons. Antigenic activity was monitored by CF and inhibition of ACIF EBNA staining. Baron et al. (1975) and Luka et al. (1977) showed that EBNA bound to DNA columns. This could be utilized for purifying EBNA. Binding to DNA-cellulose columns was an essential step in the process. The resulting product had a molecular weight of $174,000 \pm 15,000$ (Ohno et al., 1977b). In high salt (0.5–1.0 M NaCl) pieces of $98,000 \pm 8,000$ daltons were obtained. Sequential purification by DNA-cellulose, agarose, and hydroxyapatite chromatography, followed by gel filtration led to a 1200-fold purification of EBNA-CF activity (Luka et al., 1978 b). The purified product gave one band at 48,000 daltons on SDS polyacrylamide gel electrophoresis and this same molecular weight was also obtained by an independent method involving immunocomplexing with antibody and isolation of the complexes by protein A (Luka et al., 1978 b). In another approach, heat treatment was followed by $(NH_4)_2SO_3$ precipitation, preparative ultracentrifugation, and DNA-cellulose chromatography (Baron and Strominger, 1978) but this method did not lead to the same degree of purity.

Taken together, the data suggest that EBNA contains subunits of 48,000 mol. wt. that build up a 180,000 mol. wt. molecule (Table 6).

Matsuo et al. (1978) have characterized the S antigen by gel filtration and isoelectric focusing, utilizing ISRD as an assay for the antigen (Matsuo et al., 1976). They found a molecular weight of $230,000 \pm 10,000$, an isoelectric point at 4.8 pH, and the antigen was heat-resistant.

The function of EBNA can only be the subject of speculation. It is noteworthy that EBNA is the only consistently exposed viral "footprint" in cells that carry EBV DNA. It is also the first and the only detectable viral function during the primary infection of human lymphocytes (Aya and Osato, 1974; Menezes et al., 1976; Einhorn and

Table 6. Properties of the EBV nuclear antigen (EBNA)

Detected by	ACIF, CF, immunodiffusion (?), ^{125}I-labeled antibodies.
Distribution	Intranuclear antigen; present in all known EBV-infected and transformed cells.
Function	Nonstructural, not known. Autonomous expression correlated with the number of viral genomes suggests a regulatory role.
Subcomponents	Not known.
Molecular properties	Binds to DNA with preference for dsDNA.
Molecular weight	$\sim 180,000$ with 48,000 dalton subunits.

Ernberg, 1978). It is first seen in small, resting lymphocytes at 12–24 h. Subsequently the lymphocytes undergo blast transformation and some 20 h later they enter their first S phase. It is conceivable that EBNA initiates transformation and/or maintains the transformed state of the cells. In permanently growing lines, EBNA synthesis seems to precede the cellular DNA synthesis during each cell cycle (Ernberg et al., 1978). This was shown by quantitative immunofluorimetry of asynchronously growing cells and subsequent positioning of the cells in the cycle by DNA measurement (Feulgen), protein determination (dry mass), and autoradiography of ^{3}H-thymidine pulse label on individual cells.

In a comparison of cell lines with widely varying EBV-DNA genome numbers per cell, there was a positive correlation with the average amount of EBNA per cell, measured by microfluorometry (Ernberg et al., 1977). This suggests that EBNA is an autonomous function of the viral genome, expressed independently of the viral or cellular controls that limit the production of the other virally determined antigens, MA, EA, and VCA. This is particularly remarkable in relation to interspecies (mouse/human) hybrids that were completely nonpermissive for all other EBV-determined antigens, but expressed EBNA nevertheless in direct relation to their average EBV-genome numbers (Ernberg and Killander, unpublished results).

EBNA precedes the synthesis of EA during infection of EBV-negative B cell (bone marrow-derived lymphocyte) lines, and is thus presumably an early function during the lytic viral cycle (Ernberg et al., 1976). EBNA is also present in virus-producer cells of EBV-carrying cell lines. Two-color fluorescence tests have shown the simultaneous presence of EBNA and EA in such cells (Ernberg et al., 1976).

There are a number of apparent similarities between EBNA and the T antigens induced by the oncogenic papovaviruses. Like T antigens, EBNA binds to DNA and is regularly present in transformed cells. The T antigens are known to be involved in the initiation of virally induced cellular DNA synthesis. With the SV40 system, there is now evidence that T antigen is also involved in the maintenance of transformation (Martin and Chou, 1975; Tegtmeyer, 1975; Brugge and Butel, 1975; Osborn and Weber, 1975) and it is tempting to speculate that EBNA may have an analogous function. In this context it must be noted that a nontransforming EBV variant, P_3HR-1, fails to induce either EBNA or DNA synthesis in normal B lymphocytes. This virus variant does not lack the information required for EBNA induction, since it can induce the antigen in already established, EBV-susceptible but EBV-negative B lymphoma lines and convert them to permanently EBNA-positive sublines (Menezes et al., 1974).

G. LYMPHOCYTE-DETECTED MEMBRANE ANTIGEN

Human peripheral blood of healthy donors or patients with EBV-related or other diseases regularly contain nonspecifically cytotoxic, so-called natural killer (NK) cells that kill certain target lines (including established lymphoid cell lines) in an apparently quite nonspecific fashion. The presence of these, largely Fc receptor-positive cells obscures T cell-mediated cytotoxicity. In acute IM patients, Svedmyr and Jondal (1975) detected an EBV-specific killer T cell, after the removal of the nonspecifically cytotoxic cells by Fc/C3 receptor rosetting. Purified T cells killed all EBV-carrying lines, irrespective of their virus-producer or nonproducer status, but failed to kill EBV-negative lines. More recently, this finding was confirmed by a double procedure of Fc receptor-positive cell removal and positive enrichment of the T cells by E-rosetting (Bakacs et al., 1978). Surprisingly, the killer T cells lysed both allogeneic and autochthonous lymphoid lines, without any systematic distinction, as long as they were EBV-carrying. In other words, there is a curious absence of the "syngeneic or MHC restriction" that was found to characterize many other systems of T cell-mediated killing.

So far the target antigen has not been identified serologically, but it is clearly different from the fluorescence-detected membrane antigen. Since its existence can only be demonstrated by the T cell-mediated killing reaction, the antigen is temporarily designated as lymphocyte-detected membrane antigen (LYDMA) (Table 7). LYDMA appears probably at an early stage of EBV-induced B lymphocyte transformation since admixture of acute IM-derived T cells was found to prevent in vitro transformation of human lymphocytes by EBV (Rickinson et al., 1977). It is conceivable that anti-LYDMA effector cells play an important role in stopping the lymphoproliferative process in acute IM.

Killer T cells with anti-LYDMA activity appear during the acute phase of IM, in parallel with the large blast cells (of which they probably constitute an appreciable part) and disappear during convalescence (Svedmyr et al., 1978). In patients with EBV-carrying BL and NPC tumors, anti-LYDMA reactivity could not be demonstrated in the T cell fraction of the peripheral blood. However, a small number of LYDMA-reactive effector cells could be isolated from the tumor tissue and/or from the draining lymph nodes (Jondal et al., 1975; Klein et al., 1976b). They were always present as a small minority in the tumor tissue.

H. ANTIGEN EXPRESSION IN EBV-CARRYING CELL LINES

All EBV DNA-carrying cell lines express one or several of the EBV antigens described in the previous sections. EBNA is the only antigen that is universally present in EBV DNA-containing cells. Its expression is compatible with and presumably necessary for the continued growth of virus-carrying cells. The three other serologically detected antigens (MA, EA, VCA) are only expressed in lines that produce EBV. They are expressed in a variable, usually very small proportion of the cells. EA and VCA are only expressed in cells that have entered the lytic cycle, whereas MA is associated with a larger number of cells, as a rule, in most lines where it is expressed (Yata and Klein, 1969). Unlike EA- and VCA-positive cells, MA-positive cells can still continue to grow and divide, provided they are EA- and VCA-negative (Gergely et al., 1971 c; Ernberg et al., in preparation).

The frequency of EA- and VCA-producing cells is usually low, rarely exceeding 10%. Cell lines can maintain a relatively constant frequency of EA- and VCA-positive cells, although they can also change to nonproducer status in the course of time. This is more frequently observed in human lines than in nonhuman primate, EBV-carrying lines. The frequency of virus-producer cells reflects the frequency of spontaneous activation of the viral cycle which apparently occurs with a certain fixed probability within the proliferating stemline, but differing for each line.

Different lines vary not only in the frequency of virus-producing cells but also in the extent to which the virus cycle can proceed to completion before the cells die, as already mentioned (Table 8). In some lines cells tend to die around or soon after EA production and rarely go further. In other lines, they proceed to VCA, but do not necessarily make infectious virus particles. Release of biologically detectable, infectious virus into the supernatant is still a rarity, characteristic of only some human, and a larger proportion of nonhuman primate, lines (Hinuma et al., 1967; Miller and Lipman, 1973). Table 9 lists the expression of EBV antigens in some of the more widely used lines.

I. EXPRESSION OF EBV ANTIGENS DURING THE VIRAL CYCLE

The EBV genome has a size of approximately 100×10^6 daltons (Schulte-Holthausen and zur Hausen, 1970; Jehn et al., 1972). If all this genetic material were to be transcribed and translated, it could be responsible for the synthesis of 100 or 200 average-sized proteins. Since there is no lytic system that allows a convenient study of the virus cycle, definition of the viral products by, e. g., pulse-label experiments (as has been so beautifully done in lytic herpesvirus systems), and time sequence studies of their appearance have been considerably hampered. For this reason, the antigens described in the previous sections are the only relatively well-defined viral products, but they correspond only to approximately seven proteins. Moreover, it has not yet been established whether they are virally coded or virally modified cellular proteins.

Due to the random switch-on of the viral cycle in a small minority of the cells in producer lines, which is at present the only available object for the study of the viral cycle, the sequence of antigen appearance has to be studied by immunofluorescence, radioautography, and other techniques that can be applied at the cell level. Double immunofluorescence with two different labels is a particularly useful technique which has shown that EBNA preceeds the synthesis of EA (Ernberg et al., 1976). EA appears first in the nucleus but spreads later to the whole cell (Ernberg et al., 1976).

EA synthesis is independent of viral DNA synthesis (Gergely et al., 1971 c). In contrast to primary EBV infection of normal lymphocytes, EBNA synthesis in cell lines is not blocked by cytosine arabinoside (Klein et al., 1975).

Table 7. Properties of LYDMA

Detected by	Cytotoxic effect of Fc receptor-negative T cells from patients with acute IM.
Distribution	On the surface of the cells of all EBV-carrying cell lines.
Function	Not known.

Table 8. Main types of EBV-carrying cell lines with regard to antigen expression

	EBNA	MA (EMA + LMA)	EA (R + D)	VCA	LYDMA
Nonproducer	+	−	−	−	+
Virus producer	+	+	+	+	+
Abortive producer	+	+ / −	+	+ / −	+

Table 9. Expression of EBV antigens in some widely used EBV-carrying cell lines

	Origin	EBNA	MA	EA	VCA	Virus release	Inducibility[b]
Nonproducer cell lines							
Namalwa[c]	BL	100%	neg.	neg.	neg.	−	−
Rael[c]	BL	100%	neg.	neg.	neg.	−	−
AW-Ramos[a]	BL	100%	neg.	neg.	neg.	−	−
Abortive producer cell lines							
Daudi[d]	BL	100%	≤ 10%	≤ 5%	≤ 5%	−	+
Maku[e]	BL	100%	≤ 70%	≤ 5%	≤ 5%	−	+
Raji[f]	BL	100%	≤ 1%	≤ 1%	≤ 0.1%	−	+
F 265[g]	Healthy donor	100%	≤ 1%	≤ 0.01%	neg.	−	+
NC 37[g]	Healthy donor	100%	≤ 1%	≤ 1%	≤ 0.1%	−	+
LY 28[h, c]	NPC (LCL)	100%	≤ 50%	≤ 10%	≤ 5%	−	+
LY 46[h, c]	NPC (LCL)	100%	≤ 50%	≤ 5%	≤ 5%	−	+
Virus-producer cell lines							
P₃HR-1[i]	BL	100%	≤ 20%	≤ 20%	≤ 20%	+	+
B95-8[j]	IM-virus transformed marmoset cell line	100%	≤ 20%	≤ 20%	≤ 20%	+	+

[a] EBV-converted subline of an EBV-negative American BL line (Klein et al., 1975).
[b] The number of cells entering the viral cycle can be increased by adding, e. g., halogenated pyrimidines (next Sect. I).
[c] Klein and Dombos, 1973.   [g] Durr et al., 1970.
[d] Klein et al., 1968.   [h] Established by Dr. G. de-Thé.
[e] Yata and Klein, 1969.   [i] Hinuma and Grace, 1967.
[f] Pulvertaft, 1965.   [j] Miller and Lipman, 1973.

Hampar et al., (1974) studied the sequence of EA, viral DNA, and VCA synthesis after the addition and subsequent removal of 5-iododeoxyuridine (IUDR) (Gerber 1972; Hampar et al., 1972). This has led to the induction of a virus cycle that lasted ~ 12 h before the late antigen, VCA, appeared. The first EA-positive cells appeared after 6 h and viral DNA replicated 2 h later. The IUDR-induced cycle was slightly shorter than the cycle induced by P_3HR-1 viral superinfection where EA appeared after 10 h and late antigens only after approximately 24 h (Gergely et al., 1971 a). MA was induced in the majority of the cells by P_3HR-1 viral superinfection, but not after IUDR induction. A large number of the MA-positive cells failed to proceed subsequently to EA and VCA production. EMA appears at approximately the same time as EA, independently of viral or cellular DNA synthesis, but LMA is only expressed on cells that have already replicated viral DNA (Yata et al., 1970; Ernberg et al., 1974) (Table 10).

Table 10. Different patterns of EBV-host cell interaction

EB viral cycle in EBV-producing cell lines:

EBNA → EA, EMA → viral DNA synthesis → VCA,
LMA → virus release

Abortive EB viral cycle during primary infection of EBV genome-negative cell lines:

B lymphoblastoid cell + EBV → EBNA → EA (→ ?)

Events during EBV-induced transformation (immortalization) of human B lymphocytes:

B lymphocytes + EBV → EBNA → cellular DNA
synthesis → mitosis

While the productive cycle is switched on spontaneously in a small fraction of the cells in some (producer) lines only, some, but not all, nonproducer lines could be induced by a variety of treatments (Table 11), including P_3HR-1 viral infection and treatment with halogenated pyrimidines or with cycloheximide (Gergely et al., 1971 a; Gerber, 1972; Hampar et al., 1972, 1976).

It is of interest that halogenated pyrimidines of the same types can also induce a number of other latent viruses, such as the provirally integrated DNA copies of C-type viruses. The mechanism of induction is unknown; suggestions vary from derepression of viral genes due to misreading, to excision-activation type mechanisms of the integrated genome.

The control of spontaneous EA production was studied in hybrids between producer and nonproducer lines. In three different types of hybrids, Raji/Namalwa, Raji/Daudi, and Daudi/P_3HR-1, the more highly producing line imposed its pattern of spontaneous EA synthesis on the hybrid (Nyormoi et al., 1973; Klein et al., 1976 c; Ber et al., 1978).

VCA synthesis depends on EA synthesis, since VCA can only appear in EA-positive cells. However, the production of EA is a necessary but by itself insufficient requirement for VCA synthesis. As an example, in the Raji line the small number of

Table 11. EBV-inducing agents

Agents that increase/induce the number of EA (and sometimes VCA)-positive cells in producer cell lines:

TPA[a] (tumor promoting agent; phorbol ester from croton oil)
X-irradiation[b]
Mitomycin C[b]
Arginine-deficient medium[c]
Starvation[d]
Low temperature (33 °C)[d]

Agents that induce the lytic cycle in nonproducer cell lines:

Iododeoxyuridine (IUDR)[e]
Bromodeoxyuridine (BUDR)[f]
Cycloheximide[g]

---

[a] zur Hausen et al., 1978.
[b] Ernberg, unpublished results.
[c] Henle and Henle, 1968.
[d] Nagoya and Hinuma, 1972.
[e] Gerber, 1972.
[f] Hampar et al., 1972.
[g] Hampar et al., 1976.

spontaneously EA-positive cells does not progress to VCA synthesis spontaneously and even after P_3HR-1 viral superinfection it is difficult to "penetrate" the EA-VCA barrier, unless very high viral multiplicities are used. In Daudi or Jijoye, on the other hand, EA-positive cells progressed more readily to VCA synthesis (Klein et al., 1976c, 1978).

REFERENCES

Armstrong, D., Henle, G., Henle, W.: Complement fixation tests with cell lines derived from Burkitt's lymphoma and acute leukemias. J. Bacteriol. **91**, 1257–1262 (1966)

Aya, T., Osato, T.: Early events in transformation of human cord leukocytes by Epstein-Barr virus: Induction of DNA-synthesis, mitosis and virus associated nuclear antigen synthesis. Int. J. Cancer **14**, 341–347 (1974)

Bahr, G. F., Mikel, U., Klein, G.: Localization and quantitation of EBV-associated nuclear antigen (EBNA) in Raji cells. Beitr. Pathol. **155**, 72–78 (1975)

Bakacs, T., Svedmyr, E., Klein, E., Rombo, L., Weiland, O.: EBV-related cytotoxicity of Fc-receptor negative T lymphocytes separated from the blood of infectious mononucleosis patients. Cancer Letters, **4**, 185–189 (1978)

Baron, D., Strominger, J.: Partial purification and properties of the Epstein-Barr virus associated nuclear antigen, J. Biol. Chem. **253**, 2875–2881 (1978)

Baron, D., Benz, W. C., Carmichael, G., Yocum, R. R., Strominger, J. L.: Assay and partial purification of Epstein-Barr virus nuclear antigen. In: Epstein-Barr virus production, concentration and purification. IARC Internal Technical Report 75/003. pp. 257–262. Lyon: IARC 1975

Becker, Y., Weinberg, A.: Molecular events in the biosynthesis of Epstein-Barr virus in Burkitt lymphoblasts. In: Oncogenesis and herpesviruses. Biggs, P. M., de-Thé, G., Payne, L. N. (eds.), pp. 326–335. Lyon: IARC 1972

Ber, R., Klein, G., Moar, M., Povey, S., Rosén, A., Westman, A., Yefenof, E., Zeuthen, J.: Somatic cell hybrids between human lymphoma lines. IV. Establishment and characterization of a P_3HR-1/Daudi hybrid. Int. J. Cancer **21**, 701–719 (1978)

Brown, T. D. K., Ernberg, I., Lamon, E. W., Klein, G.: Detection of Epstein-Barr virus (EBV)-associated nuclear antigen in human lymphoblastoid cell lines by means of an I^{125}-IgG binding assay. Int. J. Cancer **13**, 785–794 (1974)

Brown, T. D. K., Ernberg, I., Klein, G.: Studies of Epstein-Barr virus (EBV)-associated nuclear antigen. I. Assay in human lymphoblastoid cell lines by direct and indirect determination of I^{125}-IgG binding. Int. J. Cancer **15**, 606–616 (1975)

Brugge, J. S., Butel, J. S.: Role of Simian virus 40 gene: A function in maintenance of transformation. J. Virol. **15**, 619–635 (1975)

Dalianis, T., Klein, G., Andersson, B.: Column separation of viral capsid antigen (VCA)-positive cells from VCA-negative cells in an Epstein-Barr virus (EBV)-producing lymphoid line. Int. J. Cancer **19**, 460–467 (1977)

Demissie, A.: Difference in heat stability of antigens associated with Epstein-Barr virus, demonstrated by immunodiffusion. J. Natl. Cancer Inst. **51**, 751–760 (1973)

Demissie, A., Svedmyr, A.: Difference in heat stability of antigens associated with Epstein-Barr virus, demonstrated by immunofluorescence. J. Natl. Cancer Inst. **50**, 63–67 (1973)

De Schryver, A., Klein, G., Hewetson, J., Rocchi, G., Henle, W., Henle, G., Moss, D. J., Pope, J. H.: Comparison of EBV-neutralization tests based on abortive infection or transformation of lymphoid cells and their relation to membrane reactive antibodies (anti-MA). Int. J. Cancer **13**, 353–362 (1974)

Dölken, G., Klein, G.: Expression of Epstein-Barr virus (EBV) associated membrane antigen (MA) in Raji cells superinfected with two different virus strains. Virology **70**, 210–213 (1976)

Dölken, G., Klein, G.: A solid phase radioimmunoassay for Epstein-Barr virus associated membrane antigen prepared from B95-8 cell culture supernatants. J. Natl. Cancer Inst. **58**, 1239–1245 (1977a)

Dölken, G., Klein, G.: Radioimmunoassay for Epstein-Barr virus (EBV)-associated nuclear antigen (EBNA). Binding of iodinated antibodies to antigens immobilized in polyacrylamide gel. Eur. J. Cancer **13**, 1277–1286 (1977b)

Dolyniuk, M., Pritchett, R., Kieff, E.: Proteins of Epstein-Barr virus. I. Analysis of the polypeptides of purified enveloped Epstein-Barr virus. J. Virol. **17**, 935–949 (1976a)

Dolyniuk, M., Wolff, E., Kieff, E.: Proteins of Epstein-Barr virus. II. Electrophoretic analysis of the polypeptides of the nucleocapsid and the glucosamine- and polysaccharide-containing components of enveloped virus. J. Virol. **18**, 269–287 (1976b)

Durr, F. E., Monroe, J. H., Schmitter, R., Traul, K. A., Hirshaut, Y.: Studies on the infectivity and cytopathology of Epstein-Barr virus in human lymphoblastoid cells. Int. J. Cancer **6**, 436–449 (1970)

Einhorn, L., Ernberg, I.: Induction of EBNA precedes stimulation of DNA-synthesis in EBV-infected human lymphocytes. Int. J. Cancer **21**, 157–160 (1978)

Epstein, M.A., Achong, B. G.: Specific immunofluorescence test for the herpes-type EB virus of Burkitt lymphoblasts, authenticated by electron microscopy. J. Natl. Cancer Inst. **40**, 593–603 (1968)

Epstein, M. A., Achong, B. G., Barr, Y. M.: Virus particles in cultured lymphoblasts from Burkitt's lymphoma. Lancet **1964 I**, 702–703

Ernberg, I., Brown, T. D. K.: Studies on the Epstein-Barr virus associated early antigen (EA) with I^{125}-labeled IgG. In: Oncogenesis and Herpesviruses II. de-Thé, G., Epstein, M. A., zur Hausen, H. (eds.), Part 1, pp. 339–344. Lyon: IARC, 1975

Ernberg, I., Klein, G., Kourilsky, F. M., Silvestre, D.: Differentiation between early and late membrane antigen on human lymphoblastoid cell lines infected with Epstein-Barr virus. I. Immunofluorescence. J. Natl. Cancer Inst. **53**, 61–65 (1974)

Ernberg, I., Masucci, G., Klein, G.: Persistance of Epstein-Barr viral nuclear antigen (EBNA) in cells entering the EB viral cycle. Int. J. Cancer **17**, 197–203 (1976)

Ernberg, I., Killander, D., Andersson-Anvret, M., Klein, G., Lundin, L.: Relationship between the amount of Epstein-Barr virus (EBV) determined nuclear antigen (EBNA)/cell and the number of EBV-DNA copies. Nature **266**, 269–271 (1977)

Ernberg, I., Killander, D., Lundin, L.: Quantity of Epstein-Barr viral nuclear antigen (EBNA) during different phases of the cell cycle. (Submitted for publication) (1978)

Gerber, P.: Activation of Epstein-Barr virus by 5-bromodeoxyuridine "virus-free" free human cells. Proc. Natl. Acad. Sci. USA **69**, 83–85 (1972)

Gerber, P., Birch, S. M.: Complement-fixing antibodies in sera of human and non-human primates to viral antigen derived from Burkitt's lymphoma cells. Proc. Natl. Acad. Sci. USA **58**, 478–484 (1967)

Gerber, P., Deal, D. R.: Epstein-Barr virus-induced viral and soluble complement-fixing antigens in Burkitt lymphoma cell cultures. Proc. Soc. Exp. Biol. Med. **134**, 748–751 (1970)

Gergely, L., Klein, G., Ernberg, I.: Appearance of Epstein-Barr virus associated antigens in infected Raji cells. Virology **45**, 10–21 (1971a)

Gergely, L., Klein, G., Ernberg, I.: Effect of EBV-induced early antigens on host-cell macromolecular synthesis, studied by combined immunofluorescence and radioautography. Virology **45**, 22–29 (1971 b)

Gergely, L., Klein, G., Ernberg, I.: The action of DNA-antagonists on Epstein-Barr virus (EBV)-associated early antigen (EA) in Burkitt lymphoma lines. Int. J. Cancer **7**, 293–302 (1971 c)

Hampar, B., Derge, J. G., Martos, L. M., Walker, J. L.: Synthesis of Epstein-Barr virus after activation of the viral genome in a virus negative human lymphoblastoid cell (Raji) made resistant to bromodeoxyuridine. Proc. Natl. Acad. Sci. USA **69**, 78–82 (1972)

Hampar, B., Derge, J. G., Nonoyama, M., Chang, S.-Y., Tagamets, M., Showalter, S. D.: Programming of events in Epstein-Barr virus activated cells induced by 5-iododeoxyuridine, Virology **62**, 71–89, (1974)

Hampar, B., Lenoir, G., Nonoyama, M., Derge, J. G., Chang, S. Y.: Cell cycle dependence for activation of Epstein-Barr virus by inhibitors of protein synthesis or medium deficient in arginine. Virology **69**, 660–668 (1976)

Henle, G., Henle, W.: Immunofluorescence in cells derived from Burkitt's lymphoma. J. Bacteriol. **91**, 1248–1256 (1966)

Henle, W., Henle, G.: Effect of arginine-deficient media on the herpes-type virus associated with cultured Burkitt tumor cells. J. Virol. **2**, 182–191 (1968)

Henle, W., Hummeler, K., Henle, G.: Antibody coating and agglutination of virus particles separated from the EB-3 line of Burkitt lymphoma cells. J. Bacteriol. **92**, 269–271 (1966)

Henle, W., Henle, G., Zajac, B., Pearson, G., Waubke, R., Scriba, M.: Differential reactivity of human sera with early antigens induced by Epstein-Barr virus. Science **169**, 188–190 (1970)

Henle, G., Henle, W., Klein, G.: Demonstration of two distinct components in the early antigen complex of Epstein-Barr virus infected cells. Int. J. Cancer **8**, 272–282 (1971)

Hinuma, Y., Grace, J. T.: Cloning of immunoglobulin-producing human leukemic and lymphoma cells in long term cultures. Proc. Soc. Exp. Biol. Med. **124**, 107–111 (1967)

Hinuma, Y., Ohta, R., Miyamoto, T., Ishida, N.: Evaluation of the complement method of fluorescent antibody technique with myxoviruses. J. Immunol. **89**, 19–26 (1962)

Hinuma, Y., Konn, M., Yamaguchi, J.: Immunofluorescence and herpes type virus particles in the P_3HR-1 Burkitt lymphoma cell line. J. Virol. **1**, 1045–1051 (1967)

Huang, D. P., Ho, J. H. C., Henle, W., Henle, G.: Demonstration of Epstein-Barr virus associated nuclear antigen in nasopharyngeal carcinoma cells from fresh biopsies. Int. J. Cancer **14**, 580–588 (1974)

Inoue, M., Klein, G.: Reactivity of radioiodinated serum antibody from Burkitt's lymphoma and nasopharyngeal carcinoma patients against culture lines derived from Burkitt's lymphoma. Clin. Exp. Immunol. **7**, 39–50 (1970)

Jehn, U., Lindahl, T., Klein, G.: Fate of virus DNA in the abortive infection of human lymphoid cell lines by Epstein-Barr virus. J. Gen. Virol. **16**, 409–412 (1972)

Jessel, D., Hudson, J., Landan, T., Livingston, D. M.: Interaction of partially purified Simian virus 40 T antigen with circular viral DNA molecules. Proc. Natl. Acad. Sci. USA **72**, 1960–1964 (1975)

Jondal, M., Svedmyr, E., Klein, E., Singh, S.: Killer T cells in a Burkitt's lymphoma biopsy. Nature **255**, 405–407 (1975)

Klein, E., Klein, G., Nadkarni, J. S., Nadkarni, J. J., Wigzell, H., Clifford, P.: Surface IgM kappa specificity on a Burkitt lymphoma cell in vivo and in derived culture lines. Cancer Res. **28**, 1300–1310 (1968)

Klein, E., Becker, S., Svedmyr, E., Jondal, M., Vanky, F.: Tumor infiltrating lymphocytes. Ann. NY Acad. Sci. **276**, 207–216 (1976b)

Klein, G., Dombos, L.: Relationship between the sensitivity of EBV-carrying lymphoblastoid line to superinfection and the inducibiltiy of the resident viral genome. Int. J. Cancer **11**, 327–337 (1973)

Klein, G., Vonka, V.: Brief communication: Relationship between Epstein-Barr virus determined complement-fixing antigen and nuclear antigen detected by anti-complement fluorescence. J. Natl. Cancer Inst. **53**, 1645–1646 (1974)

Klein, G., Clifford, P., Klein, E., Stjernswärd, J.: Search for tumor specific immune reactions in Burkitt lymphoma patients by the membrane immunofluorescence reaction. Proc. Natl. Acad. Sci. USA **55**, 1628–1635 (1966)

Klein, G., Clifford, P., Klein, E., Stjernswärd, J.: Membrane immunofluorescence reactions of Burkitt's lymphoma cells from biopsy specimens and tissue culture. J. Natl. Cancer Inst. **39**, 1027–1044 (1967)

Klein, G., Pearson, G., Nadkarni, J. S.: Nadkarni, J. J., Klein, E., Henle, G., Henle, W., Clifford, P.: Relation between Epstein-Barr viral and cell membrane immunofluorescence of Burkitt tumor cells.

I. Dependence of cell membrane immunofluorescence on presence of EB virus. J. Exp. Med. **128,** 1011–1020 (1968)

Klein, G., Pearson, G., Henle, G., Henle, W., Goldstein, G., Clifford, P.: Relation between Epstein-Barr virus and cell membrane immunofluorescence in Burkitt tumor cells. III. Comparison of blocking of direct membrane immunofluorescence and anti-EBV reactivities of different sera. J. Exp. Med. **129,** 697–706 (1969)

Klein, G., Gergely, L., Goldstein, G.: Two colour immunofluorescence studies on EBV determined antigens. Clin. Exp. Immunol. **8,** 593–602 (1971)

Klein, G., Giovanella, B. C., Lindahl, T., Fialkow, P. J., Singh, S., Stehlin, J. S.: Direct evidence for the presence of Epstein-Barr virus DNA and nuclear antigen in malignant epithelial cells from patients with poorly differentiated carcinoma of the nasopharynx. Proc. Natl. Acad. Sci. USA **71,** 4737–4741 (1974)

Klein, G., Giovanella, B., Westman, A., Stehlin, J. S., Mumford, D.: An EBV-genome-negative cell line established from an American Burkitt lymphoma. Receptor characteristics, EBV infectability and permanent conversion into EBV positive sublines by in vitro infection. Intervirology **5,** 319–334 (1975)

Klein, G., Svedmyr, E., Jondal, M., Persson, P. O.: EBV-determined nuclear antigen (EBNA)-positive cells in the peripheral blood of infectious mononucleosis patients. Int. J. Cancer **17,** 21–26 (1976a)

Klein, G., Clements, G., Zeuthen, J., Westman, A.: Somatic cell hybrids between human lymphoid lines. II. Spontaneous and induced pattern of the Epstein-Barr virus (EBV) cycle. Int. J. Cancer **17,** 715–724 (1976c)

Klein, G., Yefenof, E., Falk, K., Westman, A.: Relationship between Epstein-Barr virus (EBV)-production and the loss of the EBV receptor/complement receptor complex in a series of sublines derived from the same original Burkitt's lymphoma. Int. J. Cancer **21,** 552–560 (1978)

Konn, M., Yohn, D. S., Hinuma, Y., Yamaguchi, J., Grace, J. T. (Jr.): Immunogel diffusion studies with the herpes type virus (HTV) associated with Burkitt's lymphoma. Cancer Res. **27,** 2532–2534 (1967)

Lamon, E., Ernberg, I., Klein, G.: Detection of antigens determined by the Epstein-Barr virus (EBV) in human lymphoblastoid cell culture lines by elution of specific radioiodine labeled antibody. Clin. Immunol. Immunopathol. **2,** 216–233 (1974a)

Lamon, E., Ernberg, I., Klein, G.: Differential expression of Epstein-Barr virus early and membrane antigens after induction or superinfection. Cancer Biochem. Biophys. **1,** 33–38 (1974b)

Lenoir, G., Berthelon, M.-C., Favre, M.-C., de-Thé, G.: Characterization of Epstein-Barr virus antigens. I. Biochemical analysis of the complement-fixing soluble antigen and relationship with Epstein-Barr virus-associated nuclear antigen. J. Virol. **17,** 672–674 (1976)

Liabeuf, A., Nelson, K. A., Kourilsky, F. M.: The detection of the Epstein-Barr virus (EBV) nuclear antigen (EBNA) by anticomplement immunofluorescence. Immunoglobulin class of antibodies and role of complement. Int. J. Cancer **15,** 533–546 (1975)

Lindahl, T., Klein, G., Reedman, B., Johansson, B., Singh, S.: Relationship between Epstein-Barr virus (EBV)-DNA and the EBV-determined nuclear antigen (EBNA) in Burkitt lymphoma biopsies and other lymphoproliferative diseases. Int. J. Cancer **13,** 764–772 (1974)

Luka, J., Siegert, W., Klein, G.: Solubilization of the Epstein-Barr virus determined nuclear antigen and its characterization as a DNA-binding protein. J. Virol. **22,** 1–8 (1977)

Luka, J., Klein, G., Henle, W., Henle, G.: Detection of the EBV-determined nuclear antigen (EBNA) in Burkitt's lymphoma and nasopharyngeal carcinoma biopsies by the acid fixed nuclear binding (AFNB) technique. Cancer Letters **4,** 199–205 (1978a)

Luka, J., Lindahl, T., Klein, G.: Purification of the EB-virus determined nuclear antigen (EBNA) from EB-virus-transformed human lymphoid cell lines. J. Virol. **27,** 604–611 (1978b)

Martin, R. G., Chou, J. Y.: Simian virus 40 functions required for the establishment and maintenance of malignant transformation. J. Virol. **15,** 599–612 (1975)

Matsuo, T., Nishi, S., Hirai, H., Osato, T.: Studies on Epstein-Barr virus related antigens. I. Indirect single radial immunodiffusion as a useful method for detection and assay of soluble antigen. Int. J. Cancer **18,** 453–457 (1976)

Matsuo, T., Nishi, S., Hirai, H., Osato, T.: Studies on Epstein-Barr virus related antigens. II. Biochemical properties of soluble antigen in Raji Burkitt lymphoma cells. Int. J. Cancer (in press) (1978)

Mayyasi, S. A., Schidlovsky, G., Bulfone, L., Buschek, F. T.: The coating reaction of the herpes-type virus isolated from malignant tissues with an antibody present in sera. Cancer Res. **27,** 2020–2024 (1967)

Menezes, J., Leibold, W., Klein, G.: Biological differences between Epstein-Barr virus (EBV) strains with regard to lymphocyte transforming ability, superinfection and antigen induction. Exp. Cell Res. **92,** 478–484 (1974)

Menezes, J., Jondal, M., Leibold, W., Dorval, G.: Epstein-Barr virus interaction with human lymphocyte subpopulations: virus adsorption, kinetics of expression of EBV-associated nuclear antigen (EBNA) and lymphocyte transformation. Infect. Immun. **13**, 303–310 (1976)

Miller, G., Lipman, M.: Release of infectious Epstein-Barr virus by transformed marmoset leukocytes. Proc. Natl. Acad. Sci. USA **70**, 190–194 (1973)

Moar, M., Siegert, W., Klein, G.: Detection and localization of Epstein-Barr virus-associated early antigens in single cell by autoradiography using I^{125} labeled antibodies. Intervirology **8**, 226–239 (1977)

Moar, M., Siegert, W., Klein, G.: Autoradiographic detection of Epstein-Barr virus (EBV) associated early antigen (EA) in a variety of EBV-DNA containing lymphoblastoid cell lines previously designated as non-producers. Intervirology **9**, 333–343 (1978 a)

Moar, M., Klein, G., Dölken, G.: Detection of the Epstein-Barr virus (EBV)-determined viral capsid antigen (VCA) by autoradiography *in situ* using I^{125}-labeled antibodies, (Submitted for publication) (1978 b)

Nagoya, T., Hinuma, Y.: Production of infective Epstein-Barr virus in a Burkitt lymphoma cell line, P_3HR-1. Gann **63**, 87–93 (1972)

Nyormoi, O., Klein, G., Adams, A., Dombos, L.: Sensitivity to EBV superinfection and IUDR inducibility of hybrid cells formed between a sensitive and a relatively resistant Burkitt lymphoma cell line. Int. J. Cancer **12**, 396–408 (1973)

Ohno, S., Luka, J., Falk, L., Klein, G.: Detection of a nuclear, EBNA type antigen in apparently EBNA-negative Herpesvirus papio (HVP)-transformed lymphoid lines by the acid-fixed nuclear binding technique. Int. J. Cancer **20**, 941–946 (1977 a)

Ohno, S., Luka, J., Lindahl, T., Klein, G.: Identification of a purified complement fixing antigen as the Epstein-Barr virus determined nuclear antigen (EBNA) by its binding to metaphase chromosomes. Proc. Natl. Acad. Sci. USA **74**, 1605–1609 (1977 b)

Ogburn, C. A., Zajac, B. A.: Detection of Epstein-Barr virus early antigen D and its antibodies by passive haemagglutination. Int. J. Cancer **19**, 150–160 (1977)

Old, L. J., Boyse, E. A., Oettgen, H. E., de Harven, E., Geering, G., Williamson, B., Clifford, P.: Precipitating antibodies in human serum to an antigen present in cultured Burkitt's lymphoma cells. Proc. Natl. Acad. Sci. USA **56**, 1699–1704 (1966)

Osborn, M., Weber, K.: Simian virus 40 gene A function and maintenance of transformation. J. Virol. **15**, 636–644 (1975)

Pearson, G., Dewey, F., Klein, G., Henle, G., Henle, W., Relation between neutralization of Epstein-Barr virus and antibodies to cell membrane antigens induced by the virus. J. Natl. Cancer Inst. **45**, 989–997 (1970)

Pearson, G. R., Orr, T. W.: Antibody dependent lymphocyte cytotoxicity against cells expressing Epstein-Barr virus antigens. J. Natl. Cancer Inst. **56**, 485–488 (1976)

Pearson, G., Johansson, B., Klein, G.: Antibody dependent cellular cytotoxicity against Epstein-Barr virus-associated antigens in African patients with nasopharyngeal carcinoma. Int. J. Cancer **22**, 120–125 (1978)

Pope, J. H., Inoue, M. K., Wetters, E. J.: Significance of a complement-fixing antigen associated with herpes-like virus and detected in the Raji cell line. Nature **222**, 166–167 (1969)

Pulvertaft, R. J. V.: A study of malignant tumours in Nigeria in short term tissue culture. J. Clin. Pathol. **18**, 261–273 (1965)

Reed, S. I., Ferguson, J., Davis, R. W., Stark, G. R.: T antigen binds to Simian virus 40 DNA at the origin of replication. Proc. Natl. Acad. Sci. USA **72**, 1605–1609 (1975)

Reedman, B. M., Klein, G.: Cellular localization of an Epstein-Barr virus (EBV)-associated complement-fixing antigen in producer and non-producer lymphoblastoid cell lines. Int. J. Cancer **11**, 599–620 (1973)

Reedman, B. M., Pope, J. M., Moss, D. J.: Identity of the soluble EBV-associated antigens of tumor lymphoid cell lines. Int. J. Cancer **9**, 172–181 (1972)

Reedman, B. M., Klein, G., Pope, J. H., Walters, M. K., Hilgers, J., Singh, S., Johansson, B.: Epstein-Barr virus associated complement-fixing and nuclear antigens in Burkitt's lymphoma biopsies. Int. J. Cancer **13**, 755–763 (1974)

Rickinson, A. B., Crawford, D., Epstein, M. A.: Inhibition of the in vitro outgrowth of Epstein-Barr virus-transformed lymphocytes by thymus-dependent lymphocytes from infectious mononucleosis patients. Clin. Exp. Immunol. **28**, 72–79 (1977)

Sairenji, T., Hinuma, Y.: Ultraviolet inactivation of Epstein-Barr virus. Effect on synthesis of virus associated antigens. Int. J. Cancer **16**, 1–6 (1975)

Sairenji, T., Hinuma, Y., Sekizawa, T., Yoshida, M.: Appearance of early and late components of Epstein-Barr virus associated membrane antigen in Daudi cells superinfected with P_3HR-1 virus. J. Gen. Virol. **38**, 111–120 (1977)

Schulte-Holthausen, H., zur Hausen, H.: Partial purification of the Epstein-Barr virus and some properties of its DNA. Virology **40**, 776–779 (1970)

Shamoto, M., Suzubi, I.: An immunoelectron microscopic analysis of Epstein-Barr virus associated complement fixing antigen. Cancer **38**, 2057–2064 (1976)

Silvestre, D., Kourilsky, F. M., Klein, G., Yata, Y., Neauport-Sautes, C., Levy, J. P.: Relationship between the EBV-associated membrane antigen on Burkitt lymphoma cells and the viral envelope demonstrated by immunoferritin labelling. Int. J. Cancer **8**, 222–233 (1971)

Stephens, R., Traul, K., Gandrean, P., Jeh, J., Fisher, L., Mayyasi, S. A.: Comparative studies on EBV-antigens by immunofluorescence and immunoperoxidase techniques. Int. J. Cancer **19**, 305–316 (1977)

Stevens, D. A., Pry, T. W., Blackham, E. A.: Prevalence of precipitating antibody to antigens derived from Burkitt lymphoma cultures infected with herpes-type virus (EB virus). Blood **35**, 263–275 (1970a)

Stevens, D. A., Pry, T. W., Blackham, E. A., Manaker, R. A.: Immunodiffusion studies of EB virus (herpes-type virus)-infected and uninfected hemic cell lines. Int. J. Cancer **5**, 229–237 (1970b)

Sugawara, K., Osato, T.: An immunoferritin study of a Burkitt lymphoma cell line harboring EB virus particles. Gann **61**, 279 (1970).

Svedmyr, A., Demissie, A., Klein, G., Clifford, P.: Antibody patterns in different human sera against intracellular and membrane antigen complexes associated with Epstein-Barr virus. J. Natl. Cancer Inst. **44**, 595–610 (1970)

Svedmyr, E., Jondal, M.: Cytotoxic cells specific for B cell lines transformed by Epstein-Barr virus are present in patients with infectious mononucleosis. Proc. Natl. Acad. Sci. USA **72**, 1622–1626 (1975)

Svedmyr, E., Jondal, M., Henle, W., Weiland, O., Rombo, L., Klein, G.: EBV-specific killer T cells and serologic response after onset of infectious mononucleosis. (Submitted for publication) (1978)

Tegtmeyer, P.: Function of Simian virus 40 gene A in transforming infection. J. Virol. **15**, 613–618 (1975)

Vestergaard, B. F., Hesse, J., Norrild, B., Klein, G.: Production of rabbit antibodies against the viral capsid antigen (VCA) of the Epstein-Barr virus (EBV). Int. J. Cancer **21**, 323–328 (1978)

Vonka, V., Benyesh-Melnick, M., Lewis, R. T., Wimberly, I.: Some properties of the soluble (S) antigen of cultured lymphoblastoid cell lines. Arch. Ges. Virusforsch. **31**, 113–124 (1970)

Walters, M. K., Pope, J. H.: Studies of the EB virus related antigens of human leukocyte cell lines. Int. J. Cancer **8**, 32–40 (1971)

Weeke, B.: Crossed Immunoelectrophoresis. A mannual of quantitative immunoelectrophoresis. Scand. J. Immunol. Suppl **1**, 47–56 (1973)

Yata, J., Klein, G.: Some factors affecting membrane immunofluorescence reactivity of Burkitt lymphoma tissue culture cell lines. Int. J. Cancer **4**, 767–775 (1969)

Yata, J., Klein, G., Hewetson, J., Gergely, L.: Effect of metabolic inhibitors on membrane immunofluorescence reactivity of established Burkitt lymphoma cell lines. Int. J. Cancer **5**, 394–403 (1970)

Zajac, B. A., Ogburn, C. A.: Preparation of rabbit anti-sera to Epstein-Barr virus D-early antigens. In: Oncogenesis and herpesviruses II. de-Thé, G., Epstein, M. A., zur Hausen, H. (eds.), Part. 1, pp. 331–337. Lyon: IARC 1975

zur Hausen, H., Schulte-Holthausen, H.: Presence of EB virus nucleic acid homology in a "virus-free" line of Burkitt tumour cells. Nature **227**, 245–248 (1970)

zur Hausen, H., Henle, W., Hummeler, K., Diel, V., Henle, G.: Comparative study of cultured Burkitt tumor cells by immunofluorescence, autoradiography and electron microscopy. J. Virol. **1**, 830–837 (1967)

zur Hausen, H., O'Neill, F. J., Freese, U. K., Hecker, E.: Persisting oncogenic herpesvirus induced by the tumour promoter TPA. Nature **272**, 373–375 (1978)

4 Seroepidemiology of the Virus[1]

W. Henle[2] and G. Henle

Division of Virology, The Joseph Stokes, Jr. Research Institute at The Children's Hospital of Philadelphia, School of Medicine, University of Pennsylvania, 34th Street & Civic Center Boulevard, Philadelphia, PA 19104 (USA)

[1] Work by the authors was supported by research grant CA-04568 and contract NO1-CP-33272 from the National Cancer Institute, U.S. Public Health Service.

[2] W. H. is the recipient of Career Award 5-K6-AI-22683 from the National Institutes of Health, Public Health Service.

The detection of an apparently new virus in a specimen from a patient with a particular disease has to be followed by a series of immunologic and seroepidemiologic studies to determine (1) whether the virus is truly new or whether it can be identified with the aid of specific immune sera to known viruses; (2) whether the patient has or develops antibodies to the virus in the course of the disease; (3) whether other patients with the same disease also have antibodies to the new virus; (4) whether antibodies to the new virus are limited to patients with the given disease or whether they are also found in the general population which, in turn, would indicate whether infections by the new virus are invariably accompanied by signs of the disease or whether the disease is an unusual result of infection by the virus; and (5) if antibodies are found in healthy individuals, whether or not patients with the disease show higher titers and a broader spectrum of antibodies to virus-related antigens than individuals without clinical evidence of the disease. The value of these immunologic and seroepidemiologic approaches is well illustrated by the Epstein-Barr virus (EBV).

A. IDENTIFICATION OF EBV AS A NEW HUMAN HERPES GROUP VIRUS

EBV was initially discovered electron-microscopically in a small proportion of lymphoblastoid cells cultured from African Burkitt's lymphoma (BL) biopsies (Epstein et al., 1964). The virus, belonging morphologically to the herpes group, could not be transmitted to host systems known to be susceptible to herpes simplex virus (HSV), cytomegalovirus (CMV), or varicella-zoster virus (VZV) and thus appeared to be a heretofore unknown human herpes group virus (Epstein et al., 1965). Because of the inability to transmit the virus to experimental host systems, attempts to identify the virus by immunologic techniques had to rely on the virus-producing cells in the BL cultures, e. g. the application of immunofluorescence techniques.

When acetone-fixed smears of cells from the EB1 or EB2 lines of BL origin (Epstein et al., 1964) were examined by the indirect immunofluorescence technique with a serum from an African BL patient, brilliant staining was elicited in small percentages of the cells which corresponded to the percentages of cells shown electron-microscopically to contain virus particles (G. Henle and W. Henle, 1966 a). A control serum from an American child with acute lymphocytic leukemia failed to evoke immunofluorescence. The choice of this control serum proved fortuitous since many, but by no means all, American sera subsequently tested also induced staining in the same percentages of cells. However, when additional sera from African BL patients became available, they all induced brilliant fluorescence.

With the use of paired acute and convalescent phase sera from patients with primary HSV, CMV, or VZV infections the virus in the cultured BL cells was clearly shown to be antigenically distinct from these three groups of viruses; either both paired sera failed to react with the virus-containing BL cells or both elicited similar degrees of fluorescence. Commercially available human γ-globulin preparations, used either in indirect or, after coupling with fluorescein isothiocyanate, in direct immunofluorescence tests, were found to stain the appropriate numbers of BL cells. While they failed to react with CMV- or VZV-infected cells, they evoked fluorescence in HSV-infected cells. Absorption of the γ-globulin preparations with HSV abolished staining of HSV-infected cells, however, but did not diminish the fluorescence elicited in the cultured BL cells. Furthermore, immunofluorescence tests with appropriate reagents excluded various feline, canine, bovine, equine, and other animal herpesviruses (G. Henle and W. Henle, 1966 a, b, 1967). These efforts proved beyond doubt that the virus in the BL cells was a new human herpes group virus, henceforth designated the Epstein-Barr virus after the cell lines in which it was first detected.

B. SEROLOGIC ASSOCIATION OF EBV WITH BURKITT'S LYMPHOMA AND OTHER DISEASES

The immunofluorescence technique provided a convenient means to demonstrate EBV in cell cultures and, in turn, to detect and titrate antibodies to the virus in human sera. It soon became evident that the virus was not limited to cultures from African BL biopsies, but it, or a close relative, was also detected in many lymphoblastoid cell lines initiated with peripheral leukocytes of non-African patients with various diseases or of healthy donors residing in various parts of the world (Ikawata and Grace, 1966; G. Henle and W. Henle, 1966 a; Moore et al., 1966, 1967; Zeve et al., 1966; Pope, 1967; Gerber and Monroe, 1968; Diehl et al., 1968; Nilsson et al., 1971). The virus apparently had a wide distribution as was also evident from the serologic tests already mentioned.

The "anti-EBV test" of early studies was later renamed "anti-viral capsid antigen (VCA) test" to differentiate it from tests for antibodies to subsequently identified EBV-related antigens. The new designation was based on the facts that (1) immunofluorescence was elicited only in cells producing virus particles (zur Hausen et al., 1967; Epstein and Achong, 1968) and (2) sera positive in the immunofluorescence test, but not negative sera, coated the nonenveloped viral nucleocapsids extracted and concentrated from cultured BL cells, with antibodies and caused their partial

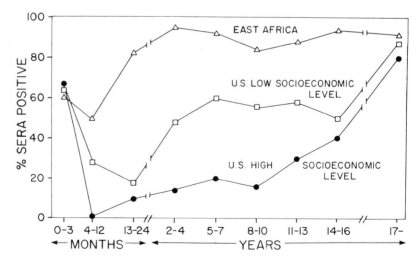

Fig. 1. Age-related incidence of antibodies to VCA in East African children and American children from different socioeconomic strata

agglutination as shown by negative-contrast electron microscopy (W. Henle et al., 1966; Mayyasi et al., 1967).

Application of the anti-VCA test to seroepidemiologic surveys soon confirmed that infections by EBV, whether a single entity or a group of antigenically closely related viruses, occur in all parts of the world, including the remotest regions and most isolated populations, such as the East African bush country (Levy and Henle G. 1967; G. Henle et al., 1969; Kafuko et al., 1972), an Aleutian island (Tischendorf et al., 1970), the Tiriyo tribe in the Amazonas basin (Black et al., 1970), and natives of New Guinea, Papua, and the New Hebrides (Lang et al., 1977). However, considerable variations in the age distribution of anti-VCA became apparent between, and also within, some of the populations surveyed (Fig. 1). In primitive societies, being one extreme, the vast majority, if not all of the children, have antibodies to VCA by the age of 3 years. In populations with high hygienic and socioeconomic standards, the opposite extreme, acquisition of antibodies to VCA is often delayed to adolescence and later (G. Henle et al., 1968; Niederman et al., 1968; Porter et al., 1969; G. Henle and W. Henle 1970). Crowded living conditions, such as those prevailing in many parts of Japan, lead to seroconversion already in early childhood (Hinuma et al., 1969). Thus, depending on hygienic standards and/or the degree of crowding, primary EBV infections occur earlier or later in life, but with advancing age all adults, with rare exceptions, acquire antibodies to VCA anywhere in the world.

The mere detection of antibodies to VCA clearly proved insufficient to link EBV with any disease with which it might be associated. It was essential therefore to titrate the antibodies and to compare the titers observed in apparently healthy donors with those obtained in patients with various diseases. By this approach, African BL remained a strong candidate for an EBV-associated disease (G. Henle et al., 1969) and other diseases were added (Fig. 2). It was noted by Old and his associates (1966, 1968) that sera from patients with undifferentiated nasopharyngeal carcinoma (NPC), like sera from BL patients, often gave one or more lines of precipitation in double diffusion tests with extracts from cultured cells of a virus-producing BL line. This observation was rapidly extended by application of the anti-VCA tests (W. Henle and G. Henle, 1968; De Schryver et al., 1969; W. Henle et al., 1970a). All African or Chinese NPC patients were found to have antibodies to VCA, usually at substantially higher titers than appropriate controls. The world-wide high rate of EBV infections suggested that the virus, besides its apparent relation to two rare malignancies, might be the unsuspected cause of a common disease. Indeed, the virus turned out to be the cause of infectious mononucleosis (IM) (G. Henle et al., 1968; Niederman et al., 1968), a disease common in Western countries but rare in most other parts of the world. It was noted that previously anti-VCA negative individuals seroconverted in the course of IM and that all patients with this disease had antibodies to VCA generally at high titers, whereas a considerable proportion of appropriate controls had no antibodies and the remainder had substantially lower titers, as a rule, than the patients (Chap. 13). Finally, an overrepresentation of high anti-VCA titers, as compared to healthy control groups, but far less striking than that seen in BL, NPC, or IM, was observed in a wide variety of malignant and nonmalignant diseases, including Hodgkin's disease, other lymphoproliferative malignancies, other types of cancers, sarcoidosis, systemic lupus erythematosus, immune-deficiency diseases, and other conditions.

With this apparent abundance of possibly EBV-associated diseases it became clear that additional serologic evidence must be adduced to link EBV with given diseases.

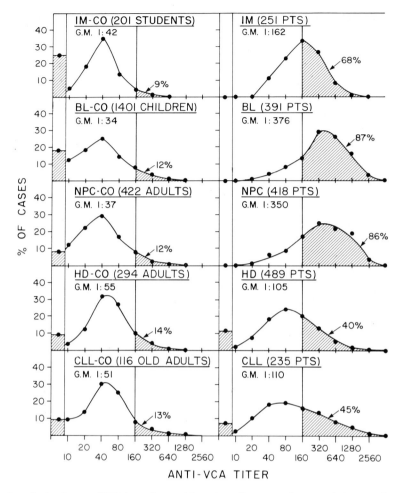

Fig. 2. Distribution of antibody titers to VCA in patients with various diseases and appropriate control groups. *IM*, infectious mononucleosis; *BL*, Burkitt's lymphoma; *NPC*, nasopharyngeal carcinoma; *HD*, Hodgkin's disease; *CLL*, chronic lymphocytic leukemia; *CO*, control; *G.M.*, geometric mean

With the inclusion of tests for antibodies to EBV-determined antigens other than VCA, especially antibodies to the EBV-induced early antigen (EA) complex (W. Henle et al., 1970b; G. Henle et al., 1971a) such evidence has been forthcoming. Since the anti-EA responses differ substantially in different diseases and the clinical conditions under consideration show in part geographic differences in prevalence, their seroepidemiologic backgrounds will be presented in separate sections. In line with the introductory remarks and the historical order of developments, BL will be discussed first, followed by NPC, IM, and the other diseases.

C. THE SEROEPIDEMIOLOGY OF BURKITT'S LYMPHOMA

Early serologic surveys in African regions of BL prevalence indicated that antibodies to VCA are acquired mostly in early childhood, yet some teenagers were found to have no antibodies detectable at a serum dilution of 1:10 (Levy and G. Henle, 1966; G. Henle et al., 1969; Kafuko et al., 1972). In more recent studies, nonreactors were limited to children $\leq$ 3 years of age (de-Thé et al., 1975; Nkrumah et al., 1976). This does not denote that the rate of infections in early childhood increased in the intervening years, but rather that the sensitivity of the anti-VCA test has been improved. In earlier studies only fluorescent anti-human globulin conjugates of low potency were available which provided no more than 2–3 antibody units at the lowest dilution suitable for the test. Thus, low titers of anti-VCA were not detectable. Furthermore, absence of staining at a serum dilution 1:10 does not necessarily denote absence of antibodies. Indeed, when the incidence of given anti-VCA titers was plotted, a bell-shape curve was obtained, permitting extrapolation to the number of sera expected to have titers of 1:5 or 1:2.5, i.e., 16% and 5%, respectively, of the children tested. These estimates were confirmed by retesting a number of sera which had been negative at 1:10 at the two lower dilutions. The anti-human globulin conjugate has been replaced by conjugates specific for human IgG of increased potency, permitting the use of at least eight antibody units in the test. Finally, dark field has been replaced by incident illumination for reading immunofluorescence that requires about 720 × instead of 150 × magnification, adding to the increased sensitivity of the test. With the improved technique, it became evident that few if any African children escape primary EBV infection within the first 3 years of life. In line with this conclusion is the fact that the geometric mean titers (GMT) of anti-VCA, calculated from the data presented by Kafuko et al. (1972), were highest in the 1-year-old group and declined gradually with advancing age to an essentially stable, persistent value by the age of 6 years and beyond (Fig. 3). The improved procedure also increased the anti-VCA titers but without

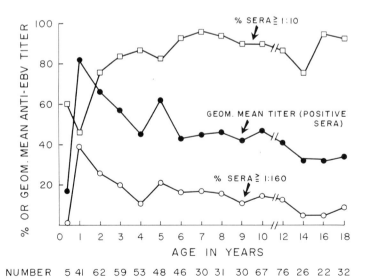

Fig. 3. Geometric mean titers of antibodies to VCA in relation to age in East African children

changing the eight to ten fold difference between the GMTs of BL patients and controls (G. Henle et al., 1969, 1971 b; Nkrumah et al., 1977).

With the introduction of tests for antibodies to EA and the differentiation of the diffuse (D) and restricted (R) components of the EA complex (W. Henle et al., 1970 b; G. Henle et al., 1971 b) a further striking difference between BL patients and controls became apparent (Table 1). Over 85% of the patients were shown to have antibodies to EA which were mostly directed against R (G. Henle et al., 1971 a; W. Henle et al., 1973 a), often at high titers which at times even exceeded the anti-VCA titers (W. Henle and G. Henle, 1976). In contrast, control children were rarely found to have antibodies to EA and if so, at generally low titers, with anti-R being more frequent than anti-D (W. Henle and G. Henle, 1973). These data provided further evidence for an association of EBV with BL. In fact, antibodies to R correlated to a considerable extent with the prognosis of the patients (G. Henle et al., 1971 b; W. Henle et al., 1973 a; Nkrumah et al., 1976). Patients brought to remission by chemotherapy were found to have a good chance of survival for 5 or more years if they had no anti-R or the anti-R titers declined gradually to low or nondetectable levels. In contrast, patients who maintained or developed high anti-R titers during remission were observed to have one or more ultimately fatal relapses even after disease-free periods of several years.

Table 1. Characteristic antibody patterns of typical cases of EBV-associated diseases

Disease	Antibodies to:					
	VCA			EA		EBNA
	IgM	IgA	IgG	D	R	
IM	+ +	0	+ +	+	0	0
BL	0	0	+ +	0	+ +	+
NPC	0	+ +	+ +	+ +	0	+ +
Controls	0	0	+	0	0	+

0 Not detectable as a rule; + Antibody titers $\leq$ 1:160; + + Antibody titers $\geq$ 1:320.

The seroepidemiologic data have shown that the primary EBV infections in regions of BL prevalence fall into the 1–3 year age range, but the peak incidence of BL is reached only by the age of 6–8 years (Burkitt, 1970). This interval between the period of seroconversions and of the peak incidence of BL denotes that the development of the tumor may be either a direct consequence of a rare delayed primary EBV infection, or the result of a secondary event occurring several years after the primary EBV infection and the establishment of a persistent viral carrier state in the lymphoreticular system. To differentiate between these possibilities, a prospective collaborative study of BL was initiated more than 8 years ago in the West Nile District of Uganda under the auspices of the International Agency for Research on Cancer (IARC). Serum was obtained from well over 42,000 children, aged 1–5 years, and stored for future reference. To date, 14 cases diagnosed as BL at $4^1/_2$–10 years of age have been detected among the pre-bled children. All of these had antibodies to VCA at least 5 and as many as 54 months prior to diagnosis of the tumor as determined in parallel at the

IARC and the authors' laboratories. These results have provided the answer that BL, if caused by EBV, must be due to a late, secondary event. The pre-sera, with two exceptions, had no antibodies to EA but after development of the tumor eight of the patients showed solely or dominantly anti-R, and two, dominantly anti-D. The anti-VCA titers had increased significantly in only three of the patients. At least three of the tumors, however, were not EBV-associated. The anti-VCA titers of these patients remained constant between the pre-bleeding and diagnosis, being low in two, but high in one of the cases, anti-EA was not detectable, and no EBV DNA was demonstrable in biopsies of the tumors. The other 11 cases were EBV-associated, all but one failed to develop antibodies to EA, and biopsies available from four contained EBV DNA.

All serologic tests were carried out under code together with numerous sera from age-, sex-, and tribe-matched controls, family members, and neighbors. The GMTs of anti-VCA calculated for given ages of the control children yielded a curve comparable to that shown in Fig. 3. The anti-VCA titers of the pre-sera from the 11 patients who developed EBV-associated BL were all substantially higher than the GMTs of anti-VCA of the control children of the corresponding ages. Occasional control children showed, however, high titers similar to those of the pre-sera of the patients. These observations denote that the persistent EBV infection of children who develop BL might be generally more 'active' than that of children who do not (Chaps. 14 and 18).

EBV-associated BL also occurs, though rarely, in Western countries, but in the majority (about 80%) of Caucasian patients with a diagnosis of BL the tumor is not associated with EBV. Such cases occur also among African BL patients but at low frequency, i. e., in no more than 3% of the cases (Lindahl et al., 1974). The Caucasian, like the African, EBV-associated cases of BL can readily be differentiated from those not associated with EBV by the EBV-related serology. They usually have high anti-VCA titers (Levine et al., 1972; Hirshaut et al., 1973) and, in addition, considerable levels of anti-R and/or anti-D (Ziegler et al., 1976; A. L. Epstein et al., 1976; Judson et al., 1977), which clearly separate them from healthy controls. Biopsies from such patients were found to contain EBV DNA or EBV nuclear antigen (EBNA)-positive tumor cells (Andersson et al., 1976; Ziegler et al., 1976; A. L. Epstein et al., 1976; Gravell et al., 1976; Bornkamm et al., 1976). Tumor specimens from patients with no or low levels of anti-VCA and no anti-EA have failed to reveal EBV DNA or EBNA-positive tumor cells (Pagano et al., 1973; Andersson et al., 1976; Ziegler et al., 1976; A. L. Epstein, 1976). Thus, two forms of BL exist, one EBV-associated, which occurs endemically in Africa and only sporadically elsewhere in the world, and the other not EBV- associated, which is observed only sporadically everywhere including Africa. It appears though that the age range of American EBV-associated BL is distinctly higher than that of African patients. While adult cases have been noted at low frequency in Africa, they seem to be more frequent in the United States. A cluster of four adult patients was recently observed in Pennsylvania (Judson et al., 1977) and two other sporadic adult BL patients have been serologically identified during the past 2 years in other regions of the state.

D. THE SEROEPIDEMIOLOGY OF NASOPHARYNGEAL CARCINOMA

In regions of enhanced prevalence of NPC (i. e., southern China, East and North Africa, or Alaska) primary EBV infections occur generally in early childhood due to crowding or low hygienic standards (W. Henle et al., 1970; de-Thé et al., 1975 a). Yet, NPC is mostly a malignancy of adults so that primary EBV infections are bound to precede the development of the tumor by numerous years.

All NPC patients observed in Hong Kong, Singapore, East Africa, or Tunisia have shown antibodies to VCA but so have healthy controls of comparable ages in these regions (W. Henle et al., 1970, 1973 b; Kawamura et al., 1970; Lin et al., 1972, 1973; Lynn et al., 1973 a, b; de-Thé et al., 1975 b). The anti-VCA titers of the patients were found, as a rule, to be substantially higher, however, than those of the control groups with the GMTs differing by factors between 8 and 10 (Fig. 2). The height of the anti-VCA titers was shown to depend to a large extent on the total tumor burden as reflected by the stage of the disease according to the classification of Ho (1970). As compared to controls, the GMT was found to be only slightly higher in stage I patients, where the tumor is limited to the nasopharynx, but to rise stepwise with invasion of lymph nodes by the tumor at increasingly greater distance from the primary site (stages II–IV) and the ultimate development of wide-spread metastases (stage V) (W. Henle et al., 1970 a, 1973 b; Lynn et al., 1973 a; de-Thé et al., 1975 b). These observations suggest that the anti-VCA titers increase over those of healthy controls only after inception of the tumor.

As in the case of BL, tests for antibodies to the D and R components of the EBV-induced EA have revealed further striking differences between NPC patients and healthy controls (G. Henle et al., 1971 a; W. Henle et al., 1973 b). In NPC, anti-D is the dominant antibody to the EA complex (Table 1), although anti-R may be observed in some of the stage I and rarely in stage II patients, when anti-D may still be absent. The incidence and titers of anti-D also increase with the total tumor burden so that this antibody becomes detectable in practically all patients in stages III–V of the disease and its GMTs rise to high levels. In contrast, anti-D is very rarely observed in healthy individuals and anti-R, only occasionally among those controls who maintain relatively high anti-VCA titers (W. Henle and G. Henle, 1973).

Another outstanding feature of NPC (Table 1) is the nearly uniform presence of serum IgA antibodies to VCA and often also to the D component of the EA complex (G. Henle and W. Henle, 1976 a, b; Ho et al., 1976). Again the titers of VCA-specific and the incidence and titers of D-specific IgA antibodies increase with the total tumor burden. EBV-related IgA antibodies are very rarely observed in healthy controls and then only anti-VCA at low titers among those with relatively high IgG antibodies to VCA.

The results discussed thus far concern NPC patients prior to therapy. Since the titers and, in part, incidence of the various antibodies were found to depend on the tumor burden, they were expected to decline again after effective therapy, and this was shown to be the case (W. Henle et al., 1973 b, 1977; Lynn et al., 1973 b; G. Henle and W. Henle, 1976 a, b; de-Thé et al., 1975 b). VCA-specific IgG antibody titers decline to lower levels whereas the corresponding IgA as well as D-specific IgG and IgA antibodies may gradually become nondetectable within 1–4 years, depending upon their initial titers (W. Henle et al., 1977). Thus, the antibody patterns of successfully treated NPC patients gradually return to those seen in healthy controls. Patients not, or only transiently responding to therapy were observed to show no or only temporary declines in the antibody spectrum and titers, followed by further or renewed broadening of the antibody spectrum and increases in antibody titers before death from widespread metastases. Increases in titers and broadening of the antibody spectrum were often noted well in advance of clinical evidence of renewed tumor activity, indicating that the serologic follow-up of patients after treatment may alert to incipient relapses and the development of metastases. Titers of antibodies to EBNA were found to be generally on the high side and to show only minor changes, as a rule, in the course of the disease.

The antibody patterns in stage I of NPC are often not clearly distinguishable from those of the occasional healthy controls who show relatively high VCA-specific IgG antibody titers, accompanied at times by barely detectable IgA antibodies to VCA, but usually not anti-D. Because of these overlaps, it seems doubtful that prospective serologic surveys would identify individuals likely to develop NPC. However, as the carcinoma develops, a broadening of the antibody spectrum and increases in antibody titers might lead to early search for and detection of the tumor. The presence of anti-D and elevated IgA antibodies would be pertinent indicators. In fact, these parameters may provide an immunologic basis for determination of the location of occult primary head and neck malignancies (Coates et al., 1978).

Another type of control group has been employed extensively in NPC studies, i. e., patients with carcinomas elswhere in the head and neck or other types of tumors in the nasopharynx (De Schryver et al., 1969, 1972; W. Henle et al., 1970 a; Andersson et al., 1977; Ho et al., unpublished). While the EBV-related antibody patterns of these control patients usually conform to those of healthy individuals, they have shown an overrepresentation of high VCA-specific IgG antibody titers, but these are not nearly as impressive as those seen in NPC. Furthermore, antibodies to the EA complex, if present, are mostly directed against R, but occasionally against D, usually at low, but at times at high titers. Also VCA-specific, but not EA-specific IgA antibodies may be found in some of the patients with malignancies of the head and neck other than NPC (G. Henle and W. Henle, 1976 a, b). It is again evident that an association of EBV with given tumors cannot be established by serology alone but requires confirmation by additional evidence, i. e., the demonstration of EBV DNA or EBNA-positive tumor cells in biopsies. This has thus far been achieved, besides BL, only in undifferentiated carcinomas of the nasopharynx and the adjacent nasal fossa, but not in any other carcinomas or tumors of the head and neck region (zur Hausen et al., 1971; Nonoyama et al., 1973; Wolf et al., 1973, 1975; Klein et al., 1974; Huang et al., 1974; Andersson et al., 1977; Ho et al., unpublished). The elevated antibody titers found among patients with carcinomas other than NPC will be discussed further in a later section.

While the above discussion was largely limited to Asian and African NPC patients, similar EBV-related serologic patterns are observed regardless of race in patients living elswhere, including the United States and Europe (Goldman et al., 1971; De Schryver et al., 1974; Henderson et al., 1974; Pearson and Orr, 1976; Levine et al., 1977). Due to the relative rarity of the disease in Caucasians, only limited numbers of patients have been appropriately studied. They included patients at various stages before therapy or tested only months or years after initiating treatment, showing no residual or recurrent tumors. When assorted according to these various criteria, the numbers of patients in individual subgroups were often too small for valid comparisons. Yet, antibody spectra and titers of IgG and IgA antibodies to VCA and D comparable to those of

Chinese or African cases of EBV-associated undifferentiated carcinomas of the nasopharynx are also found in Caucasian patients with this malignancy.

E. THE SEROEPIDEMIOLOGY OF INFECTIOUS MONONUCLEOSIS

IM is practically unknown in areas of the world where primary EBV infections generally occur in early childhood, e. g., East Africa (Diehl et al., 1969). It is a disease of economically advanced nations, occurring especially among adolescents and young adults of the middle- and upper-class population segments who often escape primary EBV infections at an earlier age (Fig. 1). Only 26% of freshman entering Yale University in the early 1950s showed antibodies to VCA, but by 1968 the percentage had doubled, reflecting a change in the admission policy to include larger numbers of students from lower socioeconomic strata (Evans, 1974).

Besides the heterophil antibody response seen in the majority of patients in the acute phase of IM, they also show a characteristic EBV-related antibody pattern seen only in primary EBV infections (Table 1). They have high titers of VCA-specific IgM and IgG antibodies, show a transient anti-D response in 85% of the cases, and no anti-EBNA, as a rule. The IgM, heterophil, and D-specific antibodies disappear in time, whereas anti-EBNA arises gradually after several weeks or months (cf. W. Henle et al., 1974). EBV-specific serodiagnostic tests are needed for identification of heterophil antibody-negative cases of IM, said to be especially frequent in childhood.

It has been assumed that primary EBV infections in early childhood remain mostly silent or are accompanied by such mild, uncharacteristic illness that a diagnosis of IM is not suspected. While this is probably to a large extent true since between 30% and 50% of primary EBV infections in college students or other groups of similar background also remain silent (Evans et al., 1968; Niederman et al., 1970; Sawyer et al., 1971; University Health Physicians and PHLS Laboratories, 1971; Hallee et al., 1974), typical IM can be identified in young children, if specifically looked for, on the basis of heterophil antibody responses and/or EBV-specific serodiagnostic tests (Tischendorf et al., 1970; Schmitz et al., 1972; Ginsburg et al., 1977). It is not known, however, how many of the primary EBV infections in early childhood are compatible with typical IM, or are submerged among the numerous mild viral infections children experience annually, or remain truly silent. It is also unknown how many of these infections occur with or without heterophil antibody responses. It seems reasonable to surmise, however, that with advancing age primary EBV infections tend to increase in severity, which is also the case with some other common viral diseases.

The same questions arise with regard to primary EBV infections in developing countries where they occur generally under the age of 4 years. The assumption that they all remain silent is probably fallacious since, in fact, no pertinent studies have been reported. It would be difficult, indeed, to examine infants under prevailing conditions at the frequent intervals required to observe them during seroconversion and to relate that event to clinical observations and pertinent laboratory data. Such studies have become essential since it has been suggested that perinatal EBV infections might set the stage for later development of BL (de-Thé, 1977). It is hard to visualize though, how perinatal infections could occur because all mothers in regions of BL prevalence are bound to have antibodies to EBV which are transmitted transplacentally to their offspring. A recent study initiated by Dr. John Biggar in Ghana confirms these doubts (unpublished). Blood was collected by finger prick at monthly intervals from 30 infants beginning 1 month after birth and continuing for 15 months. Clinical evaluations, leukocyte counts, differential blood smears, and throat swabs were obtained at each visit. Pertinent to this discussion is the fact that all the infants at 1 month of age had maternal antibodies to VCA at titers ranging from 1:20 to 1:160 with a GMT of 1:55. The antibody titers declined in subsequent months according to a half-life of about 5 weeks so that anti-VCA became nondetectable ($< 1:10$) in all infants between 3 and 7 months. Anti-VCA remained undetectable for at least the next 3 months before the first seroconversions were noted. A total of 16 infants seroconverted during the observation period, 11 thus far escaped infection and 4 were prematurely withdrawn from the study. Thus, all infants, depending on the levels of maternal antibodies, were evidently protected against primary EBV infections for the first 5–10 months after birth. The serologic patterns during serconversion and the clinical and other laboratory data are not as yet available.

F. SEROEPIDEMIOLOGIC OBSERVATIONS IN OTHER DISEASES

As mentioned earlier, an overrepresentation of high titers of VCA-specific IgG antibodies, as compared to appropriate controls, has been observed in a large variety of nonmalignant and malignant diseases. These include sarcoidosis (Hirshaut et al., 1970; Wahren et al., 1971; Byrne et al., 1973), systemic lupus erythematosus (Evans et al., 1971; Rothfield et al., 1972), chronic kidney diseases (Fiala et al., unpublished), ataxia-telangiectasia (Berkel et al., unpublished), Hodgkin's disease (HD), other malignant lymphomas, chronic lymphocytic and other leukemias (Johansson et al., 1970, 1971; Levine et al., 1971 a, b; W. Henle and G. Henle, 1973; Henderson et al., 1973; Hesse et al., 1973; Dumont et al., 1976), various carcinomas other than NPC or tumors other than carcinomas of the head and neck region (De Schryver et al., 1969, 1972; Andersson et al., 1977), Kaposi's sarcoma (Giraldo et al., 1975), and probably other conditions. In all these diseases, the overrepresentation of high anti-VCA titers is far less striking than that observed in BL, NPC, or IM (Fig. 2). Furthermore, patients without antibodies to VCA are noted in most of the disease categories, depending on age range affected, the socioeconomic conditions and the geographic regions involved. Also, the incidence of anti-EA in these various groups of patients may be somewhat higher than in appropriate controls but substantially lower than in BL, NPC, or IM (W. Henle and G. Henle, 1973). The antibodies to EA are usually of low titer and directed against the R component but in HD, other malignant lymphomas, or chronic lymphocytic leukemia they often are dominantly directed against D, reaching at times substantial titers. Antibodies to EBNA are not usually notably elevated as compared to controls; in fact the anti-EBNA titers are often of a low order. Furthermore, EBV DNA or EBNA-positive tumor cells have not been detected thus far in any tumors other than BL and NPC (Lindahl et al., 1974). It is unlikely therefore that EBV plays a role in the genesis of these various malignant or nonmalignant diseases and another explanation must be found for the elevated antibody levels.

One factor appears to be common to all the diseases mentioned in this section, i. e., they are immune deficiency conditions, or have immunosuppressive effects, or require therapy by immunosuppressive drugs. The elevated VCA-specific IgG and the occasional anti-R or anti-D titers observed may therefore be the result of an activation of the persistent viral carrier state, which regularly becomes established in the lymphoreticular system after primary EBV infections. In the lymphocyte-predominant form of HD the antibody titers are within the control range, but they are often elevated in the other types of the disease, especially the lymphocyte-depletion form (Johansson et al., 1970; Henderson et al., 1973). The high antibody titers correlate significantly with evidence of T cell (thymus-dependent lymphocyte) dysfunctions as determined by several parameters (Johansson et al., 1975). Similar observations have been made in ataxia-telangiectasia (Berkel et al., unpublished) in which, furthermore, antibodies to EBNA are often of low titer or not detectable. It has been suggested that the anti-EBNA levels might serve as another parameter for detection of T cell deficiencies (G. Henle et al., 1974). Children with genetic T cell defects may also show high anti-VCA titers accompanied by anti-D, but no anti-EBNA (Rocchi, personal communication). Likewise renal transplant or hemodialysis patients may develop elevated anti-VCA titers without parallel increases in anti-EBNA titers, which are often low or absent (unpublished). Thus, reactivation of the persistent EBV infection appears to be a reality. Further studies are needed to determine whether this interpretation holds for all diseases in which an overrepresentation of high anti-VCA titers and anti-EA reactions are observed.

G. CONCLUDING REMARKS

The immunologic and seroepidemiologic approaches to an assessment of the clinical importance of a new virus, listed in the introductory section, have proven their value in the study of EBV. The virus, originally discovered in cells cultured from African Burkitt's lymphomas, was identified serologically as a previously unknown member of the herpes group. Antibodies to EBV were detected in all African BL patients but also in all African control children above 3 years of age, suggesting that the tumor would be an uncommon result of EBV infection. The patients were, however, readily distinguishable, as a rule, from the controls by their substantially higher titers and a broader spectrum of antibodies to EBV-determined antigens, thus indicating an intimate association of EBV with BL.

Seroepidemiologic surveys established the world-wide dissemination of the virus and served to uncover in short succession two other disparate but clearly EBV-associated diseases, NPC and IM. The serologic observations leading to the implication of EBV in the development of NPC were comparable in every aspect to those regarding BL, except for differences in the preferential age ranges of the two malignancies and the characteristics of the antibody spectra of the patients. In BL, antibodies to the R component of the EA complex are the characteristic response, whereas in NPC antibodies to the D component and serum IgA antibodies to VCA and D are the distinguishing features.

IM was clearly shown to be a result of primary EBV infection. It was shown to occur only in individuals who previously had no antibodies to the virus and all IM patients were found to have high titers of IgM and IgG antibodies to VCA, often accompanied by anti-D but no anti-EBNA, whereas appropriate control individuals either had no antibodies or solely IgG antibodies to VCA and anti-EBNA at moderate titers.

The seroepidemiology of EBV has not remained free of complications. The characteristic antibody patterns are most strikingly revealed by advanced cases of BL or NPC but not necessarily at early stages of the tumors or in all BL patients for that matter. Enhanced titers and occasionally a broadening of the antibody spectrum can result from an activation of the persistent viral carrier state which regularly ensues after primary EBV infections, by immunosuppressive diseases or therapy, i.e., a number of malignant and nonmalignant diseases. Thus, the antibody patterns of controls and BL or NPC patients, and of BL or NPC and other tumor patients, may overlap to some extent. The strong lead provided by the serologic and seroepidemiologic observations has required confirmation by other evidence; this is discussed in detail in other chapters.

REFERENCES

Andersson, M., Ziegler, J. L., Klein, G., Henle, W.: Association of Epstein-Barr viral genomes with American Burkitt lymphoma. Nature **260**, 357–359 (1976)

Andersson-Anvret, M., Forsby, N., Klein, G. and Henle, W.: Studies on the occurrence of Epstein-Barr virus-DNA in nasopharyngeal carcinomas, in compasrison with tumors of other head and neck regions. Int. J. Cancer **20**, 486–494 (1977)

Black, F. L., Woodall, J. P., Evans, A. S., Liebhaber, H. Henle, G.: Prevalence of antibody against viruses in Tiriyo, an isolated Amazon tribe. Am. J. Epidemiol. **91**, 430–438 (1970)

Bornkamm, G. W., Stein, H., Lennert, K., Ruggeberg, F., Bartels, H. zur Hausen, H.: Attempts to demonstrate virus-specific sequences in human tumors. IV. EB viral DNA in European Burkitt's lymphoma and immunoblastic lymphadenopathy with excessive plasmacytes. Int. J. Cancer **17**, 177–181 (1976)

Burkitt, D. P.: General features and facial tumours. In: Burkitt's Lymphoma. Burkitt, D. P., Wright, D. H. (eds.), pp. 6–15. Edinburgh: Livingstone 1970

Byrne, E. B., Evans, A. S., Fonts, D. W., Israel, H. L.: A seroepidemiological study of Epstein-Barr virus and other viral antigens in sarcoidosis. Am. J. Epidemiol. **97**, 355–363 (1973)

Coates, H. L., Pearson, G., Neel, H. B. III, Weiland, L. H., Devine, K. D.: An immunologic basis for detection of occult primary malignancies of the head and neck. Cancer (in press) (1978)

De Schryver, A., Friberg, S. (Jr.), Klein, G., Henle, W., Henle, G., de-Thé, G., Clifford, P., Ho, H. C.: Epstein-Barr virus (EBV)-associated antibody patterns in carcinoma of the post-nasal space. Clin. Exp. Immunol. **5**, 443–459 (1969)

De Schryver, A., Klein, G., Henle, G., Henle, W., Cameron, H., Santesson, L. and Clifford, P.: EB-virus associated serology in malignant disease: Antibody levels to viral capsid antigens (VCA), membrane antigens (MA) and early antigens (EA) in patients with various neoplastic conditions. Int. J. Cancer **9**, 353–364 (1972)

De Schryver, A., Klein, G., Henle W., Henle, G.: EB virus-associated antibodies in Caucasian patients with carcinoma of the nasopharynx and in long-term survivors after treatment. Int. J. Cancer **13**, 319–325 (1974)

de-Thé, G.: Is Burkitt's lymphoma related to perinatal infection by Epstein-Barr virus. Lancet **1977 I**, 335–337

de-Thé, G., Day, N. E., Geser, A., Lavoné, M. F., Ho, J. H. C., Simons, M. J., Sohier, R., Tukei, P., Vonka, V., Zavadova, H.: Seroepidemiology of the Epstein-Barr virus: Preliminary analysis of an international study, a review. In: Oncogenesis and herpesviruses II. de-Thé, G., Epstein, M. A., zur Hausen, H. (eds.), Part 2, pp. 3–16. Lyon: IARC 1975 a

de-Thé, G., Ho, J. H. C., Ablashi, D. V., Day, N. E., Macario, A. J. L., Martin-Berthelon, M. C., Pearson, G., Sohier, R.: Nasopharyngeal carcinoma. IX. Antibodies to EBNA and correlation with response to other EBV antigens in Chinese patients. Int. J. Cancer **16**, 713–721 (1975 b)

Diehl, V., Henle, G., Henle, W., Kohn, G.: Demonstration of a herpes group virus in cultures of peripheral leukocytes from patients with infectious mononucleosis. J. Virol. **2**, 663–669 (1968)

Diehl, V., Taylor, J., Parlin, J. A., Henle, G., Henle, W.: Infectious mononucleosis in East Africa. East Afr. Med. J. **46**, 407–413 (1969)

Dumont, J., Liabeuf, A., Henle, W., Feingold, N., Kourilsky, F. M.: Anti-EBV antibody titers in non-Hodgkin lymphomas. Int. J. Cancer **18**, 14–23 (1976)

Epstein, A. L., Henle, W., Henle, G., Hewetson, J. F., Kaplan, H. S.: Surface marker characteristics and Epstein-Barr virus studies of two established North American Burkitt's lymphoma cell lines. Proc. Natl., Acad. Sci. USA **73**, 228–232 (1976)

Epstein, M. A., Achong, B. G.: Specific immunofluorescence test for the herpes-type EB virus of Burkitt lymphoblasts, authenticated by electron microscopy. J. Natl. Cancer Inst. **40**, 593–607 (1968)

Epstein, M. A., Achong, B. G., Barr, Y. M.: Virus particles in cultured lymphoblasts from Burkitt's lymphoma. Lancet **1964 I**, 702–703

Epstein, M. A., Henle, G., Achong, B. G., Barr, Y. M.: Morphological and biological studies on a virus in cultured lymphoblasts from Burkitt's lymphoma. J. Exp. Med. **121**, 761–770 (1965)

Evans, A. S., Niederman, J. C., McCollum, R. W.: Seroepidemiologic studies of infectious mononucleosis with EB virus. N. Eng. J. Med. **279**, 1121–1127 (1968)

Evans, A. S., Rothfield, N. F., Niederman, J. C.: Raised antibody titers to EB virus in systemic lupus erythematosus. Lancet **1971 I**, 167–168

Evans, A. S.: New discoveries in infectious mononucleosis. Mod. Med. **1**, 18–24 (1974)

Gerber, P., Monroe, J. H.: Studies on leukocytes growing in continuous culture derived from normal human donors. J. Natl. Cancer Inst. **40**, 855–866 (1968)

Ginsburg, C. M., Henle, W., Henle, G., Horwitz, C. A.: Infectious mononucleosis in children: evaluation of the Epstein-Barr virus-specific serology. J. Am. Med. Assoc. **237**, 781–785 (1977)

Giraldo, G., Beth, E., Kourilsky, F. M., Henle, W., Henle, G., Miké, V., Huraux, J. M., Andersen, H. K., Gharbi, M. R., Kyalwazi, S. K., Puisaant, A.: Antibody patterns to herpesviruses in Kaposi's sarcoma: serological association of European Kaposi's sarcoma with cytomegalovirus. Int. J. Cancer **15**, 839–848 (1975)

Goldman, I. M., Goodman, M. L., Miller, D.: Antibody to Epstein-Barr virus in American patients with carcinoma of the nasopharynx. J. Am. Med. Assoc. **216**, 1618–1622 (1971)

Gravell, M., Levine, P. H., McIntyre, R. F., Land, V. J., Pagano, J. S.: Epstein-Barr virus in an American patient with Burkitt's lymphoma: detection of viral genome in tumor tissue and establishment of a tumor-derived cell line (NAB). J. Natl. Cancer Inst. **56**, 701–704 (1976)

Hallee, T. J., Evans, A. S., Niederman, J. C.: Infectious mononucleosis at the United States Military Academy. A prospective study of a single class over 4 years. Yale J. Biol. Med. **3**, 182–192 (1974)

Henderson, B. E., Dworsky, R., Menck, H., Alena, B., Henle, W. Henle, G., Terasaki, P.: Case-control study of Hodgkin's disease. II. Herpesvirus group antibody titers and HL-A type. J. Natl. Cancer Inst. **51**, 1443–1447 (1973)

Henderson, B. E., Louie, E., Bogdanoff, E., Henle, W., Alena, B., Henle, G.: Antibodies to herpes group viruses in patients with nasopharyngeal and other head and neck cancers. Cancer Res. **34**, 1207–1210 (1974)

Henle, G., Henle, W.: Immunofluorescence in cells derived from Burkitt's lymphoma. J. Bacteriol. **91**, 1248–1256 (1966a)

Henle, G., Henle, W.: Studies on cell lines derived from Burkitt's lymphoma. Trans. NY Acad. Sci. **29**, 71–79 (1966b)

Henle, G., Henle, W.: Immunofluorescence, interference, and complement fixation technics in the detection of the herpes-type virus in Burkitt tumor cell lines. Cancer Res. **27**, 2442–2446 (1967)

Henle, G., Henle, W.: Observations on childhood infections with the Epstein-Barr virus. J. Infect. Dis. **121**, 303–310 (1970)

Henle, G., Henle, W.: Serum IgA antibodies to Epstein-Barr virus (EBV)-related antigens a new feature of nasopharyngeal carcinoma. Bibl. Haematol. **43**, 322–325 (1976a)

Henle, G., Henle, W.: Epstein-Barr virus-specific serum antibodies as an outstanding feature of nasopharyngeal carcinoma. Int. J. Cancer **17**, 1–7 (1976b)

Henle, G., Henle, W., Diehl, V.: Relation of Burkitt tumor associated herpes-type virus to infectious mononucleosis. Proc. Natl. Acad. Sci. USA **59**, 94–101 (1968)

Henle, G., Henle, W., Clifford, P., Diehl, V., Kafuko, G. W., Kirya, B. G., Klein, G., Morrow, R. H., Munube, G. M. R., Pike, M. C., Tukei, P. M., Ziegler, J. L.: Antibodies to EB virus in Burkitt's lymphoma and control groups. J. Natl. Cancer Inst. **43**, 1147–1157 (1969)

Henle, G., Henle, W., Klein, G.: Demonstration of two distinct components in the early antigen complex of Epstein-Barr virus infected cells. Int. J. Cancer **8**, 272–282 (1971 a)

Henle, G., Henle, W., Klein, G., Gunvén, P., Clifford, P., Morrow, R. H., Ziegler, J. L.: Antibodies to early Epstein-Barr virus-induced antigens in Burkitt's lymphoma. J. Natl. Cancer Inst. **46**, 861–871 (1971 b)

Henle, G., Henle, W., Horwitz, C. A.: Antibodies to Epstein-Barr virus-associated nuclear antigen in infectious mononucleosis. J. Infect. Dis. **130**, 231–239 (1974)

Henle, W., Henle, G.: Present status of the herpes-group virus associated with cultures of the hematopoietic system. Perspectives in virology. **6**, 105–117 (1968)

Henle, W., Henle, G.: Epstein-Barr virus-related serology in Hodgkin's disease. Natl. Cancer Inst. Monogr. **36**, 79–84 (1973)

Henle, W., Henle, G.: Antibodies to the R component of EBV-induced early antigens in Burkitt's lymphoma may exceed in titer antibodies to EB viral capsid antigen. J. Natl. Cancer Inst. **58**, 785–786 (1977)

Henle, W., Hummeler, K., Henle, G.: Antibody coating and agglutination of virus particles separated from the EB3 line of Burkitt lymphoma cells. J. Bacteriol. **92**, 269–271 (1966)

Henle, W., Henle, G., Ho, H. C., Burtin, P., Cachin, Y., Clifford, P., De Schryver, A., de-Thé, G., Diehl, V., Klein, G.: Antibodies to EB virus in nasopharyngeal carcinoma, other head and neck neoplasms and control groups. J. Natl. Cancer Inst. **44**, 225–231 (1970 a)

Henle, W., Henle, G., Zajac, B., Pearson, G., Waubke, R., Scriba, M.: Differential reactivity of human sera with EBV-induced "early antigens". Science **169**, 188–190 (1970 b)

Henle, W., Henle, G., Gunvén, P., Klein, G., Clifford, P., Singh, S.: Patterns of antibodies to Epstein-Barr virus-induced early antigens in Burkitt's lymphoma. Comparison of dying patients with long-term survivors. J. Natl. Cancer Inst. **50**, 1163–1173 (1973 a)

Henle, W., Ho, H. C., Henle, G., Kwan, H. C.: Antibodies to Epstein-Barr virus-related antigens in nasopharyngeal carcinoma. Comparison of active cases amd long term survivors. J. Natl. Cancer Inst. **51**, 361–369 (1973 b)

Henle, W., Henle, G., Horwitz, C. A.: Epstein-Barr virus-specific diagnostic tests in infectious mononu-cleosis. Hum. Pathol. **5**, 551–565 (1974)

Henle, W., Ho, H. C., Henle, G., Chau, J. C. W., Kwan, H. C.: Nasopharyngeal carcinoma: Significance of changes in Epstein-Barr virus-related antibody patterns following therapy. Int. J. Cancer **20**, 663–672 (1977)

Hesse, J., Anderson, E., Levine, P. H.: Antibodies to Epstein-Barr virus and cellular immunity in Hodgkin's disease and chronic lymphocytic leukemia. Int. J. Cancer **11**, 237–243 (1973)

Hinuma, Y., Ohta-Hatuno, R., Suto, T.: High incidence of Japanese infants with antibody to a herpes-type virus associated with cultured Burkitt lymphoma cells. Jap. J. Microbiol. **13**, 309–311 (1969)

Hirshaut, Y., Glade, P., Vieira, L. O., Ainbender, E., Dvorak, B., Siltzbach, L. E.: Sarcoidosis, another disease associated with serologic evidence for herpes-like virus infection. N. Engl. J. Med. **283**, 502–506 (1970)

Hirshaut, Y., Cohen, M., Stevens, D.: Epstein-Barr virus antibodies in American and African Burkitt's lymphoma. Lancet **1973 II**, 114–116

Ho, J. H. C.: The natural history and treatment of nasopharyngeal carcinoma. In: Oncology: Proceedings of the 10th International Cancer Congress. Clark, L. R., Crumley, R. W., McCay, J. E., Murray, M., (eds.), Vol. 4, pp. 1–14. Chicago: Year Book Publishers 1970

Ho, H. C., Ng, M. H., Kwan, H. C., Chau, J. C. W.: Epstein-Barr virus-specific IgA and IgG serum antibodies in nasopharyngeal carcinoma. Br. J. Cancer **34**, 655–660 (1976)

Huang, D. P., Ho, J. H. C., Henle, W., Henle, G.: Demonstration of EBV-associated nuclear antigen in NPC cells from fresh biopsies. Int. J. Cancer **14**, 580–588 (1974)

Ikawata, S., Grace, J. T. (Jr.): Cultivation in vitro of myeloblasts from human leukemia. NY State J. Med. **64**, 2279–2282 (1964)

Johansson, B., Klein, G., Henle, W., Henle, G.: Epstein-Barr virus (EBV) associated antibody patterns in malignant lymphoma and leukemia. I. Hodgkin's disease. Int. J. Cancer **6**, 450–462 (1970)

Johansson, B., Klein, G., Henle, W., Henle, G.: Epstein-Barr virus (EBV)-associated antibody patterns in malignant lymphoma and leukemia. II. Chronic lymphocytic leukemia and lymphocytic lymphoma. Int. J. Cancer **8**, 475–486 (1971)

Johansson, B., Holm, G., Mellstedt, H., Henle, W., Henle, G., Soderberg, G., Klein, G., Killander, D.: Epstein-Barr virus (EBV)-associated antibody patterns in relation to the deficiency of cell-mediated immunity in patients with Hodgkin's disease (HD). In: Oncogenesis and herpesviruses II. de-Thé, G., Epstein, M. A., zur Hausen, H. (eds.), Part 2, pp. 237–247. Lyon: IARC 1975

Judson, S. C., Henle, W., Henle, G.: A cluster of Epstein-Barr virus-associated American Burkitt's lymphoma. N. Engl. J. Med. **297**, 464–468 (1977)

Kafuko, G. W., Day, N. E., Henderson, B. E., Henle, G., Henle, W., Kirya, G., Munube, G., Morrow, R. H., Pike, M. C., Smith, P. G., Tukei, P., Williams, E. H.: Epstein-Barr virus antibody levels in children from the West Nile district of Uganda: Report of a field study. Lancet **1972 I**, 706–709

Kawamura, W. J., Takata, M., Gotoh, H.: Seroepidemiological studies on nasopharyngeal carcinoma by fluorescent antibody techniques with cultured Burkitt lymphoma cells. Gann **61**, 55–71 (1970)

Klein, G., Giovanella, B. C., Lindahl, T., Fialko, P. J., Singh, S., Stehlin, J. S.,: Direct evidence for the presence of Epstein-Barr virus DNA and nuclear antigen in malignant epithelial cells from patients with poorly differentiated carcinoma of the nasopharynx. Proc. Natl., Acad. Sci. USA **71**, 4737–4741 (1974)

Lang, D. J., Garruto, R. M., Gajdusek, D. C.: Early acquisition of cytomegalovirus and Epstein-Barr virus antibody in several isolated Melanesian populations. Am J. Epidemiol. **105**, 480–487 (1977)

Levine, P. H., Ablashi, D. V., Berard, C. V., Carbone, P. P., Waggoner, D. E., Malan, L.: Elevated antibody titers to Epstein-Barr virus in Hodgkin's disease. Cancer **27**, 416–421 (1971 a)

Levine, P. H., Merril, D. A., Bethlenfalvay, N., Dabich, L., Stevens, D. A., Waggoner, D. E.: A longitudinal comparison of antibodies to the Epstein-Barr virus and clinical parameters in chronic lymphocytic leukemia and chronic myelocytic leumekia. Blood **38**, 479–481 (1971b)

Levine, P. H., O'Connor, G. T., Berard, C. W.: Antibodies to Epstein-Barr virus (EBV) in American patients with Burkitt's lymphoma. Cancer **30**, 610–615 (1972)

Levine, P. H., Wallen, W. C., Ablashi, D. V., Granlund, D. J., Connelly, R.: Comparative studies on immunity to EBV-associated antigens in NPC patients in North America, Tunisia, France and Hong Kong. Int. J. Cancer **20**, 332–338 (1977)

Levy, J. A., Henle, G.: Indirect immunofluorescence tests with sera from African children and cultured Burkitt lymphoma cells. J. Bacteriol. **92**, 275–276 (1966)

Lin, T. M., Yang, C. S., Ho, S. W., Chiou, T. F., Liu, C. H., Tu, S. M., Chen, K. P., Ito, Y., Kawamura, A., Hirayama, T.: Antibodies to herpes-type virus in nasopharyngeal carcinoma and control groups. Cancer **29**, 603–609 (1972)

Lin, T. M., Yang, C. S., Chiou, J. F., Tu, S. M., Lin, C. C., Liu, C. H., Chen, K. P., Ito, Y., Kawamura, A., Hirayama, T.: Seroepidemiological studies on carcinoma of the nasopharynx. Cancer Res. **33**, 2603–2608 (1973)

Lindahl, T., Klein, G., Reedman, B. M., Johansson, B., Singh, S.: Relationship between Epstein-Barr virus (EBV) DNA and the EBV-determined nuclear antigen (EBNA) in Burkitt lymphoma biopsies and other lymphoproliferative malignancies. Int. J. Cancer **13**, 764–722 (1974)

Lynn. T. C., Tu, S. M., Hirayama, T., Kawamura, A. J.: Nasopharyngeal carcinoma and Epstein-Barr virus. I. Factors related to the anti-VCA antibody. Jap. J. Exp. Med. **43**, 121–123 (1973 a)

Lynn. T. C., Tu, S. M., Hirayama, T. Kawamura, A. J.: Nasopharyngeal carcinoma and Epstein-Barr virus. II. Clinical course and the anti-VCA antibody. Jap. J. Exp. Med. **43**, 135–144 (1973b)

Mayyasi, S. A., Schidlovsky, G., Bulfone, L. M., Buscheck, F. T.: The coating reaction of the herpes-type virus isolated from malignant tissues with antibody present in sera. Cancer Res. **27**, 2020–2024 (1967)

Moore, G., Grace, J. T. (Jr.), Citron, P., Gerner, R., Barns, A.: Leukocyte cultures of patients with leukemia and lymphomas. NY State J. Med. **66**, 2757–2764 (1966)

Moore, G. E., Gerner, R. E., Franklin, H. A.: Culture of normal human leukocytes. J. Am. Med. Assoc. **199**, 519–524 (1967)

Niederman, J. C., McCollum, R. W., Henle, G., Henle, W.: Infections mononucleosis. J. Am. Med. Assoc. **203**, 139–143 (1968)

Niederman, J. C., Evans, A. S., Subramanyan, M. S., McCollum, R. W.: Prevalance, incidence and persistence of EB virus antibody in young adults. N. Eng. J. Med. **282**, 361–365 (1970)

Nilsson, K., Klein, G., Henle, W., Henle, G.: The establishment of lymphoblastoid lines from adult and foetal human lymphoid tissue and its dependence on EBV. Int. J. Cancer **8**, 443–450 (1971)

Nkrumah, F., Henle, W., Henle, G., Herberman, R., Perkins, V., Depue, R.: Burkitt's lymphoma: its clinical course in relation to immunologic reactivities to Epstein-Barr virus and tumor related antigens. J. Natl. Cancer Inst. **57**, 1051–1056 (1976)

Nonoyama, M., Huang, C. H., Pagano, J. S., Klein, G., Singh, S.: DNA of Epstein-Barr virus detected in tissues of Burkitt's lymphoma and nasopharyngeal carcinoma. Proc. Natl. Acad. Sci. USA **70**, 3265–3268 (1973)

Old, L. J., Boyse, E. A., Oettgen, H. F., de Harven, E., Geering, G., Williamson, B., Clifford, P.: Precipitating antibody in human serum to an antigen present in cultured Burkitt's lymphoma cells. Proc. Natl. Acad. Sci. USA **56**, 1699–1704 (1966)

Old, L. J., Boyse, E. A., Geering, G., Oettgen, H. F.: Serologic approaches to the study of cancer in animals and man. Cancer Res. **28**, 1288–1299 (1968)

Pagano, J. S., Huang, C. H., Levine, P. H.: Absence of Epstein-Barr viral DNA in American Burkitt's lymphoma. N. Engl. J. Med. **289**, 1395–1399 (1973)

Pearson, G. R., Orr, T. W.: Antibody-dependent lymphocyte cytocotixity against cells expressing Epstein-Barr virus antigens. J. Natl. Cancer Inst. **56**, 485–488 (1976)

Pope, J. H.: Establishment of cell lines from peripheral leukocytes in infectious mononucleosis. Nature **216**, 810–811 (1967)

Porter, D. D., Wimberly, I., Benyesh-Melnick, M.: Prevalence of antibodies to EB virus and other herpesviruses. J. Am. Med. Assoc. **208**, 1675–1679 (1969)

Rothfield, N. F., Evans, A. S., Niederman, J. C.: Clinical and laboratory aspects of raised viral antibody titers in systemic lupus erythematosus. Ann. Rheum. Dis. **32**, 238–246 (1973)

Sawyer, R. N., Evans, A. S., Niederman, J. C., McCollum, R. W.: Prospective studies of a group of Yale University freshmen. I. Occurrence of infectious mononucleosis. J. Infect. Dis. **123**, 263–270 (1971)

Schmitz, H., Krainick-Riechert, C., Scherer, M.: Acute Epstein-Barr virus infections in children. Med. Microbiol. Immunol. **158**, 58–63 (1972)

Tischendorf, P., Shramek, G. J., Balagdas, R. C., Deinhardt, F., Knospe, W. H., Noble, G. R., Maynard, J. E.: Development and persistance of immunity to Epstein-Barr virus in man. J. Infect. Dis. **122**, 401–409 (1970)

University Health Physicians and PHLS Laboratories: Infectious mononucleosis and its relation to EB virus antibody. Br. Med. J. **1971 IV**, 643–646

Wahren, B., Carlens, E., Espmark, A., Lundbeck, H., Lofgren, S., Madar, E., Henle, G., Henle, W.: Antibodies to various herpes viruses in sera from patients with sarcoidosis. J. Natl. Cancer Inst. **47**, 747–756 (1971)

Wolf, H., zur Hausen, H., Becker, V.: EB viral genomes in epithelial nasopharyngeal carcinoma cells. Nature **244**, 245–247 (1973)

Wolf, H., zur Hausen, H., Klein, G., Becker, V., Henle, G., Henle, W.: Attempts to detect virus-specific DNA sequences in human tumors. III. Epstein-Barr viral DNA in non-lymphoid nasopharyngeal carcinoma cells. Med. Microbiol. Immunol. **161**, 15–21 (1975)

Zeve, V. H., Lucas, L. S., Manaker, R. A.: Continuous cell culture from a patient with chronic myelogenous leukemia. II. Detection of a herpes-like virus by electron microscopy. J. Natl. Cancer Inst. **37**, 761–773 (1966)

Ziegler, J. L., Andersson, M., Klein, G., Henle, W.: Detection of Epstein-Barr virus DNA in American Burkitt's lymphoma. Int. J. Cancer **17**, 701–706 (1976)

zur Hausen, H., Henle, W., Hummeler, K., Diehl, V., Henle, G.: Comparative study of cultured Burkitt tumor cells by immunofluorescence, autoradiography and electron microscopy. J. Virol. **1**, 830–837 (1967)

zur Hausen, H., Schulte-Holthausen, H., Klein, G., Henle, W., Henle, G., Clifford, P., Santesson, L.: EB-virus DNA in biopsies of Burkitt tumors and anaplastic carcinomas of the nasopharynx. Nature **228**, 1056–1058 (1970)

5 Biochemistry of the Virus and Its Effects on the Metabolism of Infected Cells[1]

Y. Becker[2]

Laboratory for Molecular Virology, The Hebrew University, Hadassah Medical School, P.O.B. 1172, Jerusalem (Israel)

---

[1] The studies on EBV in the author's laboratory were supported by a grant from the Leukemia Foundation Inc., Chicago, ILL., by contract No. NO1-CP-3-3310 with the Virus Cancer Program of the National Cancer Institute Bethesda, MD. and a grant from the Israel Cancer Association.

[2] The continous collaboration and discussions with Prof. George Klein are gratefully acknowledged. I wish to thank Dr. Julia Hadar for assistance with the manuscript and Mr. F. Marvine from the N.I.H. library Bethesda, MD, for his help with the bibliographic citations.

A. INTRODUCTION: B LYMPHOCYTES, THE NATURAL HOST OF EBV

Epstein-Barr virus (EBV) was originally found in lymphoblasts cultured from tumor biopsies of patients with Burkitt's lymphoma (BL) (Epstein and Barr, 1964; Epstein et al., 1964 a). Studies during the past 15 years have extended our knowledge of the relationship between EBV and lymphoblastoid[1] cells and established the fact that only B lymphocytes (bone marrow-derived lymphocytes) are the natural host of the virus. The lack of a permissive cell type in which EBV could replicate freely has hampered efforts to investigate the properties of this virus. No mutants could be obtained to assist in elucidating biochemical events in the virus-replication cycle, and the information available on the biochemistry of EBV and the molecular analysis of the virus components derives from studies on EB virions released from virus-producing cell lines. In some cell lines (e. g., P_3HR-1 and B95-8) the synthesis of EBV occurs spontaneously in a small percentage of the cells, while in other cell lines the synthesis of EBV requires induction. Many studies on EBV-containing lymphoblastoid cell lines provided information on the molecular process involved in virus replication as well as on control mechanisms that determine the relationship between the virus and the cell. It was realized that in most cells EBV DNA is in a latent form.

Cultivation in vitro of lymphoblastoid cells derived from tumor biopsies from patients with BL (Epstein and Barr, 1964; Epstein et al., 1964 a, b) opened the way for the study of a herpesvirus in human cancer. Epstein et al. (1964 a, b, 1965) noted the presence of herpes-like (EB) virus particles in a few cells with the morphology of dying cells. Electron microscope studies revealed that these herpesvirus particles were present in the nuclei of the lymphoblastoid cells in immature forms, while mature virions were found in the cytoplasm. Immunologic studies showed that antibodies to known herpesviruses failed to react in immunofluorescence tests with BL lymphoblasts containing EBV (Henle and Henle, 1966 a, b) while antibodies made against EBV which reacted with the virus-containing lymphoblastoid cells did not react with cells infected with known herpesviruses (Epstein and Achong, 1968).

These studies established the fact that EBV is a new herpesvirus carried in human lymphoblastoid cells. The early observations on the behavior of EBV in BL lymphoblasts suggested that the virus makes its appearance when the metabolic processes of the cells deviate from the normal and thus that the viral genetic information may be controlled by the host cell, which is capable of unrestricted growth in vitro (Epstein and Barr, 1964). A change in this control mechanism, perhaps associated with the approach of cell death, may be responsible for the appearance of the EBV particles as originally observed by Epstein et al. (1964 a, b, 1965). Since only a small percentage of BL-derived lymphoblasts produce virus particles, it was necessary to determine if there is viral genetic information in all the cell lines from BL established in vitro and if the tumor cells in biopsy samples from BL tumors contain EBV genetic information. The EBV genome was found to be double-stranded DNA with a molecular weight of 100×10^6 daltons (Weinberg and Becker, 1969; zur Hausen and Schulte-Holthausen, 1970; Nonoyama and Pagano, 1971) and has indeed been shown to be present in the cells of almost all BL-derived lines and in the tumor cells of almost all BL (Chaps. 3, 6, 7, and 14). The aim of the present analysis is to understand the biochemical processes involved in the interaction of EBV with the host cell.

---

[1] In this chapter "lymphoblastoid" is applied to cell lines of both lymphoma and nonmalignant origin – c. f. Chap. 11.

B. MOLECULAR COMPOSITION OF EB VIRIONS

The presence of EBV DNA in most of the lymphoblastoid cell lines derived from BL tumors or B lymphocytes from peripheral blood of normal donors indicated that a special relationship exists between the viral DNA and the host cell (Klein, 1973). However, the major difficulty experienced in all laboratories working with the virus was that EB virions could be found in only a few cells (up to 5% – 7%) in each culture, and most of the available information on the molecular, antigenic, and biologic properties of EBV stems from virus preparations derived from two cell lines which produce slightly more than the usual low quantities of EBV. The search for cell lines which produce larger amounts of EB virions led to the discovery that B95-8 marmoset cells, transformed in vitro by EBV derived from infectious mononucleosis (IM) (Miller et al., 1972) are good virus producers. For the same reason the P_3HR-1 line, which was selected after a crisis of cell death in the original cell culture (E. Kieff, personal communication), can also be used as a good source of virus. The reason for the increased production of EBV, which is nonetheless much lower than that in other herpesvirus-cell systems, is not well understood.

I. ISOLATION AND PURIFICATION OF EB VIRIONS

1. Isolation by Centrifugation in Sucrose Gradients

Because of the small amounts of virus made naturally by spontaneous synthesis, it was found necessary to develop techniques for inducing more cells to produce EBV.

EB virions were isolated by Weinberg and Becker (1969) from the EB3 cell line from an African BL and from the GOR cell line from a New Guinea patient with BL. In this study the virus particles were isolated from lymphoid cells incubated in an arginine-deficient culture medium. Such treatment was found to cause a marked increase in the number of cells that produce EBV antigens (Henle and Henle, 1968). However, the arginine-deficiency effect is limited to the EB3 cell line, suggesting that different lymphoblastoid lines differ markedly in their biochemical control mechanisms. After incubation of EB3 cells in an arginine-deficient medium, the virus particles were released by resuspending the cells in a buffer containing the detergent Nonidet P-40 (Weinberg and Becker, 1969). The cells were centrifuged to remove the nuclei, which are not dissolved by the detergent, and the cytoplasmic fraction was centrifuged in sucrose gradients under conditions developed for isolating herpes simplex virus (HSV). The EBV-particle band could be seen in the sucrose gradient. In addition, the lymphoblastoid cells were labeled with either ^{3}H-thymidine or radioactive amino acids during the 5-day incubation period in arginine-deficient medium. This made it possible to isolate labeled EBV particles for further analyses of EBV DNA and viral proteins.

Centrifugation of EBV in sucrose gradients after pelleting of virions released into the culture medium has also been used by Minowada et al. (1969), Schulte-Holthausen and zur Hausen (1970), Adams (1973), and Pritchett et al. (1975 a, b). Adams (1973) used a polyethylene glycol concentration step to decrease the volume of the culture fluid prior to pelleting the virus particles. These EBV particles were then used for further biochemical analyses. It should be indicated, however, that velocity centrifugation of herpes virions in sucrose gradients yields a virus preparation contaminated with membranes and other cellular debris. To separate the cellular debris and virus particles isolated from sucrose gradients it is necessary to apply density centrifugation in a second sucrose gradient, but in view of the small yields of EB virions this density centrifugation step is seldom used.

2. Characterization of the Isolated Virus Particles

Negative staining of the isolated virus revealed, through electron microscopy, particles with herpesvirus morphology (Weinberg and Becker, 1969). The enveloped virus particles had a diameter of 150 μm and the diameter of the nucleocapsid was 75 μm. Further characterization was obtained from the analyses of the viral DNA and proteins.

II. EBV DNA

1. Molecular Weight and Size of EBV DNA

EBV DNA was extracted from virions under conditions developed for the isolation of intact HSV 1 DNA (Becker et al., 1968). The EBV DNA, labeled with ^{3}H-thymidine.

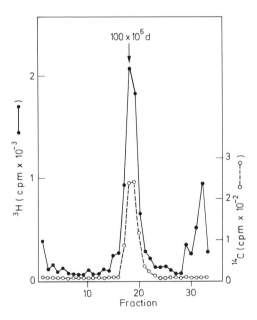

Fig. 1. Size of EBV DNA. EBV DNA was isolated from virus particles in the medium of B95-8 cells as described by Pritchett et al. (1975a). After centrifugation in 12%–52% (w/v) linear sucrose gradients at 20,000 rpm for 60 min in the SW 27 rotor of the Beckman ultracentrifuge at 4°C, the virus bands were collected, diluted in 0.025 M Tris HCl, pH 7.6, and treated with a final concentration of 5% (w/v) N-lauryl sarcosine at 63°C for 5 min. The DNA released from the virus particles was layered onto 5%–20% (w/w) sucrose gradients prepared in 0.01 M Tris HCl, pH7.8, 0.001 M EDTA, and 1.0M NaCl and centrifuged at 37,000 rpm for 2 h at 20°C in the SW41 Beckman rotor. The gradients were collected dropwise, and the trichloroacetic acid (TCA) precipitable radioactivity was determined in each fraction

was centrifuged in a sucrose gradient with HSV DNA as marker (Fig. 1) and was found to have a molecular weight of 100×10^6 daltons (Weinberg and Becker, 1969). Pritchett et al. (1975 a, b) estimated the molecular weight of EBV DNA to be $101 \pm 3 \times 10^6$ daltons, also based on centrifugation of EBV DNA in sucrose gradients. In addition, the molecular weight of EBV DNA can be determined after measurement of the contour length of the DNA molecules. Such molecules isolated from EB virions were found to have a linear conformation and a contour length of 52 ± 3 μm (Fig. 2) (Y. Becker and A. Friedmann, unpublished results). A similar value for EB virions isolated from P_3HR-1 cells (16.5 ± 0.3 times PM2 phage DNA) was reported by Pritchett et al. (1975 a, b), yielding a molecular weight of $105 \pm 3 \times 10^6$ daltons.

2. Alkali Effects on EBV DNA

Treatment of EBV DNA with alkali followed by centrifugation in a sucrose gradient led to the isolation of less than 50% of the denatured viral DNA as a band of intact single strands with a molecular weight of 50×10^6 daltons (Pritchett et al., 1975 a, b). This limited result apparently depends on the extent of nicks in the viral DNA, since in another study (Y. Becker, unpublished results) all the EBV DNA isolated from virions from P_3HR-1 cells banded as denatured intact DNA strands in an alkaline sucrose gradient.

3. Density of EBV DNA

Equilibrium centrifugation in CsCl density gradients of EBV DNA extracted from virus particles showed that the density of the viral DNA is 1.718 g/ml (Weinberg and Becker, 1969; Schulte-Holthausen and zur Hausen, 1970; Pritchett et al., 1975 b). The density of EBV DNA indicates a guanine + cytosine content of 58% in the molecule. Superinfection of Raji cells with EBV isolated from P_3HR-1 cells also resulted in the synthesis of EBV DNA with a density of 1.718 g/ml (Tanaka et al., 1976 a).

4. Organization of EBV DNA

The internal organization of herpesvirus DNA can be determined by annealing the intact single-stranded DNA molecules by the method of Sheldrick and Berthelot (1974). This self-annealing of the DNA can be visualized by electron microscopy, thus making possible the demonstration of inverted repeat sequences in the viral DNA. Electron microscope studies to determine the internal organization of EBV DNA have not yet been reported, and present information on the organization of the viral DNA is based on shear fragmentation or restriction enzyme cleavage.

a) Shear Products of Viral DNA

Shearing of EBV DNA into small DNA fragments followed by centrifugation in CsCl density gradients could provide information on the presence of sequences in the viral DNA that differ in their base composition. Pritchett et al. (1975 b) demonstrated that

Fig. 2. Electron micrograph of intact EBV DNA genome from B95-8 cells. DNA molecules isolated from virions as described in Fig. 1 were centrifuged in CsCl gradients. CsCl crystals were added to a final density of 1.70 g/ml and the tubes were centrifuged at 35,000 rpm at 20 C for 48 h in the R50 Ti rotor of the Beckman ultracentrifuge. DNA molecules from the 1.716 g/ml density region of the gradient were examined by electron microscopy as described by Shlomai et al. (1976a). The bar measures 1 μm

shearing in EBV DNA isolated from virions that were produced by B95-8 cells results in a major band of DNA fragments with a density of 1.716–1.717 g/ml (about 75% of the viral DNA) and a minor band (about 25% of the DNA) with a density of 1.720 g/ml in CsCl gradients. This finding suggests that there are EBV DNA sequences with a $G+C$ content higher than the average $G+C$ content found for the EBV genome as a whole. By analogy with HSV DNA it may be reasonable to suggest that the high $G+C$ sequences represent the inverted repeat sequences of EBV DNA.

b) Restriction Endonuclease Fragments

Fragmentation of EBV DNA with *Escherichia coli* RI endonuclease yielded 12 fragments greater than 10^6 daltons with virus preparations from P_3HR-1 cells and 11 such fragments with those from B95-8 cells. The largest fragments are present in less than 1 mole per mole of viral DNA, while other fragments are present in greater than molar quantities. This suggests the presence of repeat sequences in EBV DNA (Sugden et al., 1976). Hayward and Kieff (1977) treated EBV DNA from virions obtained from B95-8 cells with a number of endonucleases *(E. coli* RI, *Hemophilus suis* I, *Streptomyces albus* I, *Klebsiella pneumoniae* I) and analyzed the DNA fragments by electrophoresis in agarose gels. Fragments with molecular weights ranging from $1–3 \times 10^6$ daltons were obtained. Treatment of EBV DNA with lambda exonuclease prior to treatment with the restriction enzymes resulted in degradation of the DNA near the two molecular ends and the loss of two restriction fragments. The total sum of the molecular weights of the fragments was found to exceed 100×10^6 daltons, the molecular weight of the EBV genome. It is thus possible to assume that EBV DNA has two populations of DNA molecules which differ in the internal arrangement of the sequences, similar perhaps to those of HSV DNA.

5. Differences in the Organization of EBV DNA from Different Virus Strains

Using a hybridization technique, Pritchett et al. (1975 a, b) demonstrated that EBV DNA from virions originating in B95-8 cells of marmoset origin lack 15% of the sequences present in EBV DNA from P_3HR-1 (human-derived) cells. Sugden et al. (1976) reported that the DNA from the two strains of EBV share approximately 90% of their nucleotide sequences and that both DNAs contain repetitions of some of their nucleotide sequences. Comparison of the restriction fragments of EBV DNA from the two above-mentioned sources also revealed differences in the preparations (Hayward and Kieff, 1977).

Kieff and Levine (1974) reported that EBV DNA present in lymphoblastoid cells from patients with IM had 90% homology and 97% matching base pairs with EBV DNA from BL-derived lymphoblasts.

III. EB VIRION PROTEINS AND ANTIGENS

1. Electrophoresis of Viral Proteins in Polyacrylamide Gels

Isolation of partly purified EB virions labeled with radioactive amino acids made possible the analysis of the viral structural proteins. Initial studies with ^{3}H-leucine and

[14]C-arginine-labeled EBV derived from the EB3 cell line after incubation in arginine-deficient medium, revealed a peptide pattern in sodium dodecylsulfate (SDS) polyacrylamide gels similar to that obtained with the major viral peptides of HSV. The major peptide of the nucleocapsids was the viral capsid protein with a molecular weight of ~ 160,000 and six additional viral peptides (Weinberg and Becker, 1969). More detailed studies by Dolyniuk et al. (1976 a, b) revealed 18 polypeptide bands when the gels were stained with Coomassie blue, while 33 bands were resolved in fluorograms of labeled EBV purified from B95-8 cells that were subjected to electrophoresis in acrylamide gels and cross-linked with diallytartarimide. These EBV polypeptides had molecular weights similar to those of the structural peptides of HSV. The nucleocapsids were found to be composed of seven polypeptides with molecular weights ranging from $28-200 \times 10^3$. Twelve polypeptides were found to be glycoproteins.

2. Virion-Associated Antigens

The viral capsid antigen (VCA) is detected in the cytoplasm and nuclei of EBV-producing cells when certain human sera are used in direct or indirect immunofluorescence tests (Henle and Henle, 1966 a) (Chaps. 3 and 4), but antibodies to the different virion polypeptides have not yet been reported. Thus either VCA itself or the complex virion structure leads to the production of antibodies in humans infected with EBV.

C. BIOCHEMICAL CONSIDERATION OF THE RESIDENT EBV DNA IN LYMPHOBLASTOID CELLS

Multiple copies of EBV DNA occur in lymphoblastoid cells derived from BL tumors. Some of these genomes are involved in replication of EBV DNA in cells producing EB virions. In nonproducer cell lines, the multiple copies of EBV DNA are transferred to the daughter cells at the same level as present in the parental cells. It is therefore necessary to define the state of EBV DNA in the lymphoblastoid cells so as to assess the role of these viral DNA genomes in the biochemical events occurring in the cells.

I. STATE OF EBV DNA IN CELL NUCLEI

1. EBV DNA Covalently Linked to Chromosal DNA

Raji cells, which contain about 40 viral DNA genomes and do not produce EB virions even after treatment with inducers, were used to study the state of EBV DNA in nonproducer cells. Adams et al. (1973) and Adams and Lindahl (1975 a) (Chap. 8) reported that a large proportion of the intrinsic EBV DNA remains in association with cellular DNA. DNA isolated from the nuclei was centrifuged in CsCl density gradients and the position of the EBV DNA was detected by hybridization with radioactive RNA complementary to EBV DNA (cRNA); EBV DNA was found to band with the cellular DNA fraction, which is rich in dA + dT. Alkali treatment of cellular DNA released the EBV DNA. Similary it was shown by Becker et al. (1974, 1975b) that EBV DNA sequences are covalently integrated with the chromosomal DNA of Raji cells. It was suggested (Becker et al., 1974, 1975b) that fragments of EBV DNA are integrated into the chromosomal DNA, since shear products of Raji chromosomal DNA yielded DNA fragments with a density (1.710 g/ml) intermediate between that of the host cell (1.700 g/ml) and the viral EBV DNA (1.718 g/ml).

2. Episomal EBV DNA in Cell Nuclei

Nonoyama and Pagano (1972a) demonstrated that treatment of Raji cell chromosomal DNA with alkali followed by centrifugation in an alkaline sucrose gradient resulted in the separation of EBV DNA genomes from the bulk of the chromosomal DNA. In this respect the result of alkali treatment reported by Adams et al. (1973) agreed with that of Nonoyama and Pagano (1972a). However, alkali treatment may cause dissociation of EBV DNA from cellular chromosomal DNA if the former is covalently linked to the cellular DNA by alkali-sensitive phosphodiester bonds. In a subsequent study, Tanaka and Nonoyama (1975) demonstrated that EBV DNA present in Raji cells can be separated from the chromosomal DNA after treatment with 1% sarkosyl, EDTA, and pronase for 12 h at 37°C. The EBV DNA had a sedimentation coefficient of 55 S and a density of 1.717–1.718 g/ml. These experiments indicated that most of the EBV DNA present in Raji cells is situated in the nuclei as episomal DNA.

Sedimentation analysis of Raji cell DNA in neutral glycerol gradients followed by hybridization with EBV-specific labeled cRNA was reported by Adams and Lindahl (1975b), who found two distinct species of EBV DNA with sedimentation coefficients of 65 S and 100 S – higher than that of the linear EBV DNA isolated from EB virions (Chap. 8). This indicated that the nonintegrated episomal DNA molecules are circular, nicked (65 S), or supercoiled (100 S) molecules. The circular shape of the EBV DNA genomes was substantiated by direct electron microscopy of EBV DNA (Lindahl et al., 1976). In ethidium bromide CsCl density gradient centrifugation experiments, the episomal EBV DNA behaved like twisted covalently closed circular DNA molecules, and similar circular DNA molecules were isolated from tumor biopsies of BL and nasopharyngeal carcinoma (NPC) cells grown in athymic nude mice (Kaschka-Dierich et al., 1976).

These studies established that cells (like Raji) which are unable to produce EB virions contain EBV DNA genomes in the nuclei in the form of episomal viral DNA with a circular conformation and a contour length of $\sim$ 53 µm, corresponding to an average molecular weight of 106×10^6 daltons. Such circular EBV DNA molecules were not detected in BJAB-1 cells, which do not contain detectable amounts of EBV DNA or detectable EBV nuclear antigen (EBNA) (Lindahl et al., 1976). Nonintegrated EBV DNA genomes were detected in P_3HR-1 cells by electrophoresis of the nuclear DNA in polyacrylamide gels (Becker et al., 1975b).

3. Removal of Episomal EBV DNA by Cycloheximide Treatment

The presence of 50–60 EBV DNA genomes in Raji cells as circular episomal DNA led to the question of their role in transformation and maintenance of the transformed state of the lymphoblastoid cell. It is possible to postulate that the episomal EBV DNA molecules are latent viral genomes residing in the nuclei after infection of the cell but different from the EBV DNA associated with or integrated into the chromosomal DNA of the host cell. The episomal EBV DNA genomes are controlled by the host cell and only a limited amount of information is transcribed from them, possibly enough to code for the EBNA present in EBV DNA-positive cells.

An indication that episomal EBV DNA is not essential for the transformed lymphoblastoid cell has been provided by Tanaka et al. (1976 b) using P_3HR-1 cells treated with cycloheximide; such cells contain only one EBV DNA genome yet retain their transformed properties, suggesting that the episomal EBV DNA may not be essential for the transformation event and may indeed represent EBV genomes trapped in the cells and suppressed by them.

II. TRANSCRIPTION OF EBV DNA IN LYMPHOBLASTOID CELLS

1. EBV Transcripts in Lymphoblastoid Cells

Hybridization of whole-cell RNA with denatured ^{3}H-EBV DNA has been used to determine the EBV-coded RNA transcripts in virus-producing and nonproducing lymphoblastoid cells. Pritchett et al. (1975 a, b) demonstrated that in virus-producing cells (P_3HR-1 and B95-8) about 50% of the viral DNA sequences are transcribed, i. e., all the viral genetic information is expressed in these cells. Moderate amounts of EBV-specific RNA are produced in the nonproducer Namalwa and Kurgans lines where only 3% of the EBV DNA was transcribed (Hayward and Kieff, 1976).

2. RNA Polymerase II in Cells

Studies on the transcription of HSV DNA in lytically infected cells (Ben-Zeev et al., 1976; Ben-Zeev and Becker, 1977) revealed that the host-cell RNA polymerase II is responsible for the transcription of HSV DNA. This is also probably the case with the transcription of EBV DNA in lymphoblastoid cells superinfected with EBV (Yocum and Strominger, 1975). Lymphoblastoid cells have been shown to contain RNA polymerase II activity, which can be isolated by chromatography on DEAE-cellulose columns (Fig. 3) (Y. Becker, unpublished results). Synthesis of mRNA by the RNA polymerase II in lymphoblastoid cells is illustrated in Fig. 4. Most of the RNA synthesized in nuclei from Raji, P_3HR-1, and B95-8 cells was inhibited by 100 µg/ml of α-amanitin, which does not affect RNA polymerase I activity.

D. BIOCHEMICAL EVENTS LEADING TO THE RELEASE OF EBV DNA FROM CONTROL OF HOST-CELL MECHANISMS

The viral genomes in nuclei of cells that do not produce EBV are latent, and only 3% of the viral DNA sequences are transcribed (Hayward and Kieff, 1976). Since the number of viral genome equivalents per cell remains unchanged over many cell generations, it

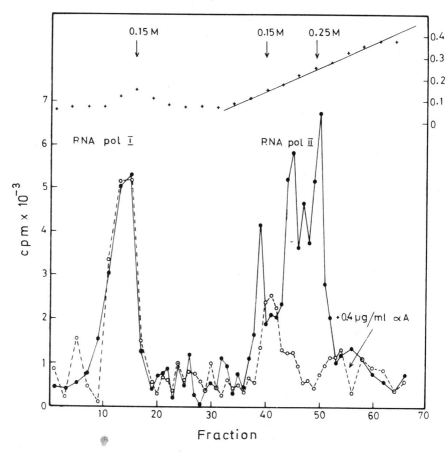

Fig. 3. RNA polymerases in B95-8 cells. 2×10^9 cells were washed and suspended in buffer A (50 mM Tris HCl pH 8.0, 0.5 mM dithiothreitol, 25% [v/v] glycerol 5 mM MgCl$_2$, 0.1 mM EDTA) containing 0.5 mM phenylmethylsulfonylfluoride (PMSF; Sigma, St. Louis, MO). Ammonium sulfate (4 M; pH 7.9) was added to a final concentration of 0.3 M. After sonication 7 times for 10-s periods at 4°C, the mixture was diluted with two volumes of buffer A containing 0.5 mM PMSF to bring the ammonium sulfate concentration to 0.1 M. The aggregated chromatin and ribosomes were removed by centrifugation at 45,000 rpm for 60 min in the SW 50.1 Beckman rotor at 4°C. The supernatant fluid containing the enzymatic activity was chromatographed on a DEAE cellulose column using buffer A containing 0.3 M ammonium sulfate. The eluate containing 1 mg/ml bovine serum albumin (buffer B) was dialysed against buffer A without MgCl$_2$ to a final concentration of 0.15 M ammonium sulfate. After centrifugation at 45,000 rpm for 60 min in the SW 50.1 rotor, the supernatant fluid was chromatographed on a DEAE Sephadex A-25 column (0.9 × 23 cm), equilibrated at 4°C with buffer B containing 0.15 M ammonium sulfate. Stepwise elution with 0.15 M ammonium sulfate in buffer B was followed by gradient elution with 0.15–0.5 M ammonium sulfate; 1-ml fractions were collected. The activity in a 50 µl sample from each fraction was determined by addition of 50 µl of a reaction mixture containing 0.8 mM each of ATP, GTP, and CTP, 0.06 mM UTP, 10 µCi of ^{3}H-UTP, 2 mM MnCl$_2$, 4 mM dithiothreitol, 40 µg native calf thymus DNA, 10 mM MgCl$_2$, and 50 mM Tris HCl pH 8.0. The reaction was carried out with or without 20 µg/ml of α-amanitin at 37°C for 30 min, and the TCA precipitable radioactivity was determined. The ammonium sulfate concentration in each fraction was determined by conductivity measurements with a CDM 3 radiometer

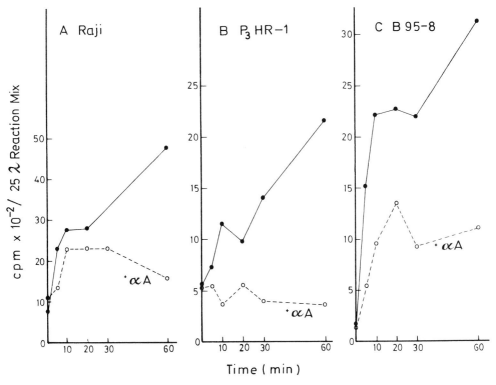

Fig. 4. In vitro RNA synthesis in nuclei from Raji **(A)**, P_3HR-1 **(B)**, and B-95-8 **(C)** cells. Nuclei from 10^7 cells were obtained by Dounce homogenization. Each 100 μl of the reaction mixture contained 12.5 mM KCl, 5 mM $MgCl_2$, 1 mM $MnCl_2$, 8% (w/v) sucrose (RNase free), 100 mM ammonium sulfate, 0.1 mM dithiothreitol, 0.4 mM each of ATP, CTP, GTP, and 12.5 μCi of ^{3}H-UTP in 50 mM Tris HCl, pH 8.0. The reaction mixture was incubated at 31° C in the absence or presence of 100 μg/ml of α-amanitin. The reaction was stopped after different time intervals by the addition of TCA, and the radioactivity was determined

may be concluded that the lymphoblastoid cells have biochemical control over EBV DNA genomes and that only when some biochemical change occurs in cells like B95-8 and P_3HR-1, spontaneous production of EB virions takes place in 10%–15% of the cells. The biochemical mechanisms involved in the control of EBV DNA may possibly be resolved by studying the process involved in the induction of EBV.

I. INDUCTION OF EBV DNA REPLICATION IN ARGININE-DEPRIVED CELLS

1. The Phenomenon

Henle and Henle (1968) noted that prolonged incubation of BL-derived lymphoblas-toid cells at 37 °C resulted in the induction of EBV antigens in 75% of all the cells, and analysis of the used medium revealed that arginine was completely depleted. Not surprisingly, culture of the same cell lines in medium lacking arginine resulted in the induction of EBV antigens, and EBV particles have in fact been concentrated from arginine-deprived EB3 cells (Weinberg and Becker, 1969). Thus, arginine deprivation markedly changed the cell metabolism, leading to activation of viral function in a majority of the cells (Henle and Henle, 1968). It should be noted that arginine deprivation of lymphoblastoid cells causes degradation of nuclear proteins, since cells prelabeled with ^{14}C-arginine before incubation in an arginine-deficient medium produced EB virions containing ^{14}C-arginine in the viral structural proteins. Arginine deprivation of cells is effective during the initial incubation period, and the initial 6 h of arginine deprivation are critical for the induction of EBV synthesis.

2. Effect of Arginine Deprivation on Macromolecular Processes in Cells

To determine if arginine deprivation has a specific effect, EB3 cells were incubated in media from which one essential amino acid was removed (Weinberg and Becker, 1970). It was found that in the absence of certain essential amino acids (except arginine) the synthesis of cellular DNA, RNA, and proteins was completely inhibited. It should be indicated that in lymphoblastoid cells, cellular DNA synthesis (the S phase of the cell cycle) is followed by protein and RNA synthesis (the G_2 phase) and cell division. However, when incubated in arginine-deficient medium, cellular DNA synthesis was slightly reduced, whereas the synthesis of cellular RNA and proteins was markedly reduced (Weinberg and Becker, 1970; Becker and Weinberg, 1971, 1972a). Thus, the synthesis of cellular DNA during the S phase does occur in arginine-deprived EB3 cells, but the synthesis of cellular RNA and proteins required for the control of cellular functions is inhibited.

3. Time Course of EBV DNA Synthesis

Centrifugation of the DNA extracted from arginine-deprived cells labeled with ^{3}H-thymidine for different time intervals in CsCl density gradients revealed that EBV DNA with a density of 1.719 g/ml was synthesized in these cells. The EBV DNA was synthesized during the initial 20 h period after incubation in arginine-deficient medium, at the same time as most of the cellular DNA was being synthesized (Becker and Weinberg, 1971). Treatment of arginine-deprived EB3 cells with distamycin A selectively inhibited the synthesis of EBV DNA (Becker and Weinberg, 1972b).

4. Arginine Deprivation: Inhibition of Cellular Protein Synthesis

Inhibition of cellular protein synthesis can change the control of cellular functions and allow the synthesis of EBV DNA, mRNA, and proteins specified by the viral DNA. Hampar et al. (1976) demonstrated that incubation of P_3HR-1 cells either in arginine-deficient medium or in the presence of cycloheximide or puromycin (potent inhibitors of protein synthesis) resulted in the induction of EBV antigens, but to be effective these treatments must be applied during the S phase of the cell cycle. In view of the marked effect that arginine deprivation has on the synthesis of cellular proteins, it is possible that it likewise affects the proteins involved in the regulation of EBV DNA, and if these are not synthesized the viral DNA can replicate.

5. Synthesis of EBV-Specific Proteins in Arginine-Deprived Cells

Inhibition of cellular proteins was found not to prevent the synthesis of viral structural proteins, since analysis of the proteins synthesized in arginine-deprived EB3 cells revealed polypeptides resembling the EBV proteins present in purified virions (Becker and Weinberg, 1971, 1972 a). Furthermore, Hampar et al. (1976) reported that 6.5% of Raji cells express only early antigen (EA), while with P_3HR-1 cells, 5.3% produced EA and 4% produced VCA; however, when the two cell lines were treated with cycloheximide a similar pattern was seen but involving more cells.

II. INDUCTION OF EBV SYNTHESIS BY HALOGENATED PYRIMIDINES (IUDR, BUDR) (Chap. 12)

1. Induction of EBV Antigen Synthesis in Treated Cells

Treatment of lymphoblastoid cell lines (Raji, NC37, and NHDL3) with 5-bromodeoxyuridine (BUDR) resulted in the activation of virus synthesis (determined by immunofluorescence tests) in about 8% of the cells (Gerber, 1972; Long et al., 1974).

2. Synthesis of EBV DNA in Cells Made Resistant to BUDR

P_3HR-1 (BU) cells, which can grow in the presence of 100 µg/ml of BUDR, lack thymidine kinase (Hampar et al., 1971, 1972 a). Under these conditions there is no synthesis of EBV DNA, proteins, or virions. However, in cells in which the synthesis of EBV DNA and viral antigens is induced, a virus-determined thymidine kinase can be detected, and the cells are capable of incorporating radioactive thymidine into both the cell and viral DNA (Hampar e al., 1971; Derge et al., 1975) as shown by radioautography. Only about 5% of the cell population could be labeled with the ^{3}H-thymidine, but extraction and analysis of the labeled DNA (Derge et al., 1975) showed that most of the DNA was EBV DNA.

3. A Critical Period During the S Phase of the Cell Cycle for EBV DNA Synthesis

Hampar et al. (1973) observed a peak of EBV activation about 1 h after initiation of cellular DNA synthesis, but the mechanism of this EBV activation by 5-iododeoxyuridine (IUDR) or BUDR is not yet fully understood.

4. Programming of Viral Events in Cells Treated with IUDR

The sequence of molecular events was studied in Raji and EB3 cells after treatment with IUDR, which was added for 60 min during the S-1 phase of the cell cycle. In activated Raji cells, only EA was detectable, while in activated EB3 cells VCA was also synthesized. Synthesis of VCA occured 3–4 h after synthesis of EA and required synthesis of DNA for $\sim$ 60 min after EA synthesis (Hampar et al., 1974 a, b, c).

III. INDUCTION OF EBV BY TREATMENT WITH HYDROXYUREA, AN INHIBITOR OF DNA SYNTHESIS

Sequence of EBV Activation in the Presence of Hydroxyurea

Virus activation was followed by the synthesis of EA, which was followed by the appearance of hydroxyurea (HU)-resistant DNA, a result of the synthesis of thymidine kinase. The HU-resistant DNA was found to contain both EBV and cellular DNA, but the synthesis of viral antigens was only detectable in cells synthesizing DNA (Hampar et al., 1972 b).

IV.INDUCTION OF EBV IN CELL HYBRIDS TREATED WITH IUDR

Fusion of a transformed cell with another cell permissive for the original transforming virus results in activation of the transforming virus. This phenomenon was studied by Glaser and O'Neill (1972), who fused BL-derived cells to mouse and human cell lines with the help of inactivated Sendai virus; the resulting heterokaryons constituted somatic cell hybrids made up of the two parent cell types.

1. Rescue of EBV in Cell Hybrids

Treatment of the somatic cell hybrids mentioned above with IUDR resulted in the continous synthesis of EBV antigens (Glaser and O'Neill, 1972; Glaser et al., 1973 a). It was also reported that treatment of a hybrid cell line (P_3 HR-1/human sternal marrow) with IUDR induced both EBV-specific antigens and virus particles (Glaser and Rapp, 1972).

2. Synthesis of EBV DNA

Hybridization with EBV DNA or specific cRNA revealed the presence of varying amounts of EBV DNA equivalents in different lines of somatic hybrids. These viral DNA genomes are repressed by the somatic cell hybrids (Glaser and Nonoyama, 1973).

3. Synthesis of EBV Antigens

Treatment of somatic cell hybrids (Raji/D98 cells) with IUDR resulted in the synthesis of EA and VCA after synthesis of EBV DNA (Glaser and Nonoyama, 1974); thymidine kinase was also increased in the activated somatic cell hybrids (Glaser et al., 1973 b). EBNA has been detected in hybrids between FL cells (EBV-negative epithelial cells from human amnion) and BL-derived lymphoblastoid cells (Yamamoto et al., 1975/76). Addition of dibutyryl cyclic AMP to the medium of IUDR-treated hybrids increased the synthesis of EA and VCA (Zimmerman et al., 1973).

4. EBV DNA in Hybrid Cells

Andersson (1975) reported that the amounts of EBV DNA in the nuclei of somatic cell hybrids between human lymphoblastoid lines are higher than in the parental cell lines. No spontaneous induction of EBV was noted in these fused cell lines.

Analysis of the chromosomes of somatic cell hybrids obtained from EBV-positive BL cell lines (P_3HR-1) and mouse CLID cells suggested that EBV DNA is not associated with the human chromosomes present in the hybrid cells (Glaser et al., 1975).

E. BIOCHEMICAL ASPECTS OF EBV DNA REPLICATION AND TRANSCRIPTION

EBV DNA genomes are present in three different conformations in lymphoblastoid cells: (a) complete genomes or fragments covalently linked to the cell chromosomal DNA; (b) episomal EBV DNA genomes with a circular conformation in transformed cells that do not produce virus; and (c) linear EBV DNA molecules not associated with the cellular DNA, in cells that produce virus particles. The biosynthesis of either integrated or episomal EBV DNA genomes occurs during the S phase of the cell cycle, while linear EBV DNA synthesis is independent of the state of the induced cell. It would appear that both integrated and episomal EBV DNA depend for replication on the cellular enzymatic mechanisms. However, in cells that produce EB virions (either spontaneously or when induced by biochemical means), linear EBV DNA may be synthesized by virus-determined enzymes similar to those involved in the synthesis of genomes of other herpesviruses.

I. BIOSYNTHESIS OF THE RESIDENT EBV DNA IN NONPRODUCER LYMPHO-BLASTOID CELLS

1. DNA Polymerases Functioning During the S Phase of the Cell Cycle

Biosynthesis of EBV DNA genomes in Raji cells takes place during the S-1 phase of the cell cycle (Hampar et al., 1974 a, b, c). Recent studies on mammalian cells have revealed three major enzymes (DNA polymerases α, β, and γ) to be responsible for the synthesis of DNA, although the DNA polymerase that replicates the chromosomal DNA was not clearly defined. Twardzik et al. (1975) found three peaks of DNA polymerase activity in P_3HR-1 cell extracts, but only two, in Raji cell extracts where the DNA polymerase sedimenting faster than 10 S was missing. Further studies will define more clearly the mechanism of EBV DNA synthesis.

2. Nature of the Expected Replicative Intermediates of EBV DNA

Since episomal EBV DNA consists of supercoiled circular DNA molecules (Sect. C I 2 above and Chap. 8) it can be expected that the replicative intermediates of such DNA molecules are relaxed circular molecules containing a replicative loop. Such EBV DNA molecules have not yet been observed.

II. REPLICATION OF EBV DNA IN VIRUS-PRODUCING CELLS

It can be assumed that the replication of linear EBV DNA molecules in virus-producing cells is by a semiconservative process and the replicative intermediates may resemble those of HSV DNA (Shlomai et al., 1976 a, b). However, replicative intermediates of EBV DNA have not yet been reported.

1. Replication of EBV in Epithelial Cells from Patients with Infectious Mononucleosis

Lemon et al. (1977), utilizing EBV-specified cRNA of a high specific activity in an in situ cytohybridization test, reported that epithelial cells in the oropharynx of IM patients contain detectable amounts of EBV DNA. These results, suggesting that EBV can infect and replicate its DNA in epithelial cells of the oropharynx, obviously need confirmation.

2. Nature of the DNA Polymerase Responsible for the Replication of EBV DNA

Phosphonoacetic acid (PAA) has been found to inhibit selectively the HSV-specific DNA polymerase (Shipkowitz et al., 1973; Mao et al., 1975). Although PAA also partly inhibits the cellular DNA polymerase, it was established that in lytically infected cells, the replication of HSV DNA is completely inhibited by PAA (Becker et al., 1977). In the case of EBV it was found (Summers and Klein, 1976; Nyormoi et al., 1976) that the replication of the episomal EBV DNA in lymphoblastoid cells was not affected by PAA, while the synthesis of EBV DNA for virus production was inhibited. This indicated that episomal EBV DNA resident in lymphoblastoid cells is replicated by a cellular DNA polymerase which is resistant to PAA, while the semiconservative replication of linear forms of EBV DNA is effected by an EBV-specific DNA polymerase. The replication of linear EBV DNA in Raji cells superinfected with EBV is prevented by treatment with PAA (100 µg/ml) (Yajima et al., 1976) and by both PAA and N-ethylmaleimide (Seebeck et al., 1977).

    Preliminary reports (Ooka et al., 1978; Goodman and Benz, 1978) describe the isolation from P_3HR-1 and B95-8 virus-producing cell lines of DNA polymerase which is resistant to $(NH_4)_2SO_4$, sensitive to $2mM$ N-ethylmaleimide, and elutes from DEAE cellulose with $190-230$ mM potassium phosphate. Miller et al. (1977) showed that PAA inhibits expression of VCA, but has no effect on EA in epithelial/Burkitt hybrid cells induced with IUDR. They also demonstrated in these cells what is probably a new EBV-determined DNA polymerase with properties similar to other herpesvirus-specified DNA polymerases.

3. In Vitro Synthesis of EBV DNA in Nuclei from Lymphoblastoid Cells

Nuclei isolated from virus-producing BL lymphoblastoid cells can continue to synthesize nuclear DNA when incubated under in vitro conditions with the four deoxyribonucleoside triphosphates in the presence of ATP and an ATP-regenerating system (Benz and Strominger, 1975; Y. Becker, unpublished results). Analysis of the

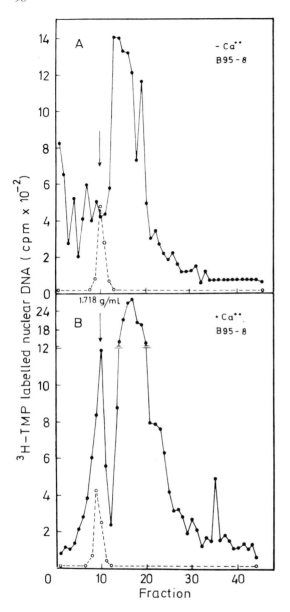

Fig. 5. CsCl gradient analysis of DNA molecules synthesized in vitro in nuclei of B95-8 cells prepared in the absence or presence of Ca$^+$. The cells were washed and fractionated in a glass Dounce homogenizer. The nuclei were washed twice in phosphate buffer (0.075 M potassium phosphate, pH 7.4, 8% (w/v) sucrose (RNase free); 1 mM dithiothreitol) without **(A)** or with **(B)** 0.5 mM CaCl$_2$, and resuspended at a concentration of 5×10^7 nuclei per 250 µl of phosphate buffer. To this was added the reaction mixture (final volume 650 µl) containing 8% (w/v) sucrose (RNase free), 6 mM MgCl$_2$, 1 mM dithiothreitol, 0.4 mM CaCl$_2$, 40 µmoles each of dATP, dGTP, dCTP, and 50 µCi of ^{3}H-TTP (specific activity 15 Ci/mole; The Radiochemical Centre, Amersham). The reaction mixture was incubated at 37°C for 30 min. The in vitro reaction was stopped by the addition of sodium dodecylsulfate (SDS) to a final concentration of 0.5% (w/w) and 20 × SSC was added to a final concentration of 1 × SSC (0.15 M NaCl; 0.015 M sodium citrate). The viscous solutions were treated with 0.3 mg/ml of pronase (free of nucleases, 90,000 units/mg, Calbiochem) for 4–5 h at 37°C. CsCl in 0.01 M Tris HCl, pH 7.5, 0.001 M EDTA was added to bring the density to 1.70 g/ml and the solutions were centrifuged in the R50 Ti rotor at 35,000 rpm for 48 h at 20° C in the Beckman ultracentrifuge as described by Shlomai et al. (1976b). DNA from virions of the HF strain of HSV 1, labeled with ^{14}C-thymidine were used as a marker (o----o)

nuclear DNA synthesized in vitro and extracted from B95-8 nuclei by centrifugation in CsCl density gradients revealed that in addition to the labeled cellular DNA, EBV DNA with a density of 1.718 g/ml was demonstrable (Fig. 5) (Y. Becker, unpublished results). Such DNA was not synthesized in nuclei isolated from nonproducer lymphoblastoid cells. In contrast, superinfected Raji cells did not require an ATP-regenerating system for the synthesis of EBV DNA in vitro (Seebeck et al., 1977).

III. TRANSCRIPTION OF EBV DNA IN VIRUS-PRODUCING CELLS

Certain genetic information encoded in EBV DNA must be fully expressed in cells permitting the synthesis of viral progeny. Indeed, Pritchett et al. (1975 b) and Hayward and Kieff (1976) reported that at least 45% of the genetic information in EBV DNA is transcribed in cultured virus-producing P$_3$HR-1 cells. The virus-coded RNA species are translated and produce the virus-specific structural and nonstructural proteins.

F. BIOCHEMICAL PROPERTIES OF EBV NUCLEAR ANTIGEN (EBNA)

I. EXTRACTION OF EBNA WITH DETERGENTS AND SALT SOLUTIONS

Reedman and Klein (1973) demonstrated that an EBV-specified protein is present in the nuclei of EBV DNA-containing lymphoid cells. Since this study, numerous experiments have confirmed that EBNA is indeed a virus-coded protein (Brown et al., 1974; Klein, 1974; Lenoir et al., 1976; Lindahl et al., 1976). The EBNA protein (Chap. 3) has been extracted from Raji cells and characterized by sucrose gradient centrifugation, gel filtration, and ion exchange chromatography; the sedimentation coefficient of the viral antigen, detected in the sucrose gradient by the complement fixation text, was estimated to be 8.5 S, corresponding to a molecular weight of 180,000 (Lenoir et al., 1976).

EBNA could be extracted from the nuclei of Raji and P$_3$HR-1 cells by solutions of either 1.0 M NaCl or 0.03 M sodium deoxycholate (Becker et al., 1975 c) which were first used for the extraction of group II histones (Smart and Bonner, 1971). This technique was chosen because EBNA was found to be bound to chromosomes in the cells. Treatment of chromatin with 0.5 M NaCl extracted 50% of the EBNA and only a minimal amount of chromosomal proteins (Pikler et al., 1977).

II. EBNA AS A DNA-BINDING PROTEIN

Klein (1978) and Pikler et al. (1978) demonstrated that EBNA preparations extracted from cells could bind to the chromosomal DNA of cells from which the chromosomal proteins were removed, indicating that EBNA can be extracted without damage to its antigenicity and that it can be rebound to DNA. This property of EBNA was utilized by Luka et al. (1977) to purify EBNA by binding it to and eluting it from double-stranded DNA cellulose columns. Centrifugation of EBNA in a sucrose gradient revealed two distinct protein peaks, one with a molecular weight of 180×10^3 daltons, similar to the finding of Lenoir et al. (1976) for the S antigen, and the other with a molecular weight of 90,000 daltons. It is possible that the latter is the monomeric form of EBNA able to form dimers.

III. POSSIBLE ROLE OF EBNA IN THE CELLS

The exact role of EBNA in cells containing EBV DNA is not yet understood. Preliminary experiments (B. Fridlender and Y. Becker, unpublished data) indicated that addition of a purified EBNA preparation to an in vitro DNA polymerase system inhibited the incorporation of the deoxyribonucleoside triphosphates into the DNA template, probably due to binding of EBNA to the DNA. Further studies on the function of EBNA are still needed.

IV. TIMING OF EBNA BIOSYNTHESIS

EBNA is synthesized in cord blood lymphocytes 12 – 25 h after infection with EBV derived from B95-8 cells. Approximately 20 h later, the cells will enter into the S phase (Einhorn and Ernberg, 1978). EBNA induction is prevented if infection by EBV is done in the presence of cytosine arabinoside but is not affected by other inhibitors of DNA synthesis (Einhorn and Ernberg, 1978). The synthesis of EBNA in infected cells (e. g., Ramos, BJAB-1) is not inhibited by cytosine arabinoside (Klein, 1978).

G. BIOCHEMICAL ASPECTS OF INFECTION OF LYMPHOBLASTOID CELLS AND LEUKOCYTES WITH EBV

I. MOLECULAR EVENTS IN EBV DNA-CONTAINING LYMPHOBLASTOID CELLS SUPERINFECTED WITH EBV

1. Synthesis of EBV DNA in Superinfected Cells

Superinfection of Raji cells with EBV prepared from P_3HR-1 cells results in the synthesis of EB virions; EBV DNA molecules are synthesized in the nuclei of such cells (Nonoyama and Pagano, 1972b; Tanaka et al., 1976 a, b; Yajima and Nonoyama, 1976; Yajima et al., 1976) to give about 5000 EBV DNA genomes in each infected cell. Virus progeny from such an infection was found to be noninfectious for Raji cells (Yajima and Nonoyama, 1976).

2. Effect of Interferon

Those EBV-containing cell lines that spontaneously produce interferon are refractory to superinfection and show inhibition of EA synthesis (Adams et al., 1975).

3. Effect of EBV Superinfection on Cellular DNA Synthesis

EBV superinfection of Raji cells resulted in a marked inhibition of cellular DNA synthesis as well as fragmentation of the chromosomal DNA (Nonoyama and Pagano, 1972b; Tanaka et al., 1976 a, b), but the mechanism involved in this inhibition of cellular DNA synthesis is not yet understood.

4. Synthesis of EBV-Specified Antigens

Gergely et al. (1971) reported on the synthesis of viral antigens in EBV-superinfected Raji cells and showed that EA inhibits cellular macromolecular synthetic processes. As regards EBNA, Menezes et al. (1978) have demonstrated that in BJAB-1 cells infected with B95-8-derived EBV, EBNA was detectable at 10 h after infection, but EA was not induced. In the same cells infected with P_3HR-1-derived virus, EBNA was detectable within $7-8$ h while EA was detectable 20 h after infection. These results confirm long recognized differences in the properties of the two EBV isolates (Chap. 1).

II. MOLECULAR EVENTS IN LEUKOCYTES INFECTED WITH EBV LEADING TO CELL TRANSFORMATION

1. Molecular Processes in the EBV-Transformed Cells

Infection of umbilical-cord leukocytes with EBV derived from B95-8 cells results in stimulation of ^{3}H-thymidine uptake into cell DNA. This does not occur with P_3HR-1-derived EBV, which is incapable of cell transformation (Gerber and Hoyer, 1971; Gerber and Lucas, 1972; Miller et al., 1974). Stimulation of cell DNA synthesis after infection with EBV may be a prerequisite for cell immortalization.

The nature of the cord blood leukocyte DNA polymerase which is responsible for the increased synthesis of cellular DNA, is not yet known. Recently Lemon et al. (1978) (Chap. 9) reported that treatment of EBV-infected mononuclear cord blood cells with PAA (200 µg/ml) totally abolished cell proliferation. However, after transformation, the cells were not affected by 200 µg/ml PAA, suggesting that a DNA polymerase α different from the PAA-sensitive enzyme is involved in the proliferation of the transformed cells. The induction of DNA synthesis in EBV-infected human umbilical-cord leukocytes is serum dependent (Robinson and Miller, 1975), likewise suggesting that a cellular DNA enzyme is involved. Since not all of the heterogeneous species of the cellular DNA polymerase α are sensitive to PAA (B. Fridlender and Y. Becker, unpublished results), it may be that the enzyme responsible for the induction of cellular DNA synthesis in EBV-infected leukocytes is indeed a DNA polymerase α.

The role of EBV in the induction of cellular DNA synthesis in EBV-infected cord blood leukocytes was determined by using UV-inactivated EBV preparations, which were found not to stimulate cellular DNA synthesis (Robinson and Miller, 1975; Sarenji and Hinuma, 1975). This finding suggests that part of the genetic information encoded in EBV DNA must be expressed to stimulate cellular DNA synthesis in infected cord blood leukocytes. The nature of this viral genetic information is not yet known.

2. Transformation of Monkey Leukocytes by EBV and Monkey EBV-Related Virus

Monkey leukocytes can be transformed both by EBV and by a simian EBV-related virus that has 50% homology with human EBV (Miller et al., 1972; Falk et al., 1976; Rabin et al., 1976, 1977) (Chap. 17). The molecular processes involved in leukocyte transformation by either human or simian EBV still need to be resolved.

H. TRANSFORMATION OF CELLS WITH DNA

Sonicated extracts from EB3 cell line of BL origin have been added to DEAE-dextran-treated human amnion cells, and foci of transformed cells were reported to appear 7–14 days later. Since the transforming agent was not neutralized by antibodies to EBV, but was degraded by DNase treatment it was concluded that the transforming agent was EBV DNA (Al-Moslih et al., 1976). The nature of this phenomenon requires further study.

I. DISCUSSION

Studies on EBV have revealed various biochemical aspects of the interaction of this herpesvirus with lymphoblastoid cells, which are its natural host. The interaction of EBV with B lymphocytes leads to a change in metabolic processes and indefinite proliferation of the cell. EBV particles attach to receptors on the surface of B lymphocytes, and after interaction between the viral envelope and the cell membrane the viral nucleocapsid is introduced into the cytoplasm where uncoating of the viral DNA takes place. Infection of human umbilical-cord leukocytes with EBV leads to a change in a small number of cells. This is expressed by acquisition of the ability to proliferate continously in vitro, corresponding in some ways to a transformation process.

The behavior of EBV in specific lymphocytes is probably dependent on processes in the cell at the time of infection which control the expression of EBV DNA. As a result, EBV DNA attains a conformation that prevents its replication, and this in turn leads to a change in the regulation of the growth properties of the cell. Such a change is expressed in enhanced proliferation of cells in vitro and the proliferation of a clone of malignantly transformed cells in vivo to form the tumors of BL.

Analyses revealed that EBV particles resemble other herpesviruses in their properties. The DNA genome has a molecular weight of 100×10^6 daltons, and the virus particle consists of a nucleocapsid enveloped by a membrane containing glycoproteins. The organization of EBV DNA is not yet known; preliminary data suggest that the DNA contains repeat sequences with a $G + C$ content higher than the average $G + C$ content (58%) of herpes viral DNA. Difficulty in propagating the virus in cell cultures has prevented the isolation of mutants, and therefore genetic studies on EBV have not yet been done.

The EBV DNA present in virions has a linear conformation. However, in transformed cells EBV DNA exists as free, episomal DNA molecules with a circular conformation. In addition, a very limited number of DNA genome equivalents seem to be associated with the chromosomal DNA, possibly by linear covalent linkages. The circular viral DNA molecules replicate in the transformed cells during the S phase of the cell cycle, the period of chromosomal DNA biosynthesis. Analogous to the duplication of the chromosomal DNA, the number of EBV DNA genomes also doubles at the end of the S period, and each of the daughter cells receives an equal number of EBV genomes. These are either separate in the form of minichromosomes (free DNA-protein complexes) or associated with the cell chromosome (Chap. 8).

It seems feasible to assume that the incoming linear EBV DNA genomes are circularized by enzymatic mechanisms present in the cell. The circular viral genomes are not efficiently transcribed by the host RNA polymerase II (possibly because the site for initiation of transcription is not available) and therefore code for a limited number of viral proteins. One of the viral proteins synthesized is EBNA, which can bind to chromosomal DNA. Suppression of EBV by circularization of the DNA and the synthesis of a viral DNA-binding protein probably prevent expression of the viral lytic properties and bring about changes in the control of cell growth. Alternatively, integration of EBV DNA into the chromosomal DNA, either as a complete genome or as DNA fragments, may be responsible for the changes in the cellular control mechanisms that lead to the establishment of the lymphocyte as a transformed lymphoblastoid cell. The biochemical processes underlying the changes in both the viral DNA and the cellular control mechanisms remain to be studied. Certain transformed lymphoblastoid cell lines respond to treatment with arginine-deficient medium, inhibitors of protein synthesis, and halogenated pyrimidines by the production of EBV. Thus, marked changes in the cellular processes (inhibition of protein synthesis or incorporation of IUDR or BUDR into DNA) lead to the conversion of circular episomal EBV DNA molecules into a linear conformation. At this stage transcription of the entire viral genome is possible (most probably by the cellular RNA polymerase II), and viral nonstructural and structural proteins are synthesized prior to cell death and the formation of EBV progeny. The mechanism leading to the linearization of EBV DNA is not yet understood, but it is a cellular enzymatic process which can be activated by treatment with inducers. EBV DNA is synthesized by a virus-specified DNA polymerase in a similar way to other herpesviruses in lytically infected cells.

The detailed mechanisms of the virus-cell interaction, in which EBV DNA is changed from a linear conformation in the virions to a circular conformation in the cell and back to a linear conformation when virus synthesis is induced, are not well understood. Studies on the organization of EBV DNA in virus strains capable of cell transformation and in those that are nontransforming may shed light on the nature of the genes or viral sequences involved in cell transformation by EBV.

REFERENCES

Adams, A.: Concentration of Epstein-Barr virus from cell culture fluids with polyethylene glycol. J. Gen Virol. **20**, 391–394 (1973)

Adams, A., Lindahl, T.: Intracellular forms of Epstein-Barr virus DNA in Raji cells. In: Oncogenesis and herpesviruses II. de-Thé, G., Epstein, M. A., zur Hausen, H. (eds.), Part 1, pp. 125–132. Lyon: IARC 1975a

Adams, A., Lindahl, T.: Epstein-Barr virus genomes with properties of circular DNA molecules in carrier cells. Proc. Natl. Acad. Sci. USA **72**, 1477–1481 (1975b)

Adams, A., Lindahl, T., Klein, G.: Linear association between cellular DNA and Epstein-Barr virus DNA in a human lymphoblastoid cell line. Proc. Natl. Acad. Sci. USA **70**, 2888–2892 (1973)

Adams, A., Lidin, B., Strander, H., Cantell, K.: Spontaneous interferon production and Epstein-Barr virus antigen expression in human lymphoid cell lines. J. Gen. Virol. **28**, 219–223 (1975)

Al-Moslih, M. I., White, R. J., Dubes, G. R.: Use of a transfection method to demonstrate a monolayer cell transforming agent from the EB3 line of Burkitt's lymphoma cells. J. Gen. Virol. **31**, 331–345 (1976)

Andersson, M.: Amounts of Epstein-Barr virus DNA in somatic cell hybrids between Burkitt lymphoma-derived cell lines. J. Virol. **16**, 1345–1347 (1975)

Becker, Y., Weinberg, A.: Burkitt lymphoblasts and their Epstein-Barr virus. Synthesis of viral DNA and proteins in arginine deprived cells. Isr. J. Med. Sci. **7,** 561–567 (1971)

Becker, Y., Weinberg, A.: Molecular events in the biosynthesis of Epstein-Barr virus in Burkitt lymphoblasts. In: Oncogenesis and herpesviruses. Biggs, P. M., de-Thé, G. Payne, L. N. (eds.), pp. 326–335. Lyon: IARC 1972a.

Becker, Y., Weinberg, A.: Distamycin A inhibition of Epstein-Barr virus replication in arginine deprived Burkitt lymphoblasts. Isr. J. Med. Sci. **8,** 75–78 (1972b)

Becker, Y., Dym. H., Sarov, I.: Herpes simplex virus DNA. Virology **36,** 184–192 (1968)

Becker, Y., Shlomai, Y., Weinberg, E., Ben-Zeev, A. Olshevsky, U.: Integration of EBV DNA into cellular DNA of Burkitt lymphoblasts (Raji cell line). Isr. J. Med. Sci. **10,** 1454–1457 (1974)

Becker, Y., Weinberg, E., Cohen, Y.: Studies on the state of EBV DNA synthesis in Burkitt lymphoblasts. In: Epstein-Barr virus production, concentration and purification. Lyon: IARC Internal Technical Report No. 75 003, 147–157 (1975a)

Becker, Y., Ben-Zeev, A., Kamincik, Y., Asher, Y., Shlomai, J.: Nucleic acid biosynthesis in nuclei of cells infected with herpesviruses (HSV and EBV). In: Oncogenesis and herpesviruses II. de-Thé, G., Epstein, M. A. zur Hausen, H. (eds.), Part 1, pp. 245–257. Lyon: IARC 1975b

Becker, Y., Weinberg, E., Cohen, Y., Klein, G.: Studies on Epstein-Barr virus specified proteins in Burkitt lymphoblasts. In: Epstein-Barr virus production, concentration and purification. Lyon: IARC Internal Technical Report No. 75 003, 285–294 (1975c)

Becker, Y., Asher, Y., Cohen, Y., Weinberg-Zahlering, E., Shlomai, J.: Phosphonoacetic acid resistant mutants of herpes simplex virus: Effect of phosphonoacetic acid on virus replication and in vitro DNA synthesis in isolated nuclei. Antimicrob. Agents Chemother. **11,** 919–922 (1977)

Benz, W. C., Strominger, J. L.: Viral and cellular DNA synthesis in nuclei from human lymphocytes transformed by Epstein-Barr virus. Proc. Natl. Acad. Sci. USA **72,** 2413–2417 (1975)

Ben-Zeev, A., Asher, Y., Becker, Y.: Synthesis of herpes simplex virus-specified RNA by an RNA polymerase II in isolated nuclei *in vitro*. Virology **71,** 302–311 (1976)

Ben-Zeev, A., Becker, Y.: Requirement of host cell RNA polymerase II in the replication of herpes simplex virus in α-amanitin-sensitive and -resistant cell lines. Virology **76,** 246–253 (1977)

Brown, T. D. K., Ernberg, I., Lamon, E. W., Klein, G.: Detection of Epstein-Barr virus-associated nuclear antigen in human lymphoblastoid cell lines by means of an ^{125}I-IgG-binding assay. Int. J. Cancer **13,** 785–794 (1974)

Derge, J. G., Birkhead, S. L., Hemmaplardh, T., Hampar, B.: DNA synthesis in cells activated for the Epstein-Barr virus. In: Oncogenesis and herpesviruses II. de-Thé, G., Epstein, M. A. zur Hausen, H. (eds.), Part 1, pp. 467–474. Lyon: IARC 1975

Dolyniuk, M., Pritchett, R., Kieff, E.: Proteins of Epstein-Barr virus. I. Analysis of the polypeptides of purified enveloped Epstein-Barr virus. J. Virol. **17,** 935–949 (1976a)

Dolyniuk, M., Wolff, E., Kieff, E.: Proteins of Epstein-Barr virus. II. Electrophoretic analysis of the polypeptides of the nucleocapsid and the glucosamine- and polysaccharide-containing components of enveloped virus. J. Virol. **18,** 289–297 (1976b)

Einhorn, L., Ernberg, I.: Induction of EBNA precedes the first cellular S-phase after EBV-infection of human lyphocytes. Int. J. Cancer **21,** 157–160 (1978)

Epstein, M. A., Achong, B. G.: Observations on the nature of the herpes-type EB virus in cultured Burkitt lymphoblasts, using a specific immunofluorescence test. J. Natl. Cancer Inst. **40,** 609–621 (1968)

Epstein, M. A., Barr, Y. M.: Cultivation *in vitro* of human lymphoblasts from Burkitt's malignant lymphoma. Lancet **1964 I,** 252–253

Epstein, M. A., Achong, B. G., Barr, Y. M.: Virus particles in cultured lymphoblasts from Burkitt's lymphoma. Lancet **1964a I,** 702–703

Epstein, M. A., Barr, Y. M., Achong, B. G.: A second virus-carrying tissue culture strain (EB2) of lymphoblasts from Burkitt's lymphoma. Pathol. Biol. (Paris) **12,** 1233–1234 (1964b)

Epstein, M. A., Henle, G., Achong, B. G., Barr, Y. M.: Morphological and biological studies on a virus in cultured lymphoblasts from Burkitt's lymphoma. J. Exp. Med. **121,** 761–770 (1965)

Falk, F., Deinhardt, F., Nonoyama, M., Wolfe, L. G., Bergholz, C., Lapin, B., Yakovleva, L., Agrba, V., Henle, G., Henle, W.: Properties of a baboon lymphotropic herpesvirus related to EBV. Int. J. Cancer **18,** 798–807 (1976)

Gerber, P.: Activation of Epstein-Barr virus by 5-bromodeoxyuridine in "virus-free" human cells. Proc. Natl. Acad. Sci. USA **69,** 83–85 (1972)

Gerber, P., Hoyer, B. H.: Induction of cellular DNA synthesis in human leukocytes by Epstein-Barr virus. Nature **231,** 46–47 (1971)

Gerber, P., Lucas, S. J.: *In vitro* stimulation of human lymphocytes by Epstein-Barr virus. Cell Immunol. **5**, 318–324 (1972)

Gergely, L., Klein, G., Ernberg, I.: Host cell macromolecular synthesis in cells containing EBV-induced early antigens studied by combined immunofluorescence and radioautography. Virology **45**, 22–29 (1971)

Glaser, R., Nonoyama, M.: Epstein-Barr virus: Detection of genome in somatic cell hybrids of Burkitt lymphoblastoid cells. Science **179**, 492–493 (1973)

Glaser, R., Nonoyama, M.: Host cell regulation of induction of Epstein-Barr virus. J. Virol. **14**, 174–176 (1974)

Glaser, R., O'Neill, F. J.: Hybridization of Burkitt lymphoblastoid cells. Science **176**, 1245–1247 (1972)

Glaser, R., Rapp, F.: Rescue of Epstein-Barr virus from somatic cell hybrids of Burkitt lymphoblastoid cells. J. Virol. **10**, 288–296 (1972)

Glaser, R., Nonoyama, M., Decker, B., Rapp. F.: Synthesis of Epstein-Barr virus antigens and DNA in activated Burkitt somatic cell hybrids. Virology **55**, 62–69 (1973a)

Glaser, R., Ogino, T., Zimmerman, J., Rapp, F.: Thymidine kinase activity in Burkitt lymphoblastoid somatic cell hybrids after induction of the EB virus. Proc. Soc. Exp. Biol. Med. **142**, 1059–1062 (1973b)

Glaser, R., Nonoyama, M., Shows, T. B., Henle, G., Henle, W.: Epstein-Barr virus studies on the association of the virus genome with human chromosomes in hybrid cells. In: Oncogenesis and herpesviruses II. de-Thé, G., Epstein, M. A., zur Hausen, H. (eds.), Part 1, pp. 457–466. Lyon: IARC 1975

Goodman, S. R., Benz, W. C.: Identification and partial purification of an Epstein-Barr virus associated DNA polymerase. In: Oncogenesis and herpesviruses III. de-Thé, G., Henle, W., Rapp, F. (eds.). Lyon: IARC (in press) 1978

Hampar, B., Derge, J. G., Martos, L. M., Walker, J. L.: Persistance of a repressed Epstein-Barr virus genome in Burkitt lymphoma cells made resistant to 5-bromodeoxyuridine. Proc. Natl. Acad. Sci. USA **68**, 3185–3189 (1971)

Hampar, B., Derge, J. G., Martos, L. M., Walker, J. L.: Synthesis of Epstein-Barr virus after activation of the viral genome in a "virus-negative" human lymphoblastoid cell (Raji) made resistant to 5-bromodeoxyuridine. Proc. Natl. Acad. Sci. USA **69**, 78–82 (1972a)

Hampar, B., Derge, J. G., Martos, L. M., Tagamets, M., Burroughs, M. A.: Sequence of spontaneous Epstein-Barr virus activation and selective DNA synthesis in activated cells in the presence of hydroxyurea. Proc. Natl. Acad. Sci. USA **69**, 2589–2593 (1972b)

Hampar, B., Derge, J. G., Martos, L. M., Tagamets, M. A., Chang, S. Y., Chakrabarty, M.: Identification of a critical period during the S phase for activation of the Epstein-Barr virus by 5-iododeoxyuridine. Nature (New Biol.) **244**, 214–217 (1973)

Hampar, B., Derge, J. G., Nonoyama, M., Chang, S. Y., Tagamets, M. A., Showalter, S. D.: Programming of events in Epstein-Barr virus-activated cells by 5-iododeoxyuridine. Virology **62**, 71–89 (1974a)

Hampar, B., Derge, J. G., Tanaka, A., Nonoyama, M.: Sequence of Epstein-Barr virus productive cycle in human lymphoblastoid cells. Cold Spring Harbor Symp. Quant. Biol. **39**, 811–815 (1974b)

Hampar, B., Tanaka, A., Nonoyama, M., Derge, J. G.: Replication of the resident repressed Epstein-Barr virus genome during the early S phase (S-1 period) of nonproducer Raji cells. Proc. Natl. Acad. Sci. USA **71**, 631–633 (1974c)

Hampar, B., Lenoir, G., Nonoyama, M., Derge, J. G., Chang, S. Y.: Cell cycle dependence for activation of Epstein-Barr virus by inhibitors of protein synthesis or medium deficient in arginine. Virology **69**, 660–668 (1976)

Hayward, S. D., Kieff, E.: Epstein-Barr virus-specific RNA. I. Analysis of viral RNA in cellular extracts and in the polyribosomal fraction of permissive and nonpermissive lymphoblastoid cell lines. J. Virol. **18**, 518–525 (1976)

Hayward, S. D., Kieff, E.: DNA of Epstein-Barr virus. II. Comparison of the molecular weights of restriction endonuclease fragments of the DNA of Epstein-Barr virus strains and identification of end fragments of the B95-8 strain. J. Virol. **23**, 421–429 (1977)

Henle, G., Henle, W.: Immunofluorescence in cells derived from Burkitt's lymphoma. J. Bacteriol **91**, 1248–1256 (1966a)

Henle, G., Henle, W.: Studies on cell lines derived from Burkitt's lymphoma. Trans. NY, Acad. Sci. **29**, 71–74 (1966b)

Henle, W., Henle, G.: Effect of arginine deficient media on the herpes-type virus associated with cultured Burkitt tumor cells. J. Virol. **2**, 182–191 (1968)

Kaschka-Dierich, C., Adams, A., Lindahl, T., Bornkamm, G. W., Bjursell, G., Klein, G., Giovanella, B. C., Singh, S.: Intracellular forms of Epstein-Barr virus DNA in human tumour cells *in vivo*. Nature **260**, 302–306 (1976)

Kieff, E., Levine, J.: Homology between Burkitt herpes viral DNA and DNA in continous lymphoblastoid cells from patients with infectious mononucleosis. Proc. Nat. Acad. Sci. USA **71**, 355–358 (1974)

Klein, G.: The Epstein-Barr virus. In: The Herpesviruses. Kaplan, A. S. (ed.), pp. 521–555. New York: Academic Press 1973

Klein, G.: Studies on the Epstein-Barr virus genome and the EBV-determined nuclear antigen in human malignant disease. Cold Spring Harbor Symp. Quant. Biol. **39**, 783–790 (1974)

Klein, G.: Studies on the EBV-determined nuclear antigen (EBNA). In: Oncogenesis and herpesviruses III. de-Thé, G., Henle, W., Rapp. F. (eds.). Lyon: IARC (in press) 1978

Lemon, S. M., Hutt, L. M., Shaw, J. E., Li, J-L. H., Pagano, J. S.: Replication of EBV in epithelial cells during infectious mononucleosis. Nature **268**, 268–270 (1977)

Lemon, S. M., Hutt, L. M., Pagano, J. S.: Epstein-Barr virus transformation of human cord lymphocytes is inhibited by phosphonoacetic acid. In: Oncogenesis and herpesviruses III. de-Thé, G., Henle, W. Rapp, F. (eds.). Lyon: IARC (in press) 1978

Lenoir, G., Berthelon, M-C., Favre, M-C., de-Thé, G.: Characterization of Epstein-Barr virus antigens. I. Biochemical analysis of the complement-fixing soluble antigen and relationship with Epstein-Barr virus-associated nuclear antigen. J. Virol. **17**, 672–674 (1976)

Lindahl, T., Adams, A., Bjursell, G., Bornkamm, G. W., Kaschka-Dierich, C., Jehn, U.: Covalently closed circular duplex DNA of Epstein-Barr virus in Raji cells. J. Mol. Biol. **102**, 511–530 (1976)

Long, C., Derge, J. G., Hampar, B.: Procedure for activating Epstein-Barr virus early antigen in nonproducer cells by 5-iododeoxyuridine. J. Natl. Cancer Inst. **52**, 1355–1357 (1974)

Luka, J., Siegert, W., Klein, G.: Solubilization of the Epstein-Barr virus-determined nuclear antigen and its characterization as a DNA-binding protein. J. Virol. **22**, 1–8 (1977)

Mao, J. G. H., Robishaw, E. E., Overby, L. R.: Inhibition of DNA polymerase from herpes simplex virus infected WI-38 cells by phosphonoacetic acid. J. Virol. **15**, 1281–1283 (1975)

Menezes, J., Patel, P., Dussault, H., Bourkas, A. E.: Comparative studies on the induction of virus-associated nuclear antigen and early antigen by lymphocyte-transforming (B95-8) and nontransforming (P3HR-1) strains of Epstein-Barr virus. Intervirology **9**, 86–94 (1978)

Miller, G., Shope, T., Lisco, H., Stitt, D., Lipman, M.: Epstein-Barr virus: Transformation, cytopathic changes and viral antigens in squirrel monkey and marmoset leukocytes. Proc. Natl. Acad. Sci. USA. **69**, 383–387 (1972)

Miller, G., Robinson, J., Heston, L., Lipman, M.: Differences between laboratory strains of Epstein-Barr virus based on immortalization, abortive infection and interference. Proc. Natl. Acad. Sci. USA **71**, 4006–4010 (1974)

Miller, R. L., Glaser, R., Rapp, F.: Studies of an Epstein-Barr virus-induced DNA polymerase. Virology **76**, 494–502 (1977)

Minowada, J., Chai, L., Moore, G. E.: Studies on Burkitt lymphoma cells. III. Equilibrium density gradient centrifugation of virus particles isolated from Burkitt lymphoma cell lines. Cancer **23**, 300–305 (1969)

Nonoyama, M., Pagano, J. S.: Detection of Epstein-Barr viral genome in nonproductive cells. Nature (New Biol.) **233**, 103–106 (1971)

Nonoyama, M., Pagano, J. S.: Separation of Epstein-Barr virus DNA from large chromosomal DNA in nonvirus-producing cells. Nature (New Biol.) **238**, 169–171 (1972a)

Nonoyama, M., Pagano, J. S.: Replication of viral deoxyribonucleic acid and breakdown of cellular deoxyribonucleic acid in Epstein-Barr virus infection. J. Virol. **9**, 714–716 (1972b)

Nyormoi, O., Thorley-Lawson, D. A., Elkington, J., Strominger, J. L.: Differential effect of phosphonoacetic acid on the expression of Epstein-Barr viral antigens and virus production. Proc. Natl. Acad. Sci. USA **73**, 1745–1748 (1976)

Ooka, T., Daillie, J., Costa, O., Lenoir, G.: Studies on Epstein-Barr virus (EBV) DNA polymerase activities in various human lymphoblastoid cell lines. In: Oncogenesis and herpesviruses III. de-Thé, G., Henle, W., Rapp, F. (eds.), pp. 389–394. Lyon: IARC 1978

Pikler, G. M., Pearson, G. R., Spelsberg, T. C.: Isolation of the Epstein-Barr virus nuclear antigen from chromatin preparations. In: Oncogenesis and herpesviruses III. de-Thé, G., Henle, W., Rapp. F. (eds.), pp. 243–248. Lyon: IARC 1978

Pritchett, R. F., Hayward, S. D., Kieff, E. D.: DNA of Epstein-Barr virus. I. Comparative studies of the DNA of Epstein-Barr virus from HR-1 and B95-8 cells: Size, structure and relatedness. J. Virol. **15**, 556–569 (1975a)

Pritchett, R. F., Hayward, S. D., Kieff, E. D.: Analysis of Epstein-Barr viruses and transcriptional products in transformed cells. In: Oncogenesis and herpesviruses II. de-Thé, G., Epstein, M. A., zur Hausen, H. (eds.), pp. 177–189. Lyon: IARC 1975b

Rabin, H., Levy, B., Neubauer, R. H., Lebowitz, H., Hopkins, R. F. III, Wallen, W. C.: Comparisons of lymphoid cell lines established from individual tumors of a cotton-topped marmoset with multiple Epstein-Barr virus induced lymphomas. In vitro 12, 288–289 (1976)

Rabin, H., Neubauer, R. H., Hopkins, R. F. III, Dzhikidze, E. K., Shevtsova, Z. V., Lapin, B. A.: Transforming activity and antigenicity of an Epstein-Barr-like virus from lymphoblastoid cell lines of baboons with lymphoid disease. Intervirology 8, 240–249 (1977)

Reedman, B. M., Klein, G.: Cellular localization of an Epstein-Barr virus (EBV)-associated complement-fixing antigen in producer and nonproducer lymphoblastoid cell lines. Int. J. Cancer 11, 499–520 (1973)

Robinson, J., Miller, G.: Assay for Epstein-Barr virus based on stimulation of DNA synthesis in mixed leukocytes from human umbilical cord blood. J. Virol. 15, 1065–1072 (1975)

Sairenji, T., Hinuma, Y.: Ultraviolet inactivation of Epstein-Barr virus: Effect on synthesis of virus-associated antigens. Int. J. Cancer 16, 1–6 (1975)

Schulte-Holthausen, H., zur Hausen, H.: Partial purification of the Epstein-Barr virus and some properties of its DNA. Virology 40, 776–779 (1970)

Seebeck, T., Shaw, J. E., Pagano, J. S.: Synthesis of Epstein-Barr virus DNA in vitro: Effects of phosphonoacetic acid, N-ethylmaleimide and ATP. J. Virol. 21, 435–438 (1977)

Sheldrick, P., Berthelot, N.: Inverted repetitions in the chromosome of herpes simplex virus. Cold Spring Harbor Symp. Quant. Biol. 39, 667–678 (1974)

Shipkowitz, N. L., Bower, R. R., Appell, R. N., Nordeen, C. W., Overby, L. R., Roderick, W. R., Schleicher, J. B., von Esch, A. M.: Suppression of herpes simplex virus infection by phosphonoacetic acid. Appl. Microb. 26, 264–267 (1973)

Shlomai, J., Friedmann, A., Becker, Y.: Replicative intermediates of herpes simplex virus DNA. Virology 69, 647–659 (1976a)

Shlomai, J., Strauss, B., Asher, Y., Friedmann, A., Becker, Y.: Analysis of herpes simplex virus DNA synthesized in infected nuclei by chromatography on benzoylated-naphthoylated DEAE cellulose columns. J. Gen. Virol. 32, 189–204 (1976b)

Smart, J. E., Bonner, J.: Selective dissociation of histones from chromatin by sodium deoxycholate. J. Mol. Biol. 58, 651–659 (1971)

Sugden, B., Summers, W. C., Klein, G.: Nucleic acid renaturation and restriction endonuclease cleavage analyses show that the DNAs of a transforming and nontransforming strain of Epstein-Barr virus share approximately 90% of their nucleotide sequences. J. Virol. 18, 765–775 (1976)

Summers, W. C., Klein, G.: Inhibition of Epstein-Barr virus DNA synthesis and late gene expression by phosphonoacetic acid. J. Virol. 18, 151–155 (1976)

Tanaka, A., Nonoyama, M.: Late genomes of Epstein-Barr virus. In: Oncogenesis and herpesviruses II. de-Thé, G., Epstein, M. A., zur Hausen, H. (eds.), Part 1, pp. 133–137. Lyon: IARC 1975

Tanaka, A., Miyagi, M., Yajima, Y., Nonoyama, M.: Improved production of Epstein-Barr virus DNA for nucleic acid hybridization studies. Virology 74, 81–85 (1976a)

Tanaka, A., Nonoyama, M., Hampar, B.: Partial elimination of latent Epstein-Barr virus genomes from virus-producing cells by cycloheximide. Virology 70, 164–170 (1976b)

Twardzik, D. R., Aaslestad, H. G., Tureckova, M. I., Gravel, N., Ablashi, D. V., Levine, P. H.: Comparison of DNA polymerase activities from an American Burkitt's lymphoma cell line and EBV producer and nonproducer cells. In: Oncogenesis and herpesviruses II. de-Thé, G., Epstein, M. A., zur Hausen, H. (eds.), Part 1. pp. 237–243, Lyon: IARC 1975.

Weinberg, A., Becker, Y.: Studies on EB virus of Burkitt lymphoblasts. Virology 39, 312–321 (1969)

Weinberg, A., Becker, Y.: Effect of arginine deprivation on macromolecular processes in Burkitt lymphoblasts. Exp. Cell Res. 60, 470–474 (1970)

Yajima, Y., Nonoyama, M.: Mechanisms of infection with Epstein-Barr virus. I. Viral DNA replication and formation of noninfectious virus particles in superinfected Raji cells. J. Virol. 19, 187–194 (1976)

Yajima, Y., Tanaka, A., Nonoyama, M.: Inhibition of productive replication of Epstein-Barr virus DNA by phosphonoacetic acid. Virology 71, 352–354 (1976)

Yamamoto, K., Matsuo, T., Osato, T.: Appearance of Epstein-Barr virus-determined nuclear antigen in human epithelial cell following fusion with lymphoid cells. Intervirology 6, 115–121 (1975/76)

Yocum, R. R., Strominger, J. L.: RNA polymerases in human lymphoblastoid cells that contain Epstein-Barr virus. In: Oncogenesis and herpesviruses II. de-Thé, G., Epstein, M. A., zur Hausen, H. (eds.), Part 1, pp. 75–83. Lyon: IARC 1975

Zimmerman, J. E., Glaser, R., Rapp, F.: Effect of dibutyryl cyclic AMP on the induction of Epstein-Barr virus in hybrid cells. J. Virol. **12**, 1442–1445 (1973)

zur Hausen, H., Schulte-Holthausen, H.: Presence of EB virus nucleic acid in a virus-free line of Burkitt tumor cells. Nature **227**, 245–248 (1970)

6 Molecular Probes and Genome Homology

J. S. Pagano and J. E. Shaw

Departments of Medicine, Bacteriology, and Immunology, Cancer Research Center, School of Medicine, University of North Carolina, Chapel Hill, NC 27514 (USA)

A. GENERAL INTRODUCTION

The Epstein-Barr Virus (EBV) offers a unique opportunity to put to test landmark concepts and technology advanced in experimental tumor virus systems in recent years. The principal concept resulting from exploration of the viral etiology of cancer is the demonstration that, at least in vitro, viral genes remain in the malignant cell after the initial infection of the normal progenitor cell. This concept has been elaborated so that we know that specific viral DNA sequences containing defined genes are integrated into the cellular genetic composition and that these viral genes are expressed in the malignant cell. This concept must occupy a central position in the elusive quest for proof of causation between virus and human cancer.

EBV continues to hold its position as the foremost candidate for a human cancer virus. In the work done during this decade with the human malignancies associated with this virus, there has been notable success in tracking the evidence that the experimental concepts hold true in vivo. This success has at once invigorated the theoretical concepts coming from the in vitro systems and bolstered the proposition that EBV causes certain cancers.

The elemental evidence at the center of theories of the viral etiology of cancer, namely, the presence of inserted viral genes, requires the technology of molecular hybridization. A number of techniques of this class has been used to advantage in the study of EBV with results at least in part as predicted by analogous studies in adenovirus and SV40 experimental systems. The technology has also, however, revealed something of a molecular departure in eukaryotic cells, namely, the novel episomal or plasmid form of the EBV genome in tumor tissue. Some of the issues involved with the physical forms of EBV DNA sequences in cells are treated by Adams in Chap. 8 and others will be touched upon in this chapter.

Molecular hybridization has made central contributions to our understanding of EBV and we will, therefore, illustrate the value of the technology. The plan of this chapter is to introduce each technique briefly, outline it and indicate its advantages and its limitations. A detailed description of several of the techniques has been published recently (Huang and Pagano, 1977). The techniques and procedures include characterization of pure viral DNA, radiolabeling of the nucleic acid probes, DNA-DNA hybridization with immobilized nucleic acids, complementary RNA-DNA hybridization, hybridization of nucleic acids in liquid medium with measurements of kinetics of reassociation, in situ cytohybridization, restriction endonuclease analysis, and the Southern transfer technique. We will recount these techniques in their application to EBV and its genome.

The experimental demands for the technology are many. Some aims have already been implied, in particular detection of cryptic viral genetic material in tumor cells and the detection and characterization of the episomal or plasmid forms of the EBV genome. Another end is to define integrated sequences. Additionally, several of the techniques are useful in disclosing the degree of sequence homology among molecules coming from different cell lines and tumor sources as well as virus strain differences at the level of DNA. Operationally, we provide enough of the details of procedures to give the flavor of what is done in the laboratory. This level of information allows us to point to special problems and pinpoint details that are critical to carrying out the work successfully. We also emphasize problems that are peculiar to the EBV systems. Since technical procedures considered in isolation tend to be bereft of meaning, we therefore select some of the contributions made by molecular hybridization to our knowledge about the biology of EBV. We conclude with a general discussion of the mainstream of EBV research from the vantage point of this technology and the prospects for further work.

B. TECHNOLOGY

I. INTRODUCTION: MOLECULAR HYBRIDIZATION

The classic expectation from experimental DNA tumor virus systems is that infectious virus is not to be found in the tumor tissue. It then becomes necessary to search for the presence of viral genetic material in the transformed cells, either experimentally produced or tissues obtained directly from patients, by molecular hybridization techniques; a whole variety of these has evolved in recent years. zur Hausen and his colleagues were the first to use molecular hybridization in an EBV system, namely, DNA-DNA hybridization (zur Hausen and Schulte-Holthausen, 1970). The general basis for hybridization is by now certainly familiar; all the techniques depend on the use under denaturing conditions of complementary strands of radiolabeled DNA as probe for the presence of corresponding or homologous strands or portions of them. For most purposes it is not necessary to use + or − strands of nucleic acid as probes, but the nucleic acid must be highly radiolabeled and consist only of viral sequences. If these requirements are met, then under the proper conditions less than a single EBV genome can be distinguished in the large mass of chromosomal DNA contained in a cell. Variations of the basic technology continue to be developed.

One of the first and most useful was to prepare a radiolabeled RNA copy (complementary RNA – cRNA) of the EBV genomic DNA as probe (Nonoyama and Pagano, 1971). The amplification by synthesis of the cRNA in vitro yielded a large amount of labeled probe from a small amount of viral template DNA, an end particularly suited to work with a virus available in scant amounts. The second landmark in the adaptation of molecular hybridization technology to EBV research was the introduction of kinetic measurements of reannealing, as in DNA-DNA renaturation kinetics analyses (Nonoyama and Pagano, 1973). The advantage of this technique is not only its greater sensitivity and the prospect of using essentially complete strands of the EBV genome itself as probe, but the technique also permits estimates of the percentage of the viral genome retained in tumor tissue if less than the intact genome is present. By extension, this technique can also be used to gauge the degree of homology between similar but not identical genomes. The use of specific fragments of EBV genome as probe is a delicate elaboration on the technique which is expected to increase sensitivity beyond the remarkable levels that are already practical (Sharp et al., 1974). Renaturation kinetics analysis also lends itself to the detection and characterization of virus-specific RNA in tumor tissue, cells, and subcellular fractions.

It is worth noting that despite the invidious comparisons sometimes made between cRNA-DNA hybridization and DNA-DNA renaturation analyses, the former technique continues to furnish accurate results in a convenient way.

The next advance was restriction endonuclease analysis of EBV DNA following the lead of SV40, adenovirus, herpes simplex virus (HSV) and human cytomegalovirus (CMV). The principle contributions of this technique, which in itself does not entail molecular hybridization, are the isolation of specific fragments that can be used in molecular hybridization techniques as mentioned above and the refinement of discrimination of degree of homology or strain differences between viral genomes. Such work is well advanced in HSV and human CMV systems (Wilkie et al., 1974; Hayward et al., 1975; Kilpatrick et al., 1976); similar work has begun with EBV systems (Sugden et al., 1976; Hayward and Kieff, 1977; Shaw et al., 1977; Lee et al., 1977).

However, the most important contribution of restriction endonucleases is just beginning to be felt by their application in the so-called Southern, or blot-transfer, technique of molecular hybridization on nitrocellulose membranes (Southern, 1975). The innovation of an ingenious transfer method and the addition of a preliminary step of digestion of the total cellular DNA with a restriction endonuclease are elements of the technique. If the cellular DNA contains EBV sequences, they are displayed in the characteristic patterns of fragments produced by digestion of the viral genome with the same enzyme. This technique is extraordinarily sensitive; nanograms or less of viral DNA can be distinguished. A single molecular fragment of the EBV genome can be detected in digests of a relatively massive amount of cellular or tumor DNA. This technique has prospects of wide use in EBV research. It has already received some attention in analysis of Burkitt's lymphomas (BL) (Sugden, 1977) and in the analysis of EBV episomes, which can be recovered only in minute amounts.

The most sensitive method of hybridization and determination of genome homology depends not upon the averaging of complementarity of many molecules as indicated by membrane or liquid methods of hybridization, but rather on direct visualization of single hybrid molecules. Such determinations properly conducted are not only unambiguous but more sensitive – able to reveal sequence homology arising from as few as 50 base pairs (Griffith, personal communication). Only direct DNA sequencing can indicate lesser degrees of homology; this is the ultimate method (Maxam and Gilbert, 1977; Sanger et al., 1977). Neither of these techniques has yet been used in EBV research.

II. VIRION DNA

To a limited extent EBV DNA can be distinguished by its density and sedimentation characteristics if enough pure DNA is available. In any case pure viral DNA has to be procured and characterized before it can be used as template for all of the other procedures.

Because small quantities of virus are spontaneously released from virus-producing cells virus purification initially requires handling large volumes of tissue-culture medium; only 1–5 μg of virus DNA are usually recovered from a liter of virus-containing fluids. The virus can be precipitated from cellular fluids with polyethylene glycol (PEG) after a low-speed removal of cellular debris (Adams, 1975). This step is followed by centrifugation through sucrose in which virus forms a band approximately one-third the distance from the bottom of the tube. As mycoplasma is also concentrated by PEG precipitation and collects in the same region as virus in the sucrose gradient, subsequent purification of the virus DNA sometimes involves working with annoyingly viscous solutions, which make it harder to recover the virus DNA in high molecular weight form.

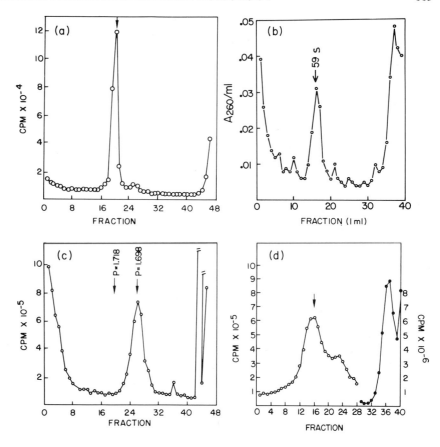

Fig. 1 a–d. Sedimentation and buoyant density characteristics of EBV DNA. **a** Density profile of the DNA of Raji cells labeled during superinfection with P_3HR-1 virus; the *arrow* indicates the position of 1.718 g-cm^{-3}, the buoyant density of EBV DNA. **b** Sedimentation in a sucrose gradient of DNA purified from P_3HR-1 virus. **c** Buoyant density profile of DNA of Raji cells labeled during mock-infection; $\varrho = 1.698$ g-cm^{-3} is the buoyant density of cellular (Raji) DNA. **d** Sedimentation profile in a sucrose gradient of the DNA of Raji cells labeled during superinfection with P_3HR-1 virus. *Closed circles*, cpm $\times$ 10^{-6}. *Arrow* indicates position of 59S. (Shaw et al., 1977)

To remove as much of the contaminating cellular DNA as possible from the virus preparation, digestion with pancreatic deoxyribonuclease is essential. This treatment does not affect the virion DNA, nor does it necessarily digest the mycoplasma DNA. The final steps of virus DNA purification are repeated equilibrium centrifugation in CsCl followed by a single velocity sedimentation centrifugation. We locate the virus DNA in CsCl gradients by mixing with it a trace quantity of ^{32}P-labeled virus DNA prepared by superinfection of Raji cells. The profile obtained is shown in Fig. 1 a. As there is little internal heterogeneity of density in EBV DNA, the ^{32}P marker can be sheared before isopyknic centrifugation with little change in its buoyant density. Shearing ensures that the labeled marker does not sediment with the unlabeled virus DNA during the subsequent velocity centrifugation step. The use of ^{32}P-labeled marker is convenient because it reduces manipulation of the virus DNA during purification and allows its location in density gradients directly. The virus DNA is located on sucrose gradients by adsorbance at 260 nm (Fig. 1b). Here care must be taken not to shear the DNA at this point.

III. RADIOLABELING OF NUCLEIC ACID PROBES

The two most critical requirements for molecular hybridization technology are the purity and specificity of the probe, i.e., its freedom from nonviral nucleic acid sequences, and adequate specific radioactivity. With the exception of an in vivo system described later the nucleic acid probes for EBV have to be prepared by labeling in vitro because of the lack of an efficient infection system for the production of virus in cell culture. The desired level of radioactivity is generally in excess of 10^6 counts per minute per microgram of nucleic acid.

A principal problem of in vitro labeling is the uniform distribution of the radiolabel in the nucleic acid to be used as probe. Bacterial DNA and RNA polymerases do not necessarily copy sequences uniformly into the probe. For in vitro labeling of DNA with DNA polymerase I the random positioning of nicks introduced by treatment with pancreatic DNase is crucial. For the synthesis of cRNA most, if not all, of the DNA template should be represented in the cRNA. These limitations make it necessary to characterize the viral nucleic acid probes that are prepared by the in vitro methods quantitatively by reconstruction or by saturation hybridization analyses.

Labeling of nucleic acids by direct or indirect iodination techniques should circumvent some of these difficulties. However, although iodination has its uses, iodinated probes have not been applied widely because of several problems that are brought out later in this chapter.

It has recently become possible to label EBV DNA to high specific radioactivity in infected cell cultures with recovery of labeled DNA in pure form suitable for use as probe (Yajima and Nonoyama, 1976; Shaw et al., 1977). This is accomplished by infection of Raji cells with EBV; the method can be used to prepare both intrinsically labeled EBV DNA of the type replicated in this system and also for the preparation of purified viral DNA that can be used as template for the synthesis in vitro of EBV-specific cRNA (Tanaka et al., 1976). The cRNA prepared by this method, however, contains labeled cellular cRNA, which is removed by cycling over nitrocellulose filters to which cellular DNA is attached. These systems have not yet been fully exploited partly because of their novelty, but also in part because the viral DNA synthesized is still being characterized in comparison with authentic virion DNA.

With this exception the best way to insure the purity of the probe is to recover viral DNA from purified extracellular virus. The recovery of intracellular EBV nucleocapsids in a manner similar to HSV nucleocapsids is not reliable; the nucleocapsids carry with them large amounts of cellular DNA that evades elimination. Even purified extracellular virus is contaminated with cellular DNA. For this reason, purified virus is treated with DNase before extraction. The viral DNA extracted from the virus must be purified to physical homogeneity on the basis of sedimentation properties and buoyant density. As a final test of purity we undertake a complete set of analyses of the behavior of probes in the presence of heterologous and homologous nucleic acids; in such tests the background radioactivity must be both low and consistent.

1. Labeling of DNA In Vivo

When Raji cells are superinfected with EBV, a new, presumably virus-specific, thymidine kinase is induced (Chen et al., 1978) and copious viral DNA is replicated (Nonoyama and Pagano, 1972a). This DNA can be labeled to high specific radioactivities with ^{32}P and can be recovered in a radiochemically pure form (Shaw et al., 1977). This is the only system in which EBV DNA can be labeled in vivo to specific activities approaching those of in vitro labeled DNA.

The viral DNA from superinfected cells can also be labeled by exposing nuclei to radioactive DNA precursors; EBV DNA appears to be labeled maximally when an ATP-regenerating system is left out of the reaction mixture (Seebeck et al., 1977). A characteristic of both in vivo and nuclear systems is that there is essentially no labeling of cellular DNA. A difference, however, lies in the low specific activity achieved in isolated nuclei probably due to the fact that most of the viral DNA has been synthesized prior to isolation of nuclei. Also, the uniformity of labeling of representative genomes in nuclei is still unsettled with this procedure which may, however, have something to offer in the future.

To label DNA in vivo with ^{32}P during superinfection, virus from P_3HR-1 cultures is concentrated approximately 250-fold by centrifugation and 3 ml of the concentrate is used to infect 10^7 Raji cells. After 1 h at 37 °C the cells are diluted with medium; incubation is continued for 3–4 h. The infected cells are washed with phosphate-free Eagle's minimal essential medium (MEM) containing 2% phosphate-free serum; 10^6 cells/ml are labeled with approximately 200 µCi/ml carrier-free ^{32}P in phosphate-free MEM. Incubation is continued for 24 h or longer. To purify ^{32}P-labeled viral DNA, a sarkosyl lysate of the infected cells is digested with pronase, mixed with solid CsCl, and centrifuged to equilibrium.

When all of the cells have been infected the acid-insoluble radioactivity can be recovered from the gradient as a well-defined band at the density of virus DNA (Fig. 1a), whereas the label from mock-infected cells manipulated similarly bands more broadly at the density of cellular DNA (Fig. 1c). If the CsCl step is omitted, and a crude cell lysate is analyzed directly by sedimentation, most of the high molecular weight DNA sediments at 58-59S (Fig. 1d). Most of the high molecular weight DNA can be isolated from nuclei 24 h after infection. The data in Table 1 and Fig. 2 show that the ^{32}P-labeled DNA from superinfected Raji cells can be used as a molecular probe for reassociation experiments.

Table 1. Determination of the number of viral genomes per cell DNA equivalent with ^{32}P-labeled EBV DNA from superinfected Raji cells as probe

DNA source	Number of viral genomes per cell DNA equivalent	
	Predicted	Determined
Raji	50–60	50
P_3HR-1	400–800	362
EBV	5.8	6.0
698[a]	<0.4	<0.4

[a] EBV DNA-negative lymphoblastoid cell line (Klein et al., 1974b; Nilsson and Sundström, 1974).

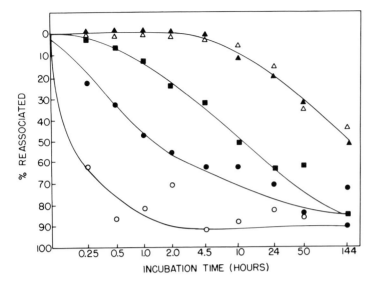

Fig. 2. Kinetics of reassociation of ^{32}P-EBV DNA from superinfected Raji cells. ^{32}P-EBV DNA was reassociated with: calf-thymus DNA (▲——▲), DNA from an EBV genome-negative lymphoblastoid cell line, U-698M (△——△), DNA from purified P_3HR-1 virus (■——■), DNA from Raji (●——●), and DNA from P_3HR-1 cells (○——○). (Shaw et al., 1977)

The efficiency of uptake of label from ^{3}H-thymidine into viral DNA during superinfection increases considerably when infected cells are labeled in phosphate-free MEM rather than RPMI-1640 medium (Yajima et al., 1976). Table 2 shows, however, that the use of MEM, phosphate-free MEM, or RPMI-1640 medium had little influence on the quantity of virus DNA made during superinfection as shown by cRNA-DNA hybridization rather than by incorporation of [3]H. The variation detected in uptake of nucleic acid precursors might occur as a result of mycoplasma contamination of the lymphoblastoid cell lines. In this respect most of the mycoplasmas studied require nucleic acid precursors for growth and interfere with cellular DNA synthesis by competitive utilization of nucleic acid precursors (Stanbridge, 1971).

2. Labeling of DNA In Vitro

The procedure described by Rigby et al. (1977) is suitable for labeling EBV DNA in vitro by nick translation. One advantage of this system, at least as shown for SV40 DNA, is that uniform labeling is achieved. Moreover, specific activities of greater than 10^8 cpm per µg can be obtained. Thus the DNA labeled by this procedure is suitable for use as a probe to detect viral sequences by in situ hybridization as well as reassociation kinetics analysis.

Monitoring of the products of the DNA polymerase reaction by evaluating their susceptibility to S_1-nuclease digestion before and after denaturation is a good practice. The kinetics of digestion of virus DNA labeled in vitro are compared to DNA labeled in superinfected cells. If there is considerable resistance to S_1 after denaturation, the

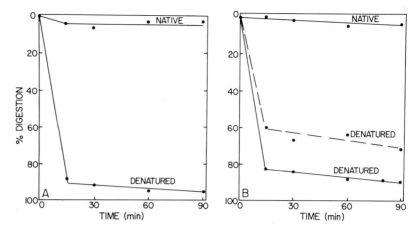

Fig. 3. Kinetics of S_1 nuclease digestion of native and denatured EBV DNA. *Left:* DNA labeled in superinfected cells. *Right:* DNA labeled in vitro with DNA polymerase I from E. coli. *Broken line,* EBV DNA labeled with DNA polymerase I with a reduced $5' \rightarrow 3'$ exonuclease activity

reaction or the polymerase itself is unsuitable. Figure 3 *(left)* shows the kinetics of S_1 hydrolysis of native and denatured viral DNA labeled during superinfection. Figure 3 *(right)* shows similar kinetics for virus DNA labeled in vitro with DNA polymerase I *(continuous line);* this is compared with a denatured product prepared with a different preparation of the polymerase *(broken line)*. The profile *(broken line)* suggests that significant strand displacement has occurred during the polymerase reaction, which created large amounts of rapidly reannealing DNA. Displacement results when the $5' \rightarrow 3'$ exonuclease activity of the enzyme is more labile than the polymerase activity. The loss of exonuclease activity increases with storage of the enzyme and should be monitored frequently. The small amount of hydrolysis that occurs with native DNA most likely is a result of "nibbling" from the ends during S_1 digestion (Rigby et al., 1977). This is not a problem, however, as it is usually less than 10% of the total radioactivity of double-stranded DNA.

Table 2. Effect of PO_4-free medium on viral DNA synthesized during superinfection

Medium	CPM of EBV-cRNA hybridized to DNA from 1.6×10^6 Raji Cells Superinfected	CPM sup./CPM mock.
MEM	45,900	25.0
MEM minus PO_4	44,542	24.3
RPMI	52,698	28.7

The assessment of specific activity is of course a crucial measurement. It can be done by optical methods, or by the diphenylamine test if there is a sufficient quantity of labeled DNA after the nick-translation reaction, or indirectly by assuming that the quantity of DNA added to the reaction mixture is the quantity that remains after nick translation.

3. Complementary RNA

The introduction of cRNA-DNA hybridization in EBV research was important because only small amounts of the virus could be recovered from the single source available at that time, P_3HR-1 BL virus-producing cells. The viral DNA in the virions recovered from these cell cultures could not be intrinsically labeled in the cell cultures to sufficiently high specific radioactivity to permit molecular hybridization except on an elementary and relatively insensitive level – which had, however, been used by zur Hausen and his colleagues to advantage (zur Hausen and Schulte-Holthausen, 1970). The amplification of radiolabeled viral sequences in the form of a cRNA probe continues to have great utility and relatively few limitations despite some early concerns over the fidelity of the copied sequences.

EBV-specific cRNA is still prepared with *E. coli* DNA-dependent RNA polymerase (Burgess, 1969). The details of this procedure are in Huang and Pagano (1977).

Briefly, the reaction (0.25 ml) is carried out at 37 °C for 2–3 h in 0.04 M Tris, pH 7.9, 0.1 M $MgCl_2$, 0.1 mM dithiothreitol, 0.15 M KCl, 0.15 mg/ml bovine serum albumin, 0.15 mM each GTP, ATP, CTP, 0.15 mM ^{3}H UTP (17–30 Ci/mM), 16 units of RNA polymerase, and 2 µg EBV DNA. The incorporation of label into TCA-precipitable material is assayed during synthesis until the level of incorporation reaches a plateau. The DNA is then digested with DNase (RNase-free), SDS is added, and protein is removed by extraction with phenol. The cRNA product is recovered from the excluded volume of G-50 Sephadex and is ready for use.

A somewhat different procedure is used by Lindahl et al. (1976). ^{3}H and ^{32}P-labeled precursors have been used to prepare EBV cRNA with specific radioactivities of 10^7– 10^8 cpm/µg or higher. Iodinated cRNA probes with specific radioactivities exceeding 10^8 cpm/µg have also been prepared (Shaw et al., 1975). The yield of RNA can be estimated from the total acid-insoluble radioactivity and the calculated specific activity. As much as 4 µg RNA can be obtained from 2 µg DNA starting material. The product, checked by velocity sedimentation analysis, is recovered in the 4S–15S range of the gradient with a prominent peak in the 12S–16S region (Nonoyama and Pagano, 1971).

Of concern in the synthesis of cRNA are the percentage of the total template that it represents and the purity of the label. Freedom of the viral DNA preparation from host DNA sequences is crucial inasmuch as they are also amplified. EBV cRNA contains sequences complementary to most or all of the EBV DNA (Lindahl et al., 1976). When hybridized to nonhomologous lymphocyte DNA attached to nitrocellulose the background radioactivity is low, in the range of 100–200 cpm per filter if the template has been purified sufficiently and is free of host-cell DNA. Higher values indicate contamination with cell DNA or the presence of extraneous matter, which causes nonspecific sticking of probe to filters. This is particularly evident if DNA from sucrose gradients is immobilized on nitrocellulose where the radioactivity resulting from nonspecific sticking can be two–four times higher than background. The use of glycerol instead of sucrose can reduce this problem somewhat as can prefiltration of reagents through nitrocellulose.

4. Labeling of DNA and RNA by Iodination Methods

In principle, iodination can yield probes of much higher specific radioactivity. Direct iodination, a chemical method of labeling, has the advantage of avoiding the need for enzymatic procedures. The method of choice for direct labeling of nucleic acids was introduced by Commerford (1971) in which ^{125}I is incorporated into DNA as 5-iodo-cytosine. Both DNA and RNA are labeled in the same way; however, the DNA must be maintained in the single-stranded state during iodination.

Indirect iodination of nucleic acids requires the preparation of iodinated derivatives of cytosine triphosphate or deoxycytosine triphosphate in vitro and insertion of the label from the precursors into the nucleic acids by enzymatic methods. This procedure has been applied to the labeling of herpesvirus nucleic acids (Shaw et al., 1975; Sudgen et al., 1976). The method follows closely that described by Commerford (1971) for direct labeling of DNA.

The reaction mixture (80 µl) is assembled at 0 °C in the following order: 0.1 M sodium acetate -0.04 M acetic acid (pH 5), 4×10^4 pmol dCTP, 17×10^2 pmol Na ^{125}I (3.8 mCi), and 17×10^3 pmol of thallium chloride prepared freshly as a 0.02 M solution. The mixture is heated to 60 °C for 15 min, chilled to 0 °C, then mixed with 20 µl of a freshly prepared solution of 90 mM sodium sulfite to reduce excess thallium chloride. After 2 min at 0 °C, 100 µl 1 M ammonium acetate -0.5 M ammonium hydroxide solution ($\sim$ pH 9) are added and the mixture is heated to 40 °C for 15 min to dissociate unstable intermediates formed during the reaction.

The product is purified by DEAE-cellulose chromatography (Shaw et al., 1975). With the volatile triethylammonium bicarbonate as the elution buffer, purification is essentially a one-step procedure, as the fractions containing the iodinated derivatives can be evaporated to dryness without buffer residue.

Two major radioactive components are resolved by DEAE-cellulose chromatography, unreacted iodine and the nucleoside triphosphate derivative; a minor component which probably represents iodinated dCDP is present as a contaminant or a breakdown product of dCTP. Unreacted nucleoside triphosphate elutes from DEAE-cellulose just before the elution of the iodinated form due to the difference in charge of the two compounds. Because there is little overlapping during elution, the specific activity of the derivative approaches that of carrier-free ^{125}I, which is 2200 Ci/milliatom.

Label from the ribo- and deoxyribonucleoside triphosphate derivatives is incorporated efficiently into RNA or DNA with the appropriate polymerase (Shaw et al., 1975). DNA (denatured) and RNA are susceptible to S_1-nuclease digestion; native DNA is resistant to S_1. RNA is completely digested by pancreatic ribonuclease. Thus the substitution of cytosine residues in RNA and DNA by iodocytosine does not significantly alter the susceptibility of these nucleic acids to nucleases. Iodinated nucleic acids are useful probes for DNA-DNA or cRNA-DNA reactions. The use of iodinated cRNA for in situ location of viral nucleic acids is discussed in Sect. B.VI.

Some of the points to keep in mind during iodination are the molar ratios of ^{125}I-labeled iodine to unlabeled iodine and cytosine, as these ratios determine the specific activity of the product. The reagents must be prepared just before use, particularly oxidizing and reducing agents, since these are less effective if left standing. An important consideration, especially if iodination is carried out in the presence of carrier-free ^{125}I, is the purity of the nucleic acid. Contaminating substances (proteins or extraneous agents in buffers) may be labeled preferentially. Such material tends to stick to columns during purification and gives the illusion that the iodination reaction did not occur.

The advantage of direct iodination is that it is fast and easy to do and yields nucleic acids of high specific radioactivity. Indirect iodination, however, has two major advantages over the direct method. It avoids exposure of the nucleic acid to oxidizing and reducing reagents, pH extremes, and high temperature, and it provides a means of labeling native DNA to high specific activity with iodine.

Several disadvantages of iodination as a means of labeling nucleic acids are: deamination of RNA and DNA which can occur at elevated temperatures and low pH; breakage of polynucleotide chains; failure of DNA to reassociate completely; change in melting profile, buoyant density and sedimentation properties; and change in net negative charge resulting in greater retention of the nucleic acid on anion exchanges. Most of these disadvantages can be minimized, however, if extensive replacement of cytosine for iodocytosine in DNA or RNA and prolonged incubation at high temperature and low pH are avoided. In this respect there were very few changes in the physical properties when bacterial DNA contained 7% of its cytosine as 5-iodocytosine. However, when 24% of the cytosine residues were iodinated the DNA no longer fully reassociated (Commerford, 1971).

IV. DNA-DNA HYBRIDIZATION ON NITROCELLULOSE FILTERS

There has been a renaissance of this classic method in EBV work because sufficient amounts of viral DNA labeled in vivo to high specific activity can now be procured relatively easily (Sect. B. III). The DNA produced by superinfection is an ideal probe for locating virus DNA sequences because it resembles the virion DNA in sedimentation characteristics, buoyant density (see below), the number and kinds of fragments produced by restriction endonucleases (although the fragments may differ in terms of their molar ratios), and the extent to which it reassociates with virus DNA, namely, 90% or more (Fig. 2).

We have used such DNA both as a marker and hybridization probe to determine the buoyant density of purified episomal DNA of Raji cells. A trace of ^{32}P-labeled EBV DNA prepared by superinfection was mixed with purified episomal DNA and run to equilibrium by isopyknic centrifugation. The marker label was located after centrifugation by counting nitrocellulose discs to which the DNA of each gradient fraction was attached. The episomal DNA sequences were located by DNA-DNA hybridization on the nitrocellulose filters. The experiment was designed so that the DNA marker alone on a gradient could not be detected by hybridization.

Coincident peaks of the marker label and hybridizing DNA should result if the purified episomal DNA and marker DNA had identical buoyant densities. This was not the case as shown in Fig. 4; the densities differ by 0.003 g/cm^3. With unlabeled DNA from superinfected Raji cells, P$_3$HR-1 cells, and purified virion DNA, each mixed with a trace quantity of the marker and centrifuged to equilibrium, the peaks were coincident with marker DNA as shown in Fig. 5. Thus, Fig. 5A shows that substitution of phosphate in DNA by ^{32}P was not sufficient to cause the density shift and Figs. 5B and C show that total viral DNA from P$_3$HR-1 cells and DNA purified from P$_3$HR-1 virus have identical buoyant densities. The small difference in buoyant

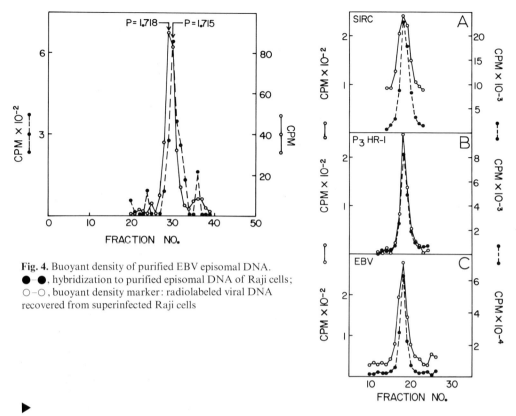

Fig. 4. Buoyant density of purified EBV episomal DNA.
●—●, hybridization to purified episomal DNA of Raji cells;
○—○, buoyant density marker: radiolabeled viral DNA
recovered from superinfected Raji cells

Fig. 5. Buoyant density of viral DNA labeled during superinfection compared with the density of unlabeled DNA from Raji cells, P₃HR-1 cells, and P₃HR-1 virus. ○—○, DNA labeled during superinfection of Raji cells with P₃HR-1 virus; ●—●, EBV DNA (cpm) hybridized to gradient fractions

density of the intrinsic EBV DNA in Raji cells from that of virion DNA observed by Adams et al. (1973) when total cellular DNA was analyzed is due, therefore, to a difference in density of the episomal DNA itself and not necessarily the result of linear virus-cell joint molecules arising from integrated viral DNA.

V. RNA-DNA HYBRIDIZATION ON NITROCELLULOSE FILTERS

Complementary RNA-DNA hybridization, first described by Gillespie and Spiegelman (1965), requires that DNA be denatured and immobilized on nitrocellulose filters. Denaturation is effected with alkali or by heating in a low salt concentration to 100 °C for 10 min and rapid cooling. The alkali-denatured DNA must be neutralized under conditions in which the DNA remains in single strands.

Denatured DNA is made 6 X with SSC (1 X SSC is 0.15 M sodium chloride -0.15 M sodium citrate) and passed through a nitrocellulose filter. The filters are washed briefly and dried before heating under vacuum at 80 °C for at least 4 h.

The filters are placed in 1 ml 6 X SSC containing $1-2 \times 10^5$ cpm of cRNA (approximately 3 ng) and heated to 66 °C (Huang and Pagano, 1977) or are placed in

50% formamide − 6 X SSC and incubated at 45 °C (Lindahl, 1976). Following incubation for 24 h or longer, the filters are washed, then exposed for 1 h at room temperature (or 37 °C for 30 min) to 20–30 µg/ml of pancreatic ribonuclease (DNase-free) in 2 X SSC, dried thoroughly and counted.

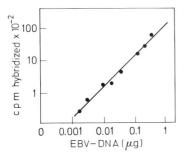

Fig. 6. Hybridization of EBV cRNA to EBV DNA (Nonoyama and Pagano, 1971)

The basis for calculation of the number of EBV genome equivalents detected by hybridization with cRNA is illustrated in Fig. 6, which shows a reconstruction curve where the number of counts/min hybridized is plotted against precisely determined amounts of EBV DNA. With such a curve it is possible to calculate the number of genome equivalents of EBV DNA per cell (Table 3).

This estimation is based on the ratio of the mass of virus and cell DNA; 10^8 daltons per virus genome divided by 4×10^{12} daltons per diploid cell is the ratio of one genome equivalent. From this ratio and knowledge of the counts/min which hybridize to the known quantities of virus DNA the amount of virus DNA in any cell preparation can be assayed reproducibly.

VI. COMPLEMENTARY RNA-DNA CYTOHYBRIDIZATION IN SITU

Cytohybridization was developed by Gall and Pardue (1971) and Jones and Corneo (1971). It was first used in EBV systems by Wolf et al. (1973) and Pagano and Huang (1974). In this procedure hybridization of the EBV cRNA is carried out directly in fixed cells or nuclei rather than to extracted cellular DNA affixed to membrane filters. The unique feature of the technique is that it makes possible the localization of viral DNA to specific cell types or intracellular location by autoradiographic techniques. The limitation of this technique is its insensitivity compared with cRNA-DNA hybridization on membrane filters. However, this insensitivity is only relative. Sixty genome equivalents of EBV DNA contained in Raji cells produce 10–15 grains per cell, perceptibly above background after a 4-week exposure with the same cRNA probe used in membrane hybridization (Pagano and Huang, 1974). The technique may actually be more sensitive than membrane hybridization if most of the viral DNA is confined to a few cells in a large mixed cell population. This procedure obviously complements the information that can be obtained by cRNA hybridization to extracted DNA.

In in situ hybridization suspended cells, nuclei or tissue sections are fit material for examination. The cellular material is fixed to a slide by acid-alcohol fixation and

Table 3. DNA-RNA hybridization tests[a, b]

DNA on filter	cRNA hybridized (cpm/50 μg DNA)	Estimated number of genome equivalents per cell
HR-1 BL	12,131	680
32 °C for 10 days	17,392	810
IF negative[c]	596	32
Raji BL		
IF negative	1126	65
Chromosomal fraction (Raji)	1099	62
EBV infected[d]	22,617	1170
6410 myelogenous leukemia	803	45
F-265 normal patient	1650	100
NC-37 healthy human donor	1343	80
HeLa human carcinoma	152	<2
HEp-2 human carcinoma	126	<2

[a] Nonoyama and Pagano, 1971.

[b] 150 cpm, the hybridized value for HeLa cell DNA, was subtracted to estimate the number of viral genome equivalents.

[c] HR-1 cell line that no longer sheds EBV.

[d] Raji cells were superinfected with EBV and the DNA was extracted after 48 h of infection.

exposed to gentle denaturation in alkali. The acid treatment also partially denatures the cellular DNA in situ. Since this treatment causes some damage to cell structure, it is important to use conditions that minimize the damage. After the DNA has been partially denatured in situ, the preparation is exposed to radiolabeled cRNA, either tritiated or iodinated. Hybridization is allowed to take place under conditions and for the length of time similar to those used for cRNA-DNA hybridization on membrane filters. After hybridization has been completed, extensive washing and treatment with RNase is carried out before autoradiography. Examples of in situ hybridization are shown in Figs. 7A–C. In situ hybridization with ^{125}I-labeled CMV cRNA has been used to locate viral DNA in infected human kidney cells (Shaw et al., 1975). Although the grain size produced by ^{125}I disintegration was approximately four times that produced by ^{3}H decay under similar conditions, ^{125}I produced visible grains within 5 days, whereas ^{3}H required 3–4 weeks of exposure.

Figure 7 A shows the use of ^{3}H-labeled cRNA in situ to distinguish cells in which there is active replication of EBV DNA in the virus-producing line, P_3HR-1.

Figure 7 B shows the result of in situ hybridization to DNA of Raji cells. There is a homogeneous distribution of grains in the cells and although the number of grains per cell is low it is still higher than the background.

Figure 7 C reveals that large amounts of EBV DNA are present in epithelial cells recovered from throat washings of patients with infectious mononucleosis (IM).

VII. DNA-DNA RENATURATION KINETICS ANALYSIS AND GENOME HOMOLOGY

Reassociation of denatured DNA follows second-order reaction kinetics in which the rate-limiting step is an in-register collision at sites along pairs of single-stranded

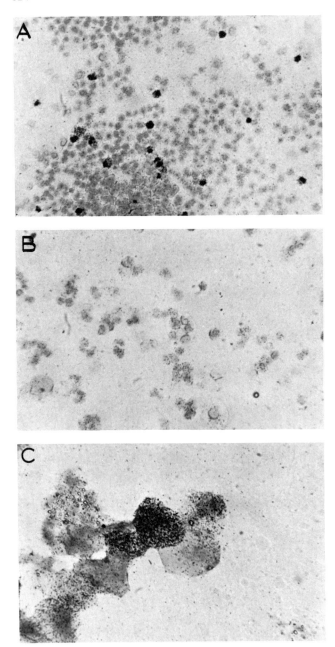

Fig. 7 A–C. In situ cytohybridization with EBV ^{3}H-cRNA. **A** P$_3$HR-1 cells; **B** Raji cells; **C** Epithelial cells from a throat washing of a patient with infectious mononucleosis (IM)

complementary segments of DNA (Wetmur and Davidson, 1968). The reaction is explained by the equation C/Co = 1/(1 + K Cot), in which C is the concentration of single-stranded DNA, Co is the total DNA concentration, K is the reassociation rate constant, and t is the time (Britten et al., 1974). The units for C and Co are moles of nucleotides per liter; t is in seconds. K, the reassociation rate constant, depends on the incubation conditions and complexity of the DNA and is the reciprocal of the Cot_{50} value (see below). The DNA complexity, DNA concentration, length of the single-stranded segments, viscosity, temperature, and salt concentration affect the rate of reassociation; usually most of these parameters are standardized so that the reaction becomes directly dependent on DNA concentration.

Hydroxyapatite has been used to measure the extent of reassociation because of its capacity to retain only double-stranded DNA at low but not high salt concentrations (Kohne and Britten, 1971). Alternatively, single-stranded DNA in the reaction can be selectively digested by a single-strand specific nuclease such as S_1 from *Aspergillus oryzae* (Ando, 1966; Vogt, 1973), which leaves only the double-stranded DNA precipitable from the digest. Nucleases of this type have the advantage that they will digest noncomplementary regions in partially double-stranded DNA, which otherwise would be retained by hydroxyapatite.

When DNAs are compared by DNA-DNA reassociation it is usually at Cot_{50}, the value obtained when 50% of the single-stranded DNA has reassociated. In a reassociation experiment, labeled virus probe is mixed with an excess of the unlabeled cellular DNA being tested for virus DNA sequences. The DNAs are sheared, denatured, and incubated at the temperature, salt concentration, and pH optimal for reassociation of the virus sequences. During reassociation, aliquots are removed to determine the percentage of the label that is resistant to S_1 or binds to hydroxyapatite in low salt solution. The results are plotted as percentage of double-stranded DNA *vs* Cot. The plots would be identical if unlabeled virus sequences were absent in the cellular DNA preparation. The presence of virus sequences, on the other hand, would increase the rate of reassociation of the labeled viral DNA in the test sample.

DNA-DNA reassociation kinetics analysis has been used to examine the degree of homology of the viral sequences in IM cell lines (Fig. 8). 30%–35% of the DNA sequences of P_3HR-1 virus could not be detected in the four cell lines derived from two patients.

Reassociation experiments are not without some pitfalls, many associated with the labeled DNA probe. Probes prepared in vitro by enzymatic methods or chemically as in direct iodination should be monitored for resistance to S_1 in the native state and susceptibility after denaturation or monitored in a similar fashion by hydroxyapatite chromatography. Hydroxyapatite varies from batch to batch and should be evaluated with a DNA the characteristics of which have been established before and after denaturation. This precaution also applies to new preparations of single-strand specific nucleases. The size of the labeled DNA should be checked routinely since the size of the DNA fragments influences their rate of reassociation. The labeled probe should fully reassociate in the presence of a large excess of unlabeled homologous DNA. Failure to do so makes the labeled DNA unsuitable for reassociation experiments in which quantitative information is needed. To obtain an accurate zero time of reassociation, especially if sequences homologous to the probe are present at a high concentration, it is necessary to dilute the DNA immediately after denaturation and determine the percentage of label which is resistant to S_1 or binds to hydroxyapatite at low salt concentration. This is a useful procedure for estimating the amount of "snap back," i.e., complementary sequences in single fragments which rapidly form double-stranded structures independent of DNA concentration.

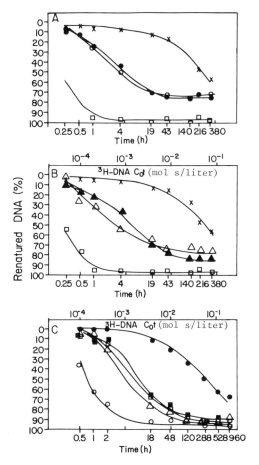

Fig. 8 A–C. Homology of EBV (P₃HR-1) DNA with viral DNA of IM cell lines. **A** Incomplete homology of EBV DNA with DNA PB20 (○ – ○), a line derived from peripheral blood, and with DNA from TW20 (●–●), a cord lymphocyte line transformed by throat washings from the same patient; (□ – □), P₃HR-1 DNA; (× – ×), calf-thymus DNA. **B** Incomplete homology of EBV DNA with DNA from PB16 (△ – △), a cell line established from peripheral blood, and with TW16 (▲– ▲), a cell line produced by exposure of cord blood to throat washings from the same patient. (□ – □) and (× – ×), same as for **A. C** Control hybridization of EBV (P₃HR-1) DNA with calf-thymus DNA (●–●), P₃HR-1 DNA (○ – ○) and increasing concentrations of Raji DNA (■–■, □ – □, △ – △). (Pagano et al., 1976)

DNA-DNA reassociation kinetics analysis has been used to show that a transforming strain of EBV (B95-8) is missing approximately 15% of the DNA sequences of P₃HR-1 virus, a nontransforming strain (Pritchett et al., 1975). In another study kinetic hybridization data suggest that B95-8 DNA may contain sequences which the P₃HR-1 DNA lacks (Sugden et al., 1976). Similar analyses were used to show that a lymphoblastoid cell line derived from a chimpanzee infected with an agent antigenically similar to human EBV lacked 55%–65% of the DNA sequences of the human virus (Gerber et al., 1976a). Rabin et al. (1978) have described "Herpesvirus pongo" isolated from an orangutang B-lymphocytic line which bears 30%–40% homology to EBV. Other isolates related to EBV have been described by Falk et al. (1976) and Rasheed et al. (1977). See also Chap. 17.

Finally, Fig. 2 shows that at least 90% of the viral DNA labeled during superinfection of Raji cells with P_3HR-1 virus reassociates with P_3HR-1 virus DNA.

VIII. RNA-DNA RENATURATION KINETICS ANALYSIS

This method has been used by Hayward and Kieff (1976) and Orellana and Kieff (1977) to determine the percentage of the EBV genome which is expressed as RNA in productive, nonproductive and abortively infected cell lines. The procedure uses virus DNA labeled in vitro as probe and unlabeled RNA extracted from lymphoblastoid cells to drive the labeled DNA into RNA-DNA hybrids. The expression, Rot (moles nucleotides of RNA × s/liters), is used to express the data quantitatively. Results of such analyses are shown in Fig. 9 and discussed later (Sect. C).

In this type of hybridization two populations of molecules reassociate, RNA with DNA and DNA with DNA. A kinetic description of RNA-DNA reassociation can only be approximated because the mere presence of RNA sequences complementary to the DNA probe influences the rate of DNA-DNA reassociation, a parameter that has to be rigorously controlled. In other words, as RNA-DNA hybrids form, the concentration of DNA sequences in the reaction that are available for hybridization decreases. Therefore, the rate of DNA-DNA reassociation in the reaction would be slower than the corresponding rate of a control which contained only homologous DNA.

To minimize the influence of self-reassociation of DNA, the DNA probe sequences are present at a very low concentration such that they do not reassociate to any

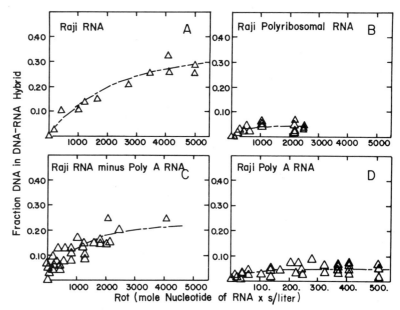

Fig. 9 A–D. RNA-driven renaturation kinetics with unlabeled EBV RNA and denatured ^{3}H-labeled EBV (P_3HR-1) DNA. **A** Total RNA; **B** Polyribosomal RNA; **C** RNA minus polyadenylated RNA; **D** Polyadenylated RNA. (Orellana and Kieff, 1977)

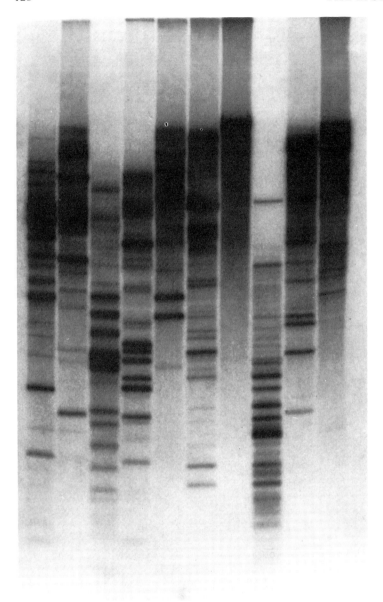

KpnI   HinbIII   SstI   XhoI   SalGI   HpaI   BamHI   SmaI   EcoRI   XbaI

Fig. 10. Restriction endonuclease digestion patterns of ³²P-EBV DNA labeled during superinfection. Patterns represent complete digests of EBV DNA with the exception of Hpa I, Bam HI, and Sma I, which show partial digestion products

appreciable extent during the period of hybridization. By this time, theoretically, the DNA sequences would have driven the probe sequences to the fullest extent possible into RNA-DNA hybrids.

Several additional controls should be included in this type of experiment. If a single-strand specific nuclease like S₁ is used to discriminate between double and single-stranded molecules, the efficiency with which it degrades single-stranded probe DNA and the resistance of native DNA to digestion with the enzyme should be monitored. Since ribonuclease is difficult to eliminate from cellular preparations, measures should be taken to limit its activity, such as including SDS during hybridization. The presence of ribonuclease can be monitored by including labeled RNA in a control mixture and assaying for the presence of acid-precipitable radioactivity during the course of hybridization. Finally, only RNA in the cellular preparation should accelerate the reassociation rate. To show that this is the case and that unlabeled DNA sequences are not an influence, a control in which the cellular preparation is treated with base to hydrolyze RNA before reassociation should be included. The rate of reassociation after base hydrolysis should be the same as that obtained when only probe sequences are reassociated.

IX. RESTRICTION ENDONUCLEASE ANALYSIS

Restriction endonucleases recognize specific cleavage sites on DNA. An expanding library of these enzymes has been used to analyze EBV genomes as well as the viral DNA of EBV genome-carrying cell lines (Hayward et al., 1976; Shaw et al., 1977; Lee et al., 1977; Sugden, 1977).

Figure 10 shows the patterns produced when ^{32}P-labeled EBV DNA produced by superinfection is digested with various restriction endonucleases and analyzed by electrophoresis on a 0.5% agarose gel. With the exception of Bam HI and Sma I endonucleases, these limit digests as determined by the complete digestion of adenovirus DNA, which was included as a control for each restriction enzyme and identified by ethidium-bromide staining before drying the gel for autoradiography.

In general, analysis of EBV DNA by restriction enzymes has shown that different cell lines can yield different patterns, indicating that diverse strains of EBV exist. Indeed differences between the restriction patterns of a transforming (B95-8) and nontransforming strain (P_3HR-1) of EBV have been reported (Sugden et al., 1976; Hayward and Kieff, 1977).

Restriction enzymes have been used in an attempt to identify putative "transforming sequences" of EBV DNA from B95-8 virus (Kieff et al., 1977) believed to represent only 2%–3% of the virus genome. Because they are apparently absent in the DNA of a nontransforming strain (P_3HR-1), these sequences were postulated to contain the genes responsible for transformation.

Linkage maps of the W-91 and B95-8 genomes have been constructed with the Hsu I, Eco RI, and Sal I enzymes (Given and Kieff, 1978) (Figs. 11 and 12).

X. SOUTHERN TRANSFER TECHNIQUE

Southern (1975) has coupled restriction endonuclease methodology and hybridization procedures with a technique that permits nanogram quantities or less of unlabeled DNA in a digest to be detected after resolution by electrophoresis on agarose gels. The Southern procedure involves transfer of electrophoretically resolved fragments directly to a sheet of nitrocellulose which serves as the solid support for the unlabeled DNA during hybridization. As only single-stranded DNA binds efficiently to nitro-

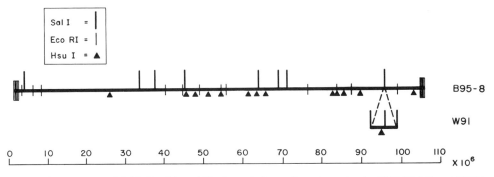

Fig. 11. Arrangement of Sal I, Eco RI, and Hsu I restriction endonuclease sites in EBV (B95-8) and (W91) DNAs. (Kieff et al., 1978)

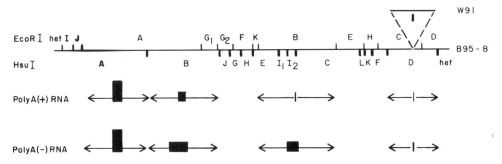

Fig. 12. Map of Eco RI and Hsu I restriction endonuclease fragments of EBV (B95-8) and (W91) DNA. The *arrows* indicate the region of the DNA in which there is homology to Namalwa poly A(+) and poly A(−) RNA. The *width of the bar* indicates the amount of DNA homologous to RNA within the region. The *height of the bar* indicates the relative abundance of homologous RNA. (Kieff et al., 1978)

cellulose the gel is exposed to alkali to denature the DNA, which is then neutralized before transfer. After transfer, the nitrocellulose is dried then heated to 80°C under vacuum for at least 3–4 h to fix the DNA to the sheet. Labeled DNA or cRNA can be used as probe to locate the unlabeled DNA sequences on the nitrocellulose sheet. Following hybridization the label is detected by autoradiographic or fluorographic procedures.

This procedure has been used to compare the restriction patterns of intracellular EBV DNA in tumor specimens and the EBV DNA of clones of transformed cells (Sugden et al., 1977) with the conclusion that the differences in cleavage patterns of viral DNA in the tumor cells and in the cells transformed in vitro were no greater than the differences found between the different clones of the cells transformed in vitro. By use of the Southern technique we compared the Xho I restriction cleavage patterns of viral DNA from P_3HR-1 cells and Raji cells (Fig. 13).

Several fragments are common to both Raji and P_3HR-1 cells. However, it is evident that fragments in the Raji digest are missing from the digest of P_3HR-1 DNA and that several fragments of P_3HR-1 DNA are missing from the Raji digest.

Micrococcal nuclease digestion, the Southern transfer technique, and molecular hybridization have been combined to probe the structure of EBV DNA in nuclei of

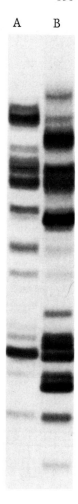

Fig. 13 A and **B.** Southern transfer and hybridization to restriction fragments of EBV DNA. **A** Total digest of Raji DNA; **B** Total digest of P$_3$HR-1 DNA

transformed cells (Shaw et al., 1979). The combination of procedures revealed quite clearly the nucleosomal arrangement of EBV DNA in Raji cells.

The Southern procedure allows remarkable resolution of most of the fragements after transfer. However, fragments which migrate very close to each other may appear as a single broad band upon hybridization since some diffusion inevitably occurs during the transfer procedure. A disadvantage of this system is that high molecular weight fragments do not transfer to nitrocellulose with the same efficiency as do the lower weight fragments. Once transferred, however, high molecular weight DNA binds much more efficiently and is less likely to be lost during hybridization than the lower molecular weight DNA. Another disadvantage lies in the impossibility of analyzing RNA by this technique since RNA does not, in general, bind to nitrocellulose efficiently.

A new procedure described by Alwine et al. (1977) permits RNA or DNA to be transferred and bound irreversibly to a solid support. In this procedure, single-stranded nucleic acids are bound covalently to diazobenzyloxymethyl-paper. Unlike the Southern technique, which is at best semi-quantitative, this procedure permits quantitation of the DNA or RNA on the diazotized paper. Both procedures, however, are limited by the inefficiency with which large fragments transfer from gels.

C. WHAT WE HAVE LEARNED

After EBV had been associated with BL and nasopharyngeal carcinoma (NPC) by immunologic means, development of the idea that the virus might be the causative agent for these two malignancies came to a standstill. Not all patients with these cancers had exceptionally high titers of EBV antibodies, and most of the population worldwide also had antibodies to the virus, so that there was no unique or even consistent association between virus infection and the lymphoma or the carcinoma. Both tumors were virus-free in vivo, and BL cell lines did not inevitably yield virus upon cultivation. NPC cells could not be cultivated in vitro except later to a limited extent after passage in nude mice.

Against this background perhaps the single most important contribution of molecular hybridization to the EBV field was the demonstration that virtually all NPCs and African BLs contain viral DNA even though they were free of detectable infectious virus or its antigens (Pagano, 1974, 1975, 1977; Klein, 1975). This demonstration established a unique relation between the genetic information of the virus and the two tumor types in a manner reminiscent of the relation between viral genes and tumor tissue in experimental systems such as SV40 and adenovirus. It established also for the first time the consistency of the associations. The few exceptions encountered in which EBV DNA has not been found in either BL or NPC probably have a trivial basis in misdiagnosis, mishandling of samples, or inadequate tumor cells in the specimen (this is not, however, the case in American BLs which only occasionally contain detectable EBV sequences [Pagano et al., 1973; Andersson et al., 1976; Gravell et al., 1976]).

From the first, however, the relatively large amount of viral sequences detectable by cRNA-DNA hybridization in tumor tissue and cell lines was surprising and unprecedented by the findings in SV40-induced tumors. As it turned out, the bulk of the viral DNA being detected in the tumor cells was the plasmid or episomal form of EBV DNA and not integrated viral sequences. To this day it is an open question as to what proportion of the viral DNA in tumor cells of either BL or NPC is actually integrated, if any. This vital question is discussed in Chap. 8 by Adams. The detection of the episomal or plasmid form of the EBV genome was achieved by cRNA-DNA hybridization (Nonoyama and Pagano, 1973). The episomes exist in the cell as supercoiled molecules and they can now be isolated in pure form (Lindahl et al., 1976).

The increased sensitivity of DNA-DNA renaturation kinetics analyses has conferred little advantage in the detection of EBV DNA in tumor tissues inasmuch as few, if any, specimens harbor less than the amount of viral DNA already detectable by the less sensitive cRNA-DNA hybridization technique. However, renaturation kinetics analyses did confirm the number of copies of EBV genomes estimated by the cRNA-DNA technique, which was used earlier, and have had some utility in confirming negative results as in the analysis of American BL. The first set of four such tumors could be said to contain less than two EBV genome equivalents per cell on the average by cRNA-DNA hybridization and less than 0.4 genome equivalent by renaturation kinetics analysis.

Principally, renaturation kinetics analysis has enlightened us about partial genomes retained in tumor or cell lines, genome homology, and possible virus-strain differences. In the case of BL, the analyses conducted to date indicate that EBV sequences are present in Ugandan as well as Kenyan tumor tissue (Olweny et al., 1977). There is at least 90% homology of the viral sequences contained in tumors from these two regions of Africa in relation to P_3HR-1 EBV DNA probe (unpublished data, Pagano, Shaw, Harris, and Olweny). More tumor samples will have to be analyzed under strictly identical conditions before we can be sure that there are no differences – indeed it would be surprising if there were none – but so far major differences in homology have not emerged. This impression is confirmed by the recent work of Sugden (1977).

In the single of seven American BLs that contained detectable amounts of EBV DNA which we have examined, there may again be at least 90% homology to the P_3HR-1 probe (Gravell et al., 1976). This result is in contrast to the lesser degree of homology that we have found in some other materials of American origin which, however, stem from IM rather than lymphomatous origin (Pagano et al., 1976). An intriguing question is whether two classes of EBV genomes can be distinguished in the USA, one associated with the rare malignancy, BL, and the other associated with IM. This classification is not expected to be a simple one inasmuch as the large spectrum of virus-strain differences found with other herpes-group viruses will probably hold true also for EBV.

In the case of NPC, we have presented evidence that not all of the viral sequences found in the P_3HR-1 probe can be detected in at least some specimens of this malignancy (Pagano et al., 1975). Since such analyses of tumor tissue containing a relatively small number of EBV genome equivalents require long annealing times, the results are subject to variations for reasons that have been indicated in Sect. B. VII. Thus we have to accumulate more results before a meaningful pattern is likely to emerge. For such analyses that purport to show incomplete homology, we cannot say whether the result is the consequence of a genome whose size is less than that of the P_3HR-1 probe, but this interpretation is not implausible in light of the work of Kaschka-Dierich et al. (1976), who have shown that the size of the episomal DNA in other NPC biopsies is slightly smaller than the circular DNA of Raji cells. Another possibility is that the episomes of NPC contain reiterated sequences in various proportions to unique sequences. A final conclusion will rest upon reciprocal analyses, which in turn require radiolabeling of EBV probe procured from NPC tissue. Up to now this type of analysis has been impossible inasmuch as NPC tumor tissue does not yield virus. However, the use as probe of episomal DNA from NPC tissue is nearing the realm of the possible.

The analysis of EBV sequences in materials from patients with IM has yielded diverse results. The initial results of analysis of cell lines from three patients seemed to show at least 90% homology to the P_3HR-1 probe (Kawai et al., 1973). However, there is some question as to whether the analyses were sensitive enough to detect relatively minor degrees of nonhomology at that time. Results obtained subsequently, in which both peripheral-blood cell lines and cord-blood cell lines that had been transformed by virus obtained from the throats of patients with IM were compared, indicated that as much as 30%–35% homology to the P_3HR-1 genome might be lacking in materials from at least some patients with IM (Pagano et al., 1976). Obviously strain differences of this magnitude could have a crucial bearing on whether or not a virus has oncogenic effects. As in the case of NPC, reciprocal analyses with a single special exception – B95-

8 virus – have not yet been conducted, but would be needed for a conclusion on a matter of such significance. In the meantime, more results need to be accumulated with analyses conducted under identical conditions and such work is in progress. Other approaches are beginning to shed light on this important question, such as the recovery of supercoiled EBV DNA from IM lines and measurement of their contour lengths (Adams et al., 1977). In this work the contour lengths of episomes obtained from three different cell lines deriving from IM were all less than the contour length of P_3HR-1 virion DNA, but the differences amounted to less than 10% and would not be enough to account for the 20%–25% nonhomology that we have observed in different cell lines. As mentioned earlier, definitive comparisons are just now becoming possible through restriction endonuclease analyses of episomes. This is an area in which heteroduplex analysis by electron microscopy should be fruitful. Denaturation mapping of EBV genomes should complement such an approach (Delius and Bornkamm, 1978).

Other work published in this area is by Kieff and Levine (1974) in which American IM cell lines with at least 90% homology to the P_3HR-1 genome were tested. In their analysis of the B95-8 cell lines, B95-8 viral DNA lacked 15% of the sequences of the P_3HR-1 probe. We had found earlier approximately 35% nonhomology – a disparity that could be due to technical factors. Pritchett et al. (1975) used the fact that the B95-8 cell line is virus-producing to conduct reciprocal DNA-DNA renaturation kinetics analyses with radiolabeled B95-8 EBV DNA as probe. In this way they concluded that B95-8 DNA lacks about 12%–15% of the DNA of P_3HR-1 EBV. The B95-8 virus originally came from a patient who had transfusion mononucleosis rather than classic acute IM. In other words, this virus originated from peripheral lymphocytes circulating in the donor of the blood transfusions and not from fresh virus coming from the throat of an acutely infected person. We now have reason to believe that the virus shed from the throat and the virus recovered from peripheral lymphocytes may differ. Furthermore, B95-8 virus has been passaged throughout its history in marmoset lymphocytes. Finally B95-8 virus, whereas it is like wild-type virus in its ability to transform cord-blood lymphocytes, differs from the P_3HR-1 virus in its inability to superinfect Raji cells (Miller et al., 1975).

Recent contour length measurements by Lindahl of episomes obtained from one of the same cell lines analyzed by Pagano et al. (1976) revealed a length corresponding to somewhat less than 100 million daltons (unpublished data). The viral DNA in this line lacked 30%–35% homology compared with the P_3HR-1 genome. If the softer aspect of this comparison, namely, the renaturation kinetics analysis, is verified, then these data comprise clear evidence that there are major strain differences between the P_3HR-1 genome and IM genome at least as reflected in peripheral-blood cells and cord-blood cells transformed by fresh IM virus.

The relation of these important biologic differences to molecular structure is quite obscure. The fine details of the genomes involved will not come from the relatively crude analysis afforded by DNA-DNA renaturation kinetics. Restriction endonuc- lease coupled with heteroduplex analyses of such molecules should furnish the critical information eventually. In short, a variety of observations are converging on EBV strain differences. However, it is too early for a full understanding. The major lines of investigation have been laid out and more work along them should lead to sound conclusions.

Two additional areas in which DNA-DNA renaturation kinetics analyses have made contributions to Epstein-Barr virology are in the analysis of EBV-like viruses from simian species (Gerber et al., 1976a; Rasheed et al., 1977) and determination of lack of homology to other human herpes-group viruses. One of the simian EBV-like agents was isolated from an orangutang with myelomonocytic leukemia (Rabin et al., 1978). Similar EBV-like agents have been isolated from a chimpanzee (Gerber et al., 1976a) and from baboons (Falk et al., 1976). The chimpanzee cell line is missing 55%–65% of the sequences of human EBV DNA.

This procedure has also been used to show that there is no detectable homology between EBV, HSV type 1 or type 2, and two strains of human CMV (Huang and Pagano, 1974).

Analyses of the EBV-specific RNA found in virus-producing cells compared with a nonvirus-producing cell line have been published by Hayward and Kieff (1977) and Orellana and Kieff (1977). This work was done by RNA-driven DNA renaturation kinetics, the probe being in vitro labeled P_3HR-1 DNA. Analysis of total RNA, polyadenylated RNA, and RNA from the polyribosomal fraction of cells by this technique revealed that productively infected cells such as P_3HR-1 contain viral RNA encoded by approximately 45% of EBV DNA, and almost all of the RNA is polyadenylated. Nonproductive cells (Raji), which express EBV nuclear antigen (EBNA) but do not produce infectious particles, contain EBV RNA encoded by only 30% of the EBV DNA; however, only 5% of the RNA is polyadenylated. The hybridization data for the Raji line are shown in Fig. 9. Abortively infected cells produced by superinfection of the Raji line with P_3HR-1 virus contain RNA encoded by approximately 41% of the viral DNA and only 20% of the viral RNA is polyadenylated.

The first results with identification of the DNA segments encoding for EBV RNA in Raji cells have been published recently (Fig. 12) (Powell et al., 1978). In any case, it is quite clear that the only virus-specified product currently identified in Raji cells, EBNA, does not account for the percentage of the genome represented in EBV-specific messenger RNA. Other viral products are probably expressed in Raji cells; one is almost certainly lymphocyte-detected membrane antigen (LYDMA) (Ernberg et al., 1976). We have some evidence that EBV-associated thymidine kinase is expressed at low levels in Raji cells (Chen, Estes, and Pagano, unpublished data). Finally, we wonder whether some of these transcripts might arise from the episomal rather than from integrated viral sequences (Pagano, 1977; Pagano and Okasinski, 1978; Pagano, 1978).

Complementary RNA-DNA hybridization carried out in cells in situ with the technique known as cytohybridization has embellished the field with a succession of results that have at once pictorial value and a quality of direct information that could be provided in no other way. zur Hausen used the technique in an attempt to show whether EBV DNA was associated with certain chromosomes (zur Hausen and Schulte-Holthausen, 1972). In metaphase-arrested chromosomes from Raji cells there appeared to be a localization of grains to several different chromosomes with a frequency greater than expected as judged from the background distribution of nonspecific grains. This impression was fortified by occasional pairs of grains in isologous regions of chromatids, a localization that seemed unlikely to occur by chance. The results of these experiments were clouded by the level of background radioactivity with the resultant scattering of grains over the cells. The sensitivity of the tests was on the borderline of being able to localize the viral DNA in this way unless many of the 60 copies contained in the Raji cells were concentrated at a single chromosomal locus. However, these experiments were quite novel and at some point they may become feasible technically. The approach needs to be repeated despite the lack of association of EBV DNA with specific chromosomes in somatic cell hybrids inasmuch as the tracer for viral sequences in the latter work was EBNA, an indirect indicator (Glaser et al., 1978).

The cytohybridization technique confirmed vividly (see Fig. 7) the notion that only a few of the P_3HR-1 cells were replicating viral DNA at any given time even though each cell has the potential for replication of viral DNA and production of virus. Similarly the technique confirmed the evidence from cloning of Raji cells that the viral DNA was evenly distributed in the Raji cell population and not concentrated in a few cells in contrast to the virus-producing lines. Interestingly, the technique also has in a sense misled – not through any fault of the technique but rather through misinterpretation. We allude to the abundant viral DNA found in cell lines established from the peripheral blood of patients with IM. Even IM cell lines that did not seem to shed virus contained such large amounts of viral DNA as visualized by this technique as to indicate that there was active DNA replication and probably production of virus, and it was thought that such blood cells were the seat of replication of the virus in vivo. There is, in fact, no evidence that EBV replicates in B cells while they are circulating in the body; viral replication apparently only takes place in such cells when they are explanted. The situation is essentially identical for BL which does not contain evidence of viral structural antigens or replicating viral DNA until BL lines are established in vitro.

One of the most fascinating searches facilitated by cytohybridization was that of zur Hausen and his colleagues who set out to determine the cell type of origin of the viral DNA sequences that had been detected in NPC. In a series of superb experiments zur Hausen and his colleagues (Wolf et al., 1975) overcame the preconception that the EBV sequences found in NPC must be in the infiltrating lymphocytes rather than in the carcinomatous cells since the latter were of epithelial origin. The first results were murky; it was hard to discern whether the grains representing hybridizable material were more heavily concentrated over epithelial cells rather than in the smaller lymphocytes in sections of NPC. Nonetheless, zur Hausen's conclusions were correct as later decisively shown by passage of NPC in nude mice. The mouse passage eliminated the human lymphocytes and generated tumors consisting of human carcinomatous cells that unequivocally contained EBV DNA (Klein et al., 1974a).

This work was the harbinger of the finding that large amounts of EBV DNA consistent with newly replicated DNA (Huang and Pagano, 1974) could be found in epithelial cells recovered by swabbing the throats of patients with acute IM (Lemon et al., 1977). Saliva collected from the Stensen's duct of the parotid gland also contained clusters of cells with very heavy concentrations of viral DNA consistent with the relatively large amount of transforming virus that could be recovered from the throats of such patients. These vivid illustrations provide novel histopathologic insights into what we would now see as the primary event in EBV infection. Features such as the asynchronous nature of the viral replication in the cells are consistent with the prolonged excretion of virus. About half of the cells do not take up trypan blue; presumably replication of these large amounts of virus has killed the cells as is often the case with herpes-group virus replication. Such cells might be more readily shed into the throat. Accumulations of viral DNA were visualized over the nucleus in many cells, an observation consistent with the nuclear site of EBV replication. Obviously, the hybridizable DNA is not restricted to the nucleus inasmuch as encapsidated viral DNA is also detected by the cytohybridization technique and mature virus is found in the cytoplasm and in the extracellular fluid. The concern that virus was being replicated in some other cell type such as the B lymphocyte and then merely adsorbed to epithelial cells is not tenable. This assessment is based on several aspects of the data, but principally through controlled experiments in which fresh transforming virus applied to epithelial cells from an EBV-negative person were also examined by cytohybridization with the result that very little evidence of hybridization was produced. These data are the principal elements in a unifying hypothesis linking EBV in a pathogenetic scheme with IM, BL, and NPC (Pagano and Okasinski, 1978).

EBV was proposed as the principal cause for IM on the basis of cogent sero-epidemiologic data (see Henle and Henle, Chap. 13). However, it took some years afterward – from 1968 to 1977 – to gather the concrete data needed to affirm the etiology. The major deficits in the data were the failure to find direct evidence of virus replication in man during IM, the organ site, and the primary cell type which was the source of the virus. Even after a filterable agent that could transform cord-blood lymphocytes was isolated from the throats of patients, the EBV-specific nature of the agent could only be inferred inasmuch as the transformed lymphocyte lines did not contain any of the EBV antigens known at that time. The virus-specific nature of the transformation was first established by cRNA-DNA hybridization on membrane filters (Pagano, 1974; Miller et al., 1976; Pagano et al., 1976). To this day this demonstration remains the principal means of determining whether EBV is present in bodily secretions, namely, transformation of cord-blood lymphocytes followed by detection of viral sequences in the lymphocytic line; the virus-specific nature of the altered cells can now also be established by the detection of EBNA. The lack of antigens associated with EBV replication in the cord-blood cell lines holds a larger interest. Not only could viral capsid antigen (VCA) and early antigen (EA) not be detected in such lines – a fact established with IM virus isolates in a number of other laboratories including Gerber's (Gerber et al., 1976b) – but the number of copies of the EBV genome was invariably low in contrast to the relatively large number of EBV genome copies that could be found in lymphocytic lines established from the peripheral blood of patients with IM. Peripheral-blood cell lines often display EA and VCA and indeed may shed transforming virus.

The question arises as to how transformation of cord-blood cell lines occurs. Does transformation require an initial round of viral DNA replication? Thorley-Lawson and Strominger (1976, 1978) believe that EBV DNA replication is needed to establish a transformed cord-blood line inasmuch as phosphonoacetic acid (PAA), an inhibitor of EBV replication, prevents transformation of cord-blood leukocytes. Lemon et al. (1978) have evidence that cellular DNA synthesis in EBV-infected cord-blood cells is not inhibited by PAA and they are inclined to attribute the failure to establish transformed lines in the presence of the drug to its effect on the α DNA polymerase of the cell. This is an intriguing question inasmuch as cord-blood lymphocytes seem to be strictly nonpermissive for EBV replication. Moreover, Miller and Robinson's evidence confirmed by Lemon (unpublished data) indicates that an input multiplicity of one is sufficient to initiate transformation of cord-blood lines. Finally, as we have pointed out recently, the scheme proposed by Thorley-Lawson and Strominger would necessitate activation of the virus-induced DNA polymerase transiently for a brief and strictly limited period of replication so that only approximately ten episomes are produced, a subversion of the usual outcome of EBV replication in which cell death is the consequence, and then deactivation of the virus-induced DNA polymerase – all of this transpiring with no EBV antigens except for EBNA being left in the cell. This question deserves the attention it is receiving inasmuch as it is directed to the phenomena of abortive viral replication and formation of the episome and the relation of these events to the enzymes involved with viral replication. This whole question is under active investigation now in this laboratory with the use of acycloguanosine (Elion et al., 1977), which has a more discrete antiviral effect without detectable suppression of cellular DNA at effective drug concentrations (Colby, Shaw, and Pagano, unpublished data).

D. PROSPECTS

From the perspective of the versatile technology illustrated here and from what we have already learned through its application spring an abundance of problems for future research. We conclude this chapter with a view of the mainstreams of current and projected research in the EBV field that, from a biochemical standpoint, are ready for significant inroads and perhaps solutions if we can bring enough imagination to the use of the ample tools at hand. Any hypothesis concerning EBV as a causative agent of disease will almost certainly have validity only if it can meet the test of drawing together in a pathogenetic sense the three quite different disease conditions, two malignant and one benign, with which it is associated. This coherence may be perceived sooner on the cellular level. At this level there are two key issues, the primary and secondary cell types with which the virus interacts and the novel molecular form of the EBV genome with which we are dealing, namely, the EBV episome. This is an attempt to select prospectively some of the key parts and pieces of the research that need to be done and to fit them together in a general outline of the intriguing biologic puzzle posed by EBV and its associated diseases and cellular effects.

We believe that the evidence is now persuasive that the primary cell infected in man by EBV is epithelial in type as brought out earlier. There is work remaining such as counterpart infections carried out in vitro with infection of human epithelial cells by EBV, a task made difficult by the unsuitability of available epithelial cell lines and the difficulty of procuring proper target cells fresh from the human host. Nevertheless, the attempt should be made because it is quite clear that the virus excreted in the throat differs biologically from some laboratory strains in the all-important property of transforming ability. Work being done on the replication of murine CMV in murine epithelial cells kept viable in tracheal organ cultures may be a forerunner of the type of work to be done with EBV (Mäntyjärvi et al., 1977). There is no question now that murine CMV, which replicates in vitro in epithelial cells rather than in fibroblasts, retains the properties essential to its biologic behavior in the intact animal, such as ability to infect or not to infect target cells and the fundamental character of virulence vs avirulence. Murine CMV grown in fibroblasts in culture is reduced to a pallid agent bearing no useful resemblance to the natural virus (Osburn and Walker, 1971; Nedrud, Collier, and Pagano, unpublished data).

Accompanying such work will have to come detailed molecular analyses of the various strains of EBV as they are isolated. DNA renaturation kinetics analyses will be insufficient; they may give an indication of degree of homology, but the genomes have to be characterized in more detail by restriction endonuclease analyses and ultimately by heteroduplex analyses; both of these undertakings should no longer be hindered by the small amounts of viral DNA available up to now. However, a broad, essentially nondirected search for sequence differences is not likely to lead to great revelations. Biologic characteristics of overriding importance such as malignant transformation *vs* benign lymphoproliferation of B cells (bone marrow-derived lymphocytes) are hardly to be traced to a single gene difference in two EBV strains. The process may be as important as the genetic basis, as we have brought out elsewhere (Pagano and Okasinski, 1978) and in Sect. E.

Another experimental aim that deals with the primary infected cell type would be the demonstration of C_3D receptors on human epithelial cells of the oropharynx and parotid ducts. The whole question of the precise nature of EBV receptors and their exact relation to complement receptors is not only interesting in and of itself, but because of what it is likely to tell us eventually about how EBV, perhaps through the capping effects engendered by the virus-receptor interaction, stimulates cellular DNA synthesis and even cell-surface changes tied to lymphoproliferation.

Another prime area should be the delineation of progenitor cells. We have postulated that the formation of progenitor cells for NPC and BL is likely to be a part of the oncogenic process for these two malignancies. In the case of NPC, the progenitor cell would contain EBV genome in an arrested circularized form. The circular form of the EBV genome has, of course, been found in NPC cells (Kaschka-Dierich et al., 1976), It will be much more difficult to find normal epithelial cells with episomes since probably in most cases infection leads to viral DNA replication and death of the cell; an abortive infection would be a rare event. This thought leads to some necessary experiments that would deal with how the EBV genome, which presumably circularizes during the process of replication, becomes fixed in the circular form with cessation of free viral DNA replication. Is the initial replication of viral DNA mediated by the virus-induced DNA polymerase? If this is the case, then the viral enzyme must become repressed inasmuch as the episomal form of the genome is replicated by host DNA polymerase; which species of DNA polymerase, α, β, or γ, is quite unknown. What is the mechanism of repression of the virus-induced polymerase and how does the episomal form of the EBV genome move into a stable association within the chromosomes of the host cell? The episomal form of EBV may be more than the state in which the genome reposes between episodes of reactivation. It may also be the molecular vehicle for the transposition of viral information to the integrated state within the DNA of the host. Presented elsewhere in this book is the mounting evidence that in addition to viral episomes there are indeed integrated viral sequences (Chap. 8). It seems perfectly reasonable that the existence of the circularized form of the EBV genome in apposition to the host genetic material would facilitate integration events.

The replication of EBV in the natural target cells of the host has other puzzling aspects. Oropharyngeal shedding of infectious virus continues for weeks or months and perhaps even for years (Niederman et al., 1976). Is this replication occurring exclusively in epithelial cells? If so, why are there so few symptoms of cell damage in the oropharynx extending over long periods? This might in part be explained by the highly asynchronous nature of the infection as visualized by relatively few cells with active viral DNA replication illustrated in Fig. 7. Perhaps only those epithelial cells that are synthesizing cellular DNA will replicate EBV DNA; there are relatively few epithelial cells that exhibit active DNA synthesis at least in tracheal organ cultures (Hu et al.,

1975). Here again recent work with murine CMV may hold some lessons for us. Under conditions in which every epithelial cell is infected with murine CMV, the tracheal organ cultures are able to replicate virus for as long as the cultures can be maintained in vitro in a viable state, as long as 8 weeks (Nedrud, Collier, and Pagano, unpublished data). In other words, epithelial cells can support viral DNA replication without destruction in utter contrast to the complete lysis that takes place in murine CMV-infected fibroblasts within a matter of days. The biologic evidence from the observations of Niederman et al. (1976) suggests that some kind of protracted infective state for EBV pertains in man. Not only may a few cells be asynchronously infected, but perhaps even infected cells can continue to replicate virus without the usual outcome of herpes-group infection, namely, cell destruction. Does this long drawn-out course of viral replication itself increase the chances for abortive replication and fixation of the episome in some epithelial cells? Insights into these mechanisms may eventually help us to understand how HSV replicates in trigeminal ganglia without apparently destroying the nerve cells (Stevens, 1978) and how chronic cytomegaloviru-ria avoids renal tubular necrosis.

For all of this work, the further definition of virus-induced enzymes and their roles in establishing and maintaining the various forms of EBV DNA in cells has much to offer. New antiviral substances, in particular acycloguanosine (Elion et al., 1977; Schaeffer et al., 1978), should help to unravel some of the issues, for example, the controversy as to whether viral DNA replication is required initially in order to set in motion the process of lymphocyte transformation by EBV, as discussed in Chap. 9. This is not an easy matter to sort out if the inhibitor of viral DNA replication also has an effect on cellular DNA polymerases, in particular α polymerase, which is active in proliferating cells (Weisbach, 1977). Clearly a perfectly discrete inhibitor of viral DNA replication has to be used to settle the question. In the meantime, we are left with two possible chains of molecular events. In the scenario outlined earlier (Sect. C), the EBV DNA polymerase is induced, causes the replication of a few copies of the genome, is then repressed, and the transformed cord cell survives. Another possibility is that the few copies of supercoiled DNA characteristically found in transformed cord-blood cells – which are nonpermissive and nonvirus-producing – represent input genomes perhaps amplified in a strictly limited fashion by host DNA polymerase before the association between episome and host DNA is stabilized, after which host DNA polymerase is certainly responsible for maintaining the episome. Yet a third possibility is that it is in the nature of the nonpermissiveness of cord-blood lymphocytes to abrogate the function of virus-induced DNA polymerase upon its appearance in the cell before viral DNA replication is freely underway and cell destruction can ensue. We do know that cord-blood lymphocytes differ in their response to virus infection compared with lymphocytes from the peripheral blood of mature persons; the latter cells can support the replication of viral DNA and production of virus at least in vitro.

de-Thé has suggested that the early age at which infection of infants occurs in Kenya may augment the chance of BL (de-Thé, 1977). On the cellular level, the fact that cord-blood lymphocytes are not destroyed but enter a stable relation with the viral genetic material would support this notion.

The episomal form of the EBV genome offers other intriguing questions which could not even be asked before in eukaryotic cell biology. These questions center on whether the episomal form of the EBV genome is expressed. According to Orellana and Kieff (1977), 5% of the coding capacity of EBV DNA of Raji is expressed as polyadenylated RNA. Only a single viral function has been unequivocally defined in Raji cells, namely, EBNA; another is suspected, LYDMA (Ernberg et al., 1976), which is defined functionally by cytotoxicity assays first applied by Hutt et al. (1975) and Svedmyr and Jondal (1975). Do these transcripts arise from integrated viral sequences or from the episomal form of the genome? Intuitively we suspect that the episome is not simply an inert repository of the viral genetic material.

One hypothesis is that IM cell lines, which are polyclonal and nonmalignant in character and contain EBNA and the episomal form of the genome, and also proliferate, are under the control of the episomal form of the EBV genome. The virus-directed effects may be dual: release of cellular DNA synthesis and alteration of cell surface, the two effects together materializing in B lymphoproliferation, which stops short of malignant change. Presumably malignant lymphoid cell lines are under the control of specific integrated EBV sequences. It is not going to be easy to sort out the origin of the transcripts, whether from episomal or integrated sequences, particularly inasmuch as with cells continued in culture transposition of viral sequences from episome to integrated state may occur. Obviously the task will be made easier if only a relatively small proportion of the EBV genome is integrated in contrast to the complete or almost complete set of sequences so far found in the episomal forms. If, however, there is substantial representation of the EBV genome in the integrated state, then the task will be rendered much more difficult and the case may have to rest upon display of active transcription on episomes by electron microscopy.

Another aspect of this hypothesis is sure to be the elucidation of the structure and function of EBNA. Is this protein (or, more likely, family of homologs) analogous to other viral proteins such as SV40 T and t antigens with their possible dual function on DNA replication and insertion in plasma membrane, where presumably one of the proteins is a mediator of cell-surface change involved with loss of contact inhibition? (Ito et al., 1977; Tijan, 1978)

Implicit in many of these investigations is the need to ascertain quantitatively integration of viral DNA sequences in both malignant and nonmalignant cell lines and to establish the identity of the inserted sequences. This straightforward aim, already impressively accomplished in adenovirus systems (Sharp et al., 1974) and materially advanced by the work of Adams and Lindahl and their colleagues, has remained elusive because of the difficulty of examining cellular DNA with its possible inserted sequences under conditions in which all remnants of nicked episomal DNA have been removed. However, this work is sure to go forward and the question should be resolved in due course.

E. UNIFYING CONCEPT

Any theory that EBV causes BL and NPC must account for the rarity of these conditions in the face of the near universality of EBV infection. The requirement for a cofactor or vector in the BL belt in Africa and a genetic predisposition in Asiatic peoples for NPC could help to explain the distribution and incidence of these malignancies as considered elsewhere in this book (Chaps. 14 and 15). Another way to view EBV in relation to BL and NPC is from the molecular standpoint with the outcome hinging more on process than on elements, i.e., infection with EBV sets in motion a cascade of cellular and molecular events which can be aborted at any step but must go to completion if malignancy is to result. In a pathogenetic scheme that we have proposed recently (Pagano and Okasinski, 1978; Pagano, 1978), the initial step is precisely the same for all three disease conditions as well as for inapparent infection.

In this conception, some of the evidence for which has been presented in other sections of this chapter, EBV infects and replicates in the epithelial cells lining the mid-pharynx. The infection may be entirely inapparent, may cause only local symptoms, or it may cause the typical syndrome of IM, which probably has its basis, at least in part, in a cell-mediated immunologic response to secondarily infected lymphocytes. The B lymphocyte is infected with transforming virus released by the infected epithelial cells. The infected B lymphocyte apparently does not generate virus and is not destroyed by virus replication while in the body. Thus, a small number of such EBV-infected cells can persist in the circulation provided that they also survive the wave of cytolysis effected by sensitized T cells (thymus-dependent lymphocyte) early in the course of infection.

On the molecular level, it is quite clear that the proliferating EBV-bearing cells carry the episomal form of the EBV genome replicated by host DNA polymerases. Although the IM cells proliferate as if they had undergone malignant transformation, they are not, in fact, believed to comprise malignant clones (Fialkow et al., 1970). We speculate that although there may be frequent crossing over and insertion of viral DNA sequences in the cellular DNA because of the proximity of the episome to the cellular DNA and its replication by the same host polymerases, the change from benign lymphoproliferation to malignant transformation requires the insertion and operation of specific viral "transforming" sequences. These molecular events themselves comprise a process. The implication is that malignant transformation is accompanied by a shift of control of cell growth from episomal sequences to integrated viral genes. The successful establishment of such a clone of cells would not automatically lead to the appearance of a lymphoma, inasmuch as cell-mediated immunologic responses already primed earlier by the proliferation of EBV-bearing lymphocytes have to be overcome.

NPC might arise in a somewhat similar fashion. Viral replication could in occasional epithelial cells be aborted with fixation of the episomal form of the EBV genome in a nonmalignant progenitor cell. Once again, there would be opportunity for insertion of viral DNA sequences from episome into the cellular DNA. With the insertion of critical transforming sequences – perhaps in selected classes of sites in the chromosomes – the emergence of a malignant clone of epithelial cells would become possible. Again, immunologic responses would have to be overcome; also, the likelihood of NPC is greatly enhanced by genetic disposition.

This theory is compatible with the frequency of IM and the infrequency of BL and NPC, the linkage of a benign condition with the two malignant states, as well as the association of the same virus with malignancies of quite different cell types. We have addressed in Sect. D some of the critical points of this hypothesis, feasible experimental approaches, and others to be devised. In one sense the association of EBV with three quite different diseases is paradoxical and complicates proof of an etiologic role. At the same time, however, this remarkable emerging mosaic of virus, cell, and disease interactions offers lines of insight that should eventually converge on an understand-ing of the meaning of the association of EBV with IM, BL, and NPC.

REFERENCES

Adams, A.: Preparation of Epstein-Barr virus from P3HR-1 cells and isolation of virus DNA. In: Epstein-Barr virus, production, concentration and purification. Internal Technical Rep. No. 75003. IARC (1975)

Adams, A., Lindahl, T.: Epstein-Barr virus genomes with properties of circular DNA molecules in carrier cells. Proc. Natl. Acad. Sci. USA **72,** 1477–1481 (1975)

Adams, A., Lindahl, T., Klein, G.: Linear association between cellular DNA and Epstein-Barr virus DNA in a human lymphoplastoid cell line. Proc. Natl. Acad. Sci USA **70,** 288–289 (1973)

Adams, A., Bjursell, G., Kaschka-Dierich, C., Lindahl, T.: Circular Epstein-Barr virus genomes of reduced size in a human lymphoid cell line of infectious mononucleosis origin. J. Virol. **22,** 373–380 (1977)

Alwine, J. C., Kemp, D. J., Stark, G. R.: Method for detection of specific RNA's in agarose gels by transfer to diazobenzyloxymethyl-paper and hybridization with DNA probes. Proc. Natl. Acad. Sci. USA **74,** 5350–5354 (1977)

Andersson, M., Klein, G., Ziegler, J. L., Henle, W.: Association of Epstein-Barr viral genomes with American Burkitt lymphoma. Nature **260,** 357–358 (1976)

Ando, T.: A nuclease specific for heat denatured DNA isolated from a product of *Aspergillus oryzae.* Biochem. Biophys. Acta **144,** 158–168 (1966)

Britten, R. J., Graham, D. E., Neufeld, B. R.: Analysis of repeating DNA sequences by reassociation. In: Methods in enzymology. Grossman, L., Moldane, K. (eds.), pp. 363–418. New York: Academic Press 1974

Burgess, R. R.: A new method for the large scale purification of *Escherichia coli* deoxyribonucleic acid-dependent ribonucleic acid polymerase. J. Biol. Chem. **244,** 6160 (1969)

Chen, S.-T., Estes, J.E., Huang, E.-S., Pagano, J. S.: EBV-associated thymidine kinase. J. Virol. **26,** 203–208 (1978)

Commerford, S. L.: Iodination of nucleic acids *in vitro.* Biochemistry **10,** 1993–2000 (1971)

Delius, H., Bornkamm, G. W.: Heterogeneity of Epstein-Barr virus. III. Comparison of a transforming and a nontransforming virus by partial denaturation mapping of their DNA's. J. Virol. **27,** 81–89 (1978)

de-Thé, G.: Is Burkitt's lymphoma related to perinatal infection by Epstein-Barr virus? Lancet **1977 I,** 335–337

Elion, G., Furman, P., Fyfe, J. A., de Miranda, P., Beauchamp, L., Schaeffer, J. J.: Selectivity of action of an antiherpetic agent, 9-(2-hydroxyethoxymethyl) guanine. Proc. Natl. Acad. Sci. USA **74,** 5616–5720 (1977)

Ernberg, I., Masucci, A., Klein, G.: Persistance of Epstein-Barr viral nuclear antigen (EBNA) in cells entering the EB viral cycle. Int. J. Cancer **17,** 197–203 (1976)

Falk, L., Deinhardt, F., Nonoyama, M., Wolfe, L. G., Bergholtz, C., Lapin, B., Yakovleva, L., Agrba, V., Henle, G., Henle, W.: Properties of a baboon lymphotropic herpesvirus related to Epstein-Barr virus. Int. J. Cancer **18,** 798–807 (1976)

Fialkow, P. J., Klein, G., Gartler, S. M., Clifford, P.: Clonal origin for individual Burkitt tumors. Lancet **1970 I,** 384–386

Gall, J. G., Pardue, M. L.: Nucleic acid hybridization in cytological preparations. In: Methods in enzymology. Grossman, L., Moldane, K. (eds.), Vol. 21, Part D, pp. 470–480. New York: Academic Press 1971

Gerber, P., Pritchett, R. F., Kieff, E. D.: Antigens and DNA of a chimpanzee agent related to Epstein-Barr virus. J. Virol. **19,** 1090–1099 (1976 a)

Gerber, P., Nkrumah, F., Pritchett, R., Kieff, E.: Comparative studies of Epstein-Barr virus strains from Ghana and the United States. Int. J. Cancer **17,** 71–81 (1976 b)

Gillespie, D., Spiegelman, S. J.: A quanitative assay for DNA-RNA hybrids with DNA immobilized on a membrane. J. Mol. Biol. **12,** 829–842 (1965)

Given, D., Kieff, E.: DNA of Epstein-Barr virus: IV. Linkage map of restrictive enzyme fragments of the B95-8 and W-91 strains of EBV. J. Virol. **28,** 524–542 (1978)

Glaser, R., Nonoyama, M., Hampar, B., Croce, C: Studies on the association of the Epstein-Barr virus genome in human chromosomes. J. Cell Physiol. **96,** 319–325 (1978).

Gravell, M., Levine, P. H., McIntyre, R. F., Land, V. J., Pagano, J. S.: Epstein-Barr virus in an American patient with Burkitt's lymphoma: detection of viral genome in tumor tissue and establishment of a tumor-derived cell line (NAB). J. Natl. Cancer Inst. **56,** 701–704 (1976)

Hayward, G. S., Frenkel, N., Roizman, B.: Anatomy of herpes simplex virus DNA; strain differences and heterogeneity in the locations of restriction endonuclease cleavage sites. Proc. Natl. Acad. Sci. USA **72,** 1768–1772 (1975)

Hayward, S. D., Kieff, E.: Epstein-Barr virus-specific RNA. I. Analysis of viral RNA in cellular extracts and in the polyribosomal fraction of permissive and nonpermissive lymphoblastoid cell lines. J. Virol. **18**, 518–525 (1976)

Hayward, S. D., Kieff, E.: DNA of Epstein-Barr virus. II. Comparison of the molecular weights of the DNA of Epstein-Barr virus strains and identification of end fragments of the B95-8 strain. J. Virol. **23**, 421–429 (1977)

Hayward, S. D., Pritchett, R., Orellana, T., King, W., Kieff, E.: The DNA of Epstein-Barr virus: fragments produced by restriction enzymes: homologous DNA and RNA in lymphoblastoid cells. In: Animal virology-Baltimore, D., Huang, E.-S., Fox, C. F. (eds.), pp. 619–639. New York: Academic Press 1976

Hu, P. C., Collier, A. M., Baseman, J. B.: Alterations in the metabolism of hamster tracheas in organ culture after infection by virulent Mycoplasma pneumoniae. Infect. Immunol. **11**, 704–710 (1975)

Huang, E.-S., Pagano, J. S.: Human CMV. II. Lack of relatedness to DNA of herpes simplex I and II, Epstein-Barr virus and nonhuman strains of CMV. J. Virol. **13**, 642–645 (1974)

Huang, E.-S., Pagano, J. S.: Nucleic acid hybridization technology and detection of proviral genomes. In: Methods in virology. Maramorosch, K., Koprowski, H. (eds.), Vol. 6, Chap. 13, pp. 457–497. New York: Academic Press 1977

Hutt, L., Huang, Y.-T., Dascomb, H., Pagano, J. S.: Enhanced destruction of lymphoid cell lines by peripheral blood leukocytes taken from patients with acute infectious mononucleosis. J. Immunol. **115**, 243–248 (1975)

Ito, Y., Brocklehurst, J. R., Dulbeco, R.: Virus-specific proteins in the plasma membrane of cells lytically infected or transformed by polyoma virus. Proc. Natl. Acad. Sci. USA **74**, 4666–4670 (1977)

Jones, K. W., Corneo, G.: Location of satellite and homogeneous DNA sequences on human chromosomes. Nature New Biol. **233**, 268–271 (1971)

Kaschka-Dierich, C., Adams, A., Lindahl, T., Bornkamm, G., Bjursell, G., Klein, G., Giovanella, B., Singh, S.: Intracellular forms of Epstein-Barr virus DNA in human tumor cell in vivo. Nature **260**, 302–306 (1976)

Kawai, Y., Nonoyama, M., Pagano, J. S.: Reassociation kinetics for Epstein-Barr virus DNA: nonhomology to mammalian DNA and homology of viral DNA in various diseases. J. Virol. **12**, 1006–1012 (1973)

Kieff, E., Levine, J.: Homology between Burkitt herpes viral DNA and DNA in continuous lymphoblastoid cells from patients with infectious mononucleosis. Proc. Natl. Acad. Sci. USA **71**, 355–358 (1974)

Kieff, E., Raab-Traub, N., Given, D., Pritchett, R., Powell, A., King, W., Dambaugh, T.: Identification of putative "transformation" DNA sequences of EBV. In: Oncogenesis and herpesviruses III. de-Thé, G., Henle, W., Rapp, F. (eds.). Lyon: IARC (in press) (1978)

Kieff, E., Given, D., Powell, A. L. T., King, W., Dambaugh, T., Raab-Traub, N.: Nucleic acid of Epstein-Barr virus. Biochem. Biophys. Acta (in press) (1978)

Kilpatrick, B. A., Huang, E.-S., Pagano, J. S.: Analysis of cytomegalovirus genomes with restriction endonucleases HinD III and EcoR-1. J. Virol. **18**, 1095–1105 (1976)

Klein, G.: Studies on the Epstein-Barr Virus genome and EBV-determined nuclear antigen in human malignant disease. Cold Spring Harbor Symp. Quant. Biol. **39**, 783–790 (1975)

Klein, G., Giovanella, B. C., Lindahl, T., Fialkow, P. J., Singh, S., Stehlin, J. S.: Direct evidence for the presence of Epstein-Barr virus DNA and nuclear antigen in malignant epithelial cells from patients with poorly differentiated carcinoma of the nasopharynx. Proc. Natl. Acad. Sci. USA **71**, 4737–4741 (1974a)

Klein, G., Lindahl, T., Jondal, M., Leibold, W., Menézes, J., Nilsson, K., and Sundström, C.: Continuous lymphoid cell lines with characteristics of B cells (bone-marrow-derived), lacking the Epstein-Barr virus genome and derived from three human lymphomas. Proc. Natl. Acad. Sci. USA **71**, 3283–3286 (1974b).

Kohne, D. E., Britten, R. J.: Hydroxyapatite techniques for nucleic acid reassociation. Prog. Nucleic Acid Res. **2**, 500–512 (1971)

Lee, Y. S., Yajima, Y., Nonoyama, M.: Mechanism of infection by Epstein-Barr virus. II. Comparison of viral DNA from HR-1 superinfected Raji cells by restriction enzymes. Virology **81**, 17–24 (1977)

Lemon, S., Hutt, L., Shaw, J., Li, J.-L. H., Pagano, J. S.: Replication of EBV in epithelial cells during infectious mononucleosis. Nature **268**, 268–270 (1977)

Lemon, S., Hutt, L., Pagano, J. S.: Cytofluorometry of lymphocytes infected with Epstein-Barr virus: effect of phosphonoacetic acid on nucleic acid. J. Virol. **25**, 138–145 (1978)

Lindahl, T., Adams, A., Bjursell. G., Bornkamm, W., Kaschka-Dierich, C., John, U.: Covalently closed circular duplex DNA of Epstein-Barr virus in a human lymphoid cell line. J. Mol. Biol. **102**, 511–530 (1976)

Mäntyjärvi, R. A., Selgrade, M. J. K., Collier, A. M., Hu, S.-C., Pagano, J. S.: Murine cytomegalovirus infection of epithelial cells in mouse tracheal ring organ culture. J. Infect. Dis. **136**, 444–448 (1977)

Maxam, A. M., Gilbert, W.: A new method for sequencing DNA. Proc. Natl. Acad. Sci. USA **74**, 560–564 (1977)

Miller, G. Robinson, J., Heston, L.: Immortalizing and nonimmortalizing laboratory strains of Epstein-Barr virus. Cold Spring Harbor Symp. Quant. Biol. **39**, 773–781 (1975)

Miller, G., Coope, D., Niederman, J., Pagano, J.: Direct comparison of biologic properties and surface antigens of transforming strains of Epstein-Barr virus from Burkitt's lymphoma and infectious mononucleosis. J. Virol. **18**, 1071–1080 (1976)

Niederman, J. C., Miller, G., Pearson, H. A., Pagano, J. S., Dowaliby, J. M.: Infectious mononucleosis; Epstein-Barr virus shedding in saliva and the oropharynx. N. Eng. J. Med. **294**, 1355–1359 (1976)

Nilsson, K. and Sunström, C. Establishment and characteristics of two unique cell lines from patients with lymphosarcoma. Int. J. Cancer **13**, 808–823 (1974).

Nonoyama, M., Pagano, J.: Complementary RNA specific to the DNA of the Epstein-Barr virus: detection of EB viral genomes in nonproductive cells. Nature New Biol. **233**, 103–106 (1971)

Nonoyama, M., Pagano, J.: Replication of viral DNA and breakdown of cellular DNA in Epstein-Barr virus infection. J. Virol. **9**, 714–716 (1972a)

Nonoyama, M., Pagano, J.: Separation of Epstein-Barr virus DNA from large chromosomal DNA in nonvirus-producing cells. Nature New Biol. **238**, 169–171 (1972b)

Nonoyama, M., Pagano, J.: Homology between Epstein-Barr virus DNA and viral DNA from Burkitt's lymphoma and nasopharyngeal carcinoma determined by DNA-DNA reassociation kinetics. Nature **242**, 44–47 (1973)

Olweny, C. L. M., Atine, I., Kaddu-Mukasa, A., Owor, R., Andersson-Anvret, M., Klein, G., Henle, W., de-Thé, G.: Epstein-Barr virus genome studies in Burkitt's and non-Burkitt's lymphomas in Uganda. J. Natl. Cancer Inst. **58**, 1191–1196 (1977)

Orellana, T., Kieff, E.: Epstein-Barr virus-specific RNA. II. Analysis of polyadenylated viral RNA in restringent, abortive and productive infections. J. Virol. **22**, 321–330 (1977)

Osborn, J. E., Walker, D. L.: Virulence and attenuation of murine cytomegalovirus. Infect. Immunol. **3**, 228–238 (1971)

Pagano, J. S.: The Epstein-Barr viral genome and its interactions with human lymphoblastoid cells and chromosomes. In: Viruses, evolution and cancer. Kurstak, E., Maramorosch, K. (eds.), Chap. 4, pp. 79–116. New York: Academic Press 1974

Pagano, J. S.: The Epstein-Barr virus and malignancy: molecular evidence. Cold Spring Harbor Symp. Quant. Biol. **39**, 797–805 (1975)

Pagano, J. S.: Molecular biological studies implicating the Epstein-Barr virus in the etiology of Burkitt's lymphoma and certain other cancers. In: Cancer research: cell biology, molecular biology and tumor virology. Gallo, R. (ed.), pp. 199–207. Cleveland (Ohio): CRC 1977

Pagano, J. S.: Epstein-Barr virus infection of epithelial cells and lymphocytes. ICN-UCLA Symposia on Molecular and Cellular Biology. (in preparation) (1978)

Pagano, J., Huang, E.-S.: The application of RNA-DNA cytohybridization to viral diagnostics. In: Viral Immunodiagnosis. Kurstak, E., Morrisset, R. (eds.). pp. 279–299. New York: Academic Press 1974

Pagano, J. S., Okasinski, G. F.: Pathogenesis of infectious mononucleosis, Burkitt's lymphoma and nasopharyngeal carcinoma, a unified scheme. In: Oncogenesis and herpesviruses III. de-Thé, G., Henle, W., Rapp, F. (eds.), pp. 687–698. Lyon: IARC (1978)

Pagano, J. S., Huang, C.-H., and Levine, P. Absence of Epstein-Barr viral DNA in American Burkitt's lymphoma. New Eng. J. Med. **289**, 1395–1399 (1973)

Pagano, J., Huang, C.-H., Klein, G., de-Thé, G., Shanmugaratnum, K., Yang, C.-S.: Homology of Epstein-Barr virus DNA in nasopharyngeal carcinomas from Kenya, Taiwan, Singapore and Tunisia. In: Oncogenesis and herpesviruses II. de-Thé, G., Epstein, M. A., zur Hausen, H. (eds.), Part 2, pp. 179–190. Lyon: IARC 1975

Pagano, J., Huang, C.-H., Huang, Y.-T.: Epstein-Barr virus genome in infectious mononucleosis. Nature **263**, 787–789 (1976)

Powell, A., King, W., Kieff, E,: Epstein-Barr virus specific RNA III mapping of DNA-encoding viral RNA in restringent infection. J. Virol. (in press), (1978)

Pritchett, R. F., Hayward, S. D., Kieff, E. D.: I. Comparative studies of the DNA of Epstein-Barr virus from HR-1 and B95-8 cells: size, structure, and relatedness. J. Virol. **15**, 556–569 (1975)

Rabin, H., Neubauer, R. H., Hopkins, R. F., III, Nonoyama, M.: Further characterization of a herpesvirus-positive orangutan cell line and comparative aspects of in vitro transformation with lymphotropic old world primate herpesviruses. Int. J. Cancer **21**, 762–767 (1978)

Rasheed, S., Rongey, R. W., Nelson-Rees, W. A., Rabin, H., Neubauer, R. H., Bruszweskij, E. G., Gardner, M. B.: Establishment of a cell line with associated Epstein-Barr-like virus from a leukemic orangutan. Science **198**, 407–409 (1977)

Rigby, P. W. J., Dieckmann, M., Rhodes, C., Berg, P.: Labeling deoxyribonucleic acid to high specific activity in vitro by nick translation with DNA polymerase I. J. Mol. Biol. **113**, 237–251 (1977)

Sanger, F., Air, G. M., Barrell, B. G., Brown, N. L., Coulson, A. R., Fiddes, J. C., Hutchinson, C. A., III, Slocombe, P. M., Smith, M.: Nucleotide sequence of bacteriophage $\Phi \times 174$ DNA. Nature **265**, 687–695 (1977)

Schaeffer, J. J., Beauchamp, L., de Miranda, P., Elion, G. B., Bauer, D. J., Collins, P.: 9-(2-Hydroxyethoxymethyl) guanine activity against viruses of the herpes group. Nature **272**, 583–585 (1978)

Seebeck, T., Shaw, J. E., Pagano, J. S.: Synthesis of Epstein-Barr virus DNA in vitro: effects of phosphonoacetic acid, N-ethylmaleimide, and ATP. J. Virol. **21**, 435–438 (1977)

Sharp, P. A., Pettersson, V., Sambrook, (Jr.): Viral DNA in transformed cells. I. A study of the sequences of adenovirus DNA in a line of transformed rat cells using specific fragments of the viral genomes. J. Mol. Biol. **86**, 709–726 (1974)

Shaw, J. E., Huang, E.-S., Pagano, J. S.: Iodination of herpesvirus nucleic acids. J. Virol. **16**, 132–140 (1975)

Shaw, J. E., Seebeck, T., Li, J.-L. H., Pagano, J. S.: The Epstein-Barr virus DNA synthesized in superinfected Raji cells. Virology **77**, 762–771 (1977)

Shaw, J. E., Levinger, L. F., Carter, C. W. (Jr.): Nucleosomal structure of Epstein-Barr virus DNA in transformed cell lines. J. Virol. (in press) 1979

Southern, E. M.: Detection of specific sequences among DNA fragments seperated by gel electrophoresis. J. Mol. Biol. **98**, 503–518 (1975)

Stanbridge, E.: Mycoplasmas and cell culture. Bacteriol. Rev. **35**, 206–227 (1971)

Stevens, J.: Herpes simplex-neuronal interaction during acute and latent infection. ICN-UCLA Symposia on Molecular and Cellular Biology. (in preparation) (1978)

Sugden, B.: Comparison of Epstein-Barr viral DNA's in Burkitt lymphoma biopsy cells and in cells clonally transformed in vitro. Proc. Natl. Acad. Sci. USA **74**, 4651–4655 (1977)

Sugden, B., Summers, W. C., Klein, G.: Nucleic acid renaturation and restriction endonuclease cleavage analysis show that the DNA's of a transforming and a nontransforming strain of Epstein-Barr virus share approximately 90% of their nucleotide sequences. J. Virol. **18**, 765–775 (1976)

Svedmyr, E., Jondal, M.: Cytotoxic effector cells specific for B cell lines transformed by Epstein-Barr virus are present in patients with infectious mononucleosis. Proc. Natl. Acad. Sci. USA **72**, 1622–1627 (1975)

Tanaka, A., Miyagi, M., Yajima, Nonoyama, M.: Improved production of Epstein-Barr virus DNA for nucleic acid hybridization studies. Virology **74**, 81–85 (1976)

Thorley-Lawson, D. A., Strominger, J. L.: Transformation of human lymphocytes by Epstein-Barr virus is inhibited by phosphonoacetic acid. Nature **263**, 332–334 (1976)

Thorley-Lawson, D. A., Strominger, J. L.: Reversible inhibition by phosphonoacetic acid of human B-lymphocyte transformation by Epstein-Barr virus. Virology **86**, 423–431 (1978)

Tijan, R.: The binding site on SV40 DNA for a T antigen-related protein. Cell **13**, 165–179 (1978)

Vogt, V.: Purification and further properties of single-strand-specific nuclease from Aspergillus oryzac. Eur. J. Biochem. **33**, 192–200 (1973)

Weisbach, A.: Eukaryotic DNA polymerases. Annu. Rev. Biochem. **46**, 25–47 (1977)

Wilkie, N. M., Clements, J. B., Macnab, J. C. M., Subak-Sharpe, J. H.: The structure and biological properties of herpes simplex virus DNA. Cold Spring Harbor Symp. Quant. Biol. **29**, 657–666 (1974)

Wolf, H., Werner, T., zur Hausen, H.: EBV DNA in nonlymphoid cells of nasopharyngeal carcinomas and in a malignant lymphoma obtained after inoculation of EBV into cottontop marmosets. Cold Spring Harbor Symp. Quant. Biol. **39**, 791–796 (1975)

Wolf, H., zur Hausen, H., Becker, Y.: Epstein-Barr viral genomes in epithelial nasopharyngeal carcinoma cells. Nature New Biol. **244**, 245–247 (1973)

Yajima, Y. and Nonoyama, M.: Mechanisms of infection with Epstein-Barr virus I. Viral DNA replication and formation of non-infectious virus particles in superinfected Raji cells. J. Virol. **19**, 187–194 (1976)

Yajima, Y., Tanaka, A., Nonoyama, M.: Inhibition of productive replication of Epstein-Barr virus by phosphonoacetic acid. Virology **71**, 353–354 (1976)

zur Hausen, H., Shulte-Holthausen, H.: Presence of EB virus nucleic acid homology in a "virus-free" line of Burkitt tumour cells. Nature **227**, 245–248 (1970)

zur Hausen, H., Shulte-Holthausen, H.: Persistence of herpesvirus nucleic acid in normal and transformed cells: A review. In: Oncogenesis and herpesviruses. Biggs, P. M., de-Thé, G., Payne, L. N. (eds.) pp. 321–325. Lyon: IARC 1972

7 Biochemical Detection of the Virus Genome[1]

H. zur Hausen[2]

Institut für Virologie, Zentrum für Hygiene der Universität Freiburg, Hermann-Herder-Straße 11, D-7800 Freiburg (FRG)

The possible involvement of a virus in the etiology of Burkitt's lymphoma (BL), as originally suggested by Burkitt (1962), gained substance by the demonstration of herpes-like particles in cells of lymphoblastoid lines derived from this tumor (Epstein et al., 1964). The development of serologic tests by Henle and Henle (1966) and their application to large groups of patients and controls revealed the presence of antibodies to Epstein-Barr virus (EBV) antigens in all populations tested (Henle et al., 1969, 1970a, 1973a, b). These tests resulted in the discovery of the etiologic role of EBV in infectious mononucleosis (IM) (Henle et al., 1968) and demonstrated clearly the prevalence of antibodies in certain groups of tumor patients. Besides BL (Henle et al., 1969) other tumors were found to be correlated with high antibody titers against EBV antigens: this was notably the case in nasopharyngeal carcinoma (NPC) (Henle et al., 1970a) and less pronounced (although still significant) in patients with Hodgkin's disease (Levine et al., 1970; Hesse et al., 1973), chronic lymphatic leukemia, lymphocytic lymphoma (Johansson et al., 1971), and occasionally also in other diseases (Evans, 1971; Papageorgiu, 1973).

Based on the speculation that tumor induction by viruses requires the persistence of at least some viral genes, nucleic acid hybridization studies were initiated with biopsy material and nonproducer cell lines derived from the respective tumors (zur Hausen and Schulte-Holthausen, 1970; zur Hausen et al., 1970). They resulted in the demonstration of multiple copies of EBV DNA in biopsies from African BL, in others from NPC, and also in the majority of lymphoblastoid cell lines (zur Hausen et al., 1973). These data have been confirmed and extended by other groups (Nonoyama and Pagano, 1971, 1973; Lindahl et al., 1974).

The demonstration of EBV-specific antigens in tumor biopsy material (Pope et al., 1969; Reedman and Klein, 1973) further underlined the close association of EBV with BL and NPC. Certain strains of the virus were found to induce efficient transformation of human B lymphocytes (bone marrow-derived lymphocytes) (Henle et al., 1967) and were also able to induce lymphomas in marmosets and owl monkeys (Shope et al., 1973; Epstein et al., 1973; Werner et al., 1975). Despite the demonstration of in vivo oncogenicity and of transforming potential some data remain puzzling and unexplained as regards induction of BL and NPC by EBV:

---

[1] Experiments cited in this review were supported by the Deutsche Forschungsgemeinschaft (Ha 449/12 and SFB 118) and by the Bundesministerium für Forschung und Technologie (BCT 99).

[2] The technical assistance of Ms. Gabriele Menzel is gratefully appreciated.

1. The geographic clustering of both diseases seems to require the postulation of yet unidentified cofactors or of a genetic predisposition.
2. At least some cases of histologically typical BL appear to be devoid of detectable EBV DNA and of the EBV nuclear antigen (EBNA). The latter correlates excellently with EBV genome persistence. In NPC the tumors are more uniformly positive.
3. BL tumor patients reveal a specific response to the restricted (R) subcomponent of an early antigen complex (EA) (Henle et al., 1970b, 1971a, b, c) presumed to be essential for EBV DNA replication (Gergely et al., 1971a, b). Patients with NPC react more often with the diffuse (D) subcomponent. In contrast to the viral capsid antigen (VCA) and EBNA, the EA antibody response reflects the prognosis of patients after chemotherapy (Henle et al., 1971b), permitting an early diagnosis of relapses in long-term survivors. In nontumor patients the EA response is irregularly observed and frequently is only transient in IM.

The present chapter summarizes current data on the persistence of EBV DNA as revealed by nucleic acid hybridizations and analyzes results on intracellular heterogeneities of EBV.

Most lymphoblastoid lines derived from tumor biopsies as well as from healthy donors do contain EBV genomes (zur Hausen and Schulte-Holthausen, 1970; Nonoyama and Pagano, 1971; zur Hausen et al., 1973). The number of genome equivalents per cell varies considerably between 2 and 125, but is most frequently in the range of 20–50.

The demonstration of EBV DNA in tumor material has thus far only been successful in BL and NPC biopsies, with the additional exception of lymph nodes from three patients with immunoblastic lymphadenopathy (Bornkamm et al., 1976; zur Hausen et al., unpublished data). EBV DNA is fairly consistently demonstrated in African BL tumors (zur Hausen et al., 1970; Nonoyama and Pagano 1973; Lindahl et al., 1974), although a few negative cases have been reported (Klein et al., 1974b). First attempts to demonstrate EBV DNA in BL cases diagnosed outside the African tumor belt failed (Pagano et al., 1973). Other groups, however, later discovered scattered cases occurring throughout the world (Bornkamm et al., 1976; Ziegler et al., 1976). In view of the small number of tumors analyzed thus far it is difficult to estimate the percentage of EBV-positive tumors of BL histology outside of Africa.

The number of genome copies in positive tumors ranges between 1–2 and 120, thus closely resembling the genome content of lymphoblastoid lines. This is in agreement with the rather uniform histology of BL, which mainly consist of tumor cells.

In NPC the situation is more complex in view of differing admixtures of lymphoid nontumor cells in the epithelial carcinoma. In situ hybridizations first indicated the localization of EBV genomes within the epithelial tumor cells (Wolf et al., 1973, 1975). This was confirmed by successful tumor transplantation into nude mice (Klein et al., 1974a), EBNA demonstration in fresh biopsy material (Wolf et al., 1973; Huang et al., 1974), and fractionation of the epithelial tumor cells followed by nucleic acid hybridization (Desgranges et al., 1975). Calculations of genome equivalents in NPC biopsies are difficult to interpret since the degree of nontumorous infiltration is hard to determine.. It seems, however, that some biopsies contain excessively high concentrations of EBV DNA (zur Hausen et al., 1974), ranging up to 200 genome copies per cell. Three cases of immunoblastic lymphadenopathy, which revealed EBV DNA when tested by reassociation kinetics hybridization, contained two to three genome copies per cell (Bornkamm et al., 1976; zur Hausen et al., unpublished data).

Attempts have been made to analyze the degree of relatedness of EBV DNA in BL and NPC biopsies as well as in lines from patients with IM (Nonoyama et al., 1973; Pagano et al., 1975).

These studies resulted in the demonstration of some differences in the reassociation behavior of EBV DNA derived from the P_3HR-1 line of BL origin and EBV DNA from NPC and IM lines. Such experiments raised the question whether the EBV DNA isolated from P_3HR-1 cells is representative for EBV in general. Differences in biologic properties of viral isolates derived from various lymphoblastoid lines when compared to P_3HR-1 EBV (Miller et al., 1972, 1976) denoted possible genomic variations. Whereas P_3HR-1 EBV induces EA efficiently upon superinfection of EBV genome-harboring B lymphoblasts, none of the other human EBV isolates appears to be capable of EA induction following superinfection. Biologic properties of most other EBV isolates are represented by the virus isolated from B95-8 cells (Miller et al., 1972). These isolates transform efficiently human umbilical cord blood lymphocytes, which are not transformed at all by EBV isolates from P_3HR-1 cells.

Comparative studies on the structure of EBV DNA from P_3HR-1 and B95-8 cells were mainly performed by Kieff and his co-workers. This group showed that both DNA isolates contain linear double-stranded molecules of equal size of about 10^8 in molecular weight (Pritchett et al., 1975). Also, in analyzing the major structural proteins of both isolates no significant differences were observed (Dolyniuk et al., 1976). This is in line with previous data failing to demonstrate differences in complement-fixation antigens, in EA, VCA, or neutralizing antigens (Miller et al., 1972, 1974, 1976; Menezes et al., 1975).

Kinetic and absorptive hybridization with in vitro labeled EBV DNA suggested the lack of 10%–15% of sequences in B95-8 EBV DNA present in the DNA of P_3HR-1 EBV (Pritchett et al., 1975). P_3HR-1 EBV DNA seemed to contain at least 90%–95% of B95-8 EBV DNA sequences (Sugden et al., 1976). The presence of a specific sequence in P_3HR-1 DNA not found in B95-8 EBV DNA was also concluded by Hayward and Kieff (1977). The analysis of the DNA of both viral prototypes was greatly facilitated by restriction endonuclease cleavage patterns after agarose gel electrophoresis. The patterns obtained revealed a remarkable heterogeneity of P_3HR-1 EBV DNA when compared with the DNA of the B95-8 viruses. In the latter case the majority of fragments was found in molar concentrations (Hayward and Kieff, 1977), whereas P_3HR-1 EBV DNA always exhibited a number of submolar bands (Hayward and Kieff, 1977; Delius and Bornkamm, 1978). This suggested a higher complexity of P_3HR-1 EBV DNA which is supported by additional biophysical and biologic experiments.

Delius and Bornkamm (1978) studied the partial denaturation pattern of B95-8 and P_3HR-1 EBV DNA. These studies showed a consistent pattern in all B95-8 EBV DNA molecules analyzed. In P_3HR-1 EBV DNA at least two different groups of denaturation patterns were recorded. Group A consisted of molecules that resemble in structure B95-8 EBV DNA if minor rearrangements of the molecules are introduced. Group B, however, showed a completely different pattern that cannot easily be reconciled with a molecular flip-flop mechanism as observed with herpes simplex virus (HSV) DNA. The ratio of the two groups of molecules within P_3HR-1 EBV isolates was approximately 3:1.

The biochemical heterogeneity of P_3HR-1 EBV DNA is paralleled by a remarkable biologic heterogeneity. Fresen and zur Hausen (1976) and Fresen et al. (1977) reported the induction of two different EBNA patterns upon infection of EBV-negative human B lymphoma cells (BJA-B and Ramos). Besides a faint granular pattern, a number of cells revealed brilliant EBNA expression. After cloning, clones with exclusively faint granular or brilliant EBNA expression were obtained.

In another set of experiments, zur Hausen and Fresen (1977) demonstrated that induction of EA by P_3HR-1 virus in EBV genome-free human B lymphoma cells follows second order kinetics. In cells harboring EBV DNA, induction of EA by P_3HR-1 virus is a single-hit event which occurs at much higher frequency. This has also been noted in other laboratories (Dalens and Adams, 1977; Henderson et al., 1978). These data argue strongly in favor of a complementation model between resident viral genomes and the superinfecting P_3HR-1 EBV. They also indicate that two P_3HR-1 EBV genomes have to enter genome-negative cells before EA synthesis is initiated.

These results seem to underline the concept of intracellular heterogeneity of EBV genomes from P_3HR-1 cells. They apparently also point to a biologic interaction between heterogeneous viral genome populations manifesting itself in EA induction. One could speculate on the role of this interaction in the consistently high spontaneous induction rate of P_3HR-1 cells, as observed for more than a decade after their original establishment (Hinuma et al., 1967).

It is possible that other EBV isolates do contain heterogeneous populations of molecules as well, although at different ratios. Evidence exists that EBV isolates from B95-8 cells do induce a "new" EBNA-like antigen in a fraction of infected Ramos cells (Fresen et al., in preparation). Comparative data on induction of specific lymphoid cell lines (Raji, NC 37, RPMI 64–10) by tumor promoters (zur Hausen et al., 1978) and on superinfection of these cells by P_3HR-1 virus denote the presence of defective EBV genomes in these cells which can be rescued by P_3HR-1 superinfection (zur Hausen et al., in preparation).

Thus, the present state of knowledge of strain variations and biologic interactions between different EBV isolates is very limited and does not permit definite conclusions. Moreover, the existence of intracellular heterogeneities of EBV isolates from individual lines renders the interpretation of biochemical differences obtained by kinetic and absorptive hybridizations extremely difficult. The detailed analysis of tumors harboring EBV DNA requires more background information on viral genome structure, on the role of strain differences in genome persistence, and on their biologic interrelationship.

REFERENCES

Bornkamm, G. W., Stein, H., Lennert, K., Rüggeberg, F., Bartels, H., zur Hausen, H.: Attempts to demonstrate virus-specific sequences in human tumors. IV. EB viral DNA in European Burkitt lymphoma and in immunoblastic lymphadenopathy with excessive plasmacytosis. Int. J. Cancer **17**, 177–181 (1976)

Burkitt, D.: A children's cancer dependent on climatic factors. Nature **194**, 232–234 (1962)

Dalens, M., Adams, A.: Induction of Epstein-Barr virus-associated early antigen in different cell lines with ultraviolet-irradiated P_3HR-1 virus. Virology **83**, 305–312 (1977)

Delius, H., Bornkamm, G. W.: Heterogeneity of Epstein-Barr virus. III. Comparison of a transforming and a non-transforming virus by partial denaturation mapping of their DNA. J. Virol. **27**, 81–89 (1978)

Desgranges, C., Wolf, H., de-Thé, G., Shanmugaratnam, K., Cammoun, N., Ellouz, R., Klein, G., Lennert, K., Muñoz, N., zur Hausen, H.: Nasopharyngeal carcinoma. X. Presence of Epstein-Barr genomes in separated epithelial cells of tumours from Singapore. Tunisia and Kenya. Int. J. Cancer **16**, 7–15 (1975)

Dolyniuk, M., Pritchett, R., Kieff, E.: Proteins of Epstein-Barr virus. I. Analysis of the polypeptides of purified enveloped Epstein-Barr virus. J. Virol. **17**, 935–949 (1976)

Epstein, M. A., Achong, B. G., Barr, Y. M.: Virus particles in cultured lymphoblasts from Burkitt's lymphoma. Lancet **1964 I**, 702–703

Epstein, M. A., Hunt, R. D., Rabin, H.: Pilot experiments with EB virus in owl monkeys *(Aotus trivirgatus)*: I. Reticuloproliferative disease in annoculated animal. Int. J. Cancer **12**, 309–318 (1973)

Evans, A. S., Rothfield, N. F., Niederman, J. C.: Raised antibody levels to EB virus in systemic lupus erythematosus. Lancet **1971 I**, 167–168

Fresen, K. O., zur Hausen, H.: Establishment of EBNA-expressing cell lines by infection of Epstein-Barr virus (EBV)-genome-negative human lymphoma cells with different EBV strains. Int. J. Cancer **17**, 161–166 (1976)

Fresen, K. O., Merkt, B., Bornkamm, G. W., zur Hausen, H.: Heterogeneity of Epstein-Barr virus originating from P$_3$HR-1 cells. I. Studies on EBNA induction. Int. J. Cancer **19**, 317–323 (1977)

Gergely, L., Klein, G., Ernberg, J.: Appearance of Epstein-Barr virus-associated antigens in infected Raji cell. Virology **45**, 10–21 (1971 a)

Gergely, L., Klein, G., Ernberg, J.: Host cell macromolecular synthesis in cells containing EBV-induced early antigens, studied by combined immunofluorescence and radioautography. Virology **45**, 22–29 (1971 b)

Hayward, S. D., Kieff, E.: The DNA of Epstein-Barr virus. II. Comparison of the molecular weights of restriction endonuclease fragments of the DNA of strains of EBV and identification of the end fragments of the B95-8 strain. J. Virol. **23**, 421–429 (1977)

Henderson, E., Heston, L., Grogan, E., Miller, G.: Radiobiological inactivation of Epstein-Barr virus. J. Virol. **25**, 51–59 (1978)

Henle, G., Henle, W.: Immunofluorescence in cells derived from Burkitt's lymphoma. J. Bacteriol. **91**, 1248–1256 (1966)

Henle, W., Diehl, V., Kohn, G., zur Hausen, H., Henle, G.: Herpes-type virus and chromosome marker in normal leucocytes after growth with irradiated Burkitt cells. Science **157**, 1064–1065 (1967)

Henle, G., Henle, W., Diehl, V.: Relation of Burkitt's tumor associated herpes-type virus to infectious mononucleosis. Proc. Natl. Acad. Sci. USA **59**, 94–101 (1968)

Henle, G., Henle, W., Clifford, P., Diehl, V., Kafuko, G. W., Kirya, B. G., Klein, G., Morrow, R. H., Manube, G. M. R., Pike, M. C., Tukei, P. M., Ziegler, J. L.: Antibodies to EB virus in Burkitt's lymphoma and control groups. J. Natl. Cancer Inst. **43**, 1147–1157 (1969)

Henle, W., Henle, G., Ho, H. C., Burtin, P., Cachin, Y., Clifford, P., De Schryver, A., de-Thé, G., Diehl, V., Klein, G.: Antibodies to Epstein-Barr virus in nasopharyngeal carcinoma, other head and neck neoplasms, and control groups. J. Natl. Cancer Inst. **44**, 225–231 (1970 a)

Henle, W., Henle, G., Zajac, B., Pearson, G., Waubke, R., Scriba, M.: Differential reactivity of human sera with EBV-induced "early antigens". Science **169**, 188–190 (1970 b)

Henle, G., Henle, W., Klein, G.: Demonstration of two distinct components in the early antigen complex of Epstein-Barr virus infected cells. Int. J. Cancer **8**, 272–282 (1971 a)

Henle, G., Henle, W., Klein, G., Gunvén, P., Clifford, P., Morrow, R. H., Ziegler, J. L.: Antibodies to early Epstein-Barr virus-induced antigens in Burkitt's lymphoma. J. Natl. Cancer Inst. **46**, 861–871 (1971 b)

Henle, W., Henle, G., Niederman, J. C., Klemola, E., Halita, K.: Antibodies to early antigens induced by Epstein-Barr virus in infectious mononucleosis. J. Infect. Dis. **124**, 58–67 (1971 c)

Henle, W., Ho, H., C., Henle, G., Kwan, H. C.: Antibodies to Epstein-Barr virus-related antigens in nasopharyngeal carcinoma. Comparison of active cases with long-term survivors. J. Natl. Cancer Inst. **51**, 361–369 (1973 a)

Henle, W., Henle, G., Gunvén, P., Klein, G., Clifford, P., Singh, S.: Patterns of antibodies to Epstein-Barr virus-induced early antigens and Burkitt's lymphoma. Comparison of dying patients with long-term survivors. J. Natl. Cancer Inst. **50**, 1163–1173 (1973 b)

Hesse, J., Andersen, E., Levine, P. H., Ebbesen, P., Halberg, P., Reisher, J. I.: Antibodies to Epstein-Barr virus and cellular immunity in Hodgkin's disease and chronic lymphatic leukemia. Int. J. Cancer **11**, 237–243 (1973)

Hinuma, Y., Konn, M., Yamaguchi, J., Wudarski, D. J., Blakeslee, J-R., Grace, J. Y.: Immunofluorescence and herpes-type virus particles in the P$_3$HR-1 Burkitt lymphoma cell line. J. Virol. **1,** 1045–1051 (1967)

Huang, D. P., Ho., J. C., Henle, G.: Demonstration of Epstein-Barr virus-associated nuclear antigen in nasopharyngeal carcinoma cells from fresh biopsies. Int. J. Cancer **14,** 580–588 (1974)

Johansson, B., Klein, G., Henle, W., Henle, G. Epstein-Barr Virus (EBV)-associated antibody patterns in malignant lymphoma and leukemia. II. Chronic lymphocytic leukemia and lymphocytic lymphoma. Int. J. Cancer **8,** 475–486 (1971)

Klein, G., Giovanella, C., Lindahl, T., Fialkow, J., Singh, S., Stehlin, S.: Direct evidence for the presence of Epstein-Barr virus DNA and nuclear antigen in malignant epithelial cells from patients with poorly differentiated carcinoma of the nasopharynx. Proc. Natl. Acad. Sci. USA **71,** 4737–4741 (1974 a)

Klein, G., Lindahl, T., Jondal, M., Leibold, W., Menézes, J., Nilsson, K., Sundström, Ch.: Continuous lymphoid cell lines with B-cell characteristics that lack the Epstein-Barr virus genome, derived from three lymphomas. Proc. Natl. Acad. Sci. USA **71,** 3283–3286 (1974b)

Levine, P. H., Ablashi, D. V., Berard, C. W., Carbone, P. P., Waggoner, D. E., Malan, L.: Elevated antibody titers to Epstein-Barr virus in Hodgkin's disease. Cancer **27,** 416–421 (1970)

Lindahl, T., Klein, G., Reedman, B. M., Johansson, B., Singh, S.: Relationship between Epstein-Barr virus (EBV) DNA and the EBV-determined nuclear antigen (EBNA) in Burkitt lymphoma biopsies and other lymphoproliferative malignancies. Int. J. Cancer **13,** 764–770 (1974)

Menezes, J., Leibold, W., Klein, G.: Biological differences between different Epstein-Barr virus (EBV) strains with regard to lymphocyte transforming ability. Exp. Cell. Res. **92,** 478–484 (1975)

Miller, G., Lipman, M.: Release of infectious Epstein-Barr virus by marmoset leucocytes. Proc. Natl. Acad. Sci. USA **70,** 190–194 (1973)

Miller, G., Shope, T., Lisco, H., Stitt, D., Lipman, M.: Epstein-Barr virus: Transformation, cytopathic changes, and viral antigens in squirrel monkey and marmoset leukocytes. Proc. Natl. Acad. Sci. USA. **69,** 383–387 (1972)

Miller, G., Robinson, J., Heston, L., Lipman, M.: Differences between laboratory strains of Epstein-Barr virus based on immortalization, abortive infection and interference. Proc. Natl. Acad. Sci. USA **71,** 4006–4010 (1974)

Miller, G., Coope, D., Niederman, J., Pagano, J.: Biological properties and viral surface antigens of Burkitt lymphoma- and mononucleosis-derived strains of Epstein-Barr virus released from transformed marmoset cells. J. Virology **18,** 1071–1080 (1976)

Nonoyama, M., Pagano, J. S.: Detection of Epstein-Barr viral genome in nonproductive cells. Nature New Biol. **233,** 103–106 (1971)

Nonoyama, M., Pagano, J. S.: Homology between Epstein-Barr virus DNA and viral DNA from Burkitt's lymphoma and nasopharyngeal carcinoma determined by DNA-DNA reassociation kinetics. Nature **242,** 44–47 (1973)

Pagano, J. S., Huang, C. H., Levine, P.: Absence of Epstein-Barr viral DNA in American Burkitt's lymphoma. New Engl. J. Med. **289,** 1395–1399 (1973)

Pagano, J. S., Huang, C. H., Klein, G., de-Thé, G., Shanmugarathnam, K., Yang, C. S.: Homology of Epstein-Barr virus DNA in nasopharyngeal carcinoma from Kenya, Taiwan, Singapore and Tunisia. In: Oncogenesis and herpesviruses II. de-Thé, G., Epstein, M. A., zur Hausen, H. (eds.), Part 2, pp. 179–190. Lyon: IARC, 1975

Papageorgiou, S., Sorokin, F., Kouzoutzakoglu, K., Bonforte, J., Workman, L., Glade, R.: Host responses to Epstein-Barr virus and cytomegalovirus infection in leprosy. Infect. Immun. **7,** 620–624 (1973)

Pope, J. H., Horne, M. K., Wetters, E. J.: Significance of a complement-fixing antigen associated with herpes-like virus and detected in the Raji cell line. Nature **222,** 186–187 (1969)

Pritchett, R. F., Hayward, S. D., Kieff, E.: DNA of Epstein-Barr virus. I. Comparison of DNA of virus purified from HR-1 and B95-8 cells. J. Virol. **15,** 556–569 (1975)

Reedman, B. M., Klein, G.: Cellular localization of an Epstein-Barr virus (EBV)-associated complement-fixing antigen in producer and non-producer lymphoblastoid cell lines. Int. J. Cancer **11,** 499–520 (1973)

Shope, T., Dechairo, D., Miller, G.: Malignant lymphoma in cotton-top marmosets following inoculation with Epstein-Barr virus. Proc. Natl. Acad. Sci. USA **70,** 2487–2491 (1973)

Sugden, B., Summers, W. C., Klein, G.: Nucleic acid renaturation and restriction endonuclease cleavage analyses show that the DNAs of a transforming and a nontransforming strain of Epstein-Barr virus share approximately 90% of their nucleotide sequences. J. Virol. **18,** 765–775 (1976)

Werner, J., Wolf, H., Apodaca, J., zur Hausen, H.: Lymphoproliferative disease in a cotton topped marmoset after inoculation with infectious mononucleosis-derived Epstein-Barr virus. Int. J. Cancer **15,** 1000–1008 (1975)

Wolf, H., zur Hausen, H., Becker, V.: EB Viral genomes in epithelial nasopharyngeal carcinoma cells. Nature New Biol. **244,** 245–247 (1973)

Wolf, H., zur Hausen, H., Klein, G. Becker, V., Henle, G., Henle, W.: Attempts to detect virus-specific DNA sequences in human tumors: III. Epstein-Barr viral DNA in nonlymphoid nasopharyngeal carcinoma cells. Med. Microbiol. Immunol. **161,** 15–21 (1975)

Ziegler, J. L., Anderson, M., Klein, G., Henle, W.: Detection of Epstein-Barr virus DNA in American Burkitt's lymphoma. Int. J. Cancer **17,** 701–706 (1976)

zur Hausen, H., Fresen, K. O.: Heterogeneity of Epstein-Barr virus. II. Induction of early antigens (EA) by complementation. Virology **81,** 138–143 (1977)

zur Hausen, H., Schulte-Holthausen, H.: Presence of EB virus nucleic acid homology in a "virus-free" line of Burkitt tumor cells. Nature **227,** 245–248 (1970)

zur Hausen, H., Schulte-Holthausen, H., Klein, G., Henle, W., Henle, G., Clifford, P., Santesson, L.: EBV DNA in biopsies of Burkitt tumours and anaplastic carcinomas of the nasopharynx. Nature **228,** 1056–1058 (1970)

zur Hausen, H., Diehl, V., Wolf, H., Schulte-Holthausen, H., Schneider, U.: Occurrence of Epstein-Barr virus genomes in human lymphoblastoid cell lines. Nature New Biol. **237,** 189–190 (1973)

zur Hausen, H., Schulte-Holthausen, H., Wolf, H., Dörries, K., Egger, H.: Attempts to detect virus specific DNA in human tumors. II. Nucleic acid hybridization with complementary RNA of human herpes group viruses. Int. J. Cancer **13,** 657–664 (1974)

zur Hausen, H., O'Neill, F. J., Freese, U. K., Hecker, H.: Induction of persisting genomes of oncogenic herpes-viruses by the tumour promotor TPA. Nature **272,** 373–375 (1978)

8 The State of the Virus Genome in Transformed Cells and Its Relationship to Host Cell DNA

A. Adams

Department of Virology, Institute of Medical Microbiology, University of Göteborg, S-413 46 Göteborg (Sweden)

A. INTRODUCTION

Cells transformed with the Epstein-Barr virus (EBV) stably maintain multiple copies of the viral genome. The number of EBV genome copies in nonvirus-producing cell lines (nonproducer cells) can vary from a few to around a hundred per cell, but each individual line has a characteristic load. This number remains constant with time and appears to be relatively insensitive to the method of cell culture employed. Table 1 summarizes some of the published data on the number of EBV genome copies per cell in a variety of human lymphoid cell lines. The most widely used line, Raji, has been found over a 5-year period to have 50–60 copies of the EBV genome per cell by researchers in different laboratories around the world. The estimated number of EBV DNA molecules per diploid quantity of cell DNA, "genome equivalents per cell", is independent of the method of nucleic acid hybridization. Thus, membrane filter hybridizations with in vitro prepared, isotopically labeled, complementary RNA (cRNA) as well as DNA-DNA reassociation kinetic studies have given comparable results. The multiple copies of the EBV genome per cell are therefore real and not an overestimation of the type initially observed with the filter hybridization technique in the SV40 system (Westphal and Dulbecco, 1968; Gelb et al., 1971). Loss of pure viral DNA from control filters, the source of error with the filter hybridization technique in the papovavirus system (Haas et al., 1972), apparently does not occur to the same extent with herpesvirus DNA of 100×10^6 mol. wt.

Nucleic acid hybridization measurements give the average number of EBV genomes per cell, but with nonproducer cells like Raji this value is equivalent to the number of viral DNA molecules in individual cells. By definition, nonproducer cells maintain multiple copies of the EBV genome in the absence of any expression of the characteristic viral functions associated with productive infection. Moreover, with Raji, in situ hybridization with isotopically labeled cRNA followed by autoradiography failed to disclose any cells in the population with an excess of EBV DNA replication (Nonoyama and Pagano, 1971, 1972a).

DNA-DNA reassociation kinetic hybridizations demonstrate that most, if not all, of the viral genetic information is present in transformed cells, i.e., there is greater than 90% homology between the intrinsic EBV DNA in cells and the labeled DNA probes prepared from DNA isolated from virus particles. The completeness of the EBV genomes maintained in transformed cells has been confirmed by the fact that in some instances the formation of morphologically identifiable herpesvirus particles can be induced even in nonproducer cells like Raji (Hampar et al., 1972; Glaser and Nonoyama, 1974). The physical state of the EBV DNA in transformed cells has been partially characterized and the present results will be reviewed in this chapter. The mechanisms that control the stable maintenance of multiple complete copies of latent herpesvirus genomes and the regulation of gene expression of this viral DNA remain problems for the future.

B. TYPES OF EBV-TRANSFORMED CELLS

Two types of EBV-transformed lymphoid cells can be grown in continuous cell culture and are convenient material for the biochemical characterization of the viral genomes. They consist of (1) the immortalized cells which can be established either from peripheral blood of EBV seropositive individuals or by exposure of unifected B-lymphocytes (bone marrow-derived lymphocyte) to the virus in cell culture and (2) the virus-transformed tumor cells obtained from Burkitt's lymphoma (BL) biopsies. A number of differences exists between these two types of transformed cells as detailed elsewhere in this volume (Chap. 11) which raises the question of differences at the level of the viral genome. A third type of EBV-transformed cell, the virus-carrying malignant epithelial cell of nasopharyngeal carcinoma (NPC) biopsies, can be propagated in nude mice and such cells have also been employed in biochemical studies.

C. MODELS FOR THE MAINTENANCE OF LATENT EBV GENOMES IN TRANS-FORMED CELLS

Animal tumor viruses have been likened to temperate phage, because these bacterial viruses can also exist in a nonproductive, latent form in the lysogenized host cell. Among the temperate bacteriophage, two types of stable association between the viral genome and the host are known: either the viral DNA is covalently integrated into the host cell genome, which assures its replication and transmission from one cell

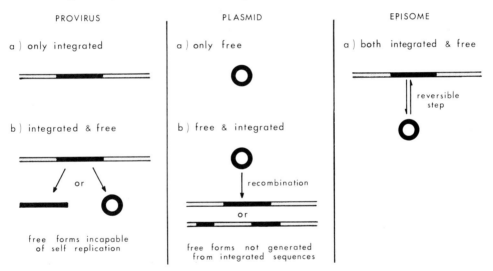

Fig. 1. Models for the maintenance of latent EBV genomes in transformed cells. Double-stranded EBV DNA molecules are depicted graphically *(solid black areas)* in various associations with cellular DNA *(clear areas)*. Concerning the terminology, provirus, plasmid, and episome are defined by Watson (1976) as follows:

Provirus: The state of a virus in which it is integrated into a host cell chromosome and is thus transmitted from one cell generation to another.

Plasmid: (Cytoplasmic), autonomously replicating chromosomal elements (found in bacteria) (parenthesis added).

Episome: A genetic element that can exist either free or as part of the normal cellular chromosome.

It is with these definitions in mind that these terms are used here and it is hoped that this does not cause undue confusion. In particular, temperate bacteriophage lambda is often referred to as the classic episome. The free circular form of λ DNA is, however, normally found associated with virus production and only what is referred to here as the provirus form is present in cells lysogenized (latently infected) with wild-type virus

Table 1. Estimated number of EBV genomes in different human cell lines[a]

Part A. Nonproducer cells[b]

Cell line	Origin[c]	No. EBV genome equivalents per cell	Method of hybridization	Reference
PE-SS[d]	BL	101	cRNA	Andersson and Lindahl, 1976
Raji	BL	65[e]	cRNA	Nonoyama and Pagano, 1971
Raji	BL	57	cRNA	Nonoyama and Pagano, 1973
Raji	BL	50—52	reassociation kinetics	Nonoyama and Pagano, 1973
Raji	BL	57	cRNA	Klein et al., 1974b
Raji	BL	50	cRNA	Klein et al., 1974c
Raji	BL	60	cRNA	Andersson and Lindahl, 1976
Raji	BL	56	reassociation kinetics	Pritchett et al., 1976
Raji	BL	54	cRNA	Klein et al., 1976
Raji	BL	50	cRNA	Yajima et al., 1976
AGR3[f]	BL	53	cRNA	Andersson, 1975
Rael	BL	56	cRNA	Andersson and Lindahl, 1976
P₃HR-1[g]	BL	32	cRNA	Nonoyama and Pagano, 1971
P₃HR-1[g]	BL	11	cRNA	Yajima et al., 1976
P₃HR-1[g]	BL	11	cRNA	Tanaka et al., 1976
TK-HR1[h]	BL	11	cRNA	Tanaka et al., 1976
Namalwa	BL	3	cRNA	Andersson, 1975
Namalwa	BL	2	reassociation kinetics	Pritchett et al., 1976
LY-1	NPC	26	cRNA	zur Hausen et al., 1972
LY-2	NPC	20	cRNA	zur Hausen et al., 1972
Kurgans	IM	23	reassociation kinetics	Pritchett et al., 1976
JHTC-33	IM	10	cRNA	Andersson and Lindahl, 1976
DSTC-4	IM	6	reassociation kinetics	Pritchett et al., 1976
F265	N	100	cRNA	Nonoyama and Pagano, 1971
F265	N	80	cRNA	Mele et al., 1974
F265	N	95	cRNA	Kaschka-Dierich et al., 1977
RPMI 1788	N	27	cRNA	Minowada et al., 1974
RPMI 7841	N	21	cRNA	Minowada et al., 1974
PG-1	N	25	cRNA	Kaschka-Dierich et al., 1977
U-303L	N	19	cRNA	Kaschka-Dierich et al., 1977
RPMI 6410	L	45	cRNA	Nonoyama and Pagano, 1971
RPMI 6410	L	23	cRNA	zur Hausen et al., 1972
RPMI 6410	L	14	cRNA	Ernberg et al., 1977
SK-L1	L	3—4	cRNA	zur Hausen et al., 1972
SK-L1	L	8	reassociation kinetics	Pritchett et al., 1976
RPMI 8235	L	5	cRNA	Minowada et al., 1974
S 84	H	31	cRNA	zur Hausen et al., 1972
S 95	H	23	cRNA	zur Hausen et al., 1972

[a] zur Hausen and Schulte-Holthausen (1970) first demonstrated EBV DNA in lymphoid cell lines. Because their values, obtained with ^{3}H-labeled EBV DNA of low specific radioactivity, are known to be underestimations they have not been included in this table.

[b] Nonproducer cells are defined here as lines in which less than 0.1% of the cells in a growing culture express antigens detectable by direct or indirect immunofluorescence with sera containing antibody to the early antigen complex.

[c] Most cell lines were established after explantation of peripheral blood cells or tumor tissue from individuals with the following diagnosis: BL = Burkitt's lymphoma, NPC = nasopharyngeal carcinoma, IM = infectious mononucleosis, N = normal healthy subject, H = Hodgkin's disease, L = leukemia, M = malignant melanoma.

[d] Lymphoblastoid cell lines established from patients with Burkitt's lymphoma. (PE-SS was established from non tumor tissue of a BL patient.)

Table 1 *(continued)*

Part B. Producer cells

Cell line	Origin	No. EBV genome equivalents per cell	Method of hybridization	Reference
P$_3$HR-1	BL	700	cRNA	Nonoyama and Pagano, 1971
P$_3$HR-1	BL	370	cRNA	zur Hausen et al., 1972
P$_3$HR-1	BL	470	cRNA	Klein et al., 1974c
P$_3$HR-1	BL	980	cRNA	Minowada et al., 1974
P$_3$HR-1	BL	280	reassociation kinetics	Pritchett et al., 1976
P$_3$HR-1	BL	350	cRNA	Tanaka et al., 1976
P$_3$HR-1	BL	304 – 340	cRNA	Yajima et al., 1976
B35M	BL	205	cRNA	Minowada et al., 1974
Daudi	BL	224	cRNA	Klein et al., 1974c
Daudi	BL	152	reassociation kinetics	Pritchett et al., 1976
Daudi	BL	118	cRNA	Andersson and Lindahl, 1976
SU-AmB-2	BL	58	cRNA	Koliais et al., 1978
Maku[d]	BL	46	reassociation kinetics	Pritchett et al., 1976
B46M	BL	36	cRNA	Minowada et al., 1974
SL-1	BL	29	cRNA	Minowada et al., 1974
LH	IM	53	cRNA	Pagano et al., 1976
Sheldon	IM	48	reassociation kinetics	Pritchett et al., 1976
KB	IM	39	cRNA	Pagano et al., 1976
MB	IM	37	cRNA	Pagano et al., 1976
ES	IM	34	cRNA	Pagano et al., 1976
NW	IM	29	cRNA	Pagano et al., 1976
DT	IM	20	cRNA	Pagano et al., 1976
Kaplan	IM	14	reassociation kinetics	Kieff and Levine, 1974
Kaplan	IM	25	reassociation kinetics	Pritchett et al., 1976
Ditzel	IM	8	reassociation kinetics	Pritchett et al., 1976
NC-37	N	80	cRNA	Nonoyama and Pagano, 1971
NC-37	N	121	cRNA	zur Hausen et al., 1972
NC-37	N	78	cRNA	Klein et al., 1974b
NC-37	N	76	cRNA	Kaschka-Dierich et al., 1977
RPMI 7281	N	40	cRNA	Minowada et al., 1974
RPMI 5287	N	34	cRNA	Minowada et al., 1974
B411-4	N	30	cRNA	Minowada et al., 1974
RPMI 7881	L	20	cRNA	Minowada et al., 1974
RPMI 7921	M	510	cRNA	Minowada et al., 1974
RPMI 7711	M	235	cRNA	Minowada et al., 1974
RPMI 7481	M	87	cRNA	Minowada et al., 1974
RPMI 7551	M	60	cRNA	Minowada et al., 1974
RPMI 7851	M	59	cRNA	Minowada et al., 1974

[e] In calculating the number of EBV genome equivalents per cell, different workers have assumed different values for the molecular weight of both the viral and host cell genomes. In the early study of Nonoyama and Pagano (1971), a molecular weight of only 60 million was assumed for EBV DNA and this, combined with an unusually low value for the amount of host DNA per cell, results in a 20% overestimation in the number of EBV genome equivalents per cell. Because the method used in calculating the number of EBV genome equivalents per cell has not always been reported, no attempt has been made to standardize the values listed in the table.

[f] An 8-azaguanine-resistant, surface-adherent variant of Raji.

[g] P$_3$HR-1 variants that have spontaneously lost the potential to produce virus.

[h] A thymidine kinase negative variant of P$_3$HR-1 which does not produce virus.

generation to the next, or, alternatively, it may exist as an autonomously replicating genetic element. These two models for the existence of latent viral DNA will be called the *provirus* and *plasmid* models, respectively, and are depicted graphically in Fig. 1. In the bacterial system, *Escherichia coli* phage lambda is the best-studied example of what I refer to here as the provirus model, while phage P1 is a good prototype for the plasmid model. Both types of association are extremely stable at a ratio of one phage genome per bacterial chromosome. Thus, in spite of the fact that there is only a single copy of the P1 genome per *E. coli* genome (Ikeda and Tomizawa, 1968), the frequency at which the virus DNA is spontaneously lost is less than 10^{-5} cured bacteria per cell division (Rosner, 1972). Finally a composite model in which the latent virus DNA can have both a free plasmid form and an integrated state may be considered. In this, the *episome* model, the viral genome can move freely between an integrated and a free state and can be replicated in either form in the latently infected cell. As indicated in Fig. 1, the episome model is to be considered distinct from either the formation of free viral DNA molecules from an integrated provirus (provirus model [b]) or an essentially irreversible recombination event between a plasmid and the host genome (plasmid model [b]). The free genomes depicted in the provirus model [b] are not plasmids since they are incapable of self-replication and the integrated sequences in the plasmid model [b] are not a provirus since they do not serve as template for the formation of free viral genomes. Finally, as shown in Fig. 1, free genomes formed from a provirus might be either linear or circular, but all independently replicating genetic elements carried in prokaryotes have a circular structure and it is assumed that an EBV plasmid or episome would also be circular in structure.

Knowledge of the mode of EBV DNA replication in transformed cells will be required before a definite assignment to either the provirus, plasmid, or episome model for the maintenance of the latent viral genomes can be made. However, the obvious question to ask first is simply if there are integrated and/or free forms of EBV DNA in transformed cells. Experimentally, the problem involves the isolation of DNA from transformed cells and determination of the physical state of the viral DNA component, i.e., whether the EBV DNA fractionates as integrated sequences together with the cellular DNA or separately with the properties expected of either linear or circular viral DNA molecules. Because of the large size of herpesvirus genomes, this becomes a difficult task and many of the methods used in analogous studies with the smaller DNA tumor viruses are simply not applicable. Techniques appropriate for the characterization of the intrinsic EBV DNA of transformed cells have been developed with the Raji cell line and these methods have subsequently been used in the study of other types of EBV-transformed cells.

D. FIRST EXPERIMENTAL EVIDENCE FOR FREE, NONINTEGRATED EBV
GENOMES IN RAJI CELLS

Nonoyama and Pagano (1972 a) provided the first experimental evidence for free, nonintegrated EBV DNA molecules in Raji cells. The approach used was sedimentation analysis of high molecular weight cellular DNA in alkaline solution, the same method originally used by Sambrook and co-workers to demonstrate covalent integration of SV40 DNA in transformed mouse cells (Sambrook et al., 1968). Isolated Raji nuclei were gently lysed directly on top of an alkaline glycerol gradient. Following centrifugation, the distribution of the bulk of the DNA was determined by ultraviolet absorption measurements while the EBV DNA was localized by nucleic acid hybridization of individual gradient fractions fixed on membrane filters. It was observed that 95% of the EBV DNA in Raji cells sedimented in the $30-70$ S region of the gradient and that no EBV DNA detectable by filter hybridization was located in the 130 S region where the bulk of the DNA sedimented. The hybridization profile with Raji was in fact nearly identical to that obtained with an artificial mixture of HeLa cell DNA and 40 ng of linear EBV DNA molecules isolated from virus particles. Nonoyama and Pagano concluded that complete or nearly complete EBV DNA molecules were present in Raji and that the majority of these were not associated with the cellular DNA by conventional covalent integration. On the basis of these results a plasmid model for the state of the EBV genomes in Raji was favored. No comment was made, however, on whether or not such free genomes might be circular in structure.

Nonoyama and Pagano (1972 a) considered the possibility that the integration of EBV DNA into Raji cell DNA might be of an unusual type which was either not covalent or otherwise sensitive to alkaline denaturation. To investigate this possibility, Tanaka and Nonoyama (1974) isolated high molecular weight DNA from Raji and analyzed the sedimentation properties of the EBV-hybridizing sequences in neutral solution. It was shown that 70%–80% of the EBV DNA sequences in Raji, as well as those of an artificial mixture made between virion DNA and, this time, Simpson cell DNA (another EBV DNA-negative human cell line like HeLa) (Kawai et al., 1973), sedimented similarly, at the approximate rate of linear EBV DNA molecules. Because of the limited capacity of neutral glycerol gradients for high molecular weight DNA, only DNA from about a half million cells could be analyzed and large fractions had to be collected in order to provide sufficient material for nucleic acid hybridization. These limitations, in combination with the absence of an internal size marker, presumably precluded the discovery of a difference in sedimentation rate between the linear virion DNA added to the Simpson cell lysate and the intrinsic EBV DNA molecules in Raji. The remaining 20%–30% of the viral DNA sequences in both the Raji lysate and the Simpson lysate mixed with EBV DNA sedimented to the bottom of the centrifuge tube, together with the bulk of the cell DNA. In the case of the artificial Simpson + EBV DNA mixture, the fast sedimenting material must have been due to trapping of viral DNA with the high molecular weight cellular DNA. However, with Raji it is likely that intrinsic EBV DNA molecules with higher sedimentation coefficients than virion DNA were also present in the fast-sedimenting material.

E. POSSIBLE FORMS OF FREE, NONINTEGRATED EBV GENOMES

In the original attempts to analyze the intracellular forms of EBV DNA in Raji cells by velocity sedimentation, it was not fully appreciated that the free, nonintegrated viral genomes can occur in an extensive variety of forms. Figure 2 depicts some of the configurations that "free" EBV genomes may assume in transformed cells. The virion DNA isolated either from P_3HR-1 or B95-8 virus particles is linear in structure (Pritchett et al., 1975). These linear EBV DNA molecules sediment $0.94-0.97$ times the rate of bacteriophage T4 DNA in neutral solution (Jehn et al., 1972; Adams and Lindahl, 1975b; Pritchett et al., 1975; Adams et al., 1977), which corresponds to a sedimentation coefficient of $58-60$ S, assuming a value of 61.8 S for T4 DNA

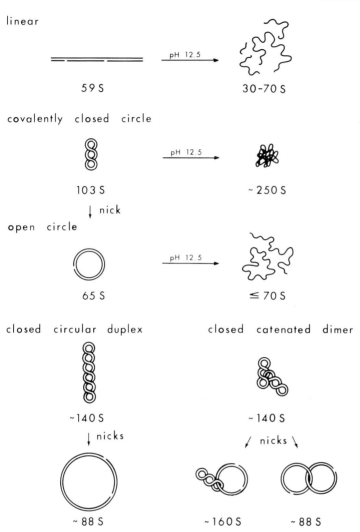

linear

59 S   pH 12.5   30–70 S

covalently closed circle

103 S   pH 12.5   ~ 250 S

| nick

open circle

65 S   pH 12.5   ≤ 70 S

closed circular duplex   closed catenated dimer

~140 S   ~140 S

| nicks   ⁄ nicks ∖

~ 88 S   ~ 160 S   ~ 88 S

Fig. 2. The various forms that the free, nonintegrated EBV genomes isolated from transformed cells might assume in solution. Sedimentation coefficients (S values) are either those experimentally observed for EBV DNA or estimated for a double-stranded DNA molecule having a molecular weight of 100×10^6

(Freifelder, 1970). The double-stranded DNA molecules isolated from virus particles contain one or more single-stranded interruptions and sediment as a broad peak from 30–70 S in alkaline solution (Nonoyama and Pagano, 1972a; Pritchett et al., 1975).

Plasmids have a circular structure and can be isolated from cells in either a covalently closed or open circular form. Natural isolates of covalently closed circles assume a compact "supercoiled" configuration in neutral solution and sediment considerably faster than linear molecules having the same molecular weight. From the relationship described by Hobom and Hogness (1974), the sedimentation coefficient of the covalently closed circular form of EBV DNA would be expected to be about 1.7 times that of the linear molecule. In alkaline solution, the two DNA strands in covalently closed circular molecules remain associated. From the sedimentation properties of other covalently closed circular DNA molecules in alkaline solution (Clayton and Vinograd, 1967), it is estimated that this form of EBV DNA would have a sedimentation coefficient of 250 S. The two DNA strands of open circular molecules can separate in alkaline solution and will sediment in a similar manner to single-stranded linear molecules. In their native state, however, open circular molecules sediment approximately 1.1 times faster than their linear counterparts (Hershey et al., 1963; Ikeda and Tomizawa, 1968).

Oligomeric forms of circular mitochondrial DNA molecules have been found in human leukocytes (Clayton and Vinograd, 1967) and it is possible that EBV DNA may likewise occur in higher than monomer forms. As shown in Fig. 2, dimers can be of two types, either a circular duplex having twice the contour length of the monomer or catenated dimers consisting of two interlocked monomer circles. The sedimentation coefficients of the various dimeric forms of circular EBV DNA are calculated according to the equations of Wang (1970). These values should be considered only rough estimates because the theoretical relationships are derived from data obtained with circular molecules considerably smaller than the EBV genome. Moreover, as noted by Wang (1970), the relative sedimentation rates of superhelical DNAs of the same superhelical density are a function of both temperature and counter ion concentration.

F. DETAILED ANALYSIS OF THE FREE, NONINTEGRATED EBV GENOMES IN RAJI CELLS

EBV DNA has a high guanine-cytosine base composition (Chap. 5) and when high molecular weight Raji DNA is fractionated in neutral CsCl density gradients, the intracellular EBV DNA sequences, localized by hybridization, form a peak at a density of $1.716 \, g/cm^3$ (Adams et al., 1973). The bulk of cellular DNA has a density of $1.700 \, g/cm^3$ under these conditions (Szybalski and Szybalski, 1971) and it is therefore possible to enrich for EBV DNA by density gradient fractionation of whole-cell DNA. With such prefractionated DNA, 10–20 times more EBV DNA can be loaded on a single velocity gradient and it is then possible to analyze in greater detail the sedimentation properties of the intrinsic viral genomes. With this approach, two peaks of EBV DNA sequences were observed on neutral glycerol gradients. Neither of these two forms, however, had the sedimentation properties of linear virion DNA (Adams and Lindahl, 1975a, b). Calculated relative to the labeled T4 DNA, which was included as an internal size marker, the faster sedimenting component had a sedimentation coefficient of 100–105 S, while the slower one had a value of 65 S. As shown in Fig. 2, these are the values expected for covalently closed and open DNA circles of 100×10^6 mol. wt. Little or no EBV DNA was found to sediment slower than the 61.8 S T4-DNA-size marker where the 59 S DNA of EBV virions is found when sedimented together with cellular DNA from virus-negative cells. The bulk of the cellular DNA sedimented as a broad peak at ~ 70 S in all these experiments.

A number of experiments have been performed to establish that the material sedimenting at 65 S and 100 S represents the open and covalently closed circular forms of EBV DNA, respectively. When material from the 100 S region of glycerol gradients was analyzed in CsCl/propidium diiodide (Adams and Lindahl, 1975b) or

CsCl/ethidium bromide (Lindahl et al., 1976), most of the EBV-hybridizing DNA sequences banded in the heavy density position expected of covalently closed DNA circles (Bauer and Vinograd, 1968). The remaining EBV DNA banded together with the bulk of the DNA. Open DNA circles fractionate together with linear DNA molecules in such dye/buoyant density gradients (Radloff et al., 1967) and the EBV DNA found in this region indicates that some single-strand nicks were inadvertently introduced in the 100 S molecules during the preparative procedures. The separation between the closed and open circular EBV DNA forms in CsCl/ethidium bromide gradients was the same as that observed for the corresponding circular forms of polyoma virus DNA, indicating that the covalently closed circular DNAs of these two viruses are of similar superhelical density (Lindahl et al., 1976). This would correspond to the presence of 700–800 superhelical turns per circular EBV DNA molecule. All EBV DNA in the 65 S region from glycerol gradients banded at low density in CsCl/propidium diiodide, which was expected for open circular molecules that do not restrict the intercalation of the dye.

When isolated 100 S material was sedimented in alkaline glycerol gradients, the EBV-hybridizing sequences sedimented considerably faster than a 53 S polyoma DNA marker (Lindahl et al., 1976). Because of the great distance between the marker and the EBV DNA peak, the sedimentation coefficient can only be estimated to be somewhere between 250 and 300 S. It is not entirely clear why Nonoyama and Pagano (1972a) failed to observe fast sedimenting EBV DNA in alkaline solution, but presumably they must have nicked any covalently closed circles present prior to centrifugation. Analysis of 65 S material in alkaline sucrose showed a broad peak consistent with the presence of small numbers of single-strand breaks in large double-stranded DNA molecules (Adams and Lindahl, 1975a).

Direct examination in the electron microscope of the DNA in the 100 S region revealed the presence of large covalently closed supercoiled DNA molecules in Raji cells (Lindahl et al., 1976). Such circular DNA molecules were not detected in lysates from the EBV-negative human lymphoid cell lines Molt-4 and BJAB after fractionation by CsCl and glycerol gradient centrifugation in the same fashion. Treatment of the 100 S form of EBV DNA with low doses of X-irradiation converts this form to the 65 S form in a direct, discontinuous fashion. The ratio of 65 S to 100 S forms in X-ray-treated DNA samples parallels the number of open circular and supercoiled large DNA circles seen in the electron microscope.

When the 100 S material from neutral glycerol gradients is further purified by CsCl/ethidium bromide, 90%–100%-pure preparations of circular EBV DNA molecules are obtained as judged by electron microscopy. Figure 3 shows two such EBV DNA molecules. One molecule is in the relaxed, open circular form, while the other is in the supercoiled, covalently closed circular form. From length measurements made on open circular forms, it is estimated that the circular EBV DNA molecules in Raji have a molecular weight of 106 million (Lindahl et al., 1976), which is very close (less than 1% difference) to that of the linear viral genomes isolated from virus particles (Pritchett et al., 1975). The size of the circular EBV genomes supports the reassociation kinetic hybridization results indicating the presence of multiple and complete viral genomes in Raji (Nonoyama and Pagano, 1973).

In addition to the 65 and 100 S forms of free EBV DNA, a third form, sedimenting at ~130 S can be observed when centrifugation times are shortened. Preliminary evidence indicates that catenated circular dimers account for at least some of this fast

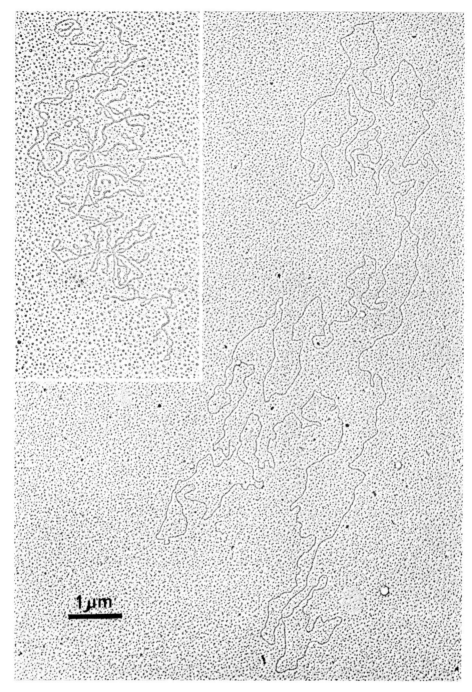

Fig. 3. Electron micrographs of a covalently closed supercoiled *(upper left)* and an open circular molecule of EBV DNA. The DNA was visualized using the formamide-modified Kleinschmidt technique (Davis et al., 1970). The superhelical conformation of the covalently closed circular DNA molecule has been partially untwisted under these spreading conditions. The micrographs were taken and kindly provided by Dr. Gunnar Bjursell, Department of Human Genetics, University of Aarhus, Aarhus, Denmark

sedimenting material (E. Gussander and A. Adams, unpublished results). Catenated dimers having one supercoiled and one open circular monomer should band between supercoiled and relaxed molecules in dye-CsCl gradients (Jaenisch and Levine, 1973). On banding 100 S DNA in CsCl/ethidium bromide, we have on occasion observed a small peak of EBV-hybridizing sequences in this intermediate position (Kaschka-Dierich et al., 1977). As estimated in Fig. 2, the mixed catenated dimer should sediment at a rate similar to that of the supercoiled monomer, so it is not unreasonable that this complex form of EBV DNA would be present when the 100 S DNA fraction from glycerol gradients is further fractionated in CsCl/ethidium bromide gradients.

G. DETECTION OF EBV DNA COVALENTLY BOUND TO HOST DNA IN RAJI CELLS

The presence of an excess of "free" circular viral genomes complicates greatly the demonstration of integrated genomes, even with small DNA tumor viruses like SV40 (Hölzel and Sokol, 1974). With a virus the size of EBV and with present technology, it will probably be impossible to demonstrate whether there are complete EBV genomes or only large fragments integrated into the host DNA in those cells with multiple, free copies of viral DNA (for a discussion of the potential applicability of various standard techniques to the characterization of integrated EBV genomes see Lindahl et al., 1978). It has, however, been possible to demonstrate that some of the EBV DNA sequences in Raji are apparently covalently bound to cellular DNA in a linear fashion (Adams et al., 1973; Adams and Lindahl, 1975a). The method that has been used is based on the complete removal of EBV genomes with a density close to 1.718 g/cm^3 in neutral CsCl solution from the less dense cellular DNA through repeated banding of high molecular weight Raji DNA in such density gradients. Some EBV-hybridizing DNA sequences cofractionate with less dense material under these conditions and the nature of this association has been studied.

The EBV DNA molecules isolated from virus particles are relatively homogeneous in base composition over their length (Pritchett et al., 1975) and the viral DNA banding at densities less than 1.71 g/cm^3 cannot be due to the isolation of a small fragment of viral DNA having an unusually low guanine-cytosine content. This is confirmed by the finding that when the DNA is sheared to approximately one-tenth of the initial size (unsheared DNA was 110×10^6 daltons and sheared material had a molecular weight of 8×10^6) prior to CsCl gradient centrifugation, the peak of EBV-hybridizing sequences shifts to a higher density (Adams et al., 1973). This result is interpreted to mean that there are fragments of EBV DNA of normal density linearly associated with less dense cellular DNA and that when the molecular weight of the hybrid DNA molecules is reduced, proportionally less host DNA will remain bound to the viral DNA. This model and the effect of shear treatment are depicted in Fig. 4. The density shift observed after shear treatment should depend on the density of the unsheared hybrid fragments and this in turn should reflect the relative proportion of viral to cellular DNA. This prediction was confirmed with DNA from Raji cells using two different pools of twice-rebanded whole-cell DNA (Adams et al., 1973).

Two trivial explanations for the isolation of EBV DNA having an aberrant density by CsCl gradient centrifugation are as follows: (1) trapping of some EBV DNA in the bulk of the high molecular weight DNA or (2) binding of some viral DNA to protein or

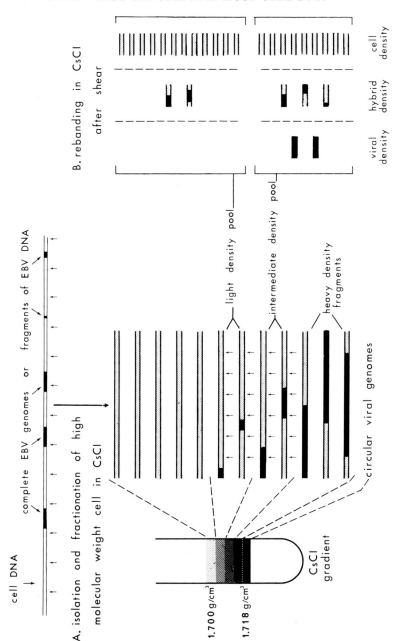

Fig. 4. Demonstration of integrated EBV DNA sequences by density gradient fraction. The hypothetical cellular DNA segment, shown in the *upper left*, with both complete integrated EBV genomes and short sequences of EBV DNA is randomly broken on isolation at the points indicated by the *small arrows*. After equilibrium density-gradient centrifugation, the high molecular weight DNA fragments distribute as indicated (fragments are shown at a $5 \times$ magnification with viral DNA being depicted as *solid black regions* and cellular DNA as *clear areas*). Material banding at densities between viral DNA (1.718 g/cm³) and cellular DNA (1.700 g/cm³) is rebanded in CsCl to give two density pools (*light* and *intermediate*). During these subsequent centrifugations to remove any circular free EBV genomes contaminating the light and intermediate density pools, most of the *heavy density* hybrid (EBV-cell) DNA fragments are also removed. DNA in the rebanded light and intermediate density pools is broken at the *arrows* by hydrodynamic shear forces. The short DNA fragments on subsequent rebanding in CsCl should distribute as indicated to the *right* of the figure

other less dense substances. Trapping seems unlikely, since EBV DNA in low density regions is not released by dilution and rebanding of the DNA (Adams et al., 1973). Moreover, trapping of labeled EBV DNA from virus particles has not been observed in reconstitution experiments at similar DNA concentrations. These include both the addition of isolated 100×10^6 mol. wt. EBV DNA at the time of cell lysis (Adams et al., 1973) and introduction of labeled virion DNA by superinfection with exogenous virus either 4 or 48 h prior to preparation of the Raji cell lysate (A. Adams, unpublished observations). It is known that most of the superinfecting DNA reaches the nucleus, is uncoated, and remains as intact but nonintegrated molecules up to 2 days after infection (Jehn et al., 1972). Finally, any objection that these reconstitution experiments are still not equivalent to the situation in Raji, either because the labeled virion DNA is linear rather than circular or that the host DNA is degraded in superinfected cells (Nonoyama and Pagano, 1972b), seems ruled out by the finding of one lymphoid cell line in which only free circular genomes and no integrated EBV sequences can be detected under analogous conditions (Adams et al., 1977). The association of EBV DNA with less dense material in Raji cells is resistant to treatment with sarkosyl, sodium dodecyl sulfate, pancreatic ribonuclease, high concentrations of pronase, proteinase K, and phenol (Adams et al., 1973).

It was initially reported that the linear association between viral and cellular DNA was sensitive to alkaline pH (Adams et al., 1973). This was based on the apparent release of hybrid density EBV DNA to a heavier density on banding in alkaline CsCl gradients. However, it was not originally appreciated that a slow salt-promoted chain scission of DNA occurs in alkaline CsCl solution (Tomizawa and Anraku, 1965; Kiger et al., 1968) and a shift to higher density is unavoidable due to reduction in the molecular weight of long single-stranded DNA during centrifugation. In subsequent studies, in which an internal density marker close to that of free EBV DNA was included, it was found that the EBV DNA fraction with properties of integrated DNA in neutral CsCl also banded at a lighter density than virion DNA in alkaline solution (Adams and Lindahl, 1975a). These data show that the alkali-induced breaks do not occur specifically at the junction between viral and cellular DNA and it is concluded that some EBV DNA in Raji is apparently covalently integrated by normal DNA phosphodiester bonds. It is noted in passing that by using a similar approach with density gradient fractionation in either neutral or alkaline CsCl, Biegeleisen and Rush (1976) have demonstrated integration of herpes simplex DNA during productive infection of monkey kidney cells.

It is not presently known if complete EBV genomes or only fragments are integrated in Raji cells. Due to the fragility of large isolated DNA, it is difficult and impractical to fractionate host DNA segments much longer than the EBV genome. Therefore, if a few complete integrated genomes bound on either end with cellular DNA were isolated, these would be predominantly of viral density and would cofractionate with the free EBV genomes in CsCl gradients (see Fig. 4). On continued fractionation, these hybrid molecules would be difficult to separate from nicked circular EBV DNA molecules. Thus, the hybrid molecules that have been studied in more detail contain only short sequences of viral DNA. It is not known if these short sequences are at the ends of the hybrid fragments, as would be expected if they are the termini of complete integrated genomes (Fig. 4). If the EBV DNA is located at the termini of the hybrid molecules, it will be of interest to determine if it represents only a portion of the viral genome, as would be predicted for a specific integration site on the EBV genome, analogous to the attachment site of the bacteriophage lambda genome.

An alternative explanation of the data indicating the presence of viral-cellular hybrid molecules is that they are EBV DNA circles which have retained the viral sequences important for self-replication and/or maintenance and have picked up varying amounts of host cell DNA. Such DNA circles would be analogous to some of the defective viral genomes produced during productive infection with SV40 or polyoma virus (Winocour et al., 1975; Yoshijke and Defendi, 1977). There is no evidence for such a hypothesis, and indeed the available data contradict it. Thus, the Raji-derived EBV DNA circles that have been measured with the electron microscope were of a homogeneous 53.0 μm length with a standard deviation of only 1.7% (Lindahl et al., 1976) and a specific search for such defective viral DNA molecules in an EBV-converted lymphoid cell line indicated that they were not present (Andersson-Anvret and Lindahl, 1978).

H. STATE OF THE EBV GENOMES IN OTHER CELLS

A number of different EBV-transformed cells have been tested for the presence of circular viral genomes and, with selected cells, the presence or absence of integrated EBV DNA sequences has been determined. The procedures that have been used are essentially those developed with the Raji cell line. The protocol is as follows: a sarkosyl-pronase lysate of 50–100 million cells is fractionated by CsCl density gradient equilibrium centrifugation. The DNA having a buoyant density greater than 1.71 g/cm^3 is analyzed for the presence of covalently closed and open circular forms of viral DNA by velocity sedimentation in neutral glycerol gradients. DNA of density 1.70–1.71 is rebanded in CsCl solution for analysis of EBV DNA having the aberrant low density expected of integrated sequences. The molecular weights of the circular EBV genomes have been estimated from the sedimentation coefficient of the covalently closed supercoiled form. In many instances, the sizes of the free viral genomes have also been confirmed by direct length measurements on electron micrographs after exposure of the covalently closed circular EBV DNA to X-irradiation; this is a much more reproducible technique than pancreatic DNase treatment to introduce 1–2 single-strand breaks per EBV DNA molecule in order to permit accurate length measurements (T. Lindahl, unpublished results). Table 2 summarizes the available data.

I. BURKITT'S LYMPHOMA CELLS

Raji, one of the first BL cell lines to be established (Pulvertaft, 1965), has been in culture for nearly 13 years and is known to be aneuploid (Jarvis et al., 1974). Nevertheless, the states of the EBV genomes in Raji are the same as in more recently established lines like Rael (Klein et al., 1972) and SU-AmB-2 (Epstein et al., 1976). Both circular and integrated EBV DNA sequences are present in Raji (Adams et al., 1973; Lindahl et al., 1976), Rael (Kaschka-Dierich et al., 1977), and SU-AmB-2 (Koliais et al., 1978). Moreover, there are no apparent differences between the sizes of the circular EBV genomes in these three lines, which were established from a Nigerian, a Kenyan, and a North American case, respectively of BL.

Both integrated and circular EBV DNA forms have been demonstrated in fresh BL biopsies (Kaschka-Dierich et al., 1976; Koliais et al., 1978). The finding of analogous forms of EBV DNA in vivo implies that neither the integrated sequences nor the circular genomes are artifacts introduced by forcing the Burkitt's tumor cells to grow in tissue culture. This is an important point because there are well-documented examples

Table 2. Properties of the intrinsic EBV DNA in different cells

	Cell	Origin	Sedimentation coefficients		Length in EM	Mol. weight × 10⁶		Integrated EBV DNA
			(closed circles)	(open circles)	(× PM2 DNA)[a]	(sedimentation)[b]	(EM)[c]	
Lymphoma cells	Raji	BL	103	65	16.6 (30)	99	106	present
	Rael	BL	102	65	16.7 (15)	98	107	present
	SU-AmB-2	BL	105	64	16.5 (28)	104	106	present
	A.O. biopsy	BL	104	65		101		present
	W.J. biopsy	BL	—	65				not tested
	J.M. biopsy	BL	104	65	16.6 (26)	101	106	present
Epithelial cells	J.G. tumor	NPC	101	64	16.2 (20)	95	104	present
	M.M. tumor	NPC	101	64		95		not tested
Lymphoblastoid cells	LY-2	NPC	106	66		106		not tested
	SK-L1	L	103	65		99		present
	F265	N	102	65	16.6 (32)	98	106	present
	NC-37	N	102	65		98		present
	PG-1	N	104	65		101		present
	U303L	N	103	65	16.8 (5)	99	108	present
	JHTC-33	IM	99	64	16.8 (9)	89	108	not tested
	Salomon	IM	105	65	16.9 (10)	104	108	
	883L	IM	98	—	14.5 (8)	89	93	present
	IM-198	IM	105	65	16.7 (7)	104	107	
	IM16	IM	104	64		101		present
In vitro transformed	cb35B1	cord cell	97	62	14.8 (14)	87	95	not tested
	cb35B3	cord cell	98	63	14.7 (28)	89	94	absent
	cb41B11	cord cell	98	63		89		not tested
	TW16	cord cell	104	63		101		present
	TW20	cord cell	104	64	16.8 (14)	99	108	present
In vitro converted	AW-Ramos	BL	circles absent			—		present
	EHRA-Ramos	BL	circles absent			—		present
	Ramos/B95-8	BL	circles absent			—		present

[a] Length of the open circular form of EBV DNA relative to bacteriophage PM2 DNA circles measured on the same grid. The figure in parenthesis is the number of EBV DNA molecules measured.

[b] Calculated using the S value of the covalently closed supercoiled form of EBV DNA and the relationship $S = 0.0312 M^{0.44}$ (Hobom and Hogness, 1974).

[c] Calculated from length measurements made in the electron microscope and assuming a molecular weight of 6.4×10^6 for the PM2 DNA circles (Pettersson et al., 1973).

of how temperate bacteriophage can be manipulated so that the latent genome will assume a state other than that characteristic of the wild-type virus. Mutants of phage P1 can be carried exclusively as an integrated prophage instead of a plasmid (Scott, 1970), and bacteriophage lambda can persist as a plasmid if the virus genome carries certain mutations (Matsubara and Kaiser, 1968; Signer, 1969; Lieb, 1970). In this regard, polyoma-transformed cells with multiple nonintegrated copies of the viral genome have recently been reported (Prasad et al., 1976; Magnusson and Nilsson, 1977). By restriction-endonuclease mapping, Magnusson and Nilsson (1977) showed that the circular free polyoma virus-genomes in their mouse 3T3 transformed cells were defective in a region close to the origin of viral DNA replication, and these cells may be more analogous to some of the lysogenized *E. coli* carrying lambda plasmids than to EBV-transformed cells.

The size of the EBV DNA circles isolated from different BL cells are, within an experimental error of 1%–2%, exactly the size of the linear genomes in virus particles. Ninety-nine BL-derived EBV DNA circles have been sized by electron microscopy, and they all have been the same length with a standard deviation of less than 2%. If these circular viral genomes are independent replicons, as required of the plasmid or episome models in Fig. 1, the uniformity in size is a striking and unexpected observation. Self-replicating genetic elements in bacteria readily acquire genes, which confer a growth advantage to the host cell. In *E. coli*, there is apparently no size limitation on the amount of genetic information which can be added, since plasmids as small as 1.5×10^6 daltons (Cozzarelli et al., 1968) and as large as 150×10^6 daltons (Sharp et al., 1972) have been isolated. Intuitively, it would seem that there should likewise be no size restrictions put on the EBV circles in transformed cells, since these DNA molecules are no longer required to remain packageable into mature virions. The EBV DNA circles in the BL-derived cells are, in fact, quite different from the herpesvirus saimiri (HVS) DNA circles isolated from a virus-transformed nonproducer cell line established from a tumor biopsy of an HVS-infected marmoset. In the HVS-transformed cells, part of the genetic information present in HVS particles has been deleted, while some of it has been duplicated, and in total the intracellular HVS DNA circles are significantly larger than virion DNA (Werner et al., 1977).

II. EPITHELIAL TUMOR CELLS OF NASOPHARYNGEAL CARCINOMA

In NPC tumors, the EBV DNA has been shown to reside in the epithelial tumor cells (Wolf et al., 1973; Klein et al., 1974a). Infiltrating nontumor human lymphoid cells in NPC biopsy specimens can be removed by passing the tumors in athymic nude mice, and two such nude-mouse NPC tumors, J. G. and M. M., have been analyzed. The state of the viral DNA in human epithelial cells appears quite analogous to that of BL cells. The size of the EBV genomes in the NPC tumor cells may, however, be very slightly smaller than those in BL cells, but more tumors must be analyzed to verify these observations (Kaschka-Dierich et al., 1976). LY-2 is a lymphoid cell line derived from an NPC tumor explant (de-Thé et al., 1970) and is clearly not of neoplastic origin; sedimentation analysis indicates that the EBV DNA circles in this line are of the large type found in both BL cells and lymphoblastoid cell lines (Kaschka-Dierich, unpublished results).

III. LYMPHOBLASTOID CELL LINES

BL cell lines differ from the lymphoblastoid cell lines obtained from presumably nonneoplastic precursors in a number of morphologic, cytogenetic, and functional parameters (Nilsson and Pontén, 1975; Manolov and Manolova, 1972; Jarvis et al. 1974; Zech et al., 1976; Nilsson et al., 1977; Chap. 11). In Table 2, LY-2, SK-L1, and the seven lines derived from normal individuals and infectious mononucleosis (IM) patients are all of the lymphoblastoid type. Circular viral genomes are found in all of these immortalized cells and, where studies have been made integrated viral sequences appear to be present as well (Kaschka-Dierich et al., 1977; Adams et al., 1977, and unpublished results). Nonoyama and Pagano (1972 a) have also reported that the F265 and NC-37 cell lines from normal individuals have free EBV genomes similar to those in Raji. At least superficially, the state of the viral DNA is the same in the neoplastic (lymphoma) cells and the cells of lymphoblastoid lines of nonneoplastic origin.

IV. IN VITRO TRANSFORMED UMBILICAL-CORD LEUKOCYTES

Circular EBV genomes have been found in cell lines established in vitro by infecting human umbilical-cord leukocytes with EBV. These include three lines (cb35B1, cb35B3, and cb41B11) established by infection with the B95-8 laboratory strain of EBV (M. Dalens, unpublished results) and two cell lines (TW16 and TW20) where the source of transforming virus was the mouth wash of two IM patients (Pagano et al., 1976). Integrated EBV DNA sequences were not detected in one of the B95-8-transformed cord-blood lines (Adams et al., 1977). However, EBV DNA with the properties of integrated sequences are clearly present in the TW16 and TW20 lines (Adams et al., 1979) and preliminary results indicate that the presence or absence of integrated B95-8 viral DNA may depend on the conditions used in the establishment of the line.

The B95-8 strain of EBV has been widely used as the laboratory prototype for the transforming virus which can be isolated from the oral cavity of recently infected individuals. This would appear to be a bad choice for a prototype strain, since both the 883L line, which was the source of EBV used in the establishment of the B95-8 marmoset producer cell (Miller et al., 1972), and all cord-blood cell lines established with B95-8 virus preparations contain atypically small circular EBV DNA molecules (Table 2). All other nonproducer lymphoid cells thus far characterized have had EBV DNA circles of a similar large size.

EBV DNA-carrying lymphoid cell lines are classified as producer or nonproducer on the basis of whether or not a few cells in growing cultures express antigens associated with the productive virus cycle (Klein et al., 1972). Moreover, some cells in nonproducer lines like Raji and F265 can be induced with 5-iododeoxyuridine (IUDR) or 5-bromodeoxyuridine (BUDR) to express antigens associated with virus production and most producer lines respond similarly with an increase in the number of cells producing virus (Gerber, 1972; Hampar, et al., 1972; Sugawara et al., 1972; Klein and Dombos, 1973). Producer and nonproducer lines as well as inducible and noninducible cell lines are included in the material analyzed in Table 2. Again, as between lymphoma and lymphoblastoid cells, there is no apparent difference between the various cell lines at the level of the physical state of their EBV DNA.

Because cord-blood cell lines are notoriously of the nonproducer, noninducible type and usually have few EBV genome equivalents per cell (Miller et al., 1976), one could speculate that these cells may lack the genetic information required for expression of antigens like early antigen (EA) and viral capsid antigen (VCA). However, the cord-blood lines in Table 2 all had approximately ten genome equivalents of EBV DNA/cell and the data in Table 2 indicate that the failure to express these antigens is not due to the loss of a substantial part of the viral genome. The size of the DNA circles in the B95-8 virus-established cord lines is the same as in the parental 883 L producer cell line. Moreover, the circles in IM 16 and TW 16 are of the same size. IM 16 is a producer cell line (the *N. W. line* in Table 1) established from the peripheral blood of an IM patient and TW 16 is a nonproducer cord-blood cell line established with the mouth wash from the same patient. The deletion of a measurable segment of the EBV genome has thus not been observed in the nonproducer cord blood lines that have been studied.

V. IN VITRO CONVERTED CELL LINES

Several unusual B type human lymphoma cell lines lacking detectable amounts of EBV DNA have been described (Klein et al., 1974b, 1975; Epstein et al., 1976). Two such B cell lymphoma lines. Ramos and BJAB, can be infected with EB virus and it is possible to isolate permanently EBV nuclear antigen (EBNA)-positive sublines after exposure of these cells in culture to either the P_3HR-1 or B95-8 laboratory strains of EBV (Clements et al., 1975; Klein et al., 1975; Fresen and zur Hausen, 1976). These converted Ramos and BJAB cells often contain only one to a few copies of the viral genome (Andersson and Lindahl, 1976; Fresen et al., 1977) and the state of the EBV DNA in three such converted lines has been investigated (Andersson-Anvret and Lindahl, 1978). Two lines, AW-Ramos and EHRA-Ramos, were converted with P_3HR-1 virus (Klein et al., 1975) and contain one and four EBV genome equivalents per cell, respectively. The third subline, Ramos/B95-8, was isolated after infection with B95-8 virus (Fresen and zur Hausen, 1976) and has two EBV DNA genome equivalents per cell. Viral DNA with the properties of circular molecules could not be demonstrated in any of these lines. Instead, all EBV DNA appears to be integrated. From the CsCl gradient hybridization profiles, it may be concluded that the viral DNA is not integrated as many small fragments at multiple locations, but it is not known if the viral DNA is integrated as whole genomes or large fragments. In addition to the standard techniques used in demonstrating integrated sequences in cells with multiple EBV DNA copies, two additional experiments, namely density analysis in actinomycin D/CsCl gradients (Kersten et al., 1966) and the Hirt fractionation method (Hirt, 1967) were employed in further substantiating that the single EBV DNA genome equivalent of AW-Ramos is integrated as part of the host DNA (Andersson-Anvret and Lindahl, 1978).

The EBV-converted Ramos and BJAB cells have altered growth properties (Steinitz and Klein, 1976) and can perhaps be compared more to SV40-transformed mouse 3T3 cells than to the other EBV-transformed cells in Table 2. Thus, the growth properties of a cell that already has the ability for unlimited passage in cell culture (Ramos or mouse 3T3 cells) have been altered by the integration of viral DNA (EBV or SV40) into the host chromosome. The SV40-transformed cells express one viral function, the T antigen, and the EBV-converted cells express an apparently analogous viral antigen, EBNA (Chap. 3).

With the clear exception of the EBV-converted Ramos cells, no marked differences have been found to date between the states of the EBV DNA in various types of cells. The tests that have been used to analyze the intracellular forms of EBV DNA are, admittedly, of limited sensitivity and there may well be profound differences between the various types of cells at the level of the viral genome. The integration of different fragments of the viral genome at specific chromosomal sites could well be an important factor influencing the phenotype of the cell. Further, in spite of the fact that length measurements show that most of the circular EBV genomes are of similar size and reassociation kinetic data indicate a high degree of nucleotide homology, important sequence differences may still exist between the EBV genomes in the different isolates.

VI. IN VIVO LATENTLY INFECTED CELLS

EBV is ubiquitous and most individuals become life-long carriers of the viral genome (Chaps. 1 and 4). It would appear that at least the immunologically competent host is resistant to any oncogenic effects of this virus. The EBV genome-carrying lymphocytes present in seropositive individuals are either (1) different from the immortalized lymphoblastoid cells growing in vitro with doubling times of 18 – 48 h or (2) these cells are held in check by immune mechanisms, either humoral or of the cell-mediated type seen in the acute phase of IM (Hutt et al., 1975; Svedmyr and Jondal, 1975; Royston et al., 1975; Rickinson et al., 1977a). A discussion of the latter immune surveillance alternative is beyond the scope of this chapter.

Rickinson and co-workers have addressed themselves to the question of whether the in vivo latently infected cells are the same or different from the immortalized lymphoblastoid cells growing in vitro. It has been demonstrated that when mononuclear blood cells from either IM patients (Rickinson et al., 1974, 1975) or healthy seropositive adults (Rickinson et al., 1977b) are placed in culture, cell lines emerge by a two-step process involving first virus production in latently EBV-infected cells and subsequent transformation of the adjacent unifected lymphocytes by the activated virus. While these results can be interpreted to mean that the EBV DNA-containing lymphocytes of normal individuals are not the same as the transformed cells growing in cell culture they do not provide information on the state of the viral genome in vivo. The same two-step process also preferentially occurs when cord blood leukocytes are cocultivated with fresh BL biopsy specimens (Dalens et al., 1975) where the state of the EBV DNA has been partially characterized.

For the time being, the question of whether the state of the EBV genome in the latently infected cell in vivo is the same or different from that in the immortalized or transformed cell growing in vitro must remain open. In the acute phase of IM, EBNA-positive blasts amount to only a few percent of the B cell population and in healthy seropositive individuals such cells can not be demonstrated (Klein et al., 1976). Because of the rarity of viral genome-carrying cells, the amount of EBV DNA in peripheral blood is below the level detectable by the most sensitive hybridization methods. Determination of the state of the EBV genome in vivo in the cells of normal individuals will therefore be technically impossible until a way is found to concentrate and collect just those few cells carrying EBV DNA.

I. REPLICATION OF THE LATENT EBV DNA IN TRANSFORMED CELLS

The finding of both integrated EBV DNA sequences and free circular viral genomes in the majority of transformed cells does not distinguish between any of the three models, provirus, plasmid, or episome presented in Fig. 1. It is important now to determine if the circular EBV genomes are self-replicating structures, and if so, to what degree the large DNA circles fluctuate between an integrated and a free state. Three studies relevant to the problem of how the latent EBV genomes of transformed cells replicate deserve mention.

I. TIME OF EBV DNA REPLICATION IN SYNCHRONIZED CELLS

With Raji cells, synchronized by the double-thymidine blocking technique, it has been observed that the amount of intrinsic EBV DNA doubles during a 1 h period early ($\sim 30-90$ min following removal of the thymidine block) in the S-1 phase of the cell cycle (Hampar et al., 1974). This is the same critical time period when IUDR must be added to induce antigen expression from the latent EBV genomes of synchronized cells of both producer and nonproducer types (Hampar et al., 1973). The maintenance of a characteristic, constant number of EBV genomes by different cells indicates that the process is tightly regulated, so the finding that the number of genomes doubles at a precise time is not in itself surprising. The state of the EBV DNA at the time of its replication, or for that matter at any other specific time during the cell cycle has not been investigated; present evidence does not distinguish between the possibility that either (1) all the free circular genomes synchronously divide once at a precise time in the cell cycle or (2) a small number of integrated genomes are used as template for the formation of a fixed number of free viral genomes in the S-1 phase. The fact that EBV DNA replication can be restricted to a specific, short time interval should, however, be useful in attempting to isolate circular viral DNA molecules in the process of replication.

It is noted that the finding of one umbilical-cord blood cell line without detectable amounts of integrated EBV DNA (Adams et al., 1977) does not prove that the circular forms are independently replicating genetic elements. If a proviral form of the EBV genome were integrated into a particularly guanine-cytosine-rich region of the host DNA of this exceptional cell, it would not have been seen by the method used to analyze for integrated EBV DNA sequences.

II. EFFECT OF PHOSPHONOACETIC ACID ON THE REPLICATION OF LATENT EBV GENOMES

Phosphonoacetic acid (PAA) is a potent inhibitor of several herpesvirus-induced DNA polymerases (see for example for herpes simplex virus, Mao et al., 1975: for human cytomegalovirus, Huang, 1975; for Marek's disease virus, Lee et al., 1976; and for equine abortion virus, Allen et al., 1977). PAA inhibits the spontaneous EBV production of B95-8 cells and greatly reduces the number of VCA-positive cells in both B95-8 and P_3HR-1 cell cultures (Nyormoi et al., 1976). It appears, however, that PAA only inhibits productive EBV DNA synthesis and has no effect on the replication of the latent viral genomes. With Raji, the number of viral genome copies per cell remains unchanged after long-term culture in the presence of PAA at concentrations sufficient to inhibit the productive EBV DNA replication that can be induced in these cells following superinfection with P_3HR-1 virus (Yajima et al., 1976; Summers and Klein, 1976). When producer cells are grown in the presence of PAA the number of EBV genome copies decreases to a constant low number, which for P_3HR-1 cells is approximately ten EBV genome equivalents per cell (Yajima et al., 1976). This is the same number of latent EBV genomes as retained by P_3HR-1 cells which have lost the ability to produce virus spontaneously (Table 1) and the decrease from an average of several hundred EBV DNA molecules per cell to only ten presumably is due to the elimination of those few cells producing large quantities of linear viral genomes in untreated cultures of producer P_3HR-1 cells.

The number of latent EBV genomes in the B95-8 virus-producing cell line is about 40 (Summers and Klein, 1976). The state of the EBV genomes in PAA-treated B95-8 cells has been characterized and both integrated and circular forms of EBV DNA have been found (Gussander and Adams, 1979). The DNA polymerase induced by EBV is apparently not used in the replication or formation of the latent circular EBV genomes. On removal of PAA, B95-8 cells will again produce transforming virus, but whether the linear genomes encapsulated in virus particles are copied from an integrated provirus template or from the free circular EBV genomes is not known.

III. CURING OF LATENT EBV GENOMES

With the polyoma-transformed rat cells which have multiple copies of the viral genome in both integrated and free circular forms, it has been possible to establish that the circles most probably arise from an integrated provirus (Prasad et al., 1976). The method used was first to cure the cells of the circular viral genomes and then follow their reformation. In this system it was possible to eliminate the circular forms of virus DNA by shifting cells, transformed with the ts-a mutant of polyoma at the permissive temperature, to the nonpermissive temperature of 40 °C. At the high temperature only integrated polyoma genomes remained, but when the temperature was lowered to 33 °C the circular genomes reappeared.

While mutants of EBV analogous to the polyoma ts-a mutant are not available, it has been reported that the number of latent viral genomes can be reduced by exposing EBV-carrying cells to cycloheximide (Pagano et al., 1973; Tanaka et al., 1976). Cycloheximide, an inhibitor of protein synthesis, also blocks cellular DNA synthesis by more than 80%. In cycloheximide-treated Raji cells, the number of EBV DNA copies/µg cellular DNA remains constant and replication of the latent EBV genomes must be inhibited in parallel with the host DNA (Pagano et al., 1973). (In EBV-superinfected Raji cells virus DNA replication can proceed in the presence of cycloheximide if the drug is added after early virus-induced enzymes have been synthesized, ibid. Thus in this situation the replication of latent EBV genomes is different from that of productive EBV DNA replication, just as with PAA). However, when cycloheximide was washed away after 1–2 days, the number of EBV genome equivalents per Raji cell first increased to about twice the normal load by day 4 and then the amount of EBV DNA was reported to have dropped to an average of only 10–20 copies per cell. The early increase in amount of EBV DNA after removal of cycloheximide could simply be due to the induction of virus production in a few of the cells (Hampar et al., 1976). However, the decrease in the number of viral genomes must be due to the loss of some latent EBV DNA sequences from the majority of the cells.

The number of EBV genome copies in cycloheximide-treated Raji cells will, with time, return to the characteristic number of 50–60 copies per cell (Pagano et al., 1973). However, if the cycloheximide treatment is repeated at weekly intervals the number of

EBV genomes apparently remains at 10–20 copies per cell, and it should be possible to study the state of the EBV DNA in such cultures. Growth in the presence of cycloheximide or puromycin is known to alter the superhelical density of the covalently closed supercoiled forms of SV40 and polyoma DNA (Jaenisch and Levine, 1973; Bourgaux and Bourgaux-Ramoisy, 1972) and similar changes in EBV DNA circles might well lead to the elimination of these latent forms.

The number of EBV genomes in P₃HR-1-producer cells can also be greatly reduced by exposure to cycloheximide (Tanaka et al., 1976) and by cloning these cells shortly after removal of cycloheximide it was possible to isolate a P₃HR-1 variant that stably maintains only a single EBV genome equivalent. The state of the EBV DNA in this cell, which grows at the same rate as normal P₃HR-1 cells, is not known.

J. ASSOCIATION OF EBV DNA WITH CHROMOSOMES

It has been reported and often quoted that all of the 50–60 EBV genome copies in Raji are associated with metaphase chromosomes (Nonoyama and Pagano, 1971). It is unfortunate that no details concerning controls and the purity of the Raji metaphase chromosomes used in this important experiment have been published. Assuming the statement to be correct, it is of interest to determine if circular EBV genomes are bound to the chromosomes at metaphase, and if so, in which fashion. The DNA extracted from chromosomes isolated by the standard technique of Maio and Schildkraut (1969) is partially degraded and contains many single-strand nicks. If covalently closed circular forms of EBV DNA are associated with metaphase chromosomes they will, in all probability, be destroyed during this chromosome isolation procedure. Wray (1973) has reported an improved method of isolating metaphase chromosomes at pH 10.5 by which it is possible to obtain DNA of higher molecular weight. This method may, therefore, be more useful in attempting to demonstrate whether the circular forms of EBV DNA are associated with the chromosomes at metaphase.

In situ hybridization indicates that the EBV DNA of Raji may be associated with specific chromosomes (zur Hausen and Schulte-Holthausen, 1972). If either an integrated proviral genome or a specific host-cell function is required for the maintenance of the latent EBV genomes, it was thought possible to localize this chromosome(s) by the somatic cell hybridization method that has been used in the SV40 system. In that case, it has been possible to assign the integration site of the SV40 DNA to specific human chromosomes in different transformed cell lines by following the segregation of human chromosomes and viral T antigen in mouse/man cell hybrids that preferentially lose human chromosomes (Croce et al., 1973; Croce, 1977). Four different mouse/man hybrids have been used in an attempt to localize the human chromosome(s) required for the maintenance of EBV DNA. These include the following hybrid combinations: mouse fibroblast line A9/BL producer cell line Daudi (Klein et al., 1974c); mouse CLID cells/BL producer cell line P₃HR-1 (Glaser et al., 1975); mouse TA3Ha mammary carcinoma cells/BL producer cell line Daudi (Spira et al., 1977); and several different mouse cells/human NPC tumor cells from biopsies or nude-mouse propagated tumors (Steplewski et al., 1978). All hybrid combinations expressed the EBNA antigen and this was used as a convenient, rapid assay for the presence or absence of the viral genome. EBNA expression, like SV40 T antigen, is known to be directly correlated with the presence of viral DNA (Lindahl et al., 1974). With selected somatic cell hybrid clones, nucleic acid hybridization tests have confirmed that the presence or absence of EBV DNA followed that of EBNA. Human chromosomes were identified in all four investigations by both isoenzyme markers and Giemsa banding techniques.

The uniformly disappointing conclusion of these four somatic cell hybridization studies is that the presence of EBV DNA is associated with some but not all human chromosomes and that no specific human chromosome responsible for the maintenance of EBV DNA could be identified. One likely explanation for these results is that EBV DNA has some degree of motility and has integrated on different chromosomes after the hybrids were formed. The original human cells that were fused with the various mouse cells presumably had multiple free, circular viral genome copies, which might well have randomly integrated with time. It is still possible that there is a specific human chromosome required for the maintenance of the free viral genomes. It is, however, technically impossible to determine when the hybrids lose this form of latent EBV DNA, since it is known from the studies on the EBV-converted Ramos cells that EBNA can be expressed from integrated EBV DNA sequences.

K. THE EBV GENOME AND THE EVOLUTION OF BURKITT'S LYMPHOMA

Irrespective of which of the three models, provirus, plasmid, or episome, is normally employed in the maintenance of the EBV genome in transformed cells, the circular viral DNA molecules most likely recombine randomly with the cell DNA at a low frequency. The entire EBV genome could thus be likened to the structurally defined, evolutionary important transposable genetic elements in prokaryotes (for reviews see Cohen, 1976; Kleckner, 1977). By analogy, the viral genome of lymphoblastoid cells could function not only as the immortalizing agent but also as a cofactor in the evolution of these nonmalignant cells to a tumor cell. By randomly integrating and creating new homology sites on different chromosomes, the virus genome could play a part in causing chromosome translocations as well as in augmenting gene expression in regions adjacent to the site of integration.

Tumor evolution is obviously a multistep process, as has been discussed by Klein and Klein (1977), and in the absence of strong in vivo selective pressures it is not surprising that the specific changes associated with lymphoma cells have not been reproduced in vitro. Nevertheless, if the presence of intracellular EBV genomes may have a tendency to facilitate the introduction of the BL-associated chromosomal changes, there is hope that evidence of the virus can be found in the form of integrated viral DNA sequences at certain sites in the host genomes of these rapidly growing monoclonal tumor cells.

REFERENCES

Adams, A., Lindahl, T.: Intracellular forms of Epstein-Barr virus DNA in Raji cells. In: Oncogenesis and herpesviruses II. de-Thé, G., Epstein, M. A., zur Hausen, H. (eds.), Part 1, pp. 125–132. Lyon: IARC, 1975a

Adams, A., Lindahl, T.: Epstein-Barr virus genomes with properties of circular DNA molecules in carrier cells. Proc. Natl. Acad. Sci. USA **72**, 1477–1481 (1975b)

Adams, A., Lindahl, T., Klein, G.: Linear association between cellular DNA and Epstein-Barr virus DNA in a human lymphoblastoid cell line. Proc. Natl. Acad. Sci. USA **70**, 2888–2892 (1973)

Adams, A., Bjursell, G., Kaschka-Dierich, C., Lindahl, T.: Circular Epstein-Barr virus genomes of reduced size in a human lymphoid cell line of infectious mononucleosis origin. J. Virol. **22**, 373–380 (1977)

Adams, A., Bjursell, G., Gussander, E., Koliais, S., Falk, L., Lindahl, T.: Size of the intracellular circular Epstein-Barr virus DNA molecules in infectious mononucleosis-derived human lymphoid cell lines. J. Virol. **29** (in press) (1979)

Allen, G. P., O'Callaghan, D. J., Randall, C. C.: Purification and characterization of equine herpesvirus-induced DNA polymerase. Virology **76**, 395–408 (1977)

Andersson, M.: Amounts of Epstein-Barr virus DNA in somatic cell hybrids between Burkitt lymphoma-derived cell lines. J. Virol. **16**, 1345–1347 (1975)

Andersson, M., Lindahl, T.: Epstein-Barr virus DNA in human lymphoid cell lines: *in vitro* conversion. Virology **73**, 96–105 (1976)

Andersson-Anvret, A., Lindahl, T.: Integrated viral DNA in EB virus-converted human lymphoma lines J. Virol. **25**, 710–718 (1978)

Bauer, W., Vinograd, J.: The interaction of closed circular DNA with intercalative dyes. I. The superhelix density of SV40 DNA in the presence and absence of dye. J. Mol. Biol. **33**, 144–171 (1968)

Biegeleisen, K., Rush, M. G.: Association of *Herpes simplex* virus type 1 DNA with host chromosomal DNA during productive infection. Virology **69**, 246–259 (1976)

Bourgaux, P., Bourgaux-Ramoisy, D.: Is a specific protein responsible for the supercoiling of polyoma DNA? Nature **253**, 105–107 (1972)

Clayton, D. A., Vinograd, J.: Circular dimer and catenate forms of mitochondrial DNA in human leukaemic leucocytes. Nature **216**, 652–657 (1967)

Clements, G. B., Klein, G., Povey, S.: Production by EBV infection of an EBNA-positive subline from an EBNA-negative human lymphoma cell line without detectable EBV DNA. Int. J. Cancer **16**, 125–133 (1975)

Cohen, S. N.: Transposable genetic elements and plasmid evolution. Nature **263**, 731–738 (1976)

Cozzarelli, N. R., Kelly, R. B., Kornberg, A.: A minute circular DNA from *Escherichia coli* 15. Proc. Natl. Acad. Sci. USA **60**, 992–999 (1968)

Croce, C. M.: Assignment of the simian virus 40 integration site to chromosome 17 in the SV40-transformed human cell line GM54VA. Proc. Natl. Acad. Sci. USA **74**, 315–318 (1977)

Croce, C. M., Girardi, A. J., Koprowski, H.: Assignment of the T antigen gene of simian virus 40 to human chromosome C-7. Proc. Natl. Acad. Sci. USA **70**, 3617–3620 (1973)

Dalens, M., Zech, L., Klein, G.: Origin of lymphoid lines established from mixed cultures of cord-blood lymphocytes and explants from infectious mononucleosis, Burkitt lymphoma and healthy donors. Int. J. Cancer **16**, 1008–1014 (1975)

Davis, R. W., Simon, M., Davidson, N.: Electron microscope heteroduplex methods for mapping regions of base sequence homology in nucleic acids. Methods Enzymol. **21D**, 413–428 (1971)

de-Thé, G., Ho, H. C., Kwan, H. C., Desgranges, C., Favre, M. C.: Nasopharyngeal carcinoma (NPC) 1. Types of cultures derived from tumour biopsies and non-tumorous tissues of Chinese patients with special reference to lymphoblastoid transformation. Int. J. Cancer **6**, 189–206 (1970)

Epstein, A. L., Henle, W., Henle, G., Hewetson, J. F., Kaplan, H. S.: Surface marker characteristics and Epstein-Barr virus studies of two established North American Burkitt's lymphoma cell lines. Proc. Natl. Acad. Sci. USA **73**, 228–232 (1976)

Ernberg, I., Andersson-Anvret, M., Klein, G., Lundin, L., Killander, D.: Relationship between amount of Epstein-Barr virus-determined nuclear antigen per cell and number of EBV-DNA copies per cell. Nature **266**, 269–270 (1977)

Freifelder, D.: Molecular weights of coliphages and coliphage DNA. IV. Molecular weights of DNA from bacteriophages T4, T5 and T7 and the general problem of determination of M. J. Mol. Biol. **54**, 567–577 (1970)

Fresen, K.-O., zur Hausen, H.: Establishment of EBNA-expressing cell lines by infection of Epstein-Barr virus (EBV)-genome-negative human lymphoma cells with different EBV strains. Int. J. Cancer **17**, 161–166 (1976)

Fresen, K.-O., Merkt, B., Bornkamm, G. W., zur Hausen, H.: Heterogeneity of Epstein-Barr virus originating from P3HR-1 cells. Int. J. Cancer **19**, 317–323 (1977)

Gelb, L. D., Kohne, D. E., Martin, M. A.: Quantitation of simian virus 40 sequences in African green monkey, mouse and virus transformed cell genomes. J. Mol. Biol. **57**, 129–145 (1971)

Gerber, P.: Activation of Epstein-Barr virus by 5-bromodeoxyuridine in "virus-free" human cells. Proc. Natl. Acad. Sci. USA **69**, 82–85 (1972)

Glaser, R., Nonoyama, M.: Host cell regulation of induction of Epstein-Barr virus. J. Virol. **14**, 174–176 (1974)

Glaser, R., Nonoyama, M., Shows, T. B., Henle, G., Henle, W.: Epstein-Barr virus: Studies on the association of virus genome with human chromosomes in hybrid cells. In: Oncogenesis and herpesviruses II. de-Thé, G., Epstein, M. A., zur Hausen, H. (eds.), Part 1, pp. 457–466. Lyon: IARC, 1975

Gussander, E., Adams, A.: Intracellular state of Epstein-Barr virus DNA in producer cell lines. J. Gen. Virol. (in press)

Haas, M., Vogt, M., Dulbecco, R.: Loss of simian virus 40 DNA-RNA hybrids from nitrocellulose membranes; implications for study of virus-host DNA interactions. Proc. Natl. Acad. Sci. USA **69**, 2160–2164 (1972)

Hampar, B., Derge, J. G., Martos, L. M., Walker, J. L.: Synthesis of Epstein-Barr virus after activation of the viral genome in a "virus-negative" human lymphoblastoid cell (Raji) made resistant to 5-bromodeoxyuridine. Proc. Natl. Acad. Sci. USA **69**, 78–82 (1972)

Hampar, B., Derge, J. G., Martos, L. M., Tagamets, M. A., Chang, S.-Y., Chagrabarty, M.: Identification of a critical period during the S phase for activation of the Epstein-Barr virus by 5-iododeoxyuridine. Nature New Biol. **244**, 214–217 (1973)

Hampar, B., Tanaka, A., Nonoyama, M., Derge, J.: Replication of the resident repressed Epstein-Barr virus genome during the early S phase (S-1 period) of non-producer Raji cells. Proc. Natl. Acad. Sci. USA **71**, 631–633 (1974)

Hampar, B., Lenoir, G., Nonoyama, M., Derge, J. G., Chang, S.-Y.: Cell cycle dependence for activation of Epstein-Barr virus by inhibitors of protein synthesis or medium deficient in arginine. Virology **69**, 660–668 (1976)

Hershey, A. D., Burgi, E., Ingraham, L.: Cohension of DNA molecules isolated from phage lambda. Proc. Natl. Acad. Sci. USA **49**, 748–755 (1963)

Hirt, B.: Selective extraction of polyoma DNA from infected mouse cell cultures. J. Mol. Biol. **26**, 365–369 (1967)

Hobom, G., Hogness, D. S.: The role of recombination in the formation of circular oligomers of the $\lambda\,dv\,1$ plasmid. J. Mol. Biol. **88**, 65–87 (1974)

Huang, E.-S.: Human cytomegalovirus. IV. Specific inhibition of virus-induced DNA polymerase activity and viral DNA replication by phosphonoacetic acid. J. Virol. **16**, 1560–1565 (1975)

Hutt, L. M., Huang, Y. T., Dascomb, H. E., Pagano, J. S.: Enhanced destruction of lymphoid cell lines by peripheral blood leukocytes taken from patients with acute infectious mononucleosis. J. Immunol. **115**, 243–248 (1975)

Hölzel, F., Sokol, F.: Integration of progeny simian virus 40 DNA into the host cell genome. J. Mol. Biol. **84**, 423–444 (1974)

Ikeda, H., Tomizawa, J.: Prophage P1, an extrachromosomal replication unit. Cold Spring Harbor Symp. Quant. Biol. **33**, 791–798 (1968)

Jaenisch, R., Levine, A. J.: DNA replication of SV40-infected cells. VII. Formation of SV40 catenated and circular dimers. J. Mol. Biol. **73**, 199–212 (1973)

Jarvis, J. E., Ball, G., Rickinson, A. B., Epstein, M. A.: Cytogenetic studies on human lymphoblastoid cell lines from Burkitt's lymphomas and other sources. Int. J. Cancer **14**, 716–721 (1974)

Jehn, U., Lindahl, T., Klein, G.: Fate of virus DNA in the abortive infection of human lymphoid cell lines by Epstein-Barr virus. J. Gen. Virol. **16**, 409–412 (1972)

Kaschka-Dierich, C., Adams, A., Lindahl, T., Bornkamm, G. W., Bjursell, G., Klein, G., Giovanella, B. C., Singh, S.: Intracellular forms of Epstein-Barr virus DNA in human tumour cells *in vivo*. Nature **260**, 302–306 (1976)

Kaschka-Dierich, C., Falk, L., Bjursell, G., Adams, A., Lindahl, T.: Human lymphoblastoid cell lines derived from individuals without lymphoproliferative disease contain the same latent forms of Epstein-Barr virus DNA as those found in tumor cells. Int. J. Cancer **20**, 173–180 (1977)

Kawai, Y., Nonoyama, M., Pagano, J. S.: Reassociation kinetics for Epstein-Barr virus DNA: Nonhomology to mammalian DNA and homology of viral DNA in various dieseases. J. Virol. **12**, 1006–1012 (1973)

Kersten, W., Kersten, H., Szybalski, W.: Physico-chemical properties of complexes between DNA and antibiotics which affect RNA synthesis (actinomycin, daunomycin, cinerubin, nogalamycin, chromomycin, mithramycin, and olivomycin). Biochemistry **5**, 236–242 (1966)

Kieff, E., Levine, J.: Homology between Burkitt herpes viral DNA and DNA in continuous lymphoblastoid cells from patients with infectious mononucleosis. Proc. Natl. Acad. Sci. USA **71**, 355–358 (1974)

Kiger, J. A., Young, E. T., Sinsheimer, R. L.: Purification and properties of intracellular lambda DNA rings. J. Mol. Biol. **33**, 395–413 (1968)

Kleckner, N.: Translocatable elements in procaryotes. Cell **11**, 11–23 (1977)

Klein, G., Dombos, L.: Relationship between the sensitivity of EBV-carrying lymphoblastoid lines to superinfection and the inducibility of the resident viral genome. Int. J. Cancer **11**, 327–337 (1973)

Klein, G., Klein, E.: Immune surveillance against virus-induced tumors and nonrejectability of spontaneous tumors: Contrasting consequences of host versus tumor evolution. Proc. Natl. Acad. Sci. USA **74**, 2121–2125 (1977)

Klein, G., Dombos, L., Gothoskar, B.: Sensivity of Epstein-Barr virus (EBV) producer and non-producer human lymphoblastoid cell lines to superinfection with EB-virus. Int. J. Cancer **10**, 44–57 (1972)

Klein, G., Giovanella, B. C., Lindahl, T., Fialkow, P. J., Singh, S., Stehlin, J. S.: Direct evidence for the presence of Epstein-Barr virus DNA and nuclear antigen in malignant epithelial cells from patients with poorly differentiated carcinoma of the nasopharynx. Proc. Natl. Acad. Sci. USA **71**, 4737–4741 (1974a)

Klein, G., Lindahl, T., Jondal, M., Leibold, W., Menezes, J., Nilsson, K., Sundström, C.: Continuous lymphoid cell lines with characteristics of B cells (bone marrow-derived), lacking the EBV genome and derived from three human lymphomas. Proc. Natl. Acad. Sci. USA **71**, 3283–3286 (1974b)

Klein, G., Wiener, F., Zech, L., zur Hausen, H., Reedman, B.: Segregation of the EBV-determined nuclear antigen (EBNA) in somatic cell hybrids derived from the fusion of a mouse fibroblast and a human Burkitt lymphoma line. Int. J. Cancer **14**, 54–64 (1974c)

Klein, G., Giovanella, B., Westman, A., Stehlin, J. S., Mumford, D.: An EBV-genome-negative cell line established from an American Burkitt lymphoma; receptor characteristics, EBV infectibility, and permanent conversion into EBV-positive sublines by *in vitro* infection. Intervirology **5**, 319–334 (1975)

Klein, G., Svedmyr, E., Jondal, M., Persson, P. O.: EBV-determined nuclear antigen (EBNA)-positive cells in the peripheral blood of infectious mononucleosis patients. Int. J. Cancer **17**, 21–26 (1976)

Koliais, S., Bjursell, G., Adams, A., Lindahl, T., Klein, G.: State of Epstein-Barr virus DNA in an American Burkitt lymphoma line. J. Natl. Cancer Inst. **60**, 991–993 (1978)

Lee, L. F., Nazerian, K., Leinbach, S. S., Reno, J. M., Boezi, J. A.: Effect of phosphonoacetate on Marek's disease virus replication. J. Natl. Cancer Inst. **56**, 823–827 (1976)

Lieb, M.: Lambda mutants which persist as plasmids. J. Virol. **6**, 218–225 (1970)

Lindahl, T., Klein, G., Reedman, B. M., Johansson, B., Singh, S.: Relationship between Epstein-Barr virus (EBV) DNA and the EBV-determined nuclear antigen (EBNA) in Burkitt lymphoma biopsies and other lymphoproliferative malignancies. Int. J. Cancer **13**, 764–772 (1974)

Lindahl, T., Adams, A., Bjursell, G., Bornkamm, G. W., Kaschka-Dierich, C., Jehn, U.: Covalently closed circular duplex DNA of Epstein-Barr virus in a human lymphoid cell line. J. Mol. Biol. **102**, 511–530 (1976)

Lindahl, T., Adams, A., Andersson-Anvret, M., Falk, L.: Integration of Epstein-Barr virus DNA. In: Oncogenesis and herpesviruses III. de-Thé, G., Henle, W., Rapp, F. (eds.). Lyon: IARC, (in press, 1978)

Magnusson, G., Nilsson, M.-G.: Multiple free viral DNA copies in polyoma virus-transformed mouse cells surviving productive infection. J. Virol. **22**, 646–653 (1977)

Maio, J. J., Schildkraut, C. L.: Isolated mammalian metaphase chromosomes II. Fractionated chromosomes of mouse and chinese hamster cells. J. Mol. Biol. **40**, 203–216 (1969)

Manolov, G., Manolova, Y.: Marker band in one chromosome 14 from Burkitt lymphomas. Nature **237**, 33–34 (1972)

Mao, J. G.-H., Robishaw, E. E., Overby, L. R.: Inhibition of DNA polymerase from herpes simplex virus-infected WI-38 cells by phosphonoacetic acid. J. Virol. **15**, 1281–1283 (1975)

Matsubara, K., Kaiser, A. D.: λ dv: An autonomously replicating DNA fragment. Cold Spring Harbor Symp. Quant. Biol. **33**, 769–775 (1968)

Mele, J., Glaser, R., Nonoyama, M., Zimmerman, J., Rapp, F.: Observations on the resistance of Epstein-Barr virus DNA synthesis to hydroxyurea. Virology **62**, 102–111 (1974)

Miller, G., Shope, T., Lisco, H., Stitt, D., Lipman, M.: Epstein-Barr virus: transformation, cytopathic changes, and viral antigens in squirrel monkey and marmoset leukocytes. Proc. Natl. Acad. Sci. USA **69**, 383–387 (1972)

Miller, G., Coope, D., Niederman, J., Pagano, J.: Biological properties and viral surface antigens of Burkitt lymphoma and mononucleosis-derived strains of Epstein-Barr virus released from transformed marmoset cells. J. Virol. **18**, 1071–1080 (1976)

Minowada, J., Nonoyama, M., Moore, G. E., Rauch, A. M., Pagano, J. S.: The presence of the Epstein-Barr viral genome in human lymphoblastoid B-cell lines and its absence in a myeloma cell line. Cancer Res. **34**, 1898–1903 (1974)

Nilsson, K., Pontén, J.: Classification and biological nature of established human hematopoietic cell lines. Int. J. Cancer **15**, 321–341 (1975)

Nilsson, K., Giovanella, B. C., Stehlin, J. S., Klein, G.: Tumorigenicity of human hematopoietic cell lines in athymic nude mice. Int. J. Cancer **19**, 337–344 (1977)

Nonoyama, M., Pagano, J. S.: Detection of Epstein-Barr viral genome in nonproductive cells. Nature New Biol. **233**, 103–106 (1971)

Nonoyama, M., Pagano, J. S.: Separation of Epstein-Barr virus DNA from large chromosomal DNA in non-virus-producing cells. Nature New Biol. **238**, 169–171 (1972a)

Nonoyama, M., Pagano, J. S.: Replication of viral deoxyribonucleic acid and breakdown of cellular deoxyribonucleic acid in Epstein-Barr virus infection. J. Virol. **9**, 714–716 (1972b)

Nonoyama, M., Pagano, J. S.: Homology between Epstein-Barr virus DNA and viral DNA from Burkitt's lymphoma and nasopharyngeal carcinoma determined by DNA-DNA reassociation kinetics. Nature **242**, 44–47 (1973)

Nyormoi, O., Thorley-Lawson, D. A., Elkington, J., Strominger, J.: Differential effect of phosphonoacetic acid on the expression of Epstein-Barr viral antigens and virus production. Proc. Natl. Acad. Sci. USA **73**, 1745–1748 (1976)

Pagano, J. S., Nonoyama, M., Huang, C. H.: Epstein-Barr virus in human cells. In: Possible Episomes in Eukaryotes. Silvestri, L. (ed.), pp. 218–228. Amsterdam: North-Holland 1973

Pagano, J. S., Huang, C.-H., Huang, Y.-T.: Epstein-Barr virus genone in infectious mononucleosis. Nature **263**, 787–789 (1976)

Pettersson, U., Mulder, C., Delius, H., Sharp, P.: Cleavage of adenovirus type 2 DNA into six unique fragments by endonuclease R. Rl. Proc. Natl. Acad. Sci. USA **70**, 200–204 (1973)

Prasad, I., Zouzias, D., Basilico, C.: State of the viral DNA in rat cells transformed by polyoma virus. I. Virus rescue and the presence of nonintegrated viral DNA molecules. J. Virol. **18**, 436–444 (1976)

Pritchett, R. F., Hayward, S. D., Kieff, E. D.: DNA of Epstein-Barr virus I. Comparative studies of the DNA of Epstein-Barr virus from HR-1 and B95-8 cells: size, structure, and relatedness. J. Virol. **15**, 556–569 (1975)

Pritchett, R., Pedersen, M., Kieff, E.: Complexity of EBV homologous DNA in continuous lymphoblastoid cell lines. Virology **74**, 227–231 (1976)

Pulvertaft, R. J. V.: A study of malignant tumours in Nigeria by short term tissue culture. J. Clin. Path. **18**, 261–273 (1965)

Radloff, R., Bauer, W., Vinograd, J.: A dye-buoyant-density method for the detection and isolation of closed circular duplex DNA: The closed circular DNA in HeLa cells. Proc. Natl. Acad. Sci. USA **57**, 1514–1521 (1967)

Rickinson, A. B., Jarvis, J. E., Crawford, D. H., Epstein, M. A.: Observations on the type of infection by Epstein-Barr virus in peripheral lymphoid cells of patients with infectious mononucleosis. Int. J. Cancer **14**, 704–715 (1974)

Rickinson, A. B., Epstein, M. A., Crawford, D. H.: Absence of infectious Epstein-Barr virus in blood in acute infectious mononucleosis. Nature **258**, 236–238 (1975)

Rickinson, A. B., Crawford, D., Epstein, M. A.: Inhibition of the *in vitro* outgrowth of Epstein-Barr virus-transformed lymphocytes by thymus-dependent lymphocytes from infectious mononucleosis patients. Clin. Exp. Immunol. **28**, 72–79 (1977a)

Rickinson, A. B., Finerty, S., Epstein, M. A.: Comparative studies on adult donor lymphocytes infected by EB virus *in vivo* or *in vitro:* Origin of transformed cells arising in co-cultures with foetal lymphocytes. Int. J. Cancer **19**, 775–782 (1977b)

Rosner, J. L.: Formation, induction, and curing of bacteriophage P1 lysogens. Virology **48**, 679–689 (1972)

Royston, I., Sullivan, J. L., Periman, P. O., Perlin, E.: Cell-mediated immunity to Epstein-Barr-virus-transformed lymphoblastoid cells in acute infectious mononucleosis. New Engl. J. Med. **293**, 1159–1163 (1975)

Sambrook, J., Westphal, H., Srinivasan, P. R., Dulbecco, R.: The integrated state of viral DNA in SV40-transformed cells. Proc. Natl. Acad. Sci. USA **60**, 1288–1295 (1968)

Scott, J. R.: A defective P1 prophage with a chromosomal location. Virology **40**, 144–151 (1970)

Sharp, P. A., Hsu, M.-T., Ohtsubo, E., Davidson, N.: Electron microscope heteroduplex studies of sequence relations among plasmids of *Escherichia coli* I. Structure of F-prime factors. J. Mol. Biol. **71**, 471–497 (1972)

Signer, E.: Plasmid formation, a new mode of lysogeny by phage lambda. Nature **223**, 158–160 (1969)

Spira, J., Povey, S., Wiener, F., Klein, G., Andersson-Anvret, M.: Chromosome banding, isoenzyme studies and determination of Epstein-Barr virus DNA content on human Burkitt lymphoma/mouse hybrids. Int. J. Cancer **20**, 849–853 (1977)

Steinitz, M., Klein, G.: Epstein-Barr virus (EBV)-induced change in the saturation sensitivity and serum dependence of established, EBV-negative lymphoma lines *in vitro*. Virology **70**, 570–573 (1976)

Steplewski, Z., Koprowski, H., Andersson-Anvret, M., Klein, G.: Epstein-Barr virus in somatic cell hybrids between mouse cell and human nasopharyngeal carcinoma cells. J. Cell. Physiol. (in press)

Sugawara, K., Mizuno, F., Osato, T.: Epstein-Barr virus associated antigens in non-producing clones of human lymphoblastoid cell lines. Nature New Biol. **239**, 242–243 (1972)

Summers, W. C., Klein, G.: Inhibition of Epstein-Barr virus DNA synthesis and late gene expression by phosphonoacetic acid. J. Virol. **18**, 151–155 (1976)

Svedmyr, E., Jondal, M.: Cytotoxic effector cells specific for B cell lines transformed by Epstein-Barr virus are present in patients with infectious mononucleosis. Proc. Natl. Acad. Sci. USA **72**, 1622–1626 (1975)

Szybalski, W., Szybalski, E. H.: Equilibrium density gradient centrifugation. In: Procedures in nucleic acid research. Vol. 2. Cantoni, G. L., Davies, D. R. (eds.), pp. 311–354. New York: Harper & Row 1971

Tanaka, A., Nonoyama, M.: Latent DNA of Epstein-Barr virus: Separation from high-molecular weight cell DNA in a neutral glycerol gradient. Proc. Natl. Acad. Sci. USA **71**, 4658–4661 (1974)

Tanaka, A., Nonoyama, M., Hampar, B.: Partial elimination of latent Epstein-Barr virus genomes from virus-producing cells by cyclohexamide. Virology **70**, 164–170 (1976)

Tomizawa, J.-I., Anraku, N.: Molecular mechanisms of genetic recombination in bacteriphage. IV. Absence of polynucleotide interruption in DNA of T4 and lambda phage particles, with special reference to heterozygosis. J. Mol. Biol. **11**, 509–527 (1965)

Wang, J. C.: Interlocked DNA rings. II. Physicochemical studies. Biopolymers **9**, 489–502 (1970)

Watson, J. D.: Molecular biology of the gene. 3rd ed. Menlo Park (California): Benjamin 1976

Werner, F.-J., Bornkamm, G. W., Fleckenstein, B.: Episomal viral DNA in a *Herpesvirus saimiri*-transformed lymphoid cell line. J. Virol. **22**, 794–803 (1977)

Westphal, H., Dulbecco, R.: Viral DNA in polyoma- and SV40-transformed cell lines. Proc. Natl. Acad. Sci. USA **59**, 1158–1165 (1968)

Winocour, E., Frenkel, N., Lavi, S., Osenholts, M., Rozenblatt, S.: Host substitution in SV40 and polyoma DNA. Cold Spring Harbor Symp. Quant. Biol. **39**, 101–108 (1975)

Wolf, H., zur Hausen, H., Becker, V.: EB viral genomes in epithelial nasopharyngeal carcinoma cells. Nature New Biol. **244**, 246–247 (1973)

Wray, W.: Isolation of metaphase chromosomes with high molecular weigth DNA at pH 10.5. In: Methods in cell biology, Vol. VI. Prescott, D. M. (ed.), pp. 307–315. New York: Academic Press 1973

Yajima, Y., Tanaka, A., Nonoyama, M.: Inhibition of productive replication of Epstein-Barr virus DNA by phosphonoacetic acid. Virology **71**, 352–354 (1976)

Yoshiike, K., Defendi, V.: Addition of extra DNA sequences to Simian virus 40 DNA *in vivo*. J. Virol. **23**, 323–337 (1977)

Zech, L., Haglund, U., Nilsson, K., Klein, G.: Characteristic chromosomal abnormalities in biopsies and lymphoid cell lines from patients with Burkitt and non-Burkitt lymphomas. Int. J. Cancer **17**, 47–56 (1976)

zur Hausen, H., Schulte-Holthausen, H.: Presence of EB virus nucleic acid homology in a "virus free" line of Burkitt tumour cells. Nature **227**, 245–248 (1970)

zur Hausen, H., Schulte-Holthausen, H.: Detection of Epstein-Barr viral genomes in human tumour cells by nucleic acid hybridization. In: Oncogenesis and Herpesviruses. Biggs, P. M., de-Thé, G., Payne, L. N. (eds.), pp. 321–325. Lyon: IARC 1972

zur Hausen, H., Diehl, V., Wolf, H., Schulte-Holthausen, H., Schneider, U.: Occurrence of Epstein-Barr virus genomes in human lymphoblastoid cell lines. Nature New Biol. **237**, 189–190 (1972)

9 Early Events in Transformation of Human Lymphocytes by the Virus[1]

J. L. Strominger and D. Thorley-Lawson

Sidney Farber Cancer Institute, Charles A. Dana Cancer Center, Harvard Medical School, 44 Binney Street, Boston, MA 02115 (USA)

[1] Work from the authors' laboratory was supported by research grants from the National Institutes of Health AI 15669; CA 21082; AICA 15310; and the National Science Foundation PCM 7801422.

Epstein-Barr virus (EBV) is unusually adapted for transformation of human B lymphocytes (bone marrow-derived lymphocyte). In this chapter, presently available information on the events leading to transformation will be reviewed. For reasons which will become apparent, we will assume that some event occurs at about 3 days after infection of human B lymphocytes with EBV in vitro, following which the cells are transformed into permanently established lines. It is assumed that this event is the integration of one or more genomes or fractional genomes of EBV into cellular DNA. In other systems which may be regarded as models for the transformation of lymphocytes by EBV, integration has been established. The integration of viral genomes or fractional genomes into the host genome, occurs, for example, in the transformation of appropriate cells by SV40 (Sambrook et al., 1975; Botchan et al., 1976), by adenovirus (Sambrook et al., 1975; Green et al., 1976; van der Eb and Houweling, 1977), by ultra violet-inactivated or temperature-sensitive mutants of herpes simplex viruses 1 and 2 (HSV) (Macnab, 1974; Rapp and Li, 1975; Galloway et al., in preparation), which are related to EBV, and by RNA tumor viruses in which a form of the DNA provirus is the intermediate for integration (Guntaka et al., 1975; Weinberg, 1977). A more general model for this kind of process is the lysogenization of *Escherichia coli* by phage lambda or phage mu.

Transformation can be divided into four distinct processes: (1) recognition of some cell receptor by the virus and adsorption of virus; (2) penetration of the virus through the cell membrane and uncoating; (3) expression of some viral information encoded by early viral genes; and (4) integration. The last process may in some cases where unit length genomes are integrated be followed by a fifth process, expression of viral genes required for maintenance of the repressed state. Information available on these processes during transformation by EBV is very limited. One function of this chapter is to highlight areas in which additional information might be obtained.

A. RECOGNITION AND ADSORPTION

Recognition and adsorption of EBV involves an interaction between the viral envelope and the membrane of the infected cell. Thus, both viral envelope protein(s) and some protein(s) on the surface of the cell must be involved in this initial process. Although the proteins of EBV have been examined by SDS gel electrophoresis (Weinberg and Becker, 1969; Dolyniuk et al., 1976 a, b), limited information is presently available and it is not known which of the viral protein(s) observed in gels participate in the recognition process. HSV contains several envelope glycoproteins which may be involved in recognition (Roizman et al., 1977; Spear, 1979). As a first assumption, one might examine the possibility that envelope glycoprotein(s) are involved in recognition by EBV. For example, antibodies could be prepared against these EBV proteins separated by SDS gel electrophoresis and the effects of such antibodies on adsorption of EBV could then be examined.

It has been known for several years that the receptor for EBV is present on peripheral B lymphocytes but not on T lymphocytes (thymus-dependent lymphocyte) (Jondal and Klein, 1973; Mizuno et al., 1974; Greaves and Brown, 1975). It is noteworthy that the P_3HR-1 strain of EBV, a nontransforming strain, can apparently bind to the EBV receptor of peripheral B cells since its adsorption prevents the subsequent effect of the addition of the transforming B95-8 strain of EBV (Steinitz et al., 1978). A variety of experiments has suggested that this receptor for EBV on B cells is either identical to or closely associated with the receptor for the C3 component of complement (Jondal et al., 1976; Yefenof et al., 1976, 1977; Yefenof and Klein, 1977; Trowbridge et al., 1977; Einhorn et al., 1978; Klein et al., 1978). In the first place, the occurrence of the EBV receptor is closely correlated with the occurrence of the complement receptor in both normal B cells and a variety of B lymphoid cell lines. The cell line Jijoye is an EBV receptor and complement receptor positive line from which a virus-producing subclone, P_3HR-1, was isolated. P_3HR-1 cells are EBV receptor and complement receptor negative. In spontaneous, nonproducing revertants of P_3HR-1 the reappearance of EBV receptors and complement receptors are closely linked (Klein et al., 1978). Moreover, there is complete overlap of the two receptors by immuno-fluorescence and cocapping of these receptors, and the binding of C3 prevents binding of EBV (Jondal et al., 1976; Yefenof et al., 1976).

Nevertheless, several experiments indicate that the EBV receptor either includes components in addition to the complement receptor or is closely linked to but separate from the complement receptor. A number of cell types including a subset of peripheral T cells, red blood cells, macrophages, and granulocytes express complement receptors even though they do not adsorb EBV (Einhorn et al., 1978). Some peripheral null cells (presumably those which are immature cells in the B cell lineage) express both complement receptors and EBV receptors to a limited extent, although the adsorption of EBV by these cells is unable to effect induction of EBV nuclear antigen (EBNA), DNA synthesis, or transformation. Similarly, the T lymphoid cell line, Molt 4, expresses complement receptors on about 65% of cells, and adsorbs EBV, but the adsorbed virus does not induce EBNA or stimulate DNA synthesis (Menezes et al., 1977). It is possible that complement receptors on different cell types are structurally and functionally distinct. Moreover, adsorption of EBV to B cells inhibits formation of erythrocyte-antibody-complement rosettes, but it does not inhibit C3 binding (Jondal et al., 1976). Finally, antisera against the B cell specific protein, a product of the HLA-D locus, which is the human analog of the murine Ia region, also blocks EBV adsorption, but some cell lines containing this antigen do not bind EBV (Trowbridge et al., 1977). Is the B cell antigen (and the complement receptor) part of the EBV receptor or does the binding of antibody to the B cell antigen (and of C3 to the complement receptor) prevent EBV adsorption for "steric" reasons? At the moment it is difficult to combine these observations to form a complete picture and it seems likely that the demonstration of the chemical nature of the EBV receptor and of the complement receptor will be necessary to further clarify their relationship.

Related to the question of the nature of the EBV receptor is the question of the nature of the cell that is transformed by EBV. It has been known for several years that all EBV-transformed cell lines are B lymphoblastoid cell lines and that essentially all peripheral B cells bind EBV. However, a number of more recent experiments has suggested the possibility that only a small fraction of B cells which binds EBV can be transformed. Several experiments have indicated that a maximum of 5% of peripheral B cells are transformable even at high multiplicity of infection and that the fraction transformed may have surface IgM or secrete IgM or contain an unusually high density of HLA antigens (McCune et al., 1975; Robinson and Miller, 1975; Katsuki and Hinuma, 1976; Rosen et al., 1977; Steel et al., 1977; Thorley-Lawson et al., 1977; Thorley-Lawson and Strominger, 1978; Katsuki et al., 1978; Steinitz et al., 1978). The increase in number of IgM-bearing cells in infectious mononucleosis (IM) (a disease caused by EBV) may be related to these facts (Aiuti et al., 1973). Another possibility is that only the subset of B cells which expresses the human equivalent of the murine I-C antigen (one product of the Ia region) is transformable. This suggestion derives from the fact that all EBV-transformed B cell lines examined thus far express an HLA-D (Ia)-region product which has structural homology to murine I-C antigen; no structural equivalent of murine I-A antigen has been seen so far (Strominger et al., 1978; Orr et al., 1978). One problem in exploring this possibility further is that while subsets of B cells in the mouse are beginning to be defined, no comparable progress has been made with definition of subsets of human B cells.

B. PENETRATION OF VIRUS

Following recognition and adsorption to the cell membrane, the virus enters the cell and is uncoated. Two processes have been suggested for penetration of cell membranes by viruses, viropexis (or pinocytosis of the virus), and fusion of the viral membrane with the membrane of the host cell with subsequent opening of the interior of the virion to the cell interior (Dales, 1973). Which of these processes occurs with EBV has not yet been established, although electron microscope observations suggest that fusion does in fact occur (Seigneurin et al., 1977). A new method of examining the interaction of enveloped viruses with cell membranes which may allow measurement of the fusion event has been developed (Rosenthal et al., 1978). This method depends upon the polarization of fluorescence of the dye, diphenylhexatriene, in a lipid environment. The degree of polarization is dependent on the rigidity or fluidity of the particular membrane. This fluorescence probe indicates that the membrane of EBV (both the P_3HR-1 and the B95-8 strains) is quite rigid, while the membrane of its targets, peripheral B cells or B lymphoid cell lines, is relatively fluid. Thus, when the dye is included in the membrane of the enveloped EBV particle, a high polarization of fluorescence is recorded. When such fluorescence-labeled virions are mixed with unlabeled target cells (peripheral B lymphocytes in a transformation assay or the Raji cell line in a superinfection assay), the polarization of fluorescence rapidly drops to the value found when the dye is introduced directly into the cell membrane. The half-time for dye transfer at $25°$ C is 10 minutes. If C3 is first adsorbed to the cell, no such decrease is observed, and moreover, the polarization of fluorescence changes only slightly when the fluorescence-labeled EBV is mixed either with peripheral human T cells or with rabbit B or T cells, neither of which is infectable by this virus (Fig. 1). The rapid drop in fluorescence is almost certainly due to the diffusion of the dye into a membrane of lower rigidity. Further work will be required to establish whether this transfer occurs simply when the virus is adsorbed specifically to its receptor or follows upon fusion of the two membranes.

    The time of penetration of virus is less than 1 h, as measured by loss of ability of anti-EBV serum to inhibit transformation or by the ability to abort transformation by separation of cells and virus by centrifugation (Thorley-Lawson and Strominger, 1978). Either during or immediately after penetration, the virus is uncoated and some "membrane antigens" may represent a viral envelope left at the cell surface (see below). A multitude of phenomena may occur after uncoating: (1) release of enzymes

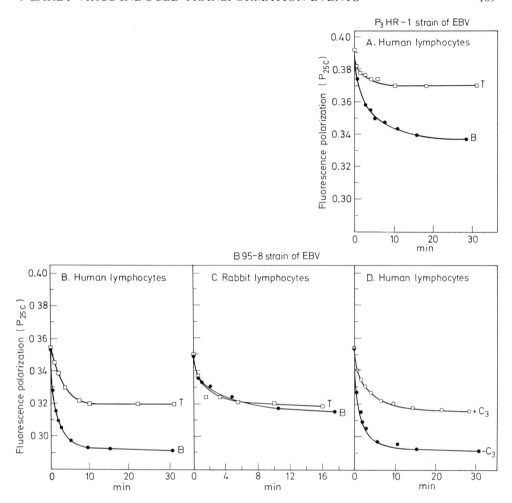

Fig. 1 A–D. Translocation of DPH from EBV to human and rabbit lymphocytes (Rosenthal et al., 1978). EBV was labeled with diphenylhexatriene (DPH). Subpopulations of normal human B and T lymphocytes were isolated from the peripheral blood of normal donors by Ficoll-hypaque density gradient centrifugation followed by a B-cell immunoabsorbent column. Rabbit B and T lymphocyte subpopulations were separated using a nylon wool column. An aliquot of DPH labeled EBV was added to the nonlabeled cells and the fluorescence polarization at 25 °C recorded at different time intervals in a microviscosimeter. **A** Addition of DPH-P₃HR-1 strain of EBV to human B (*B*) and T (*T*) lymphocytes. **B** Addition of DPH-B95-8 strain of EBV to human B (*B*) and T (*T*) lymphocytes. **C** Addition of DPH-B95-8-strain of EBV to rabbit B (*B*) and T (*T*) lymphocytes. **D** Inhibition of EBV interaction with human B lymphocytes by the C3 component of complement, (+C3) B cells with C3; (−C3) B cells without C3

contained in the virion into the cell interior; (2) further movement of the nucleocapsid through the cytoplasm to the nucleus; (3) dissociation of the nucleocapsid and subsequent transcription of some early viral genes followed by export of these messages to the cytoplasm for translation; and (4) degradation of viral DNA in the nucleus to pieces which are less than genome length. If the model for transformation by HSV is applicable, it seems likely that only a fraction of the genome would be needed for transformation, but in the case of EBV the size of this fraction is unknown.

C. EXPRESSION OF VIRAL INFORMATION

I. EBV NUCLEAR ANTIGEN

Presumably a number of new proteins are synthesized in the presence of EBV which are required for transformation. The complexity of the messenger RNA in Raji cells (which are not producers of EBV) suggests that as many as 20 new proteins may be synthesized in this virus-transformed cell (Hayward and Kieff, 1976). However, only one new protein has been identified in virus-transformed cells, EBNA. This protein is a DNA-binding protein and some preliminary characterization and purification of it has recently been carried out (Baron and Strominger, 1978; Luka et al., 1978). It appears to be a tetramer consisting of four subunits of 49,000 daltons each. There is, however, evidence that proteins of other sizes may also have EBV-specific complement fixing activity (Luka and Edson, unpublished observation). Moreover, careful studies of the in vitro conversion of the Ramos cell line (an EBV-negative B cell line) by the P_3HR-1 strain of EBV suggest the possibility that more than one EBNA may occur in the nuclei of transformed cells (Fresen et al., 1977). Superficially at least, the nuclear protein EBNA is analogous to nuclear proteins associated with the transformation of cells by DNA tumor viruses, i. e., the T antigens associated with the transformation of cells by SV40, polyoma, or adenovirus. Recently, additional complexity has been introduced by the finding that a number of different proteins (called T, t, and middle t) are found in cells transformed by SV40 or polyoma and that these different proteins are encoded in the same genetic region, the A gene, and share common DNA templates (Schaffhausen et al., 1978). Since SV40 T antigen is a DNA-binding protein, which induces mitogenesis and stimulates DNA synthesis when the purified protein is introduced into non-virus-containing cells (Kriegler et al., 1978; Tjian et al., 1978), it has been natural to speculate that EBNA may have a similar function. Studies of the early events occurring after transformation of lymphocytes by EBV have indicated that EBNA is synthesized very early after addition of virus, after $\sim$ 12–18 h (Aya and Osato, 1974; Yata et al., 1975; Einhorn and Ernberg, 1978; Takada and Osato, 1979). The appearance of EBNA is followed at 24 h by morphologic changes characteristic of blast cells without an increase in cell number. Blast cells are identified by their large size and large nuclei with diffuse chromatin staining, as compared to smaller-sized, normal lymphocytes containing nuclei with compact chromatin staining. At 36 h, the initiation of DNA synthesis can be detected by radioautography in the presence of ^{3}H-thymidine, occurring simultaneously with the beginning of cell proliferation. Thus, in the present model the appearance of EBNA induces blastogenesis, which is followed by DNA synthesis and then cell division. However, no information is available as to how EBNA (or T antigens) might function, if indeed their role is as described.

Moreover, in view of our present knowledge of the complexity of the products of the early gene of SV40 and polyoma (T antigens) together with the knowledge that several nuclear proteins are synthesized in cells transformed by larger DNA viruses (both adenovirus and HSV) (van der Vliet and Levine, 1972; Kit et al., 1978), it seems likely that either the material now defined as EBNA consists of more than one protein or that other proteins not defined by methods presently used also occur in the nuclei of EBV-transformed cells.

II. ENZYMES FOR NUCLEIC ACID SYNTHESIS OR MODIFICATION

The EBV genome infecting a cell is a double-stranded linear molecule. It seems likely that this molecule must be processed in some way before it is replicated and integrated into the host genome. For reasons that will become apparent below, the possibility that replication of EBV must precede transformation is a plausible hypothesis. Essentially nothing is known about the replication of EBV and there is very little information even about the replication of the much more thoroughly studied HSV. In the case of EBV it is difficult to study what happens to the virion after infection of purified B cells because only a small fraction of these cells becomes transformed. As a beginning, studies of the fate of the linear virus DNA after superinfection of Raji cells (where over 90% of cells can be superinfected) have been initiated on the hypothesis that a similar process would occur in peripheral B cells infected by EBV. After superinfection, both linear (55S) and circular (65S, a size characteristic of nicked double-stranded circles) EBV DNA molecules are synthesized (Fig. 2) (Siegel, unpublished observation). The prominent shoulder (about 80S) may represent other replicative intermediates. A small amount of material may also appear at 100S, the sedimentation velocity of a closed circular DNA. The circular and closed circular forms have been observed in Raji cells themselves, which contain 50–60 episomal EBV DNA molecules per cell (Lindahl et al., 1976). Early antigens (EA) appearing in Raji cells after superinfection are defined immunologically by utilizing immunofluorescence. Two forms of EA, diffuse (D) and restricted (R), have been seen, but each of these forms may quite possibly include a variety of enzymes of DNA metabolism.

What kinds of enzymes are required for replication of EBV DNA? It is certain that the replication of a DNA molecule of this size requires a very large number of enzymes. Phage T4 is of comparable size and at least 20 phage-specific enzymes of DNA metabolism have been implicated in its synthesis (Mathews, 1971). A similar situation may pertain for HSV since temperature-sensitive mutants in $\sim 30\%$ of viral cistrons

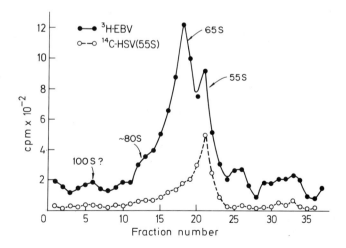

Fig. 2. Sizing gradient of EBV DNA from superinfected Raji cells (% EA > 90%) (Siegel, unpublished observation). ^{3}H-thymidine was added at 14 h, cells were harvested at 18 h post infection, pronase treated, and directly layered onto a 10%–30% high salt neutral glycerol gradient. HSV DNA was added as a 55S marker

identified to date in both HSV 1 and HSV 2 are unable to synthesize DNA at the nonpermissive temperature (Schaffer et al., 1978). As a minimum, these enzymes are likely to include both RNA and DNA polymerases (to initiate and extend the DNA molecules), thymidine kinase (TK), endonucleases (to open closed circular DNA molecules and to generate unit length viral DNA strands from concatemers), DNA ligases, DNA methylases, and nucleases (to shut down host DNA synthesis and degrade host DNA). Only a few of these have so far been found associated with EBV. The occurrence of an EBV-specific DNA polymerase was inferred from the sensitivity of EBV-replication to phosphonoacetic acid (PAA) (Nyormoi et al., 1976; Summers and Klein, 1976; Yajima et al., 1976; Lemon et al., 1978). An EBV-specific DNA polymerase has been identified in an EBV-producer line and has been purified (Miller et al., 1977; Goodman et al., 1978). In addition, some evidence has been obtained that a different virus-specific DNA polymerase is associated with the virion (Goodman et al., 1978). Similarly HSV is known to code for a PAA-sensitive DNA polymerase as well as for a TK (Keir and Gold, 1963; Kit and Dubbs, 1963). EBV probably codes for a TK, since a new TK was recently identified after superinfection of Raji cells with EBV (Chen et al., 1978). Whether or not the expression of the DNA polymerase and the TK are also required as an early event in transformation remains to be established. Methylation of replicative forms of HSV has been observed, the methylation of HSV being competed by the methyl trap, nicotinamide (Sharma and Biswal, 1977). Since the linear HSV DNA molecules in the virion are not methylated, demethylation must occur before packaging of the DNA. The observation that nicotinamide also inhibits replication of EBV (Siegel, unpublished observation) suggests that a similar process may occur with this virus, but the phenomenon remains to be further explored. Conceivably methylation of the replicative form serves to distinguish host DNA and viral DNA for enzymes that specifically degrade host DNA.

In addition to the variety of genes which encode information for structural polypeptides of the virion or for enzymes used for viral replication, the viral DNA must contain a variety of genes that encode information for polypeptides, required for the expression of other genes, i.e., regulatory proteins. Several such genes are known to be required for HSV gene expression (Roizman et al., 1977). One of these (the B gene of HSV) has been shown to be specifically required for synthesis of the HSV TK (Kit et al., 1978). These experiments were carried out with temperature-sensitive mutants of HSV, i.e., infection was carried out with an intact viral DNA molecule. It is noteworthy that biochemical transformation of a TK mouse cell line has also been accomplished utilizing relatively small segments of HSV DNA which were obtained with a restriction endonuclease (Pellicer et al., 1978). The TK gene is expressed after transfection with this small segment of DNA and therefore, if a regulatory protein is required for its expression, that protein must also be encoded in the fragment of DNA used for the transfection or the expression of this gene must be under cellular control. The size of the fragment used in the transfection, 3.4 kilobases, is enough to encode a single polypeptide of 100,000 daltons or, of course, several smaller polypeptides (without making assumptions about gene splicing). The low efficiency of transfection is contrasted to the higher degree of transfection when the same TK gene is recovered from host DNA (Pellicer et al., 1978) and may indeed suggest that integration at only certain sites yields a TK gene which can be transcribed (under control of a host cellular element?).

Since a TK activity has now been found after infection with EBV (Chen et al., 1978), similar experiments with this virus might now be contemplated.

III. MEMBRANE ANTIGENS

Upon infection with EBV, lymphocytes express membrane-associated antigens. The study of these antigens is important because they elicit the immune responses which limit lymphoproliferation during IM and which, presumably, fail in Burkitt's lymphoma (BL) and nasopharyngeal carcinoma. There has also been a great deal of speculation about the involvement of surface antigens in the transformation event, i. e., are surface changes important in the change from controlled to uncontrolled growth? A number of phenomena related to membrane antigens have been described:

1. All EBV-transformed cells seem to express the lymphocyte-detected membrane antigen (LYDMA), which is recognized by killer T cells present during the acute phase of IM (Svedmyr and Jondal, 1975). It is not known at what stage of infection this antigen is first expressed. However, it has been suggested that it may occur even before EBNA (18–24 h in vitro). This suggestion is based on the claim that during acute IM the EBV-infected, presumably LYDMA-positive cells, are EBNA-negative (Crawford et al., 1978); however, this claim has been disputed (Klein et al.,

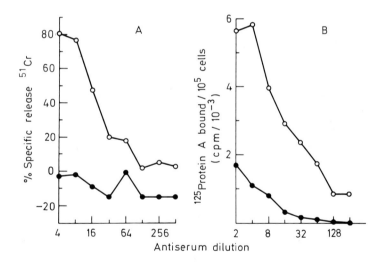

Fig. 3 A and B. Activity of anti-EHRB-Ramos sera (Rosenthal and Shuman, 1978).
A Complement Mediated Lysis of Antibody Treated Cells. Ramos ($\bullet$——$\bullet$) and EHRB-Ramos ($\bigcirc$——$\bigcirc$) were incubated with ^{51}Cr and then treated with varying dilutions of anti-EHRB-Ramos sera. This was then incubated with rabbit complement for 10 h at 37 °C. Release of ^{51}Cr to the supernatant was indicative of complement lysis of antibody binding cells.
B Specificity of Anti-EHRB-Ramos Antiserum by Radioimmunoassay. Absorption of anti-EHRB-Ramos serum by Ramos and EHRB-Ramos cells was measured using the ^{125}I-Staphylococcal protein A assay. Suspensions of 3×10^5 cells fixed with glutaraldehyde were allowed to absorb varying concentrations of antisera for 1 h at 4 °C. After removal of excess antibody by successive washings, ^{125}I-Staphylococcal protein A was incubated with the cells for 1 h at 4 °C. Cells were washed free of excess ^{125}I-Staphylococcal protein A, dissolved in 1 M NaOH, and counted in a γ-counter

1976). LYDMA has not been defined in a biochemical sense and indeed the methods (reagents) for doing so are not presently available.

2. An attempt has been made to define EBV-specific surface antigens by immunizing rabbits with EBV-transformed cells and absorbing nonspecific antibodies with a syngeneic EBV-negative cell line. For this purpose, the EBV-negative lymphoma cell line Ramos has been employed together with EHRB-Ramos, an EBV-containing line derived by infection of Ramos in vitro. The rabbit antiserum resulting from immunization with EHRB-Ramos and absorption of the resulting antiserum with Ramos has been characterized (Rosenthal and Shuman, 1978). It recognizes an antigen defined by cytotoxicity, immunofluorescence, fluorescence-activated cell sorter, or the ^{125}I-staphylococcal protein A binding assay, which is present on EHRB-Ramos but not on Ramos (Fig. 3). The antigen is also present in a second Ramos converted cell line, EHRA-Ramos, but is either not found or is present in only very small amounts on several other converted sublines containing fewer EBV genomes per cell. Similarly it is present in only small amounts or not at all on a variety of other EBV-transformed cell lines (e. g., Raji). The antigen is not due to infection with mycoplasma and is not an expression of C-type virus particles. Its significance is still unknown. The most recent information suggests that it represents the unusual expression of a normal cellular antigen, a T-lymphocyte specific antigen, on a cell type abnormal for this antigen (Rosenthal, unpublished observation).

3. The EBV virion itself possesses antigens recognized by neutralizing antibodies in sera from seropositive individuals. There is a strong correlation between the virus-neutralizing titer of these sera and the titer of antibodies against the late membrane antigens (defined by immunofluorescence) expressed on producer cells, suggesting cross-reactivity (De Schryver et al., 1974). This conclusion is strongly supported by the following recent experiments (Thorley-Lawson, 1979). A rabbit anti-EBV neutralizing antiserum has been produced which also reacts by immunofluorescence with a small percentage (3%–5%) of cells in a producer culture (the same % as that of viral capsid antigen (VCA)-positive producer cells in this culture) but not with cells in a nonproducer culture (Fig. 4). The neutralizing antibody may be absorbed out with the producer B95-8 cell line but not with the nonproducer Raji cell line. Similarly, B95-8 cells pretreated with PAA, known to block expression of late viral functions (VCA) (Nyormoi et al., 1976; Summers and Klein, 1976; Yajima et al., 1976), do not absorb the antiserum. Thus, the expression of this membrane antigen, like that of VCA, is a late viral function and occurs only when EBV is being replicated for virus production (in contrast to the replication of episomal EBV DNA which is apparently carried out by the host DNA synthetic machinery). With this serum it has been possible to detect the antigen in preparations of detergent (Triton X-100)-solubilized plasma membranes from a producer cell line (P_3HR-1). Immunoprecipitation experiments suggest that this antiserum recognizes two major polypeptides of approximate molecular weights, 150,000 and 75,000. Further characterization of these antigens may be of considerable importance, since they are probably responsible for eliciting the immune responses which prevent reinfection with EBV, and therefore, could theoretically be used in immunization programs. Several lines of experimentation have similarly suggested that glycoproteins of about 60,000 and 120,000 mol. wt. found in the virion of HSV are expressed on the

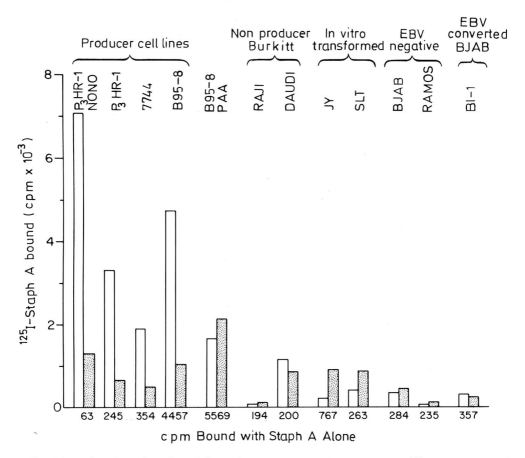

Fig. 4. Screening of a variety of B cell lines using the rabbit anti-EBV Serum in the ^{125}I-Protein A Assay (Thorley-Lawson, 1978).

12 cell lines were screened at an antibody dilution of 1:40 using the ^{125}I-Protein A Radioimmunoassay. □, counts bound after incubation with immune serum; ▨, counts bound after incubation with preimmune serum. In each case a background of counts bound after incubation of each cell line with medium followed by ^{125}I-Protein A was subtracted. The amount subtracted for each cell line is written on the *abscissa*. Note extremely high background for B95-8

    surface of transformed cells and that the expression of these glycoproteins may be essential for tumorigenicity (Roizman et al., 1977; Cohen et al., 1978; Camacho and Spear,1978; Spear, 1979).

4. When an enveloped virus infects a cell, the envelope is left on the surface and thus newly infected cells express membrane antigens for a few hours. This antigen is observed early after superinfection of Raji cells with EBV and it can be removed by papain (Dölken and Klein, 1976). During superinfection of Raji, a second and new membrane antigen is expressed 48–72 h postinfection. However, there is disagreement as to whether this second antigen is late (inhibited by PAA) or early (not inhibited by Ara C) and perhaps equivalent to the membrane antigen seen in fresh BL biopsies (defined by immunofluorescence using patient antisera) (Klein et al., 1966).

5. The transitory expression of membrane antigens on newly infected cells may be responsible for inducing a third kind of immune response (antibody production and killer T cells being the first two). It has been observed that T cells from healthy adult individuals can suppress EBV infection in vitro (Thorley-Lawson et al., 1977; Thorley-Lawson et al., 1978). It was observed that fetal B lymphocytes transformed equally efficiently if by themselves or in a mixture of 20% B cells and 80% autologous T (Ig-negative) cells or if unseparated lymphocytes were used. By comparison, transformation of adult B lymphocytes was strongly inhibited by the presence of 80% autologous T lymphocytes (the ratio which is found in vivo) and were slightly inhibited by 50% T lymphocytes (the ratio found in vivo with fetal cord blood). Similarly, in another study lymphocytes from seropositive individuals were shown to inhibit transformation by EBV (Moss et al., 1977). In this latter system it was necessary to infect the cells while cultured on an adult fibroblast feeder layer.

Time-course experiments on the suppression event indicate that the B cells are effectively suppressed within 2 days postinfection (Fig. 5) (Thorley-Lawson et al., 1978). Furthermore, experiments in which the T cells were added at various times postinfection suggest that they are only effective if added within 24 h, although they do not interfere with the initial infection and penetration. These results strongly suggest that the T lymphocytes respond to viral antigens left on the cell surface and that the response is not effective once transformation is complete (appearance of EBNA and DNA synthesis, both requiring ∼ 24 h). More recent experiments using double

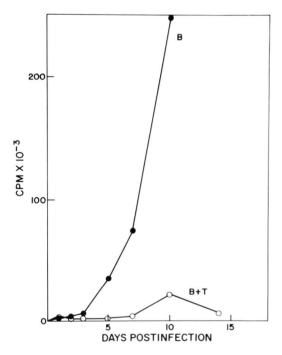

Fig. 5. Time course of suppression of outgrowth of EBV-infected B lymphocytes by autologous adult T lymphocytes (Thorley-Lawson et al., 1978). At various times postinfection, B lymphocytes were reisolated from the infection mixtures by passage over a rabbit anti-human Fab' immunoabsorbent column and DNA synthesis was assayed by pulsing with ³H-thymidine

chambers separated by a membrane have led to the finding that this response is mediated, at least in part, by a soluble factor (Thorley-Lawson, 1978). Attempts to isolate this factor have proved unsuccessful so far. It appears, therefore, that these T cells are part of a mechanism for suppressing B cell proliferation. Such a mechanism may play a role in recovery from EBV infection since it is known that individuals who have recovered from IM carry EBV-infected cells which are suppressed in vivo in the absence of cytotoxic lymphocytes.

Thus, a variety of membrane antigens have been described in the EBV system including the following:

1. An antigen recognized by killer T cells (LYDMA).
2. An antigen present on an EBV-infected clone, EHRB-Ramos, but not on its non-EBV-containing parent, Ramos. This antigen has been defined serologically.
3. An antigen expressed late in the infection process and the appearance of which is blocked by PAA. This antigen is packaged in the virion.
4. An antigen expressed only early in the infection process and which is probably the remnants of viral envelopes that were left at the cell surface. This antigen may be the same as that recognized by suppressor T cells and leading to inhibition of transformation.

How many proteins does this variety of phenomena define? Are any of these essential for the conversion of a nonproliferating lymphocyte into an "immortalized" cell? Which if any of these antigens is expressed early in the infectious process, in the sense that it is expressed before the cell is immortalized? These questions and characterization of the various proteins remain open for the future.

D. INTEGRATION OF EBV GENOMES

A number of proteins discussed in the preceding section may be expressed prior to integration of viral genomes and, more specifically, some of them would certainly be required for the integration of viral genomes. Whether or not genomes are actually integrated in the case of EBV is still a controversial question. Part of the controversy arises from the difficulty of measuring a relatively small number of integrated genomes in cell lines which contain a much larger number of complete viral DNA molecules present as episomes. Recent data utilizing a cell line which contains relatively small amounts of viral DNA seem to point to the occurrence of integrated genomes (Andersson-Anvret and Lindahl, 1978). Such integrated genomes have been observed with other oncogenic DNA viruses including SV40, polyoma, adenovirus, and HSV and in all of these cases fractional genomes are adequate for transformation. For example, in the case of adenovirus, 6% of the genome at the left-hand end is sufficient for transformation of rat embryo fibroblasts into cells giving rise to metastasizing tumors in the rat (Chen et al., 1976). This fractional genome is sufficient to code for $\sim$ 150,000 daltons of protein (without considering the important problem of gene splicing). The two T antigens of adenovirus (72,000 and 48,000 daltons) are encoded in the same DNA sequence and thus there may be sufficient coding capacity for at least one additional protein. There is some evidence that one of the T antigens may be a tumor-specific transplantation antigen, i. e., a membrane protein. Recent studies with both HSV 1 and HSV 2 have similarly suggested that a small fraction of the genome close to the TK gene may be sufficient for transformation (Camacho and Spear, 1978; Galloway et al., in preparation). These precedents clearly suggest that a similar situation could pertain for EBV, i.e., that genomes are integrated and, moreover, that integration of fractional genomes may be sufficient for transformation. Methods presently available with EBV may not be adequate clearly to detect fractional genomes.

Moreover, the study of the effect of PAA on transformation is most readily interpreted by assuming that integration is the critical event required for immortalization of B lymphocytes by EBV. PAA at appropriate concentrations inhibits transformation of human B lymphocytes by EBV in vitro (Thorley-Lawson and Strominger, 1976, 1978). In the presence of these concentrations of PAA, EBNA is expressed and morphologically the cells undergo a blast transformation (i. e., they enlarge and contain nuclei with diffusely staining chromatin). However, they do not proliferate logarithmically and no outgrowth of cultures is observed. This phenomenon is observed if PAA is added at any time up to 3 days after addition of virus. After 3 days, the cells are immortalized and thereafter addition of PAA has no effect on outgrowth. This phenomenon has been termed "abortive transformation" (Thorley-Lawson and Strominger, 1978). The cells have many of the phenotypic characteristics of transformed cells including blast transformation, DNA synthesis, expression of EBNA, and long life in culture. Normal B lymphocytes in culture die within 5 days, but in the presence of PAA such abortively transformed lymphocytes remain viable and continue to synthesize DNA at a steady rate for up to a month (Fig. 6). After removal

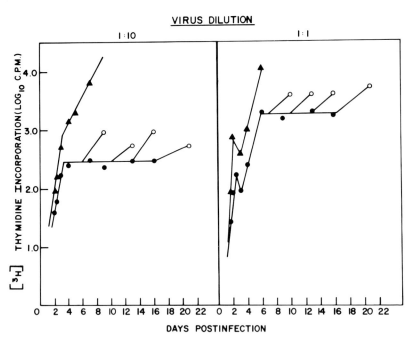

Fig. 6. The kinetics of DNA synthesis in the presence and absence of PAA (Thorley-Lawson and Strominger, 1978). Cells were infected in the presence or absence of PAA at a concentration known to inhibit transformation. Cultures were fed every 3–4 days and PAA was removed by replacing 75% of the medium with fresh medium lacking PAA. ▲, control infection; ●, infection in the presence of 200 µg/ml PAA; ○, level of incorporation after removal of PAA

of the inhibitor, DNA synthesis accelerates logarithmically and the cells proliferate. The simplest interpretation of these experiments is that no replication of EBV DNA occurs in the presence of PAA, but the cell receiving an EBV particle is transformed by the viral DNA. Viral information (e. g., EBNA) is expressed and the cell divides. However, at division only one of the daughters receives the EBV DNA copy. Only that cell can divide again and its sister dies. Thus, no proliferation is seen in the culture, but DNA synthesis continues at a steady rate and cell number remains constant. The cells become resistant to the effect of PAA if it is added after 3 days because at that time integration occurs. When integration occurs, integrated genomes replicate with the cellular DNA, becoming independent of replicative functions specified by independently replicating genomes.

What viral functions are required for integration? It is reasonable to suppose that the linear EBV DNA molecules packaged in the virion are not competent for integration of unit length viral DNA (and clearly must be processed if only a fraction of a genome is integrated). What form of DNA is the intermediate for integration? Virtually nothing is known as regards this question concerning any eukaryotic virus. Even in the case of the most extensively studied system, phage lambda, the information is still incomplete (Nash, 1978). Phage lambda is linearly integrated into the *Escherichia coli* genome as a unit length genome. There are specific phage and host attachment sites on each DNA for integration. Integration can also occur at secondary sites but with much reduced efficiency. Lambda contains a specific gene, *int,* which specifies a protein needed for the site-specific recombination, but the function of this protein is not known. It appears that the substrate for integration is covalently closed, double-stranded, supercoiled DNA. This form is generated by DNA gyrase, which requires ATP. It is possible that supercoiling may alter the secondary structure of attachment sites and thus make them accessible for the enzymes catalyzing the integration event.

If this model, or anything like it, applies to eukaryotic DNA and specifically to EBV DNA, a number of viral functions may be required to generate this closed circular form. These would include exonucleases to generate sticky ends (assuming there is terminal redundancy in EBV as there is in HSV), and other enzymes required to circularize the linear EBV DNA molecules. However, it seems likely that some modifications of the linear DNA molecules are essential for integration. In addition, most transformed cell lines contain ten or more plasmid EBV DNA molecules per cell. Are these generated prior to integration and immortalization, or are they generated subsequently? Thus, it is possible that replication of EBV DNA may occur prior to integration, either to generate the form of the DNA molecule required for the integration step or to generate a number of copies of EBV DNA molecules. When one considers the integration of relatively small fractional genomes, the kinds of mechanisms operating in its integration may be similar to the mechanism operating in the recombination of genes in general.

What is the PAA-sensitive function that occurs at about 3 days? The simplest interpretation of the sensitivity of immortalization to PAA is that EBV DNA replication must precede integration and that this replication requires a specific EBV DNA polymerase. Several other viral DNA polymerases have been found to be inhibited by PAA, including the DNA polymerases of HSV, cytomegalovirus, and Marek's disease virus (Mao et al., 1975; Huang, 1975; Leinbach et al., 1976). It has been suggested that PAA is an analog of inorganic pyrophosphate, one of the products of the polymerase reaction (Leinbach et al., 1976). If so, there are a number of possible enzymes of DNA metabolism which could be involved in integration in addition to the DNA polymerase and which might be sensitive to PAA. In one study the EBV DNA polymerase was found to be sensitive to PAA (Miller et al., 1977), but surprisingly in another the isolated EBV DNA polymerase was relatively insensitive to PAA (Goodman et al., 1978) (although it was tested with calf-thymus DNA substrate and not with EBV DNA itself). The result, however, warns of the possibility that the PAA-sensitive step could be something other than a DNA polymerase.

E. EXPRESSION OF INFORMATION FROM INTEGRATED GENOMES

What functions maintain the episomal EBV DNA molecules in a repressed state? Clearly not all of the approximately 100 genes encoded by the EBV DNA molecule are expressed in transformed cell lines. An analysis of messenger RNA synthesized by such cell lines suggests that only 10% or less of the genes are expressed (Hayward and Kieff, 1976). However, we are certain of the product of only one of these genes, EBNA. What are the functions of the remainder? Among them may be repressors such as those associated with phage lambda (Ptashne et al., 1976). These repressors may be synthesized from genes expressed only from the integrated genome. Their function would be to prevent the replication of EBV which would lead to cell death.

The occurrence of a strong repressor(s) for middle and/or late viral functions among the early gene products of EBV might be sufficient to account for the difficulty of finding a fully permissive cell line for this virus or of inducing it with high efficiency. Of course, no similar repressor would be required if only a small fractional genome were integrated, unless intact episomal EBV DNA molecules were also present. It is important, however, to point out that no eukaryotic repressor has been identified yet and other possible mechanisms which could account for inactive genes also have to be considered (e. g., absence of a positive regulatory factor or presence of promoters which are not recognized by the lymphocyte DNA-dependent RNA polymerase).

In summary, the early events in transformation of human B lymphocytes by EBV are certain to be quite complex. They include:

1. Recognition by a viral envelope protein of a cell receptor and the subsequent uncoating of the virus at the cell surface.
2. Penetration of the virus which may involve fusion of the viral and cellular membrane and may be followed by further uncoating and movement of the EBV DNA through the cytoplasm to the nucleus.
3. Expression of viral information, i. e., transcription and translation, of some viral gene(s) required early in the transformation process. These genes certainly include the gene(s) for EBNA synthesis and are likely also to include a variety of genes required to modify the linear EBV DNA molecule to a form which is a substrate for integration as well as gene(s) for synthesis of virus-specific membrane proteins (LYDMA and other membrane antigens).
4. The integration event itself about which comparatively little is known, even in a system as extensively studied as phage lambda; and finally,
5. The expression of some functions which may be necessary for maintenance of the transformed state if unit length viral genomes are integrated or present as episomes.

Since comparatively little is known about these various functions, a fascinating, fertile field awaits further investigation.

REFERENCES

Aiuti, F., Ciarla, M. V., D'Asero, C., D'Amelio, R., Garofalo, J. A.: Surface markers on lymphocytes of patients with infectious diseases. Infect. Immun. **8,** 110–117 (1973)

Andersson-Anvret, M., Lindahl, T.: Integrated viral DNA sequences in Epstein-Barr virus-converted human lymphoma lines. J. Virol. **25,** 710–718 (1978)

Aya, T., Osato, T.: Early events in transformation of human cord lymphocytes by Epstein-Barr virus: Induction of DNA synthesis, mitosis and the virus-associated nuclear antigen synthesis. Int. J. Cancer **14,** 341–347 (1974)

Baron, D., Strominger, J. L.: Partial purification and properties of the Epstein-Barr virus-associated nuclear antigen. J. Biol. Chem. **253,** 2875–2881 (1978)

Botchan, M., Topp, D., Sambrook, J.: The arrangement of simian virus 40 sequences in the DNA of transformed cells. Cell **9,** 269–287 (1976)

Camacho, A., Spear, P. G.: Transformation of hamster embryo fibroblasts by a specific fragment of the herpes simplex virus genome. Cell **15,** 993–1002 (1978)

Chen, L. B., Gallimore, P. H., McDougall, J. K.: Correlation between tumor induction and the large external transformation sensitive protein on the cell surface. Proc. Natl. Acad. Sci. USA **73,** 3570–3574 (1976)

Chen, S.-T., Estes, J. E., Huang, E.-S., Pagano, J. S.: Epstein-Barr virus-associated thymidine kinase. J. Virol. **26,** 203–208 (1978)

Cohen, G. H., Katze, M., Hydrean-Stern, C., and Eisenberg, R. J.: Type-common CP-1 antigen of herpes simplex virus is associated with a 59.000-molecular-weight envelope glycoprotein. J. Virol. **27,** 172–181 (1978)

Crawford, D. H., Rickinson, A. B., Finerty, S., Epstein, M. A.: Epstein-Barr (EB) virus genome-containing, EB nuclear antigen-negative B-lymphocyte populations in blood in acute infectious mononucleosis. J. Gen. Virol. **38,** 449–460 (1978)

Dales, S.: Early events in cell-animal virus interactions. Bacteriol. Rev. **37,** 103–135 (1973)

De Schryver, A., Klein, G., Hewetson, J., Rocchi, G., Henle, W., Henle, G., Moss, D. J., Pope, J. H.: Comparison of EBV neutralization tests based on abortive infection or transformation of lymphoid cells and their relation to membrane-reactive antibodies (anti-MA). Int. J. Cancer **13,** 353–362 (1974)

Dölken, G., Klein, G.: Expression of Epstein-Barr-virus-associated membrane antigen in Raji cells superinfected with two different virus strains. Virology **70,** 210–213 (1976)

Dolyniuk, M., Pritchett, R., Kieff, E. D.: Proteins of Epstein-Barr virus. I. Analysis of the polypeptides of purified enveloped Epstein-Barr virus. J. Virol **17,** 935–949 (1976 a)

Dolyniuk, M., Wolff, E., Kieff, E.: Proteins of Epstein-Barr virus II. Electrophoretic analysis of the polypeptides of the nucleocapsid and glucosamine and polysaccharide-containing components of enveloped virus. J. Virol. **18,** 289–297 (1976 b)

Einhorn, L., Ernberg, I.: Induction of EBNA precedes the first cellular S-phase after EBV-induction of human lymphocytes. Int. J. Cancer **21,** 157–160 (1978)

Einhorn, L., Steinitz, M., Yefenof, E., Ernberg, I., Bakacs, T., Klein, G.: Epstein-Barr Virus (EBV) receptors, complement receptors, and EBV infectivity of different lymphocyte fractions of human peripheral blood, II. Epstein-Barr virus studies. Cell. Immunol. **35,** 43–58 (1978)

Fresen, K. O., Merkt, B., Bornkamm, G. W., zur Hausen, H.: Heterogeneity of Epstein-Barr virus originating from P_3HR-1 cells. I. Studies on EBNA induction. Int. J. Cancer **19,** 317–323 (1977)

Galloway, D., Copple, D., McDougal, J. K.: in preraration

Goodman, S. R., Prezyna, C., Benz, W. C.: Two Epstein-Barr virus associated DNA polymerase activities. J. Biol. Chem. **253,** 8617–8628 (1978)

Greaves, M. F., Brown, G.: Epstein-Barr virus binding sites on lymphocyte subpopulations and the origin of lymphoblasts in cultured lymphoid cell lines and in the blood of patients with infectious mononucleosis. Clin. Immunol. Immunopathol. **3,** 514–524 (1975)

Green, M. R., Chinnadurai, G., Mackey, J. K., Green, M.: A unique pattern of integrated viral genes in hamster cells transformed by highly oncogenic human adenovirus 12. Cell **7,** 419–428 (1976)

Guntaka, R. V., Mahy, B. W. J., Bishop, J. M., Varmus, H. E.: Ethidium bromide inhibits appearance of closed circular viral DNA and integration of virus-specific DNA in duck cells infected by avian sarcoma virus. Nature **253**, 507–511 (1975)

Hayward, S. D., Kieff, E. D.: Epstein-Barr virus-specific RNA. I. Analysis of viral RNA in cellular extracts and in the polyribosomal fraction of permissive lymphoblastoid cell lines. J. Virol. **18**, 518–525 (1976)

Huang, E.-S.: Human cytomegalovirus IV. Specific inhibition of virus-induced DNA polymerase activity and viral DNA replication by phosphonoacetic acid. J. Virol. **16**, 1560–1565 (1975)

Jondal, M., Klein, G., Oldstone, M. B. A., Bokish, V., Yefenof, E.: Surface markers on human B and T lymphocytes. Scand. J. Immunol. **5**, 401–410 (1976)

Jondal, M., Klein, G.: Surface markers on human B and T lymphocytes II. Presence of Epstein-Barr virus receptors on B lymphocytes. J. Exp. Med. **138**, 1365–1378 (1973)

Katsuki, T., Hinuma, Y.: A quantitative analysis of the susceptibility of human leukocytes to transformation by Epstein-Barr virus. Int. J. Cancer **18**, 7–13 (1976)

Katsuki, T., Hinuma, Y., Yamamoto, N., Abo, T., Kumagai, K.: Identification of the target cells in human B lymphocytes for transformation by Epstein-Barr virus. Virology, **83**, 287–294 (1977)

Keir, H., Gold, E.: Deoxyribunucleic acid nucleotidyltansferase deoxyribonuclease from cultured cells infected with herpes simplex cells. Biochim. Biophys. Acta **72**, 263–273 (1963)

Kit, S., Dubbs, D.: Acquisition of thymidine kinase activity by herpessimplex infected mouse fibroblast cells. Biochim. Biophys. Acta **71**, 55–59 (1963)

Kit, S., Kurchak, M., Wray, W., Dubbs, D. R.: Binding to chromosomes of herpes simplex-related antigens in biochemically transformed cells. Proc. Natl. Acad. Sci. USA **75**, 3288–3291 (1978)

Kit, S., Dubbs, D. R., Schaffer, P. A.: Thymidine kinase activity of biochemically transformed mouse cells after superinfection by thymidine kinase-negative, temperature-sensitive, herpes simplex virus mutants. Virology **85**, 456–463 (1978)

Klein, G., Clifford, P., Klein, E., Stjernswärd, J.: Search for tumor-specific immune reactions in Burkitt lymphoma patients by the membrane immunofluorescence reaction. Proc. Natl. Acad. Sci. USA **55**, 1628–1635 (1966)

Klein, G., Svedmyr, E., Jondal, M., Persson, P. O.: EBV-determined nuclear antigen (EBNA) positive cells in the peripheral blood of infectious mononucleosis patients. Int. J. Cancer **17**, 21–26 (1976)

Klein, G., Yefenof, E., Falk, K., Westman, A.: Relationship between Epstein-Barr virus (EBV)-production and the loss of the EBV receptor/complement receptor complex in a series of sublines derived from the same original Burkitt's lymphoma. Int. J. Cancer **21**, 552–560 (1978)

Kriegler, M. P., Griffin, J. D., Livingston, D. M.: Phenotypic complementation of the SV40 *tsA* mutant defect in viral DNA synthesis following microinjection of SV40 T antigen. Cell **14**, 983–994 (1978)

Leinbach, S. S., Reno, J. M., Lee, L. F., Isbell, A. F., Boezi, J. A.: Mechanism of phosphonoacetate inhibition of herpesvirus-induced DNA polymerase. Biochemistry **15**, 420–430 (1976)

Lemon, S. M., Hutt, L. M., Pagano, J. S.: Cytofluorometry of lymphocytes infected with Epstein-Barr virus: Effect of phosphonoacetic acid on nucleic acid. J. Virol. **25**, 138–145 (1978)

Lindahl, T., Adams, A., Bjursell, G., Bornkamm, G. W., Kaschka-Dierich, C., Jehn, U.: Covalently closed circular duplex DNA of Epstein-Barr virus in a human lymphoid cell line. J. Mol. Biol. **102**, 511–530 (1976)

Luka, J., Lindahl, T., Klein, G.: Purification of the EB virus-determined nuclear antigen (EBNA) from EB virus-transformed human lymphoid cell lines. J. Virol. **27**, 604–611 (1978)

Macnab, J. C. M.: Transformation of rat embryo cells by temperature-sensitive mutants of herpes simplex virus. J. Gen. Virol. **24**, 143–153 (1974)

Mathews, C. K.: Bacteriophage biochemistry. New York: Van Nostrand Reinhold 1971

Mao, J. C.-H., Robishaw, E. E., Overby, L. R.: Inhibition of DNA polymerase from herpes simplex virus-infected WI-38 cells by phosphonoacetic acid. J. Virol. **15**, 1281–1283 (1975)

McCune, J. M., Humphreys, R. E., Yocum, R. R., Strominger, J. L.: Enhanced representation of HL-A antigens on human lymphocytes after mitogenesis induced by phytohemagglutinin or Epstein-Barr virus. Proc. Natl. Acad. Sci. USA **72**, 3206–3209 (1975)

Menezes, J., Siegneurin, J. M., Patel, P., Bourkas, A., Lenoir, G.: Presence of Epstein-Barr virus receptors, but absence of virus penetration, in cells of an Epstein-Barr virus genome-negative human lymphoblastoid T line (Molt 4). J. Virol. **22**, 816–821 (1977)

Miller, R. L., Glaser, R., Rapp, F.: Studies of an Epstein-Barr virus-induced DNA polymerase. Virology **76**, 494–502 (1977)

Mizuno, F., Aya, T., Osato, T.: B-lymphocytes as target cells for EB virus transformation. Br. Med. J. **1974 III**, 689

Moss, D. J., Scott, W., Pope, J. H.: An immunological basis for inhibition of transformation of human lymphocytes by EB virus. Nature **268**, 735–736 (1977)

Nash, H. A.: Integration and excision of bacteriophage λ. Curr. Top. Microbiol. Immunol. **78**, 171–199 (1978)

Nyormoi, O., Thorley-Lawson, D. A., Elkington, J., Strominger, J. L.: Differential effect of phosphonoacetic acid on the expression of Epstein-Barr viral antigens and virus production. Proc. Natl. Acad. Sci. USA **73**, 1745–1748 (1976)

Orr, H., Fuks, A., Kaufmann, J., Lancet, D., Ploegh, H., Robb, R., Strominger, J. L.: Structural studies of the membrane associated products of the human major histocompatibility complex. In: Advances in Pathobiology: Cell Membranes. Fenoglio, C. M., King, D. W., (eds.). New York: Intercontinental Medical Book 1978

Pellicer, A., Wigler, M., Axel, R., Silverstein, S.: The transfer and stable integration of the HSV thymidine kinase gene into mouse cells. Cell **14**, 133–141 (1978)

Ptashne, M., Backman, K., Humayun, M. Z., Jeffrey, A., Maurer, R., Meyer, B., Sauer, R. T.: Autoregulation and function of a repressor in bacteriophage lambda. Science **194**, 156–161 (1976)

Rapp, F., Li, J.: Demonstration of the oncogenic potential of herpes simplex viruses and human cytomegalovirus. In: Herpesviruses, Cold Spring Harbor Symp. Quant. Biol. **39**, 747–763 (1974)

Robinson, J., Miller, G.: Assay for Epstein-Barr virus based on stimulation of DNA synthesis in mixed leukocytes from human umbilical cord blood. J. Virol. **15**, 1065–1072 (1975)

Roizman, B., Frenkel, N., Kieff, E. D., Spear, P. G.: The structure and expression of human herpesvirus DNAs in productive infection and in transformed cells. In: Origins of human cancer. Hiatt, H. H., Watson, J. D., Winsten, J. A. (eds.), pp. 1069–1111. Cold Spring Harbor Laboratory 1977

Rosen, A., Gergely, P., Jondal, M., Klein, G., Britton, S.: Polyclonal Ig production after Epstein-Barr virus infection of human lymphocytes *in vitro*. Nature **267**, 52–56 (1977)

Rosenthal, K., Yanovich, S., Inbar, M., Strominger, J. L.: Translocation of a hydrocarbon fluorescent probe between Epstein-Barr virus and lymphoid cells: An assay for early events in viral infection. Proc. Natl. Acad. Sci. USA **75**, 5076–5080 (1978)

Rosenthal, K. S., Shuman, H.: A new Epstein-Barr virus (EBV) associated cell surface antigen. Fed. Proc. **37**, 1561 (1978) (Abs.)

Sambrook, J., Botchan, M., Gallimore, P., Ozanne, B., Pettersson, U., Williams, J.: Viral DNA sequences in cells transformed by simian virus 40, adenovirus type 2 and adenovirus type 5. Cold Spring Harbor Symp. Quant. Biol. **39**, 615–633 (1974)

Schaffer, P. A., Carter, V. C., Timbury, M. C.: A collaborative complementation study of temperature-sensitive mutants of herpes simplex virus types 1 and 2. J. Virol. **27**, 490–504 (1978)

Schaffhausen, B. S., Silver, J. E., Benjamin, T. L.: Tumor antigen(s) in cells productively infected by wild-type polyoma virus and mutant NG-18. Proc. Natl. Acad. Sci. USA **75**, 79–83 (1978)

Seigneurin, J.-M., Vuillaume, M., Lenoir, G., de-Thé, G.: Replication of Epstein-Barr virus: Ultrastructural and immunofluorescent Studies of P_3HR-1-superinfected Raji cells. J. Virol. **24**, 836–845 (1977)

Sharma, S., Biswal, N.: Studies on the *in vivo* methylation of replicating herpes simplex virus type 1 DNA. Virology **82**, 265–274 (1977)

Spear, P. G.: Herpesvirion envelopes and infected cell membranes. In: Cell membranes and viral envelopes. Blough, H. A., Tiffany, J. M. (eds.). New York: Academic Press 1979 (in press)

Steel, C. M., Philipson, J., Arthur, E., Gardiner, S., Newton, M. S., McIntosh, R. V.: Possibility of EB virus preferentially transforming a subpopulation of human B lymphocytes. Nature **270**, 729–731 (1977)

Steinitz, M., Bakacs, T., Klein, G.: Interaction of the B95-8 and P_3HR-1 substrains of Epstein-Barr virus (EBV) with peripheral human lymphocytes. Int. J. Cancer **22**, 251–258 (1978)

Strominger, J. L., Ferguson, W., Fuks, A., Giphart, M., Kaufman, J., Mann, D., Orr, H., Parham, P., Robb, R., Terhorst, C.: Isolation and structure of HLA antigens. In: Differentiation of normal and neoplastic hematopoietic cells, pp. 467–478. Cold Spring Harbor Laboratory Press: Cold Spring Harbor, New York 1978

Summers, W. C., Klein, G.: Inhibition of Epstein-Barr virus DNA synthesis and late gene expression by phosphonoacetic acid. J. Virol. **18**, 151–155 (1976)

Svedmyr, E., Jondal, M.: Cytotoxic effector cells specific for B cell lines transformed by Epstein-Barr virus are present in patients with infectious mononucleosis. Proc. Natl. Acad. Sci. USA **72**, 1622–1626 (1975)

Takada, K., Osato, T.: Analysis of the transformation of human lymphocytes by Epstein-Barr virus. I. Sequential occurrence from the virus-determined nuclear antigen synthesis, to blastogenesis, to DNA synthesis. Intervirology, **11**, 30–39 (1979)

Thorley-Lawson, D. A.: Characterization of cross-reacting antigens on the Epstein-Barr virus envelope and plasma membranes of producer cells. Cell **16**, 33–42 (1979)

Thorley-Lawson, D. A.: Studies on the mechanism by which T cells suppress EBV infection *in vitro*. Herpes Virus Workshop. Cambridge (GB), 1978 Abs.

Thorley-Lawson, D. A., Strominger, J. L.: Transformation of human lymphocytes by Epstein-Barr virus is inhibited by phosphonoacetic acid. Nature **263**, 332–334 (1976)

Thorley-Lawson, D. A., Strominger, J. L.: Reversible inhibition by phosphonoacetic acid of human B lymphocyte transformation by Epstein-Barr virus. Virology **86**, 432–431 (1978)

Thorley-Lawson, D. A., Chess, L., Strominger, J. L.: Suppression of in vitro Epstein-Barr virus infection. J. Exp. Med. **146**, 495–508 (1977)

Thorley-Lawson, D., Chess, L., Strominger, J. L.: Suppression of *in vitro* Epstein-Barr virus infection: A new role for adult human T lymphocytes. In: Advances in comparative leukemia research. Bentvelzen, et al. (eds.), pp. 219–222. Amsterdam: Elsevier, North-Holland Biomedical Press 1978

Tjian, R., Fey, G., Graessmann, A.: Biological activity of purified simian virus 40 T antigen proteins. Proc. Natl. Acad. Sci. USA **73**, 1279–1283 (1978)

Trowbridge, I. S., Hyman, R., Klein, G.: Human B cell line deficient in the expression of B-cell specific glycoproteins (GP 27, 35). Eur. J. Immunol. **7**, 640–645 (1977)

van der Eb, A. J., Houweling, A.: Transformation with specific fragments of adenovirus DNAs II. Analysis of the viral DNA sequences present in cells transformed with a 7% fragment of adenovirus 5 DNA. Gene **2**, 133–146 (1977)

van der Vliet, P. C., Levine, A. J.: DNA-binding proteins specific for cells infected by adenovirus. Nature New Biol. **246**, 170–174 (1972)

Weinberg, R. A.: Structure of the intermediate leading to the integrated provirus. Biochim. Biophys. Acta **473**, 39 (1977)

Weinberg, A., Becker, Y.: Studies on EB virus of Burkitt's lymphoblasts. Virology **39**, 312–321 (1969)

Yajima, Y., Tanaka, A., Nonoyama, M.: Inhibition of productive replication of Epstein-Barr virus DNA by phosphonoacetic acid. Virology **73**, 352–354 (1976)

Yata, J., Desgranges, C., Nakagawa, T., Favre, M. C., de-Thé, G.: Lymphoblastoid transformation and kinetics of appearance of viral nuclear antigen (EBNA) in cord-blood lymphocytes infected by Epstein-Barr virus (EBV). Int. J. Cancer **15**, 377–384 (1975)

Yefenof, E., Klein, G.: Membrane receptor stripping confirms the association between EBV receptors and complement receptors on the surface of human B lymphoma lines. Int. J. Cancer **20**, 347–352 (1977)

Yefenof, E., Klein, G., Jondal, M., Oldstone, M. B. A.: Surface markers of human B- and T-lymphocytes. IX. Two-color immunofluorescence studies on the association between EBV receptors and complement receptors on the surface of lymphoid cell lines. Int. J. Cancer **17**, 693–700 (1976)

Yefenof, E., Klein, G., Kvarnung, K.: Relationships between complement activation, complement binding, and EBV absorption by human hematopoietic cell lines. Cell. Immunol. **31**, 225–233 (1977)

10 Transformation by the Virus In Vitro

J. H. Pope

Queensland Institute of Medical Research, Bramston Terrace, Herston, Brisbane 4006 (Australia)

A. INTRODUCTION

Transformation of human cells by Epstein-Barr virus (EBV) in vitro is of considerable interest for several major reasons. It provides a basic virologic tool in the form of a practical assay of infectivity of the virus. It allows detailed study of virus-cell relationships, which can be expected to have at least some parallels with the activity of the virus in vivo. It is a useful model for the study of control of cell proliferation and, in addition, cell lines may be readily established from specific donors to provide material for the study of genetic or other diseases.

Transformation is used here in the sense usual in tumor virology and refers to virus-induced alterations to cells, including morphologic changes, unrestricted cellular proliferation, and persistence of viral genome with restricted expression. The history of EBV transformation in vitro is generally considered to begin with the observation by Henle et al. (1967) that cocultivation of X-irradiated EBV-carrying lymphoblastoid cells with normal leukocytes resulted in the establishment of lymphoblastoid cell lines. Pope et al. (1968) also observed transformation during the course of attempts to transmit filtered EBV from the QIMR-WIL lymphoblastoid line to fetal bone-marrow cells. The transforming factor was identified as EBV on the basis of its typical herpesvirus characteristics and its specific neutralization by human sera with antibody to EBV (Pope et al., 1969). Subsequent reports confirmed these basic findings (Miller et al., 1969; Gerber et al., 1969; Baumal et al., 1971; Chang, 1971; Nilsson et al., 1971) and there has since been considerable interest in the basic nature of the transformation phenomenon. The intention here is to assess present knowledge in this field and to try to indicate areas of interest or neglect.

B. GENERAL DESCRIPTION OF TRANSFORMATION

The literature on transformation by EBV refers almost solely to studies based on lymphocytes. Lymphocytes are prepared from peripheral blood or other tissue, usually by some form of separation on density gradients, and are set up in tissue culture. Infection with most strains of EBV results in proliferation of cells which are commonly referred to as lymphoblastoid. These cells characteristically grow in suspension, are irregular, and form large but loosely bound aggregates. Almost invariably proliferation continues and a cell line becomes established. These transformed cell lines fall into the category of lymphoblastoid cell lines as defined by Nilsson and Pontén (1975) and it has been stressed that they do not resemble lymphoid cells of the type established from Burkitt's lymphoma (BL) (Pope, 1975 a).

Under ideal tissue-culture conditions, virus-induced changes may be detected microscopically as early as 4–5 days post inoculation in the form of small clusters of irregular cells which may be observed to proliferate (Figs. 1–4). Important cultural factors include the use of nontoxic fetal-calf serum and avoidance of undue increases in pH. Hepes buffer or a feeder layer of fibroblasts or amnion cells are sometimes used to help maintain steady conditions. Microtiter plates with 0.15 ml cultures are the smallest practicable cultures since, below this level, control of conditions over the long periods required becomes more difficult.

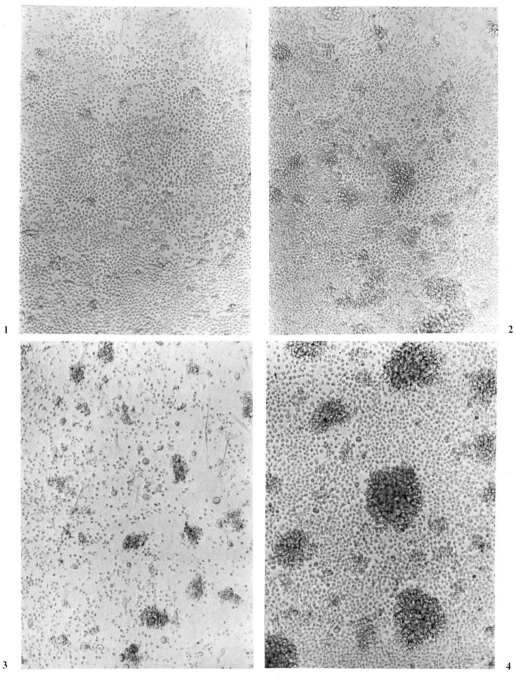

Fig. 1. Uninfected culture of viable mononuclear cells from an adult donor without antibody to EBV; 7 days; small aggregates of leukocytes are present. (× 90)

Fig. 2. Culture infected with filtered QIMR-WIL EBV preparation (multiplicity of infection 0.0001); 7 days; more and larger aggregates are present, reflecting the active proliferation already in progress. (× 90)

Fig. 3. Uninfected culture at 15 days; the majority of the aggregates show marked cell mortality. (× 90)

Fig. 4. EBV-infected culture at 15 days; typical enlargement of numerous aggregates leading to establishment of lymphoblastoid cell line. (× 90)

C. VIRAL CHARACTERISTICS

In some lymphoblastoid and lymphoid cell lines the expression of the EBV genome is such that a proportion of the cells produces infective virus and such lines are the most common source of EBV; titers of about 10^5–10^6 TD_{50}/ml can be obtained. Throat washings, particularly from patients with infectious mononucleosis (IM), constitute a second major source of transforming EBV, which is of much greater significance from the epidemiologic point of view.

Miller et al. (1976) found some evidence of heterogeneity of surface antigens of EBV strains from IM and BL; sera taken early after onset of IM contained low levels of antibody neutralizing IM-derived but not BL-derived EBV. This is an area for further exploration, but the general body of serologic evidence, based on neutralization, complement fixation (CF), and immunofluorescence tests, indicates that there is a considerable degree of antigenic homogeneity among EBV strains.

Transformation by various strains of EBV has shown remarkable similarities as far as general morphologic and proliferative aspects of the cellular response are concerned. Few detailed studies have been made, but one report suggested that with two strains of EBV (QIMR-WIL and B95-8) some consistent differences could be detected in the transformed cell lines (Katsuki and Hinuma, 1975). The QIMR-WIL-derived lines grew in larger flake-like aggregates while those of the B95-8-derived lines were smaller and rounded. The QIMR-WIL lines consistently reached higher maximal cell numbers. Differences occurred also in Ig production, the proportion of cells with cytoplasmic μ or γ chains being higher in the B95-8 group and the proportion with surface κ chains higher in the QIMR-WIL group. Both groups of transformed lines had similar levels of viral capsid antigen (VCA)-positive cells, but the proportion of membrane antigen-positive cells and the level of virus production were higher in the QIMR-WIL group. These are marked differences and it would be worthwhile to determine whether variations in viruses or receptors lead to selective infection of target cells or whether the individual viral replication processes result in variations in the expression of cellular properties. Menezes et al. (1976 a) also found that the level of EBV antigen expression, both early antigen (EA) and VCA, in lymphoblastoid cell lines established from cord leukocytes by B95-8 virus was lower than that in lines derived from the QIMR-WIL or 833L viruses. A third study (Gerber et al., 1976 a) detected a difference in the expression of orally excreted EBV strains of African (BL) and United States (IM) origin. Cord lymphocytes transformed by BL strains produced low levels of EA and VCA as well as infective virus, but the lines derived from IM strains produced only EBV-associated nuclear antigen (EBNA) and soluble CF antigen. Such biologic studies need to differentiate between qualitative and quantitative effects. This touches on an attractive area for study, the search for a correlation between the molecular structure of the genome of EBV strains and their biologic activities.

So far, only a single strain of EBV has been detected which fails to transform lymphocytes in the usual manner, that present in the P_3HR-1 cell line (Hinuma et al., 1967; Miller et al., 1974). The viral antigens present in the P_3HR-1 line are not detectably distinct from those of cell lines producing transforming virus, and the P_3HR-1 virus is neutralized, similarly to transforming strains, by human convalescent sera (de Schryver et al., 1974). Though it does not transform human lymphocytes, the P_3HR-1 virus is able to superinfect a range of EBV genome-carrying lymphoid lines (such as Raji) in which subsequent viral expression is usually limited to production of EA (Henle et al., 1970; Miller et al., 1974; Menezes et al., 1975). In phosphate-free medium Raji cells superinfected with P_3HR-1 virus produced large amounts of virus which differed from the original inoculum in not being infectious for Raji cells (Yajima and Nonoyama, 1976). Intact P_3HR-1 virus interfered with transformation by the B95-8 strain, but heat- or ultraviolet (UV)-inactivated or neutralized virus did not (Miller et al., 1974). Although interference was associated with the P_3HR-1 virion, the interference mechanism was not defined. There are some curious aspects about the history of the P_3HR-1 strain, particularly the fact that it was derived from a BL line which originally yielded transforming virus (Henle et al., 1967; Gerber et al., 1969). The processes resulting in this highly significant change remain an enigma. Infection of EBV genome-negative cell lines by P_3HR-1 virus revealed evidence of heterogeneity in the viral populations (Fresen et al., 1977). A recent report described a possible variant of the P_3HR-1 virus (Osato et al., 1976). Obtained by cocultivation of frozen and thawed P_3HR-1 cells with cord lymphocytes, the EBV recovered was found to induce a transient blast response in cord lymphocytes. EBNA was not detectable in these cells unless treated with pokeweed mitogen and 5-iododeoxyuridine. These results, which should be further explored, suggest the detection of a new virus-lymphocyte relationship.

An EBV-related virus from the baboon transformed lymphocytes from five primate species as well as human cord lymphocytes and, in fact, had a wider host range for transformation than B95-8 virus (Rabin et al., 1977). The chimpanzee EBV-related virus (Landon et al., 1968) was tested for transformation of human cord-blood or marmoset lymphocytes by means of cell lysates or concentrated culture fluid of chimpanzee cell lines and by cocultivation of X-irradiated chimpanzee cells with human cord lymphocytes, with negative results (Gerber et al., 1976b).

D. TARGET CELLS AND THEIR PROPERTIES

As already indicated, lymphocytes are used in EBV transformation work; transformed cell lines consistently showed the characteristics of B (bone marrow-derived lymphocyte) rather than T (thymus-dependent) lymphocytes (Shevach et al., 1972; Jondal and Klein, 1973; Moore and Minowada, 1973; Pattengale et al., 1974). Transformation of lymphocytes from other primates including chimpanzees (Gerber et al., 1976b), gibbons (Werner et al., 1972), and marmosets and squirrel, owl and cebus monkeys (Deinhardt et al., 1974; Falk et al., 1974) also yielded lymphoblastoid lines of B cell type.

Transformation of partially purified populations of human B and T lymphocytes confirmed that only the B lymphocyte was the target cell specifically transformed (Schneider and zur Hausen, 1975; Yata et al., 1975; Menezes et al., 1976b). Other cells shown to be unlikely target cells for EBV included K cells (Peter et al., 1975), null cells (Robinson et al., 1977), and macrophages (Pope et al., 1974; Schneider and zur Hausen, 1975). The target role of B cells was supported by the detection of EBV receptors on B but not T lymphocytes by Jondal and Klein (1973) using a combination of cellular adherence and immunofluorescence techniques. The proportion of B cells with receptors was not determined. Greaves et al. (1975) used a high titer preparation of the QIMR-WIL virus and an antiviral fluorescent conjugate to detect attachment of EBV to receptors on tonsillar lymphocytes. It was considered that virtually all B lymphocytes carried EBV receptors.

Menezes et al. (1976 b) also used P_3HR-1 viral preparations and an immuno-fluorescence test to detect adsorption of EBV to lymphocytes. Although the technique showed EBV receptors on over 90% of Raji cells, only 3%–6.5% of unfractionated lymphocytes reacted and the authors estimated that only $\sim$ 31% of the B cells carried receptors detectable in this way. T lymphocytes showed no evidence of EBV receptors. Menezes et al. (1977) made the additional unexpected observation that a subline of the MOLT-4 lymphoid cell line (Minowada et al., 1972), which has T cell characteristics was able to adsorb EBV although it did not allow virus penetration.

Considerable progress has been made in the study of the EBV receptors. The presence of receptors for EBV and for C3 was found to correlate in established lymphoid cell lines (Jondal et al., 1976) in experiments where concentrated EBV was found to block complement receptor-detecting rosette formation by cell lines with C3 receptors, and complement blocked binding of EBV, but the sites were not actually identical. Yefenof et al. (1976) showed by double-fluorescence staining that the distribution of EBV and C3 receptors on lymphoid lines was almost identical in capping experiments in which the EBV and C3 receptors showed a direct association while other markers (Fc receptors, IgM, and β_2 microglobulin) were unrelated to EBV receptors. Yefenof and Klein (1977) found that selective removal of EBV or C3 receptors from cell lines significantly reduced the cells' capacity to adsorb EBV, while removal of Fc receptors, IgM, or β_2 microglobulin did not. Complement consumption by a wide range of lymphoid cell lines with or without EBV genome was found to be independent of deposition of C3 onto its receptors and EBV receptors again correlated with C3 receptors but not with complement consumption (Yefenof et al., 1977). These findings on cell lines were extended to peripheral blood lymphocytes by Robinson et al. (1977), who found that the efficiency of transformation of both human and marmoset lymphocytes correlated with the presence of cells with complement receptors. Einhorn et al. (1978) fractionated peripheral blood lymphocytes and found a close association between the frequency of B cells with surface Ig or complement receptors and adsorption of EBV, which correlated with the frequency of EBNA-positive cells at 2–3 days and cellular DNA synthesis at 7–8 days. Of the non-B cell fractions, the null cell component carried some complement receptors, and adsorbed EBV but failed to respond to it. In contrast, the T cell fraction had a low frequency of complement receptors but failed to adsorb EBV. It is evident that not all complement receptors play the same role as EBV receptors and these observations appear to preclude infection of cells without receptors by an alternative process such as pinocytosis.

Lymphoid target cells susceptible to transformation by EBV survived quite well in tissue culture; transformation occurred in fetal bone-marrow cells cultivated for 15 days before infection (Pope et al., 1971) and in cord lymphocytes cultivated for 18 days (Pope, unpublished).

Although the target cell role of B lymphocytes has been established, little or no detail on the relative susceptibility of lymphocytes in different stages of differentiation has been recorded. Some evidence suggested that the B lymphocytes of chronic lymphocytic leukemia were highly resistant to EBV transformation (Chang et al., 1976) and it would be interesting to know whether this was due to lack of EBV receptors or to some other perhaps disease-related mechanism. It is generally accepted that lymphocytes from children and cord blood are more readily transformed than from adult (Diehl et al., 1968) and in a quantitative study Henderson et al. (1977) found adult lymphocytes a hundredfold less susceptible to transformation than cord lymphocytes. The explanation for this may lie in the observation that adult but not fetal T lymphocytes were inhibitory to transformation of partially purified B lymphocytes (Thorley-Lawson et al., 1977). Hinuma et al. (1976) found no relationship between the efficiency of transformation of adult leukocytes and the titer of antibody to VCA. Addition of cord to adult leukocytes improved the transformation efficiency, suggesting that some samples of adult leukocytes may be deficient in susceptible cells. Marmoset leukocytes had about 2000 times lower frequency of transformation than human cord leukocytes (Robinson et al., 1977).

A second type of target cell susceptible to EBV is the EBV genome-negative lymphoid cell line with B cell characteristics (Klein et al., 1974a). Several such cell lines studied have been found to be converted to EBV genome-positive and EBNA-positive status by infection with various strains of EBV, including P_3HR-1 (Klein et al., 1974b; Klein et al., 1975; Clements et al., 1975; Steinitz and Klein, 1975; Fresen and zur Hausen, 1976; Steinitz and Klein, 1976; Fresen et al., 1977). This type of EBV infection is characterized by persistence of the viral genome, expression of a viral-induced nonstructural antigen (EBNA) apparently equivalent to the tumor antigens of classic oncogenic viruses, and failure to produce infectious virus.

By analogy with Marek's disease infection in chickens, it has long been suspected that lytic EBV infection may occur in epithelial tissue in man and because of the excretion of virus in the oropharynx, this is thought to be a likely site. Two observations suggest that epithelial tissue might indeed be susceptible to EBV. First, epithelial cells of one of three EBNA-positive nasopharyngeal carcinomas (NPC's) carried receptors for P_3HR-1 virus and responded by production of EA in 10%–25% of cells (Glaser et al., 1976). From this it can be assumed that normal epithelium may carry receptors, but direct proof that EBV is adsorbed and leads to lytic or abortive infection is required. Second, it has been reported that B95-8 infection of non-neoplastic nasopharyngeal epithelium in tissue culture resulted in changes suggestive of transformation (Huang et al., 1977). Growth of epithelial-like cells was stimulated in 19 out of 20 biopsy samples within 12 days and continued in several cases during subculture for $\sim$ 1 year. Results on the EBV status of these long-term cultures are not yet available, but, no doubt, a full evaluation of this finding will rapidly be made. Al-Moslih et al. (1976) recently reported that inoculation of sonicated EB3 lymphoid cells onto human amnion cultures resulted in outgrowth of foci of altered cells carrying EBV antigens. This was interpreted as due to transfection by the EBV genome, but other possibilities such as outgrowth of altered EB3 cells or hybrid cells were apparently not eliminated.

E. INFECTIVITY ASSAYS

The infectivity of an EBV preparation can be assessed relatively quickly by simply observing the rapidity of onset of the cellular proliferative response, higher virus concentrations giving an earlier response. The proportion of inoculated lymphocytes carrying EBNA can also be used as an indicator of the activity of EBV in the inoculum.

The observation has to be made early enough (3–5 days) to detect cells initially infected before they proliferate. The uptake of ^{3}H-thymidine following inoculation was also found to reflect the viral concentration; with high concentrations stimulation of cells was evident in 3–10 days (Robinson and Miller, 1975).

The infectivity of a preparation can be more accurately estimated by a quantitative assay. If conducted in microtiter plates to provide enough replicates, the 50% end point of the titration can be calculated by regular virologic methods (Moss and Pope, 1972). The necessity of clearly establishing whether or not each culture has transformed requires an observation period of at least 1 month.

The most accurate estimate of the infectivity of a lytic virus is obtained by an enumeration assay using plaque techniques. The equivalent with EBV transformation of lymphocytes would be a colony-forming technique using a semisolid gel in which, ideally, each infected B lymphocyte would proliferate to yield a colony. Several groups have approached this problem with some success. Yamamoto and Hinuma (1976) noted formation of colonies of cord lymphocytes transformed by B95-8 EBV, with a "one-hit" dose response. However, 10^4 cord cells yielded only 1–4 colonies and adult peripheral-blood lymphocytes were much less responsive. Essentially similar results (one colony per 10^3 cord lymphocytes infected with B95-8 virus) were obtained by the second group (Mizuno et al., 1976). Comparison of these results using colony-forming techniques with the usual suspension-culture technique indicates that the former are relatively insensitive with regard to the proportion of cells responding; this is perhaps not surprising since the plating efficiency of transformed cell lines would have to be taken into account. Katsuki and Hinuma (1976) using two methods estimated that $\sim 4.4\%$ of cord cells in suspension were initially transformed. In one method, sufficient virus to obtain maximum response was inoculated; growth curves of transformed cells were obtained and extrapolated to the time of infection, taking into account an estimated 24 h lag-phase. The other test was based on measuring the amount of virus required for transformation, as used by Schneider and zur Hausen (1975). Henderson et al. (1977) considered the figure to be at least 10% of the T-cell depleted lymphocyte population. This estimate was made using data from both a limiting dilution assay and a transformed center assay, with corrections for the plating efficiency of transformed cord cells and for an inhibitory effect of T cells. In all such studies it is difficult to determine whether failure of infected B cells to transform is due to suboptimal cultural conditions for small cell populations (population effects) or to inherent inability of all infected B lymphocytes to transform. If the sensitivity of the colony formation assay can be increased, the technique should provide a useful tool for application to several problems in the biology of EBV. Transformation by EBV in mass culture is polyclonal and the colony technique would provide a ready means of selecting clones.

F. VIRUS-CELL RELATIONSHIPS

In transformation of lymphocytes the viral replication cycle is arrested or modified and the lack of a lytic system has made difficult the detailed biochemical study of EBV replication. So far most investigation into the status of the viral genome has used established, transformed cell lines, where multiple copies are distributed between episomal and integrated components. These aspects are considered elsewhere in this volume (Chap. 8).

With the advent of infectivity assays it became possible to record the multiplicity of infection (MOI) in transformation experiments. This has provided a general idea of the virus input, but to be more accurate it would be necessary to estimate the MOI for the B lymphocyte target cell population itself. Transformation occurred quite satisfactorily with QIMR-WIL virus at a MOI in the range of 0.01–15 (Moss et al., 1976) while for B95-8 virus a MOI of 0.02–0.2 was sufficient to induce maximum transformation of cord cells (Katsuki and Hinuma, 1976), although in another laboratory a MOI of ~ 6 was required (Henderson et al., 1977). There is evidence that EBV transformation follows "one-hit" kinetics (Yamamoto and Hinuma, 1976; Henderson et al., 1977).

One of the earliest effects of EBV on lymphocytes appears to be the stimulation of cellular DNA synthesis. Thus, Pope et al. (1971) observed an increase in uptake of ^{3}H-thymidine between 7 and 11 days in fetal bone-marrow cells infected with the QIMR-WIL virus, while Gerber and Hoyer (1971) observed increasing synthesis of DNA at 3–12 days following inoculation of adult peripheral blood lymphocytes with the AV strain of EBV, with the subsequent establishment of cell lines. UV-inactivated AV strain of EBV specifically stimulated DNA synthesis, with a peak at 6–7 days, in lymphocytes from donors with antibody to EBV (Gerber and Lucas, 1972). Heat-inactivated P$_3$HR-1 virus appeared to be still capable of inducing DNA synthesis at 6 days in lymphocytes from 5 out of 5 EBV-seropositive and 11 out of 14 seronegative donors but not from 15 neonates (Chang and Spina, 1976); the control inoculum in this study was prepared from MOLT-4, a T cell line, but it would have been of interest to include a control extract from a B cell line as well. The stimulating factor in this work was not identified. Aya and Osato (1974) found that P$_3$HR-1 virus induced early DNA synthesis with a peak of 7.5% of cord lymphocytes at 15 h, and $\sim 18\%$ of these labeled cells proceeded into mitosis. EBNA-positive cells were detected as early as 2 days (2.5%) and after 5 days increased rapidly in numbers. Although these cultures were not observed for more than 1 month, growth was apparently still continuing and this seems to be a rare report of transformation by P$_3$HR-1 virus. Using a different virus (B95-8), Einhorn and Ernberg (1978) found that cellular DNA synthesis in infected cord lymphocytes followed, rather than preceded, the appearance of EBNA. Because of the variety of virus strains and of cultural conditions used in these studies it is difficult to assess how much of the DNA synthesis response observed in the early stages of infection is contributed by replication of viral DNA or by replication of DNA of cells transformed by EBV or stimulated by EBV-related antigens. After a certain point in the infection, however, DNA synthesis due to proliferation of transformed cells is clearly recognizable.

In early studies on transformation, proliferation commonly began 3 weeks or more after infection (Henle et al., 1967; Pope et al., 1968, 1969). Titration of virus in fetal bone-marrow cells showed that the lag period before the beginning of proliferation increased up to about 3 months as the virus concentration decreased (Pope et al., 1971). In these experiments it was clear from microscopy that the infected cells remained quite inactive for many weeks before suddenly beginning to proliferate. These observations revealed an interesting aspect of the EBV-cell relationship, i. e., that infection of cells may be followed by a long lag period before proliferation. This relationship between viral inoculum and outgrowth of transformed cells was confirmed by Robinson and Miller (1975) using a different EBV strain and uptake of ^{3}H-thymidine as the indicator of cellular activity; delays of up to 40–50 days occurred with higher virus dilutions. In subsequent work by various groups, infection was followed by proliferation of lymphocytes as early as 4–7 days later. This apparent alteration in EBV response over the years was probably due to a combination of higher virus titers and better culture conditions. In any event, this type of prompt response highlights to a greater extent the lag period seen under certain conditions with low virus concentrations.

A second important aspect of the virus-cell relationship is the production of virus-induced antigens. It was shown quite early that low levels of an EBV antigen could be detected in transformed lines by immunofluorescence (Henle et al., 1967) and that an EBV-associated CF antigen was produced in transformed fetal leukocyte cell lines (Pope et al., 1969). Subsequently, several groups have studied EBNA production following EBV infection of lymphocytes from cord blood; as already mentioned, Aya and Osato (1974) used P_3HR-1 virus and detected EBNA in 2.5% of lymphocytes at 2 days, with the proportion of EBNA-positive cells increasing slowly until 5 days, then rapidly to 50% at 10 days. Yata et al. (1975) infected cord cells with the B95-8 strain and observed EBNA production at 2–3 days in unfractionated and B cell populations; 50–80% of cells were EBNA-positive in 7 days. Leibold et al. (1975) also used the B95-8 strain and obtained similar results with lymphocytes from cord blood or adult peripheral blood regardless of the EBV-antibody status, and found that the addition of pokeweed mitogen enhanced EBNA formation, while concanavalin A was inhibitory and phytohemagglutinin (PHA) had little effect. Moss and Pope (1975) inoculated the QIMR-WIL strain of virus onto lymphocytes from peripheral blood of EBV seropositive adults; EBNA-positive cells were detected usually at 3 days and proliferated to yield cell lines. Overall, this body of information showed that with a sufficiently high inoculum of various strains of EBV, EBNA-positive cells appeared in a few days and a high proportion proliferated to yield lymphoblastoid cell lines.

The degree of expression of the EBV genome beyond the synthesis of EBNA has been found to vary with the origin of the cells transformed. Neither VCA nor infectious virus was produced in four transformed lines derived from cord leukocytes but VCA occurred at a low level in three out of four lines produced from adult peripheral blood lymphocytes by the same virus strain B95-8; four marmoset-derived lines expressed high levels of both VCA and infectious virus (Miller and Lipman, 1973 a). Similarly, nonhuman primate transformed cell lines (B84-15, squirrel monkey, and B95-8, cotton-top marmoset) showed a consistently higher degree of viral antigen expression and of virus production than the human 883L line, which was the source of the transforming EBV strain (Miller and Lipman, 1973 b). These results indicate that a strong genetic influence in the target cell controls viral genome expression following transformation, but its nature remains unknown. Klein et al. (1975) showed also that the strain of virus could affect the expression of viral antigens in the same cells. Another interesting and relevant point is that viral antigen expression was much less restricted in spontaneously established lymphoblastoid cell lines than in those obtained by inoculation of EBV (Menezes et al., 1976 a). This observation seems highly significant and should be further explored.

Other characteristics of B lymphocytes, including Fc receptors, complement receptors, and synthesis of Ig, have also been studied in relation to transformation by EBV. Expression of the receptors for Fc and for complement was similar on fresh lymphocytes from man, woolly monkey, and marmoset. Following transformation by the B95-8 strain of EBV, human cells expressed predominantly complement receptors, monkey cells expressed both, but marmoset cells expressed neither (Robinson et al., 1977). This is further evidence of the important role of the host cell in determining the properties of transformed cell lines. Surface Ig was expressed in the majority of transformed lines, but one negative result has been recorded (Menezes et al., 1976 b). Transformed lines were derived from tonsillar lymphocytes by infection with the B95-8 or QIMR-WIL viruses and 6 out of 11 and 2 out of 11, respectively, showed a high proportion of cells (15%–45%) synthesizing IgA, in contrast to the absence of IgA in cord-derived cell lines (Yamamoto et al., 1976). Study of the early period (3–7 days) after infection of lymphocytes from EBV-seropositive or seronegative donors by the B95-8 strain of EBV showed that polyclonal B cell stimulation occurred and that IgG and IgM (19S) were synthesized (Rosén et al., 1977). Although heterophil antibody was not detectable in the culture fluid, individual cells were detected which formed plaques with sheep red blood cells (SRBC) and haptenated SRBC. The possibility of obtaining lymphoblastoid cell lines synthesizing antibody to a particular antigen has been recognized for some time and this field of research has considerable potential practical application. An important step in this direction has been taken with the recent establishment of an EBV-transformed cell line synthesizing specific IgM antibody to the synthetic hapten 4-hydroxy-3,5-dinitrophenacetic acid (Steinitz et al., 1978). This was achieved by selection of the appropriate B cell population by adherence to antigen-coated RBC followed by transformation by EBV, a method that should find general application.

G. CELLULAR INTERACTIONS

As already noted, B lymphocytes are the target cells for EBV. Macrophage depletion of mononuclear preparations from EBV-seropositive donors by adherence to a plastic surface resulted in a marked reduction in the response to the QIMR-WIL strain of EBV (Pope et al., 1973). The response was enhanced by addition of the nonadherent macrophage-depleted population to macrophages. Similar results were reported by Furukawa (1975), but other studies suggested that macrophages may not be essential for transformation but perhaps provide optimal culture conditions (Schneider and zur Hausen, 1975; Gergely and Ernberg, 1977).

   In experiments with lymphocytes from EBV-seropositive donors, active transformation by EBV was observed in some cultures in the first week or two, only to be followed by deterioration and failure to establish cell lines (Moss and Pope, 1972, 1975). This effect was observed with higher virus concentrations and higher lymphocyte concentrations and may possibly be due to induction of an active cytotoxic immune response in vitro.

H. INHIBITION OF TRANSFORMATION

Studies of the cell relationships in transformation led to the discovery that transformation could be inhibited in vitro (Pope et al., 1974). The basic observation was that a nonadherent lymphocyte population from an EBV-seropositive donor underwent typical EBV transformation when cultivated alone or on a feeder layer of human fetal fibroblasts, but failed to transform on fibroblasts of adult origin (Pope et al., 1974; Moss et al., 1976). Many lymphocytes in such inhibited cultures remained viable but failed to proliferate during periods of up to 3 months (Pope, 1975 b).

Inhibition of transformation was found to be reversible at 1 month either by adding PHA or by removing the nonadherent cells to clean tissue culture vessels (Pope, 1975 b). This finding, together with the presence of EBNA in a significant proportion of the inhibited lymphocytes, showed that inhibition was not due to inactivation of the viral inoculum. Addition of adult fibroblasts to infected nonadherent lymphocytes after 2–4 days did not result in inhibition of transformation, suggesting that the transformation process was already complete. The evidence suggests that a block in transformation occurred between induction of EBNA and the onset of proliferation (Moss et al., 1976). This is interesting in view of the finding that in EBV-transformation synthesis of EBNA was found to precede that of cellular DNA (Einhorn and Ernberg, 1978). It has been suggested previously that a stimulus to DNA synthesis in the form of a blast transformation may be required to enhance completion of the EBV-transformation process (Pope et al., 1972, 1974; Moss et al., 1976).

A significant advance was made when it was found that inhibition of transformation occurred with lymphocytes from donors with prior EBV infection, but not with those from seronegative donors or from cord blood (Moss et al., 1977). This suggests that inhibition has an immunologic basis, but the details of the mechanism are not known at present. Such complete inhibition has so far been observed only with nonadherent lymphocytes under the particular conditions described, and we and other researchers have shown that successful transformation of lymphocytes from seropositive donors readily occurs under standard conditions.

If this inhibition model reflects events in vivo then its study may help elucidate both the manner in which primary EBV infection is brought under control and the mechanisms by which the virus persists indefinitely. In particular, a most important question in maintaining virus persistence in vivo concerns the roles played by transformed cells perhaps controlled immunologically, by infected nonproliferating cells exhibiting a latent or abortive infection, and by a smouldering lytic infection; the in vitro inhibition system shows that the second of these situations is biologically feasible. This basic type of inhibition may well be the explanation of the lag period seen in vitro with inoculation of low virus doses.

Other reported studies are relevant to inhibition of transformation. Lai et al. (1977) studied a factor with properties similar to those of interferon which was produced by cultures of sensitized lymphocytes in response to inoculation of specific antigen, either UV-irradiated QIMR-WIL EBV, or tuberculin purified protein-derivative; treatment of cord lymphocytes with this factor for 12 h prevented subsequent transformation by infectious QIMR-WIL EBV. This work, which has not yet been confirmed, may also prove relevant to the pathogenesis of EBV infection, but it should be noted that Menezes et al. (1976 c) were unable to detect any effect of exogenous interferon on transformation of cord-blood lymphocytes by B95-8 virus.

Following up the lower susceptibility of adult leukocytes to transformation by EBV in culture under the usual conditions, Thorley-Lawson et al. (1977) reported evidence that a T lymphocyte population from adult but not cord blood partially suppressed transformation of EBV-infected purified B lymphocytes. The B cells from cord and adult blood showed similar susceptibility to transformation once the T cells were removed. It remains to be seen whether this was related to the serologic status of these adult donors or was a nonspecific effect of T cells. A detailed study by Rickinson et al. (1977 a) showed that purified T lymphocytes from peripheral blood in acute IM were able to inhibit the outgrowth of cord lymphocytes transformed by EBV. Inhibition occurred when the T lymphocytes were added immediately postinfection or up to 7 days later. In contrast to the results of Thorley-Lawson et al. (1977), no inhibitory effect of T lymphocytes from control donors was noted, regardless of whether or not the donor had antibody to EBV. Robinson et al. (1977) also found no evidence of a suppressor effect of T lymphocytes. Leibold et al. (1975) observed no difference in EBNA production, an early marker of transformation, in lymphocytes from adult donors with or without EBV antibody.

Conflicting results have been obtained in experiments on the effects of phosphonoacetic acid (PAA) on transformation by EBV in vitro. PAA, which inhibits synthesis of herpes viral DNA, was reported at concentrations of 50–200 μg/ml to inhibit transformation by B95-8 EBV, but not by PHA. Addition of PAA was most effective up to 3 days after infection, but less so thereafter (Thorley-Lawson and Strominger, 1976). Rickinson and Epstein (1978) found that the response of cord cells to B95-8 EBV in the first week was no more sensitive to PAA than was the response to pokeweed mitogen, but levels above 100 μg/ml were significantly inhibitory. Furthermore, virus transformation was no more sensitive to PAA than was colony formation by cells already transformed by EBV. Thus, although there is general agreement that PAA inhibits EBV replication, further study of its effects on EBV transformation is required.

A genuine inhibition of EBV transformation has to be distinguished from simple explanations such as toxicity or defective cultural conditions. However, evidence is building up to show that inhibition can result from a range of factors. It will be of considerable interest to determine whether or not these factors operate through a common pathway.

I. ROLE OF IN VITRO TRANSFORMATION BY EBV IN THE ESTABLISHMENT OF LYMPHOBLASTOID CELL LINES IN PRIMARY CULTURE OF HUMAN TISSUES

It has been suggested before (Pope et al., 1972) that when tumor material or IM peripheral blood is cultivated in vitro, outgrowth of lymphoblastoid cell lines may occur due to EBV transformation in vitro. A considerable body of evidence has accumulated to show that this actually does occur when lymphocytes from peripheral blood of IM cases or normal seropositive donors are cultivated in vitro. Establishment of cell lines from this material appears to involve two phases. In the first, some of the EBV-infected cells undergo lytic infection with release of infectious virus; only a very low proportion of cells, if any, proliferate to yield cell lines. In the second phase, virus released in culture transforms other B lymphocytes and it is these transformed cells that predominantly lead to establishment of lymphoblastoid cell lines (Rickinson et al., 1974, 1977b). Henderson et al. (1975) recently reported that exposure to N-methyl-N'-nitro-N-nitrosoguanidine (MNNG) for 2 h on the 3rd day of culture significantly increased the proportion of lymphoblastoid cell lines established from lymphocytes from peripheral blood of seropositive donors. Establishment of cell lines was completely inhibited by autologous human serum with antibody to EBV, suggesting that the two-phase phenomenon applied here also. The action of MNNG may have been either to induce more EBV-infected cells into the lytic cycle or to improve the efficiency of transformation in the second phase. In view of this phenomenon, it is highly desirable that any lymphoid line obtained by in vitro cultivation of lymphoma or other neoplastic tissue is confirmed as being of tumor origin.

J. EFFECTS OF EBV TRANSFORMATION ON KARYOTYPE

In general, EBV-transformed cells were diploid but tended to become aneuploid on continued culture (Nilsson and Pontén, 1975). The occurrence of a subterminal constriction on the long arms of a group C chromosome (probably No. 10) was detected in some metaphase plates of lymphoblastoid cell lines (Kohn et al., 1967; Miles and O'Neill, 1967). This aberration was also detected in lymphoblastoid cell lines established by transformation of normal cells by EBV, which usually had a diploid karyotype (Henle et al., 1967; Pope et al., 1968; Gerber et al., 1969). Several studies failed to establish a relationship between the No. 10 marker and EBV (Whang-Peng et al., 1970; Huang et al., 1970). Inoculation of the EBNA-positive RPMI 6410 cell line with a high concentration of P_3HR-1 virus resulted in numerous random breaks and constrictions (Huang et al., 1971). It is considered that the No. 10 constriction is probably not specifically associated with the presence of the EBV genome.

The No. 10 marker was clearly not specific for BL. A No. 14 marker (Manolov and Manolova, 1972) was detected in BL and was subsequently shown to be an 8–14 translocation (Zech et al., 1976). The No. 14 marker was also found in other forms of lymphoma (Zech et al., 1976), and in a BL-lymphoid cell line without EBV genome (Kaiser-McMaw et al., 1977). The No. 14 marker was clearly not related to EBV as it was not seen in 18 cell lines of fetal origin transformed in vitro by EBV or in 31 lymphoblastoid lines of IM origin (Jarvis et al., 1974).

K. CONCLUSION

Transformation of human lymphocytes by EBV in vitro is such a readily reproducible phenomenon that it is difficult to believe that a similar process would not sometimes occur in vivo. In the meantime, EBV transformation must be viewed as a fascinating subject which contributes directly to knowledge of the biology of the virus.

The majority of strains of EBV encountered so far, whether under natural conditions in the throat or in the somewhat artificial situation in tissue culture, has the capacity to transform lymphocytes and establish lymphoblastoid cell lines and these lines invariably have B lymphocyte characteristics; only one virus strain appears not to have this transforming capacity. As mentioned above, the target cell for EBV transformation is the B lymphocyte, and such transformation may be relevant to the etiology of BL.

Adsorption of EBV to B lymphocytes has been shown to involve receptors which are closely associated with the receptors for C3. Infection of lymphocytes apparently results in induction of EBNA, followed by synthesis of cellular DNA. The EBV genome persists in the transformed cells, but its expression is limited and is largely dependent on the source of the lymphocytes. An increasing level of viral genome expression is shown by transformed lines derived from cord lymphocytes (low), adult human lymphocytes (low but variable), and marmoset lymphocytes (high, with infectious virus).

Transformation in vitro of lymphocytes from seropositive donors may be inhibited by the presence of a feeder layer of adult human fibroblasts and such inhibition is manifested as a block between synthesis of EBNA and cellular proliferation. Since this inhibition is reversible at least up to 1 month after infection, it appears to be highly relevant to the persistance of the virus in lymphocytes.

One of the most important aspects of EBV transformation for future study is the chain of events, involving the viral genome, which begins with infection of the lymphocyte and culminates in the establishment of the fully transformed state in 3–4 days. The investigation of target cells, and in particular the search for further types of susceptible cells, is sure to attract continuing attention. Host- and virus-determined factors influencing the expression of the viral genome and of various cellular characteristics also require clarification. Progress can likewise be expected in the definition of cell-virus relationships with particular emphasis on the mechanisms of persistence of the virus in cells. Immunologic parameters affecting EBV transformation will have to be taken into account and a beginning has been made in this direction. Many of these aspects are highly relevant to the pathogenesis of IM, BL, and NPC.

Knowledge of EBV transformation has reached a stage at which further research will increasingly be made at the molecular level. Elucidation of the mechanism by which EBV induces and maintains proliferation of lymphocytes may well make a significant contribution to the understanding of the neoplastic process.

REFERENCES

Al-Moslih, M. I., White, R. J., Dubes, G. R.: Use of a transfection method to demonstrate a monolayer cell transforming agent from the EB3 line of Burkitt's lymphoma cells. J. Gen. Virol. **31,** 331–345 (1976)

Aya, T., Osato, T.: Early events in transformation of human cord leukocytes by Epstein-Barr virus: induction of DNA synthesis, mitosis and the virus-associated nuclear antigen synthesis. Int. J. Cancer **14,** 341–347 (1974)

Baumal, R., Bloom, B., Scharff, M. D.: Induction of long term lymphocyte lines from delayed hypersensitive human donors using specific antigen plus Epstein-Barr virus. Nature (New Biol.) **230,** 20–21 (1971)

Chang, R. S.: Umbilical cord leucocytes transformed by lymphoid cell filtrates from healthy people. Nature (New Biol.) **233,** 124 (1971)

Chang, R. S., Fillingame, R. A., Paglieroni, T., Glassy, F. J.: A procedure for quantifying susceptibility of human lymphocytes to transformation by Epstein-Barr viruses. Proc. Soc. Exp. Biol. Med. **153,** 193–196 (1976)

Chang, R. S., Spina, C. A.: *In vitro* stimulation of lymphocytes of donors seronegative for Epstein-Barr virus by preparations of inactivated Epstein-Barr virus. J. Infect. Dis. **133,** 676–680 (1976)

Clements, G. B., Klein, G., Povey, S.: Production by EBV infection of an EBNA-positive subline from an EBNA-negative human lymphoma cell line without detectable EBV DNA. Int. J. Cancer **16,** 125–133 (1975)

Deinhardt, F., Falk, L. A., Wolfe, L. G.: Transformation of nonhuman primate lymphocytes by Epstein-Barr virus. Cancer Res. **34,** 1241–1244 (1974)

De Schryver, A., Klein, G., Hewetson, J., Rocchi, G., Henle, W., Henle, G., Moss, D. J., Pope, J. H.: Comparison of EBV neutralization tests based on abortive infection or transformation of lymphoid cells and their relation to membrane reactive antibodies (ANTI-MA). Int. J. Cancer **13,** 353–362 (1974)

Diehl, V., Henle, G., Henle, W.: Effect of a herpes-type (EBV) on growth of peripheral leukocyte cultures. Fed. Proc. **27,** 682 (1968)

Einhorn, L., Ernberg, I.: Induction of EBNA precedes the first cellular S-phase after EBV infection of human lymphocytes. Int. J. Cancer **21,** 157–160 (1978)

Einhorn, L., Steinitz, M., Yefenof, E., Ernberg, I., Bakacs, T., Klein, G.: Epstein-Barr virus (EBV) receptors, complement receptors and EBV-infectability of different lymphocyte fractions of human peripheral blood. II. EBV studies. Cell. Immunol. (in press) (1978)

Falk, L., Wolfe, L., Deinhardt, F., Paciga, J., Dombos, L., Klein, G., Henle, W., Henle, G.: Epstein-Barr virus: transformation of non-human primate lymphocytes *in vitro*. Int. J. Cancer **13,** 363–376 (1974)

Fresen, K-O., zur Hausen, H.: Establishment of EBNA-expressing cell lines by infection of Epstein-Barr virus (EBV)-genome-negative human lymphoma cells with different EBV strains. Int. J. Cancer **17,** 161–166 (1976)

Fresen, K-O., Merkt, B., Bornkamm, G. W., zur Hausen, H.: Heterogeneity of Epstein-Barr virus originating from P_3HR-1 cells. I. Studies on EBNA induction. Int. J. Cancer **19,** 317–323 (1977)

Furukawa, T.: Cellular cooperation in transformation by EB virus. Res. Commun. Chem. Pathol. Pharmacol. **10,** 554–558 (1975)

Gerber, P., Hoyer, B. H.: Induction of cellular DNA synthesis in human leucocytes by Epstein-Barr virus. Nature **231,** 46–47 (1971)

Gerber, P., Lucas, S. J.: *In vitro* stimulation of human lymphocytes by Epstein-Barr virus. Cell. Immunol. **5,** 318–324 (1972)

Gerber, P., Whang-Peng, J., Monroe, J. H.: Transformation and chromosome changes induced by Epstein-Barr virus in normal human leukocyte cultures. Proc. Natl. Acad. Sci. USA **63,** 740–747 (1969)

Gerber, P., Nkrumah, F. K., Pritchett, R., Kieff, E.: Comparative studies of Epstein-Barr virus strains from Ghana and the United States. Int. J. Cancer **17,** 71–81 (1976 a)

Gerber, P., Pritchett, R. F., Kieff, E.: Antigens and DNA of a chimpanzee agent related to Epstein-Barr virus. J. Virol. **19,** 1090–1099 (1976 b)

Gergely, P., Ernberg, I.: Blastogenic response and EBNA induction in human lymphocytes by Epstein-Barr virus only requires B cells but not macrophages. Cancer Letters **2,** 217–220 (1977)

Glaser, R., de-Thé, G., Lenoir, G., Ho, J. H. C.: Superinfection of epithelial nasopharyngeal carcinoma cells with Epstein-Barr virus. Proc. Natl. Acad. Sci. USA **73,** 960–963 (1976)

Greaves, M. F., Brown, G., Rickinson, A. B.: Epstein-Barr virus binding sites on lymphocyte subpopulations and the origin of lymphoblasts in cultured lymphoid cell lines and in the blood of patients with infectious mononucleosis. Clin. Immunol. Immunopathol. **3,** 514–524 (1975)

Henderson, E. E., Norin, A. J., Strauss, B. S.: Induction of permanently proliferating human lymphoblastoid lines by N-methyl-N′-nitro-N-nitrosoguanidine. Cancer Res. **35,** 358–363 (1975)

Henderson, E., Miller, G., Robinson, J., Heston, L.: Efficiency of transformation of lymphocytes by Epstein-Barr virus. Virology **76,** 152–163 (1977)

Henle, W., Diehl, V., Kohn, G., zur Hausen, H., Henle, G.: Herpes-type virus and chromosome marker in normal leukocytes after growth with irradiated Burkitt cells. Science **157,** 1064–1065 (1967)

Henle, W., Henle, G., Zajac, B. A., Pearson, G., Waubke, R., Scriba, M.: Differential reactivity of human serums with early antigens induced by Epstein-Barr virus. Science **169,** 188–190 (1970)

Hinuma, Y., Konn, M. Yamaguchi, J., Grace, J. T., (Jr): Replication of herpes-type virus in a Burkitt lymphoma cell line. J. Virol. **1,** 1203–1206 (1967)

Hinuma, Y., Katsuki, T., Yamamoto, N.: Transformation of leukocytes from seropositive individuals by Epstein-Barr virus. Bibl. Haematol. **43,** 403–405 (1976)

Huang, C. C., Minowada, J., Smith, R. T., Osunkoya, B. O.: Reevaluation of relationship between C chromosome marker and Epstein-Barr virus: chromosome and immunofluorescence analyses of 16 human hematopoietic cell lines. J. Natl. Cancer Inst. **45,** 815–829 (1970)

Huang, C. C., Minowada, J., Horoszewicz, J. S.: Chromosome lesions induced in a human hematopoietic cell line by infection with Epstein-Barr virus. Proc. Soc. Exp. Biol. Med. **137,** 183–190 (1971)

Huang, D. P., Ho, H. C., Ng, M. H., Lui, M.: Possible transformation of nasopharyngeal epithelial cells in culture with Epstein-Barr virus from B95-8 cells. Br. J. Cancer **35,** 630–634 (1977)

Jarvis, J. E., Ball, G., Rickinson, A. B., Epstein, M. A.: Cytogenetic studies on human lymphoblastoid cell lines from Burkitt's lymphomas and other sources. Int. J. Cancer **14**, 716–721 (1974)

Jondal, M., Klein, G.: Surface markers of human B and T lymphocytes. II. Presence of Epstein-Barr virus receptors on B lymphocytes. J. Exp. Med. **138**, 1365–1378 (1973)

Jondal, M., Klein, G., Oldstone, M. B. A., Bokish, V., Yefenof, E.: Surface markers on human B and T lymphocytes. VIII. Association between complement and Epstein-Barr virus receptors on human lymphoid cells. Scand. J. Immunol. **5**, 401–410 (1976)

Kaiser-McCaw, B., Epstein, A. L., Kaplan, H. S., Hecht, F.: Chromosome 14 translocation in African and North American Burkitt's lymphoma. Int. J. Cancer **19**, 482–486 (1977)

Katsuki, T., Hinuma, Y.: Characteristics of cell lines derived from human leukocytes transformed by different strains of Epstein-Barr virus. Int. J. Cancer **15**, 203–210 (1975)

Katsuki, T., Hinuma, Y.: A quantitative analysis of the susceptibility of human leukocytes to transformation by Epstein-Barr virus. Int. J. Cancer **18**, 7–13 (1976)

Klein, G., Lindahl, T., Jondal, M., Leibold, W., Menézes, J., Nilsson, K., Sundstrom, C.: Continous lymphoid cell lines with characteristics of B cells (bone-marrow-derived), lacking the Epstein-Barr virus genome and derived from three human lymphomas. Proc. Natl. Acad. Sci. USA **71**, 3283–3286 (1974a)

Klein, G., Sugden, B., Leibold, W., Menezes, J.: Infection of EBV-genome-negative and -positive human lymphoblastoid cell lines with biologically different preparations of EBV. Intervirology **3**, 232–244 (1974b)

Klein, G., Giovanella, B., Westman, A., Stehlin, J. S., Mumford, D.: An EBV-genome-negative cell line established from an American Burkitt lymphoma; receptor characteristics. EBV infectibility and permanent conversion into EBV-positive sublines by *in vitro* infection. Intervirology **5**, 319–334 (1975)

Kohn, G., Mellman, W. J., Moorhead, P. S., Loftus, J., Henle, G.: Involvement of C group chromosomes in five Burkitt lymphoma cell lines. J. Natl. Cancer Inst. **38**, 209–222 (1967)

Lai, P. K., Alpers, M. P., Mackay-Scollay, E. M.: Epstein-Barr herpesvirus infection: inhibition by immunologically induced mediators with interferon-like properties. Int. J. Cancer **20**, 21–29 (1977)

Landon, J. C., Ellis, L. B. Zeve, V. H., Fabrizio, D. P. A.: Herpes-type virus in cultured leukocytes from chimpanzees. J. Natl. Cancer Inst. **40**, 181–192 (1968)

Leibold, W., Flanagan, T. D., Menezes, J., Klein, G.: Induction of Epstein-Barr virus-associated nuclear antigen during in vitro transformation of human lymphoid cells. J. Natl. Cancer Inst. **54**, 65–68 (1975)

Manolov, G., Manolova, Y.: Marker band in one chromosome 14 from Burkitt lymphomas. Nature **237**, 33–34 (1972)

Menezes, J., Leibold, W., Klein, G.: Biological differences between Epstein-Barr virus (EBV) strains with regard to lymphocyte transforming ability, superinfection and antigen induction. Exp. Cell Res. **92**, 478–484 (1975)

Menezes, J., Joncas, J. H., Patel, P., Leibold, W.: Epstein-Barr virus (EBV) expression in transformed human lymphoblastoid cell lines from different sources. Bibl. Haematol. **43**, 406–408 (1976a)

Menezes, J., Jondal, M., Leibold, W., Dorval, G.: Epstein-Barr virus interactions with human lymphocyte subpopulations: virus adsorptions, kinetics of expression of Epstein-Barr virus-associated nuclear antigen, and lymphocyte transformation. Infect. Immun. **13**, 303–310 (1976b)

Menezes, J., Patel, P., Dussault, H., Joncas, J.: Effect of interferon on lymphocyte transformation and nuclear antigen production by Epstein-Barr virus. Nature **260**, 430–432 (1976c)

Menezes, J., Seigneurin, J. M., Patel, P., Bourkas, A., Lenoir, G.: Presence of Epstein-Barr virus receptors, but absence of virus penetration, in cells of an Epstein-Barr virus genome-negative human lymphoblastoid T line (Molt 4). J. Virol. **22**, 816–821 (1977)

Miles, C. P., O'Neill, F.: Chromosome studies of 8 in vitro lines of Burkitt's lymphoma. Cancer Res. **27**, 392–402 (1967)

Miller, G., Enders, J. F., Lisco, H. I.: Establishment of lines from normal human blood leukocytes by co-cultivation with a leukocyte line derived from a leukemic child. Proc. Soc. Exp. Biol. Med. **132**, 247–252 (1969)

Miller, G., Lipman, M.: Release of infectious Epstein-Barr virus by transformed marmoset leukocytes. Proc. Natl. Acad. Sci. USA **70**, 190–194 (1973a)

Miller, G., Lipman, M.: Comparison of the yield of infectious virus from clones of human and simian lymphoblastoid lines transformed by Epstein-Barr virus. J. Exp. Med. **138**, 1398–1412 (1973b)

Miller, G., Robinson, J., Heston, L., Lipman, M.: Differences between laboratory strains of Epstein-Barr virus based on immortalization, abortive infection, and interference. Proc. Natl. Acad. Sci. USA **71**, 4006–4010 (1974)

Miller, G., Coope, D., Niederman, J., Pagano, J.: Biological properties and viral surface antigens of Burkitt lymphoma- and mononucleosis-derived strains of Epstein-Barr virus released from transformed marmoset cells. J. Virol. **18**, 1071–1080 (1976)

Minowada, J., Ohnuma, T., Moore, G. E.: Rosette-forming human lymphoid cell lines. I. Establishment and evidence for origin of thymus-derived lymphocytes. J. Natl. Cancer Inst. **49**, 891–895 (1972)

Mizuno, F., Aya, T., Osato, T.: Growth in semisolid agar medium of human cord leukocytes freshly transformed by Epstein-Barr virus. J. Natl. Cancer Inst. **56**, 171–173 (1976)

Moore, G. E. Minowada, J.: B and T lymphoid cell lines. N. Engl. J. Med. **288**, 106 (1973)

Moss, D. J., Pope, J. H.: Assay of the infectivity of Epstein-Barr virus by transformation of human leucocytes *in vitro*. J. Gen. Virol. **17**, 233–236 (1972)

Moss, D. J., Pope, J. H.: EB virus-associated nuclear antigen production and cell proliferation in adult peripheral blood leukocytes inoculated with the QIMR-WIL strain of EB virus. Int. J. Cancer **15**, 503–511 (1975)

Moss, D. J., Pope, J. H., Scott, W.: Inhibition of EB virus transformation of non-adherent human lymphocytes by co-cultivation with adult fibroblasts. Med. Microbiol. Immunol. **162**, 159–167 (1976)

Moss, D. J., Scott, W., Pope, J. H.: An immunological basis for the inhibition of transformation of human lymphocytes by EB virus. Nature **268**, 735–736 (1977)

Nilsson, K., Pontén, J.: Classification and biological nature of established human hematopoietic cell lines. Int. J. Cancer **15**, 321–341 (1975)

Nilsson, K. Klein, G. Henle, W., Henle, G.: The establishment of lymphoblastoid lines from adult and fetal human lymphoid tissue and its dependence on EBV. Int. J. Cancer **8**, 443–450 (1971)

Osato, T., Aya, T., Mizuno, F.: Indefinite and temporary growths of human cord lymphocytes *in vitro* by Epstein-Barr virus. Bibl. Haematol **43**, 302–307 (1976)

Pattengale, P. K., Smith, R. W., Gerber, P.: B-cell characteristics of human peripheral and cord blood lymphocytes transformed by Epstein-Barr virus. J. Nat. Cancer Inst. **52**, 1081–1086 (1974)

Peter, H. H., Diehl, V., Knoop, F., Kalden, J. R.: Inability of human 'K' cells to transform with Epstein-Barr-virus (EBV). Fed. Proc. **34**, 987 (1975)

Pope, J. H.: Transformation *in vitro* by herpesviruses, a review. In: Oncogenesis and herpesviruses II. de-Thé, G., Epstein, M. A., zur Hausen, H. (eds.), Part 1, pp. 367–378. Lyon: IARC 1975 a

Pope, J. H.: Cell co-operation involved in transformation of leukocytes by the QIMR-WIL strain of EBV. In: Oncogenesis and herpesviruses II. de-Thé, G., Epstein, M. A., zur Hausen, H. (eds.), Part 1, pp. 385–388. Lyon: IARC 1975 b

Pope, J. H., Horne, M. K., Scott, W.: Transformation of foetal human leukocytes in vitro by filtrates of a human leukaemic cell line containing herpes-like virus. Int. J. Cancer **3**, 857–866 (1968)

Pope, J. H., Horne, M. K., Scott, W.: Identification of the filtrable leukocyte-transforming factor of QIMR-WIL cells as herpes-like virus. Int. J. Cancer **4**, 255–260 (1969)

Pope, J. H., Scott, W., Reedman, B. M., Walters, M. K.: EB virus as a biologically active agent. In: Recent advances in human tumor virology and immunology. Proceedings of the 1st International Symposium of the Princess Takamatsu Cancer Research Fund. Tokyo, November, 1970. Nakahara, W. *et al.* (eds.) pp. 177–188. University of Tokyo Press 1971

Pope, J. H., Walters, M. K., Reedman, B. M.: Virological and immunological aspects of the role of EBV in the proliferation of lymphoid cells. In: The nature of leukaemia. Proceedings of the Intern. Cancer Conference. Sydney,13–17 March 1972. Vincent, P. D. (ed.), pp. 47–60. Sydney: Government Press 1972

Pope, J. H., Scott, W., Moss, D. J.: Human lymphoid cell transformation by Epstein-Barr virus. Nature (New Biol.) **246**, 140–141 (1973)

Pope, J. H., Scott, W., Moss, D. J.: Cell relationships in transformation of human leukocytes by Epstein-Barr virus. Int. J. Cancer **14**, 122–129 (1974)

Rabin, H., Neubauer, R. H., Hopkins, III, R. F., Dzhikindze, E. K., Shevtsova, Z. V., Lapin, B. A.: Transforming activity and antigenicity of an Epstein-Barr-like virus from lymphoblastoid cell lines of baboons with lymphoid disease. Intervirology **8**, 240–249 (1977)

Rickinson, A. B., Epstein, M. A.: Sensitivity of the transforming and replicative functions of Epstein-Barr virus to inhibition by phosphonoacetate J. Gen. Virol. **40**, 409–420 (1978)

Rickinson, A. B., Jarvis, J. E., Crawford, D. H., Epstein, M. A.: Observations on the type of infection by Epstein-Barr virus in peripheral lymphoid cells of patients with infectious mononucleosis. Int. J. Cancer **14**, 704–715 (1974)

Rickinson, A. B., Crawford, D., Epstein, M. A.: Inhibition of the *in vitro* outgrowth of Epstein-Barr virus-transformed lymphocytes by thymus-dependent lymphocytes from infectious mononucleosis patients. Clin. Exp. Immunol. **28**, 72–79 (1977 a)

Rickinson, A. B., Finerty, S., Epstein, M. A.: Comparative studies on adult donor lymphocytes infected by EB virus *in vivo* or *in vitro:* Origin of transformed cells arising in co-cultures with foetal lymphocytes. Int. J. Cancer **19,** 775–782 (1977b)

Robinson, J., Miller, G.: Assay for Epstein-Barr virus based on stimulation of DNA synthesis in mixed leukocytes from human umbilical cord blood. J. Virol. **15,** 1065–1072 (1975)

Robinson, J. E., Andiman, W. A. Henderson, E., Miller, G.: Host determined differences in expression of surface marker characteristics on human and simian lymphoblastoid cell lines transformed by Epstein-Barr virus. Proc. Natl. Acad. Sci. USA **74,** 749–753 (1977)

Rosén, A., Gergely, P., Jondal, M., Klein, G.: Polyclonal Ig production after Epstein-Barr virus infection of human lymphocytes *in vitro.* Nature **267,** 52–54 (1977)

Schneider, U., zur Hausen, H.: Epstein-Barr virus-inducted transformation of human leukocytes after cell fractionation. Int. J. Cancer **15,** 59–66 (1975)

Shevach, E. M., Herberman, R., Frank, M. M., Green, I.: Receptors for complement and immunoglobulin on human leukemic cells and human lymphoblastoid cell lines. J. Clin. Invest. **51,** 1933–1938 (1972)

Steinitz, M., Klein, G.: Comparison between growth characteristics of an Epstein-Barr virus (EBV)-genome-negative lymphoma line and its EBV-converted subline *in vitro.* Proc. Natl. Acad. Sci. USA **72,** 3518–3520 (1975)

Steinitz, M., Klein, G.: Epstein-Barr virus (EBV)-induced change in the saturation sensitivity and serum dependence of established, EBV-negative lymphoma lines *in vitro.* Virology **70,** 570–573 (1976)

Steinitz, M., Koskimies, S., Klein, G., Mäkela, O.: Epstein-Barr virus (EBV) induced immortalization of B lymphocytes with specific anti-hapten antibody production. Nature (in press) (1978)

Thorley-Lawson, D., Strominger, J. L.: Transformation of human lymphocytes by Epstein-Barr virus is inhibited by phosphonoacetic acid. Nature **263,** 332–334 (1976)

Thorley-Lawson, D. A., Chess, L., Strominger, J. L.: Suppression of *in vitro* Epstein-Barr virus infection, a new role for adult human T lymphocytes. J. Exp. Med. **146,** 495–508 (1977)

Werner, J., Henle, G., Pinto, C. A., Haff, R. F., Henle, W.: Establishment of continuous lymphoblast cultures from leukocytes of gibbons *(Hylobates lar).* Int. J. Cancer **10,** 557–567 (1972)

Whang-Peng, J., Gerber, P., Knutsen, T.: So-called C marker chromosome and Epstein-Barr virus. J. Natl. Cancer Inst. **45,** 831–839 (1970)

Yajima, Y., Nonoyama, M.: Mechanisms of infection with Epstein-Barr virus. I. Viral DNA replication and formation of noninfectious wirus particles in superinfected Raji cells. J. Virol. **19,** 187–194 (1976)

Yamamoto, N., Hinuma, Y.: Clonal transformation of human leukocytes by Epstein-Barr virus in soft agar. Int. J. Cancer **17,** 191–196 (1976)

Yamamoto, N., Katsuki, T., Hinuma, Y.: Transformation of tonsil lymphocytes by Epstein-Barr virus. J. Natl. Cancer Inst. **56,** 1105–1107 (1976)

Yata, J., Desgranges, C., Nakagawa, T., Favre, M. C., de-Thé, G.: Lymphoblastoid transformation and kinetics of appearance of viral nuclear antigen (EBNA) in cordblood lymphocytes infected by Epstein-Barr virus (EBV). Int. J. Cancer **15,** 377–384 (1975)

Yefenof, E., Klein, G.: Membrane receptor stripping confirms the association between EBV receptors and complement receptors on the surface of human B lymphoma lines. Int. J. Cancer **20,** 347–352 (1977)

Yefenof, E., Klein, G., Jondal, M., Oldstone, M. B. A.: Surface markers on human B-and T-lymphocytes. IX. Two-color immunofluorescence studies on the association between EBV receptors and complement receptors on the surface of lymphoid cell lines. Int. J. Cancer **17,** 693–700 (1976)

Yefenof, E., Klein, G., Kvarnung, K.: Relationship between complement activation, complement binding, and EBV absorption by human hematopoietic cell lines. Cell. Immunol. **31,** 225–233 (1977)

Zech, L., Haglund, U., Nilsson, K., Klein, G.: Characteristic chromosomal abnormalities in biopsies and lymphoid cell lines from patients with Burkitt and non-Burkitt lymphomas. Int. J. Cancer **17,** 47–56 (1976)

11 The Nature of Lymphoid Cell Lines and Their Relationship to the Virus

K. Nilsson[1]

Department of Tumor Biology, The Wallenberg Laboratory, University of Uppsala, P. O. Box 562, S-751 22 Uppsala (Sweden)

---

[1] The author is indebted to Ms. Kerstin Lindberg, Ms. Anna-Greta Lundquist, Ms. Gunilla Aberg, and Ms. Ingalill Sjö for excellent help with the preparation of the manuscript.

A. INTRODUCTION

Lymphoid cell lines have been invaluable tools not only in studies of the biologic properties of Epstein-Barr virus (EBV), but also in the fields of oncology, hematology, immunology, genetics, and cell biology. In 1964, Pulvertaft (1964a) and Epstein and Barr (1964) independently described the first cell lines from tumor biopsies of patients with Burkitt's lymphoma (BL). Before this, attempts to cultivate normal and malignant hematopoietic tissue in vitro had usually led to a gradual deterioration and subsequent death of the various cell types within weeks or months (Osgood, 1958; Reisner, 1959). Only rarely had permanent cell lines been established from leukemic blood (Osgood and Broke, 1955) and bone marrow (Benyesh-Melnick et al., 1963). In the latter report, the sudden outgrowth of permanent cell lines with a lymphoblastoid morphology was described at a low frequency in fibroblastoid monolayers several weeks after initiation of bone-marrow cultures derived from children with leukemia, infectious mononucleosis (IM) and hemolytic anemia. This remarkable event was termed "lymphoblastoid transformation of fibroblastic bone-marrow cultures." The meaning of the term "lymphoblastoid transformation" here was thus different from the "lymphoblastoid transformation" used to describe the morphologic changes of normal lymphocytes after exposure to phytohemagglutinin (PHA) (Nowell, 1960).

These early papers were soon followed by numerous reports on successful establishment of "leukemia" and "lymphoma" cell lines (Iwakata and Grace, 1964; Epstein et al., 1965a; Epstein et al., 1965b; Foley et al., 1965; O'Conor and Rabson, 1965; Pulvertaft, 1965; Armstrong, 1966; Epstein et al., 1966a; Moore et al., 1966a; Trujillo et al., 1966; Clarkson et al., 1967; Minowada et al., 1967; Osunkoya, 1967; Sinkovics et al., 1967; Belpomme et al., 1969).

Attempts to develop permanent lymphoid cell lines from normal donors were, however, unsuccessful (Bichel, 1952; Trowell, 1965; Moore et al., 1966a; Clarkson et al., 1967; Pope, 1967) and cells of normal lymphoid tissue were generally considered to have a very short life span in vitro (for a review see Trowell, 1965). Therefore, until 1967 when Moore et al. reported continuous lymphoid cell lines from healthy individuals it was a widely held view that all lines derived from malignant hematopoietic tissue were progeny of the neoplastic cell population in vivo. The results of Moore et al. (1967) were soon confirmed by other laboratories (Clarkson, 1967; Gerber and Monroe, 1968; Nilsson et al., 1968) and with the reports of Pope (1967), Glade et al. (1968a), Diehl et al. (1968), it became apparent that lymphoid lines could be established with particular ease from peripheral blood of patients with acute IM. It was now clear that blood and hematopoietic tissue of donors without neoplastic disease contained cells – normal or preneoplastic – with the capacity for infinite proliferation in vitro and that the morphology and growth properties of lymphoid lines were essentially similar regardless of normal or malignant derivation. Consequently, the neoplastic nature of the "leukemia" and "lymphoma" lines came to be questioned (Clarkson, 1967; Nilsson et al., 1968).

The assumption that the biologic nature of most lymphoid lines was identical was further strengthened by the studies on the relationship of EBV to the establishment of such lines in vitro. Work with the first BL lines led to the discovery of virus particles (Epstein et al., 1964a, 1965c). The virus was subsequently characterized as a new herpesvirus and became known as Epstein-Barr virus. Some of the earlier established lymphoid lines were examined by the time-consuming electron microscopy (EM) technique and most, but not all, lines were found to contain EBV particles in a small fraction of the cells. However, with the development of an immunofluorescence test for detection of EB viral capsid antigen (VCA) (Henle and Henle, 1966) hematopoietic cell lines could be screened for the presence of EBV more easily than by EM. With some exceptions cell lines of both normal and malignant derivation were found to contain a low fraction of VCA-positive cells (Diehl et al., 1968; Moses et al., 1968; Moore and Minowada, 1969; Nilsson et al., 1971; Paltrowitz et al., 1971; Steel and Edmond, 1971). Further experiments with EBV clarified the lymphoproliferative role of the virus. In cocultivation experiments, Henle et al. (1967), Diehl et al. (1969), and Miller et al. (1969) demonstrated that X-irradiated EBV-producing lymphoid cells induced the capacity for infinite growth in vitro in leukocytes from adults and newborns. Addition of EBV-containing cell lysate to fetal blood lymphocytes and lymphoid tissue resulted in the development of permanent lymphoid lines (Pope et al., 1968; Chang et al., 1971 a; Nilsson et al., 1971); uninfected control cells always failed to grow.

Cell lines could be established spontaneously from peripheral blood and lymphoid tissue only from EBV-seropositive donors (Diehl et al., 1968; Gerber et al., 1969; Chang et al., 1971; Nilsson et al., 1971). The observation that lymphoid cell lines were easily established from blood of patients with acute IM also became an argument for the immortalizing role of EBV when Henle et al. (1968) and Niederman et al. (1968) demonstrated that heterophil antibody-positive IM was caused by EBV infection. With the development of more sensitive techniques, particularly nucleic acid hybridization (zur Hausen et al., 1970; Nonoyama and Pagano, 1971; zur Hausen et al., 1972) and immunofluorescence staining for EBV nuclear antigen (EBNA) (Reedman and Klein, 1973), it was found that even the seemingly EBV-negative lines in fact carried EBV genomes.

This, together with the cytologic similarity between the many lymphoid cell lines suggested that all lines, regardless of origin, might represent the same type of EBV-immortalized lymphoid cell that for proliferation in vitro was strictly dependent on the presence of the EBV genome. In recent years, however, comparative phenotypic and chromosome studies have provided evidence for a heterogeneity in the large group of EBV-carrying cell lines. Two biologically distinct types of such lines can be distinguished, BL lines of true malignant derivation and lymphoblastoid lines of presumed non-neoplastic derivation (Nilsson and Pontén, 1975). In addition to the BL and lymphoblastoid lines a few EBV genome-negative, neoplastic lymphoma, leukemia, and myeloma lines have recently been reported with phenotypic properties different from those of the EBV-carrying lines (Sect. H).

Several reviews, concentrating on different aspects of human lymphoid cell lines have been published previously (Moore and Minowada, 1969; Miller, 1971; Nilsson, 1971 a; Moore, 1972; Papageorgiou and Glade, 1972; Nilsson and Pontén, 1975; Glade and Beratis, 1976; Nilsson, 1977). The purpose of this review is to summarize the phenotypic and chromosomal characteristics of human lymphoid cell lines with particular emphasis on the differences between the two types of EBV-carrying lines.

The methods for transforming B lymphocytes (bone marrow-derived lymphocytes) in vitro by EBV and the expression of EBV-related antigens in established lines, which are important aspects of human lymphoid cell lines, are described elsewhere (Chaps. 10 and 3 respectively).

B. PROVISIONAL CLASSIFICATIONS OF HEMATOPOIETIC CELL LINES

During the last decade the possibilities of making a meaningful and discriminative characterization of various types of lymphoid, myeloid and histiocytic cells have increased considerably by use of the following techniques: (a) detection of surface markers on lymphoid cells to complement conventional cytology (for a review see Möller, 1973); (b) cytochemical methods (for a review see Stuart et al., 1975); (c) use of heteroantisera against various surface antigens (Greaves et al., 1977); (d) surface glycoprotein labeling methods (Trowbridge et al., 1975; Andersson et al., 1976; Trowbridge et al., 1976; Andersson et al., 1977; Nilsson et al., 1977 a); (e) reliable tests for the presence of EBV genomes (zur Hausen et al., 1970; Reedman and Klein, 1973); (f) discriminative chromosome analysis using banding techniques (Caspersson et al., 1970; Dutrillaux and Lejeune, 1971; Sumner et al., 1971; Seabright, 1972); (g) testing for the malignancy of human cells in vivo by heterotransplantation to athymic nude mice, a comparatively reliable test compared to heterotransplantation to strongly immunosuppressed or newborn animals (Pantelouris, 1968; Rygaard, 1969; Rygaard and Povlsen, 1969; Povlsen and Rygaard, 1971; Giovanella et al., 1972; Giovanella and Stehlin, 1973); and (h) use of the enzymatic marker glucose-6-phosphate dehydrogenase (G-6-PD) to determine the clonality of cell lines (Fialkow, 1976, 1977).

The above techniques have confirmed that there are two main types of EBV-carrying cell lines – BL and lymphoblastoid lines (Table 1). The BL lines are derived from the malignant cells in BL-tumor biopsies, have a monoclonal origin (Sect. D), are aneuploid with a chromosome 14 marker in the vast majority of the cases (Sect. F), are tumorigenic when injected subcutaneously into nude mice with few exceptions (Sect. E.VII) and have a characteristic surface glycoprotein profile (Sect. E.III.4). The lymphoblastoid lines, which may be derived both from normal and neoplastic hematopoietic tissue, are polyclonal, normal diploid and nontumorigenic shortly after establishment (Sect. D, F, and E.VII), and have a surface glycoprotein pattern similar to mitogen-stimulated B blasts and clearly distinct from that of BL and other hematopoietic cell lines (Sect. E.III.4).

Table 1. Defining features of the two types of EBV-carrying cell lines – Burkitt's lymphoma (BL) and lymphoblastoid (BED) lines[a]

Characteristic	BL lines	BED lines	References
Clonality	Monoclonal	Polyclonal	Fialkow et al., 1970; van Furth et al., 1972; Fialkow et al., 1973; Béchet et al., 1974
Karyotype	Aneuploid, 14 marker	Normal diploid	Manolov and Manolova, 1972; Jarvis et al., 1974; Zech et al., 1976; Hellriegel et al., 1977
Tumorigenicity[b]	Pos., rarely neg.	Neg.	Nilsson et al., 1977b
Surface glycoprotein pattern	GP 210, GP87/85, GP 71/69	GP 160, GP 115	Nilsson et al., 1977a; Gahmberg et al., 1978

[a] Examination should be done shortly (< 6 months) after establishment (also Sect. G).
[b] Tested subcutaneously in nude mice.

The relatively rare EBV genome-negative B cell lines have always been derived from malignant hematopoietic tissue and never from normal donors. They are always monoclonal, aneuploid, and mostly tumorigenic. Just as in the case of the BL lines described above, these EBV genome-negative lines usually keep the characteristic features of the corresponding in vivo tumor as has been shown by comparative marker studies on the tumor cell population and the derived cell line (Sect. H).

Unfortunately, no accepted classification of hematopoietic cell lines exists. This has led to a very confusing terminology involving many vague terms such as lymphoblastoid-, lymphoblast-, lymphocytoid, lymphocyte-, lymphocytic, lymphoid-, leukocyte-, leukocytic cell lines. With the discovery of lymphocyte surface markers, lines were designated B lines, B lymphoid, B lymphoblastoid, T (thymus-dependent lymphocyte) lines, etc. By use of newer techniques for characterizing the phenotype and chromosomes it is now possible to make some provisional classifications of hematopoietic cell lines. A definitive classification, based on the origin of the proliferating cells, is not at present possible since the different cells within the lymphoid, myeloid, and monocytic series from which cell lines may be derived are to a great extent undefined.

A provisional classification scheme for all types of hematopoietic cell lines useful for researchers in oncology, hematology, and viral oncogenesis is presented in Table 2. This classification is based on the most widely used morphologic definitions of lymphoma and leukemia and on the presence of EBV. The lines have been categorized in two main groups – EBV-carrying and EBV-negative lines. Examples of the numerous EBV-carrying lines have been selected from those that have been examined for the most important defining features i. e., clonality, karyotype, tumorigenicity, and morphology (Table 1). It should be stressed that the many lines established "spontaneously" (without the experimental addition of EBV) by Moore and co-workers (Moore and Minowada, 1969; Moore, 1972) and in many other laboratories (Benyesh-Melnick et al., 1963; Rabson et al., 1966; Clarkson et al., 1967; Osunkoya and Mottram, 1967; Pope et al., 1967; Sinkovics et al., 1967; Belpomme et al., 1969; Nadkarni et al., 1969; Rosenfeld and Macieira-Coelho, 1969; Stevens et al., 1969; de-Thé et al., 1970; Chang et al., 1971 a, 1971 b; Steel and Edmund, 1971; Gerber, 1974; v. Heyden and v. Heyden, 1974; Glade and Beratis, 1976; Diehl and Johansson, 1977; Karpas et al., 1977) are probably lymphoblastoid lines and as representative as the lines listed but data on all the "defining features" are not available. Cell lines established by the experimental addition of exogenous EBV in vitro (Chap. 10) seem to be of the same type as lymphoblastoid lines established "spontaneously", at least when EBV from the B95-8 line (Miller and Lipman, 1973) is used.

In the context of classification, EBV genome-negative lines are still so few that all that have been published are included in Table 2, which thus serves as a catalogue for the malignant, EBV-negative lymphoma, leukemia, and myeloma lines. It is notable that among common hematopoietic tumors, only chronic lymphocytic leukemia, acute myeloid leukemia, and perhaps chronic myeloid leukemia are unrepresented.

For studies of lymphocyte differentiation and function, a classification based on the expression of lymphocyte surface markers may be useful. Such a classification, restricted only to lines of lymphoid origin is presented in Table 3. Four main groups can be distinguished: B lines, T lines, non-B, non-T lines (null lines), and plasma cell lines (myeloma lines).

Table 2. Classification and catalogue of human hematopoietic cell lines according to presence of EBV and histologic diagnosis (Rappaport, 1966 and others)

Type of cell line	Cell type	Representative cell lines
1. EBV genome-carrying lines [a]		
Burkitt's lymphoma (BL) lines	B cell	Raji (Pulvertaft, 1964a), EB3 (Epstein et al., 1966), Daudi (Klein et al., 1968), P_3HR-I (Hinuma and Grace, 1967)
Lymphoblastoid lines	B cell (B blast?)	833L (Miller et al., 1971), U-303 (Nilsson, 1971c), IM lines (Jarvis et al., 1974), 2c (Hellriegel et al., 1977), CCRF-SB (Royston et al., 1974)
Not yet classifiable		S 95 (zur Hausen et al., 1972; Nilsson et al., 1975), Balm-2 (Minowada et al., 1977a)
2. EBV genome-negative lines [b]		
Lymphoma lines		
Lymphocytic lymphoma	B cell	U-698, U-715 (Nilsson and Sundström, 1974)
Exceptional BL	B cell	BJAB (Klein et al., 1974), Ramos (Klein et al., 1975), SU-AmB-1 (Epstein et al., 1976), JBL (Miyoshi et al., 1977b) DG-75 (Ben-Bassat et al., 1977)
Histiocytic lymphoma		
Lymphoid type	B cell	SU-DHL-3-7, SU-DHL-10 (Epstein et al., 1978)
Histiocytic type	Histiocyte	SU-DHL-1-2 (Epstein and Kaplan, 1974), U-937 (Sundström and Nilsson, 1976)
Null cell type	Non-T, non-B cell	SU-DHL-8-9 (Epstein et al., 1978)
Hodgkin's disease	Histiocyte?	Fq and RY (Long et al., 1977)
Leukemia lines		
Acute lymphocytic leukemia	T cell	CCRF-CEM (Foley et al., 1965), CCRF-H-SB2 (Adams et al., 1968), MOLT-4 (Minowada et al., 1972), RPMI 8402 (Minowada and Moore, 1975), JM (Schwenk and Schneider, 1975), HPB-ALL, HPB-MLT (Minowada et al., 1977b), 45 (Karpas et al., 1977)
Acute lymphocytic leukemia	B cell	Balm-1 (Minowada et al., 1977a), BALL-1 (Hiraki et al., 1977)
Acute lymphocytic leukemia	Non-T, non-B cell	Nalm 6, Nalm 13 (Minowada, pers. com.), NALL-1 (Miyoshi et al., 1977a), Reh (Rosenfeld et al., 1977), KM3, SH-2 (Schneider et al., 1977)
Chronic myeloid leukemia, blast crisis		
Lymphoid type	Non-T, non-B cell	NALM-1 (Minowada et al., 1977c)
Not yet fully defined type	Myeloid (?) cell	K562 (Lozzio and Lozzio 1975; Klein et al., 1976; Minowada et al., 1977)
Myeloma lines	Plasma cell	RPMI 8226 (Matsouka et al., 1967), U-266 (Nilsson et al., 1970a)

[a] Burkitt's lymphoma lines are of malignant origin; lymphoblastoid lines of presumed non-neoplastic derivation. [b] All lines are progeny of the malignant cell population of the donor.

Table 3. Classification of lymphoid lines according to lymphocyte surface marker expression

Designation	Short designation	Representative lines (References to surface marker studies)
1. B lines		
EBV-carrying		
Burkitt's lymphoma	B lymphoma (BL^{EBV+})	Daudi (Jondal and Klein, 1973; Huber et al., 1976)
		Raji (Jondal and Klein, 1973; Huber et al., 1976)
Lymphoblastoid	*B*-lymphoblastoid, *E*BV carrying, *D*iploid (BED)	CCRF-SB (Royston et al., 1974), U-303L (Huber et al., 1976), SU-LB-2 (Epstein et al., 1976)
Not yet classifiable		S 95 Nilsson et al., 1975) Balm-2 (Minowada et al., 1977)
EBV genome-negative		
Lymphocytic lymphoma	B lymphoma (BLL)	U-698, U-715 (Huber et al., 1976)
Exceptional Burkitt's lymphoma	B lymphoma (BL^{EBV-})	BJAB (Menezes et al., 1975), Ramos (Klein et al., 1975), SU-AmB-1 (Epstein et al., 1976), JBL (Miyoshi et al., 1977b), DG75 (Ben-Bassat et al., 1977),
Histiocytic lymphoma, B cell type	B lymphoma (BHL)	SU-DHL-3-7 (Epstein et al., 1978)
Acute lymphocytic leukemia	B leukemia (BALL)	Balm-1 (Minowada et al., 1977b), BALL-1 (Hiraki et al., 1977)
2. T lines		
Acute lymphocytic leukemia	T leukemia (TALL)	MOLT-3 (Huber et al., 1976), JM (Schwenk and Schneider, 1975), TALL-1 (Miyoshi et al., 1977a), HPB-ALL, HPB-MLT, RPMI 8402 (Minowada et al., 1977b)
3. Non-B, non-T ("null") lines		
Histiocytic lymphoma, null cell type	0 lymphoma (NHL)	SU-DHL-8-9 (Epstein et al., 1977)
Acute lymphocytic leukemia	0 leukemia (NALL)	NALL-1 (Miyoshi et al., 1977), KM3, SH-2 (Schneider et al., 1977), Reh (Rosenfeld et al., 1977), Nalm-6, Nalm-13 (Minowada, pers. com.)
Chronic myeloid leukemia, blast crisis, lymphoid type	0 leukemia (NCML)	Nalm-1 (Minowada et al., 1977c)
4. Plasma cell lines	Myeloma	RPMI 8226 (Matsouka et al., 1967), U-266 (Nilsson et al., 1970a)

In this review, since so many different types of cell lines will be described, the abbreviation BL will be used to indicate a line originating from the BL-tumor cell population, and the purely descriptive abbreviation BED (*B*-lymphoblastoid, *E*BV-carrying, diploid line), to designate the other common polyclonal, B-lymphoblastoid, normal diploid, nontumorigenic type of EBV-carrying line. These BED lines share many features such as morphology, type of immunoglobulin (Ig) production (surface expression and secretion), lymphokine secretion, surface glycoprotein pattern, and expression of β_2-microglobulin and HL-A, with mitogen stimulated B lymphocytes (B blasts), but their normalcy, although they are nontumorigenic subcutaneously in nude mice, can still be questioned since heterologous transplantation is not an "absolute" test for malignancy. It should also be remembered that the BED lines have an infinite life span in vitro, a feature assumed to be typical for malignantly transformed cells (see Pontén, 1971).

It should be noted that two as yet unclassified EBV-carrying cell lines, the S 95 (zur Hausen et al., 1972; Nilsson et al., 1975) and Balm-2 (Minowada et al., 1977 b), have been included in Tables 2 and 3. It should also be noted in Table 3 that among the EBV genome-negative B lines some lines derived from lymphomas, which are classified as histiocytic according to Rappaport (1966) express B cell markers or features indicating an origin from a B or null lymphoid cell and not a histiocytic cell (Epstein et al., 1977). No T cell lines have as yet been reported from lymphocytic lymphomas, while from lymphocytic leukemia many B, T, and null lines have been documented.

C. "SPONTANEOUS" ESTABLISHMENT OF PERMANENT EBV-CARRYING LYMPHOID CELL LINES

It is well established that EBV when added experimentelly in vitro to lymphocytes from humans and some nonhuman primates can convert such cells to lymphoblastoid lines with an unlimited life span (Gerber, 1974; Klein, 1974; Miller, 1974; Epstein, 1975; zur Hausen, 1975; Pope, 1975). The principal target cell for EBV seems to be a complement and EBV receptor-bearing B lymphocyte (Pattengale et al. 1973; Jondal and Klein, 1973; Greaves et al., 1975), but the molecular mechanism(s) by which the B lymphocytes acquire the capacity for infinite growth in vitro after exposure to EBV is still to a large extent unknown (Chaps. 9 and 10). The contrasting "spontaneous" establishment of lines is discussed below.

I. ESTABLISHMENT OF B LYMPHOBLASTOID, EBV-CARRYING, DIPLOID (BED) CELL LINES

This type of line can be established "spontaneously" from blood and hematopoietic tissue provided that the donor has previously been infected by EBV (Gerber et al., 1969; Chang et al., 1971 b; Nilsson et al., 1971). Once it had been clarified that establishment in vitro of BED lines was dependent on the presence of EBV it was assumed that "spontaneously" established lines were derived from EBV-carrying precursor cells present in small numbers mainly in normal and malignant blood and hematopoietic tissue but also among lymphocytes infiltrating nonlymphoid tumors such as nasopharyngeal carcinoma (NPC) (de-Thé et al., 1970) and glioma (Nilsson and Pontén, 1975). BED precursor cells, although thought to be immortalized by EBV, were assumed to be under physiologic growth-control mechanisms in vivo (Nilsson et al., 1971) and only after explantation in vitro to be able to display their potential for unlimited growth. The BED lines would, if this reasoning were correct, become established by a process of selection and/or adaptation in vitro of cells already immortalized in vivo (Sinkovics et al., 1967; Nilsson, 1971 b; Klein, 1973). A dissenting view has recently been presented by Epstein and co-workers (Epstein, 1975; Rickinson et al., 1974, 1975, 1977), who have shown that the process of "spontaneous" establishment may always be a two-step in vitro event rather than a direct outgrowth of in vivo immortalized lymphoblastoid cells. Their experiments suggest that lymphocytes, latently infected by EBV in vivo, will liberate EBV during a lytic cycle when explanted in vitro and that the establishment of a BED line is the result of a polyclonal outgrowth of B lymphocytes, immortalized in vitro by the released EBV. The rate of success in attempts to establish BED lines from seropositive donors would thus be dependent on the number of in vivo EBV-latently infected lymphoid cells, and also on the number of normal B lymphocytes in the explant.

Depending on the type of biopsy material, different methods have been used to initiate BED lines without addition of exogenous EBV in vitro. They have all provided a high cell density with opportunity for intimate cell contacts, which seem necessary for successful establishment. From peripheral blood, BED lines were originally established by a technique, developed by Iwakata and Grace (1964) and Moore et al. (1966 a). This technique involves the initiation, from each donor, of multiple nonstirred suspension cultures from a large volume (500–1000 ml) of blood. Successful establishment of BED lines requires a high initial cell density ($5–15 \times 10^6$ cells/ml) and maintenance of a minimal concentration of viable cells ($> 5 \times 10^5$ cells/ml) during a typical lag period of 30–100 days. In this type of suspension culture permanent growth is heralded by a fall in pH and the occurrence of rapidly proliferating cells growing mainly in dense clumps. The success rate with this technique is 30%–50% from normal individuals (Gerber and Monroe, 1968) and 40%–75% from patients with myelogenous leukemia, "leukemoid reactions," or lymphomas (Moore and Minowada, 1969). With smaller volumes of blood (10–50 ml), the frequency of spontaneous establishment has been high only when donors had acute IM or recent histories of it (Pope, 1967; Glade et al., 1968 a; Diehl et al., 1968, 1969; Steel and Edmond, 1971) or infectious hepatitis (Glade et al., 1968 b; Stevens et al., 1969), while from healthy donors no lines were derived except after the addition of small doses of PHA (Broder et al., 1970; Brodsky and Hurd, 1974) or by use of a grid organ culture and presence of allogeneic feeder fibrolasts (Nilsson, 1971 b).

From hematopoietic tissue most lines have been derived from biopsies which were dispersed and cultivated in suspension culture (Benyesh-Melnick et al., 1963; Trujillo et al., 1966; Sinkovics et al., 1967; Jensen et al., 1967; Ito et al., 1968; Benyesh-Melnick et al., 1968 a, b; Oboshi, 1969; Moore and Minowada, 1969). The success rate has been high ($\sim 50\%$) in these mixed fibroblast-lymphoid cell cultures when they were derived from patients with acute IM, low, ($\sim 10\%$) from leukemia and lymphoma patients, and zero when obtained from normal individuals (Benyesh-Melnick et al., 1968 a). For lymph nodes from cancer patients the corresponding figure was 15% according to Jensen et al. (1967). Pontén (1967), Levy et al. (1968), and Nilsson et al. (1968) introduced the use of modified Trowell-type organ cultures (Jensen et al., 1964) to cultivate fragmented lymph node and spleen biopsies. This technique gave even better results from non-IM patients than the method described above. Hence Pontén (1967) and Nilsson et al. (1968) reported establishment of BED lines in 50% of 21 explanted normal and malignant lymph-node biopsies.

The most efficient method of establishing BED lines from normal and malignant hematopoietic tissue seems to be the Spongostan grid culture (Nilsson, 1971 c), which is a further improvement of the grid culture originally used by Jensen et al. (1964) (Fig. 1). With this type of grid culture, BED lines were established from lymph nodes of 21 out of 22 consecutive, unselected individuals without manifest malignancy or IM (Nilsson, 1971 c). The technique has also been found useful for establishing BL and

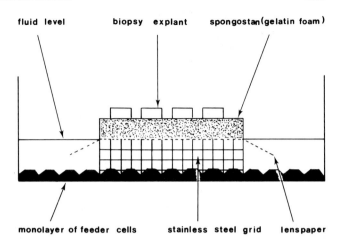

Fig. 1. The Spongostan grid assembly. (Nilsson, 1977a)

other types of malignant hematopoietic cell lines (Nilsson et al., 1970a; Nilsson and Sundström, 1974; Sundström and Nilsson, 1976; Nilsson, 1977; Schneider et al., 1977). The rate of successful spontaneous establishment of BED and tumor lines with the Spongostan grid culture over the past years in our laboratory is found in Table 4.

Table 4. Establishment of permanent cell lines with the Spongostan grid technique[a]

Type of biopsy	No. of biopsies	No. of established cell lines: –			
		Lymphoblastoid (BED) lines	(%)	Tumor cell line	(%)
Myeloma	53	19	36	1	2
Lymphocytic lymphoma	26	9	35	2	8
Burkitt's lymphoma	46	2	4	24	52
Histiocytic lymphoma	19	1	5	1	5
Hodgkin's disease	41	35	85	0	
Normal lymph node	34	30	88	0	
Ca-draining lymph node	14	11	78	0	
Tonsillitis	51	45	88	0	
Spleen, hemolytic anemia	6	4	66	0	
Blood, healthy donor	10	4	40	0	
Blood, patient with malignancy	12	6	50	0	
Total	312	166	53	28	9

[a] Data from Nilsson and Pontén (1975); Nilsson and Sundström (1974); Sundström and Nilsson (1976); (Nilsson, 1977) and unpublished.

II. ESTABLISHMENT OF BURKITT'S LYMPHOMA CELL LINES

BL lines are relatively easy to establish in suspension cultures from dispersed BL-tumor tissue (Epstein and Barr, 1964; Pulvertaft, 1964a, b; Epstein et al., 1965a, b; O' Conor and Rabson, 1965; Stewart et al., 1965; Epstein et al., 1966a; Rabson et al., 1966; Minowada et al., 1967; Osunkoya, 1967; Pope et al., 1967; Nadkarni et al.,

1969; van Furth et al., 1972; Béchet et al., 1974; Klein et al., 1975; Menezes et al., 1975; Ben-Bassat et al., 1976; Epstein et al., 1976; Goldblum et al., 1977) or from fragmented tumor tissue cultivated in grid cultures (Nilsson and Pontén, 1975). The frequency of establishment is similar to that of BED lines by the Spongostan grid culture (Table 4) and is higher than for BED lines when suspension cultures are employed. In rare cases, the BED type of line may become established also from BL-tumor tissue (Nilsson and Pontén, 1975; Nilsson, unpublished observations), but then only after the lag phase of 30–100 days, which is always so characteristic for the spontaneous initiation of BED lines. The lag phase for BL lines is shorter than for the establishment of BED lines, usually 2–4 weeks (Nadkarni et al., 1969). BL lines sometimes become established without this short lag phase, but when this occurs pronounced cell death is observed during the first few weeks of culture in parallel with survival and active proliferation of a fraction of the biopsy cells (Klein et al., 1975; Nilsson and Pontén, 1975). The presence of feeder cells has sometimes been a prerequisite for establishment, but usually BL cells are less exacting than BED cells in their nutritional requirements (Nilsson, unpublished observations). The culture events during establishment seem to be more variable for BL than for BED lines, which accords with the commonly observed individuality of human tumors (Sect. E).

D. MARKERS FOR CLONALITY

Several genetic markers have been used to trace the cellular origin of human tumors (Fialkow, 1976). The most extensively employed marker on cellular mosaicism is the X-linked G-6-PD locus. Females who are heterozygous at this locus and carry one gene for the usual B phenotype of G-6-PD on one X-chromosome and one variant gene (for the A phenotype) on the other, have two distinct cell populations, one producing G-6-PD B and one, G-6-PD A. Thus, monoclonal tumors or cell lines from G-6-PD heterozygotes should contain cells producing only one of the two G-6-PD phenotypes. The presence of both G-6-PD A and G-6-PD B variants, on the other hand, would be suggestive of a multicellular origin. Analyses of the G-6-PD in BL-tumor biopsy cells from G-6-PD heterozygotes have strongly indicated that BL has a monoclonal origin (Fialkow et al., 1970, 1971, 1973; Béchet et al., 1974; Fialkow, 1977).

A second marker is Ig synthesis. The basis for the use of this marker is that the production of Ig is stable and restricted to one, or at most two, heavy chains and one light chain in normal and neoplastic B lymphoid cells both in vivo and in derived cell lines in vitro (Sect. E.V.1). Results from several studies with the Ig-synthesis marker on BL-tumor biopsy cells are in accordance with those obtained with G-6-PD marker studies (van Furth et al., 1972; Fialkow et al., 1973; Béchet et al., 1974).

Finally, chromosome analyses have provided additional evidence that BL is monoclonal (Gripenberg et al., 1969; Manolov and Manolova, 1972; Zech et al., 1976).

The above cell markers have also been used (a) to examine whether EBV-carrying, BL cell lines have originated from the tumor cell population or from non-neoplastic cells in the biopsy, and (b) in attempts to understand the nature of the BED lines.

Van Furth et al. (1972) demonstrated that the pattern of Ig synthesis was essentially identical in BL-tumor biopsy cells and the derived cell lines. The small differences noted in a few cases can most likely be ascribed to methodologic imperfections. Similar results have been reported by Béchet et al. (1972), who found an identical and

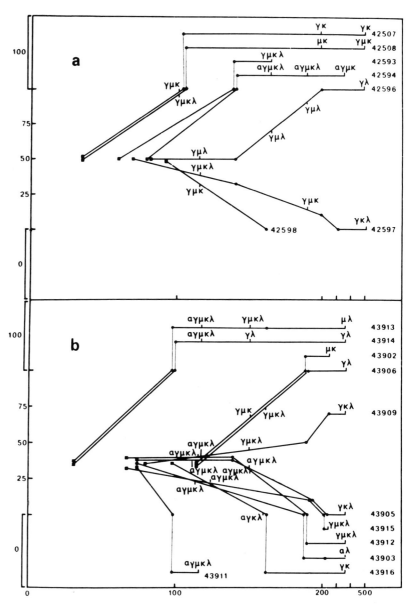

Fig. 2 a and b. G-6-PD phenotypes and Ig synthesis in BED lines from tonsils of G-6-PD heterozygotes: evolution in long-term cultures. *Abscissa:* time after biopsy (days); *ordinate:* % type A-G-6-PD. *a* Biopsy no. 425; **b** Biopsy no. 439. ■ establishment of culture as continuously growing BED; ●——●, G-6-PD assays; ⌐⌐, Ig assays. (Béchet et al., 1974)

monoclonal Ig synthesis in all of the multiple lymphoid lines that were established from each BL biopsy. Béchet et al. (1974) employed both the Ig synthesis and G-6-PD marker on the same panel of newly established BL lines and found agreement between the results with the two markers. It can therefore be concluded that BL lines almost without exception are representative of the tumor cell population in vivo which agrees with results of chromosome studies (Sect. F).

Several early studies on the pattern of Ig synthesis indicated that some BED lines, derived from patients with IM (Glade and Chessin, 1968 a), leukemia (Tanigaki et al., 1966; Wakefield et al., 1967; Finegold et al., 1967), and lymph nodes from patients with and without malignancy (Nilsson, 1971 c), might be of multicellular derivation. Béchet et al. (1973) established multiple BED lines from different parts of normal and two non-BL lymphoma lymph nodes and found a polyclonal Ig-synthesis pattern shortly after establishment in *all* the 23 lines. The most conclusive study concerning the cellular origin of BED lines, however, was performed by Béchet et al. (1974) using Ig synthesis and G-6-PD variants as cell markers. They demonstrated not only a multicellular origin of tonsil-derived BED lines but also a gradual evolution towards uniclonality in all the multiple BED lines that had been established in parallel from each of the two tonsils. Figure 2 illustrates the progressive selection of single-cell clones in the different lines. It should be noted that this selection seems to occur at random since no apparent preference for any of the two G-6-PD phenotypes is noted. The rate of clonal evolution differs. Most lines become homogeneous with respect to G-6-PD production within 12–18 months. This rate agrees with earlier findings on the gradual alteration of the Ig-secretion pattern in lymph node-derived BED lines (Nilsson, 1971 c; Béchet et al., 1973).

The difference in clonality between the BED and BL type of lymphoid cell line is an important distinguishing feature provided that the line is examined shortly after establishment (Table 1). Furthermore, the polyclonal origin of BED lines favors the view that they are derived from non-neoplastic, EBV "immortalized" B lymphocytes, whether infected by EBV in vivo or in vitro.

E. PHENOTYPIC CHARACTERISTICS OF EBV-CARRYING LYMPHOID CELL LINES

Documented phenotypic differences between the BL and BED type of lymphoid line will be described in this section. Table 5 summarizes the properties of over 200 *newly established* BL and BED lines examined by our group.

I. MORPHOLOGY

The predominant cell type in BED lines has generally been described as lymphoblastoid (Benyesh-Melnick et al., 1963; Sinkovics, 1968; Levy et al., 1968; Moore et al., 1968) with a considerable pleomorphism. Its cytologic appearance is closely similar to PHA-, pokeweed mitogen (PWM)-, or antigen-stimulated peripheral lymphocytes (Douglas et al., 1969). The cell diameter varies considerably (8–22 μ, mean 12–13 μ) (Nilsson, 1971 d). The nucleus is immature and contains 2–5 large nucleoli. The nucleocytopla-

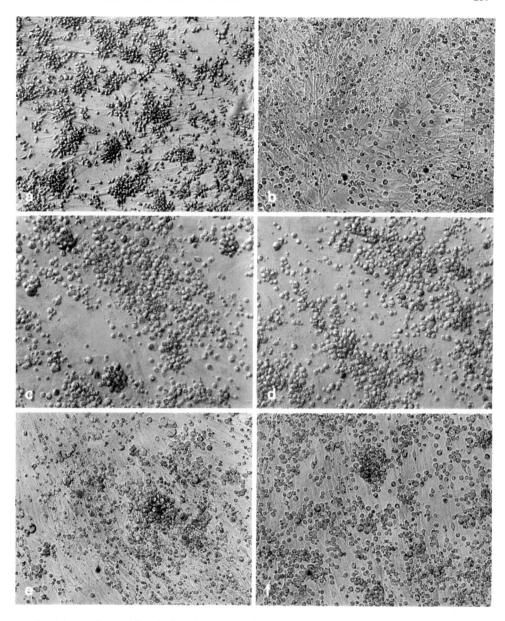

Fig. 3. a A human lymphoblastoid (BED) cell line on feeder cells. Between the BED cells, mainly assembled in dense clumps, isolated cells engaged in peripolesis may be seen. Inverted microscope × 150. **b** Secondarily altered BED line (NC 37) on feeder cells; peripolesis, but no clumps; nonadherent cells are mainly round. Inverted microscope × 200. **c** Burkitt's lymphoma cells (Raji); picture almost identical to the secondarily altered lymphoblasts of Fig. 3 **b**. Inverted microscope × 200. **d.** Burkitt's llymphoma cells (Daudi); monomorphic morphology; no peripolesis; a few loose clumps. Inverted microscope × 100. **e** Burkitt's lymphoma cells (U-47703 BL); picture as 3 **c** and 3 **d** except for a higher rate of cell death and differences in cell size; a few adhering cells but no peripolesis. Inverted microscope × 200. **f** Burkitt's lymphoma line (P3) grows almost without any clumps; a few cells are elongated. (Nilsson and Pontén, 1975). Inverted microscope × 200

Table 5. Properties of newly established human EBV-carrying lymphoid Uppsala (U-) cell lines

Characteristics	BED lines	BL lines	References
Morphology			Nilsson and Pontén, 1975
Cell type (diameter, μ)	Lymphoblastoid (12–13)	Lymphoblastoid (10–11)	
Morphologic diversity			
between lines	None	Present	
within lines	Prominent	Slight	
Ultrastructure (TEM)	Moderate development of endoplasmic reticulum and Golgi apparatus	Sparsely developed Golgi apparatus and endoplasmic reticulum. Fat droplets	
Surface morphology (SEM)	Long villi often with assymmetric (uropod) location	Thin, short villi covering the entire surface	
Motility			
Time lapse cinematography	Highly motile. Translocation.	Low motility. No translocation	Nilsson and Pontén, 1975
Location of actin	Surface villi. Uropod.	Diffuse, submembranous	Fagreus et al., 1975
Growth characteristics			Nilsson and Pontén, 1975
Efficiency of establishment	High	High	
Length of lag phase during establishment (days)[a]	30–100	0–30	
Attachment to feeder cells	Strong and rapid, most cells	Loose and slow, only some cells	
Growth in suspension	Large, dense clumps	Single cells or usually small, loose clumps	
Dependence on rich medium for maintenance in suspension	Yes	Yes or no	
Population doubling time (h)	24–48	18–30	
Maximal cell density (cells/μl)	$1–1.2 \times 10^6$	$1–3 \times 10^6$	
Colony formation in agarose	Yes, low cloning efficiency. Microscopic colonies	Yes or no. Often high cloning efficiency. Sometimes macroscopic colonies	

Table 5 *(continued)*

Characteristics	BED lines	BL lines	References
Surface characteristics			
Lymphocyte markers (% pos. cells)			Huber et al., 1976
SRBC	0	0	
C3	60–95	0–95	
Fc	0–5	0–60	
Fc (Agg. Ig)	2+	2–3+	
Ig	70–100	70–100	
Surface glycoprotein pattern	B blast-like	B cell-like. B lymphoma pattern GP 87/85, GP 71/69	Gahmberg et al., 1978 Nilsson et al., 1977 a
Lectin agglutinability	3+	4+	Glimelius et al., 1975
HLA antigens	Present	Present with one exception	Welsh et al., 1977
B$_2$-microglobulin			Nilsson et al., 1974;
No. molecules/cell	10^6	Variable, 0–10^6	
Secretion (ng/10^6 cells/24 h)	200–250	Variable 0–80	
Human Ia-like antigens	Present	Present	Gahmberg et al., 1978 Mc Conahey et al., 1971
Functional markers			
Ig, surface Molecules/cell	IgG, IgM, IgA, IgD 2 × 10^4	IgM predominantly 8 × 10^4	Ghetie et al., 1974
Ig, secretion (μg/10^6 cells/24 h)	1–3	0 (exceptions)	
Interferon production	Yes	Yes	Zajac et al., 1969 Adams et al., 1975
Phagocytosis			Sundström, 1977
Tumorigenicity (subcutaneously in nude mice)	No	Mostly but not always	Nilsson et al., 1977b
Karyotype	Normal diploid	Aneuploid. 14 marker	Zech et al., 1976

[a] "Spontaneous" establishment with the Spongostan grid culture.

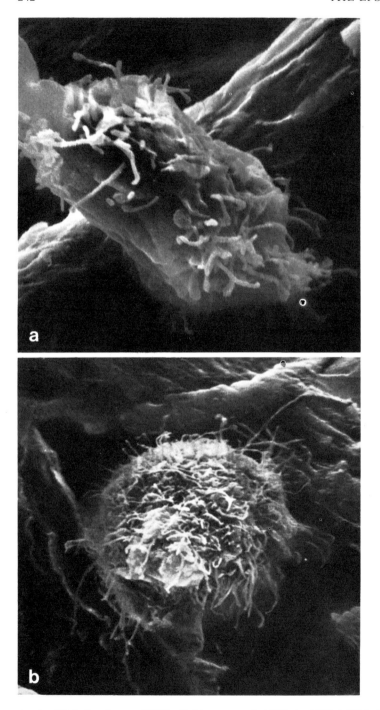

Fig. 4. a SEM of an elongated BED cell. (Fagraeus et al., 1975). (× 5500). **b** SEM of a round villous BED cell.
(Nilsson and Pontén, 1975). (× 5000)

smic ratio is moderately high. The cytoplasm is strongly basophilic, shows a marked pyroninophilia, and stains bright red-orange in acridine orange, indicating a high RNA content (Nilsson, 1971 d). Within each line a spectrum of cell types can be identified. Thus, in addition to the above lymphoblastoid cell type, which constitutes ~ 85% of the cells in suspension cultures, the lines contain medium- and small-sized lymphocytes (10%) and multinucleate cells (5%) (Moore et al., 1968). Examination by inverted microscopy of BED cell cultures containing allogeneic feeder fibroblasts (Nilsson and Pontén, 1975) (Fig. 3 a) and studies with scanning electron microscopy (SEM) (Nilsson and Pontén, 1975; Fagraeus et al., 1975; Ben-Bassat et al., 1977) (Figs. 4 a, 4 b) have confirmed the morphologic heterogeneity. This heterogeneity is due to the wide morphologic flexibility of individual BED cells observed even in longestablished cloned lines by phase-contrast time-lapse cinematography (Fig. 6) (Sect. E.II). The general static and dynamic morphology is similar in all BED lines shortly after establishment, but with prolonged continuous culture changes may occur (Fig. 3 b) (Sect. G).

In transmission electron microscopy (TEM), the BED cells usually contain a round or often irregularly shaped nucleus with finely granular chromatin and one or a few prominent nucleoli. The cytoplasm is moderately extensive and contains a fairly well-developed Golgi apparatus, numerous mitochondria, short cisternae of rough and smooth endoplasmic reticulum, and abundant polyribosomes (Chandra et al., 1968; Moore et al., 1968; Belpomme et al., 1969; Oboshi, 1969; Recher et al., 1969; Levy et al., 1971; Heyden and Heyden, 1974; Nilsson and Pontén, 1975). Fat droplets have been found, but usually only a few. EBV is sometimes found in a small percentage of the cells (Moore et al., 1966 b; Jensen et al., 1967; Moore et al., 1967; Gerber et al., 1968; Moses et al., 1968; Levy et al., 1971; Steel and Edmond, 1971). Some special ultrastructural features have been noted: granules in the nuclei (Gerber et al., 1968); projections or doublings of the nuclear membrane (Recher et al., 1968; Gerber, 1968); cytoplasmic annulate lamellae (Gerber et al., 1968; Recher et al., 1969); aggregates of particles within the rough endoplasmic reticulum (Moses et al., 1968). These features are, however, not unique for BED cells but have been found also in BL and T leukemia lines (Epstein and Achong, 1965; Uzman et al., 1966).

The basic cell type in BL lines, which is similar to that observed in short-term cultured BL biopsy cells (Pulvertaft, 1965; Osunkoya, 1967), was originally described as an immature lymphoid cell with strong resemblance to PHA-stimulated lymphocytes (Pulvertaft, 1964 b). Cytologically the cells thus superficially resemble BED cells, but some fairly consistent differences have been found (Epstein and Barr, 1964; Pulvertaft, 1964 a, b; Epstein and Barr, 1965; Epstein et al., 1965 a; Stewart et al., 1965; O'Conor and Rabson, 1965; Epstein et al., 1966 a, b; Rabson et al., 1966; Pope et al., 1967; Nilsson and Pontén, 1975):

1. BL cells almost without exception contain numerous fat droplets.

2. BL cells are usually somewhat smaller than BED cells and the variability in cell size within each line is less pronounced (range 9–13 µ, mean 10–11 µ). Cells in most BL lines are round and have only a very slight morphologic flexibility (Figs. 3 c and 6).

3. The morphologic heterogeneity within each BL line is very slight.

4. The diversity between different BL lines is sometimes pronounced in contrast to the morphologic homogeneity among the BED lines.

SEM studies (Fig. 5) have confirmed the above differences and also demonstrated that surface villi on BL cells are more numerous, shorter, and more symmetrically distributed over the cell surface than on BED cells (Klein et al., 1975; Nilsson and Pontén, 1975; Fagraeus et al., 1975).

TEM studies (Epstein and Achong, 1965; Epstein et al., 1966b; Pope et al., 1967; Moore et al., 1968; Hammond, 1970) have revealed a few, quite regular additional differences: (1) the ribosomes are abundant but, unlike in BED cells, they are almost never attached to the endoplasmic reticulum; and (2) the Golgi apparatus is comparatively scanty in BL cells. Atypical features like annulate lamellae and projections of the nuclear envelope seem to be as frequent in BL as in BED lines.

It can thus be concluded that morphologic differences do exist between the two types of EBV-carrying lymphoid lines. However, since some diversity has been noted in the group of BL lines it is possible that morphology will not be discriminatory in some cases. Observations on the dynamic morphology of living cells cocultivated with skin fibroblasts is probably the most simple and reliable type of morphology (Sect. E.II).

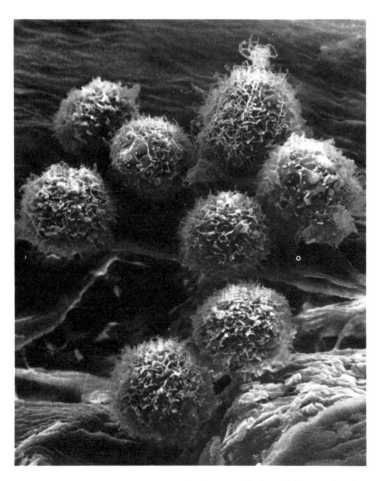

Fig. 5. SEM of BL cells (Daudi). Note the homogeneity in cell shape and surface morphology. (Klein et al., 1975). (× 2900)

II. MOTILITY AND DISTRIBUTION OF ACTIN

Studies with phase-contrast time-lapse cinematography of EBV-carrying lymphoid cell lines have disclosed marked differences between the two types of lines in pattern and intensity of motility (Pulvertaft, 1964a, 1965; Clarkson, 1967; Clarkson et al., 1967; Nilsson et al., 1970b; Nilsson, 1971d; Nilsson and Pontén, 1975; Fagraeus et al., 1975). The type of motility found in suspension cultures and feeder cell-containing cultures of BED and BL cells is schematically summarized in Figure 6. The BED cells are highly motile with the shape of individual cells changing constantly. In suspension, the spectrum of interchangeable forms is limited; single, free-floating cells are mostly round and have multiple short and long surface villi covering the entire surface symmetrically (Fig. 4b). Most cells, however, grow in dense aggregates. Cells at the surface of these clumps are pear ("hand-mirror")-shaped. The typical uropod has a few long, surface villi pointing centrifugally. When feeder cells (skin fibroblasts or glia cells) are present at the bottom of the culture dish most BED cells adhere quickly to the feeder cell surface where they display a rapid and very complex motility (peripolesis). The spectrum of interchangeable forms is wide; individual cells may reversibly attach to the feeder cells for some hours, while other cells remain adherent to the surface of the feeder cell or even reside within the feeder cell (emperipolesis) for several days. A few typical patterns of motility have been noted (Fig. 6):

1. The most common type of cell is pear-shaped with many long (up to $7\,\mu$) thin villi and sometimes a few undulating surface lamellae. This cell can translocate efficiently with its multiple lamellipodia as the leading part of the cell. The speed of translocation has been estimated to reach 2000 μm/h, and the direction of locomotion can change abruptly. The rear end of the cell will then rapidly organize lamellipodia and become the leading part of the cell. The former leading part is simultaneously changed into a nonvillous rear end. Such cycles of change in the direction of the translocation, when they occur in rapid succession, have been termed "ping-pong" locomotion (Pontén, 1975), indicating that during the repetitive changes of the leading cell pole the nucleus will travel like a ping-pong ball within the elongated cell.

2. A minority of cells attain a fibroblast like shape for some hours during which time very little cell surface motility and no translocation occurs.

3. Postmitotic cells, but also a minority of other cells, may show a rapid surface "blebbing." It should be stressed that individual cells may change form and type of motility within a quite short period of time (minutes).

Cells of BL lines are comparatively immobile. The spectrum of possible cell shapes is very limited and most lines contain uniformly round cells (Figs. 3 c–e, 5, and 6). In suspension, the tendency for clumping is restricted and in some lines nonexistent. Even where clumps occur, cells seem to keep short surface villi symmetrically distributed. In cultures with feeder cells, attachment is very slow (weeks) or does not occur at all. Attached cells may be peri- or emperipoletic. Translocation cells are not observed in BL lines with a few possible exceptions. The motility seems to be confined entirely to the surface villi or sometimes to other parts of the plasma membrane where some "blebbing" or slow undulating movements of a larger part of the cell surface are noted.

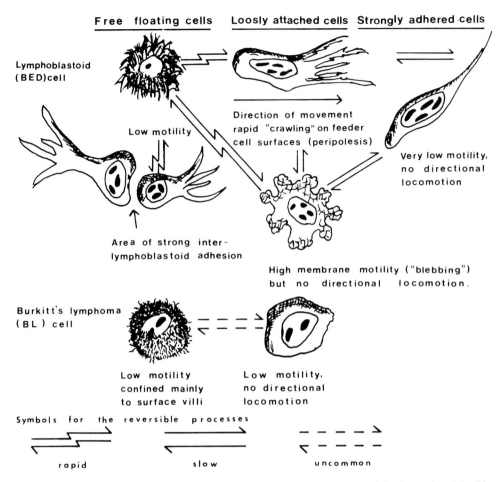

Fig. 6. Morphologic dynamics in human lymphoid cell lines cocultivated with allogeneic adult skin fibroblasts. BED and BL cells observed in time-lapse cinematography. (Nilsson and Pontén, 1975)

The general surface morphology and the degree of motility in the two types of EBV-carrying cell lines have been found to correlate with the distribution and amount of actin as visualized by immunofluorescence studies with anti-actin antibodies (Fagraeus et al., 1975). The nine lines of BED type examined all contained a proportion of cells with brilliantly stained, long, thin villi, most often distributed at one pole of the cell but sometimes over the entire surface (Fig. 7a), while in the two BL lines studied, only membrane staining of low intensity was found but not fluorescent villi (Fig. 7b) (Fagraeus et al., 1975). Several additional BL lines have been examined (Fagraeus and Nilsson, unpublished) and have displayed essentially the same distribution of actin.

Taken together, the studies on motility and actin distribution demonstrate a general difference in motility and organization of one of the contractile proteins, actin. The morphologic pleomorphism in BED lines and the morphologic homogeneity in BL lines seem to be due to the difference in morphologic flexibility between the two types of lines, and not to the fact that BED lines, at least for some months after establishment, are polyclonal while BL lines are monoclonal.

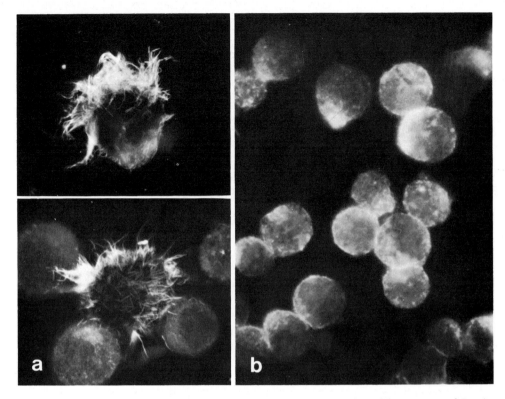

Fig. 7. a Cells of the BED line U-704 with brilliantly stained, long, surface villi. (Courtesy of Dr. A. Fagraeus). (× 800). **b** BL line (Ramos) with membrane staining. (Fagraeus et al., 1975). (× 1000)

III. CELL SURFACE CHARACTERISTICS

1. Lymphocyte Surface Markers

The presence of surface immunoglobulin (S-Ig) and receptors for complement (C3), EBV, the Fc part of IgG(Fc), and sheep red blood cells (SRBC) on the surface of EBV-carrying lymphoid lines has been studied in many laboratories (Schevach et al., 1972; Jondal and Klein, 1973; Kaplan et al., 1974; Royston et al., 1974; Theofilopoulos et al., 1974; Greaves et al., 1975; Papenhausen et al., 1975; Epstein et al., 1976; Huber et al., 1976; Jondal et al., 1976; Yefenof et al., 1976; Yount et al., 1976; Karpas et al., 1977; Robinson et al., 1977; Siegert et al., 1977; Yefenof and Klein, 1977; Yefenof et al., 1977 a).

Apart from the study of Huber et al. (1976), the EBV-carrying cell lines had not been categorized with regard to cell type and age, and although it is well known that the various methods for surface-marker detection differ in sensitivity and are difficult to standardize, nevertheless a clear picture of the expression of the various markers has emerged.

The group of BED lines is qualitatively homogeneous with only few exceptions, and these were found by Huber et al. (1976) to be old lines with secondary chromosomal aberrations. Cells of newly established BED lines (spontaneously or by use of exogenous EBV in vitro) express S-Ig (Sect. E.V.1), C3, EBV, and Fc receptors (Table 5). Both C3b and C3d receptors are found (Theofilopoulos et al., 1974; Huber et al., 1976). The fraction of C3 receptor-positive cells in logarithmically growing cultures, as determined by rosette assays with complement-coated erythrocytes (EAC) or Zymosan beads, ranges from 55%–95%. The expression of C3 receptor has been found to be unrelated to any particular phase of the cell cycle (Papenhausen et al., 1975). The percentage of Fc receptor-bearing cells is zero or very low (0–20) when assayed by the erythrocyte adherence test, but high (20–100) when uptake of radio- or fluorescein-labeled aggregated Ig is recorded. No BED line has been found to bind SRBC.

Among the group of BL lines some heterogeneity in surface-marker expression is found, which agrees with the commonly observed individuality of BL lines (Nilsson and Pontén, 1975). Cells in most lines carry S-Ig (Sect. E.V.1). A few lines, most notably the P_3HR-1, have no detectable C3 and EBV receptors while other lines (e. g., Raji) seem to express exceptionally high amounts of C3 receptor. There is also a heterogeneity with regard to the type of C3 receptor in the group of BL lines (Jondal et al., 1976), and in such lines the C3 receptor seems to be equally well expressed throughout the cell cycle (Huber et al., 1976; Yount et al., 1976). Only a minority (0%–13%) of BL cells bind IgG-coated erythrocytes. However, as in the case of BED cells, more sensitive techniques with aggregated cells reveal the presence of Fc receptors. In fact, no BL line has been found consistently negative. Tests for SRBC binding have always been negative.

Taken together, both BL and BED lines express B lymphocyte surface markers. The expression of the various markers is homogeneous among newly established BED lines while some individuality is noted among new and old BL lines and old BED lines.

Several lines of evidence, suggesting a close relationship between the C3 and EBV receptor, have been presented in recent years. Jondal and Klein (1973) showed co-expression or simultaneous absence of both receptors in a large number of EBV-genome positive and negative human lymphoid cell lines. The EAC rosette formation could be blocked by EBV-containing supernatant, and EBV absorbtion was blocked by preincubation with C3 and anti-C3 antibodies (Jondal et al., 1976). Yefenof et al. (1976) demonstrated that C3 and EBV receptors capped and redistributed together, while no association was detected between either of the two receptors and some other surface markers [S-Ig, β_2-microglobulin (β_2-μ), Fc receptor, and Ia-like antigen]. Furthermore, stripping of C3 and EBV receptors from the surface of two EBV-genome negative BL lines reduced their EBV-absorbing ability. Stripping of IgM, β_2-μ, or Fc receptors did not affect the EBV-absorptive capacity of the cells (Yefenof and Klein, 1976). Finally, Yefenof et al. (1977a) showed correlation between EBV absorption, complement membrane fluorescence, and EAC rosetting in a panel of lymphoid lines. As in the study of Yefenof and Klein (1976), a quantitative bioassay was used to measure EBV absorption. It was therefore possible to exclude that EBV antigenic material and not infectious EBV particles had bound to C3 receptor-associated surface structures. A close association between the EBV and C3 receptor has thus been demonstrated. However, it should be stressed that so far only the C3 receptor on B lymphocytes has been functional in EBV binding as evidenced by the absence of EBV receptors in all other C3 receptor bearing cell types tested.

2. HL-A, β_2-Microglobulin, and Ia-Like Antigen

EBV-carrying lymphoid cell lines and, in particular, BED lines derived from normal donors have been used extensively in studies on the structure and function of products of the major histocompatibility complex. It has, for instance, been possible to isolate HL-A, β_2-μ, and B-alloantigens (human Ia-like antigens ["Ia"]) not only from the cell surface by 3 M KCl extraction, papain digestion, sonication, and detergents, but also from culture supernatants (see Möller, 1974, 1976). Intact lymphoid cells have also been invaluable tools in the characterization and absorption of allo- and heteroantisera against HL-A, β_2-μ, and "Ia."

The first studies indicating that established lymphoid cells retained the expression of HL-A qualitatively unaltered after establishment were reported by Bernoco et al. (1969), Papermaster et al (1969), and Rogentine and Gerber (1969, 1970). In addition to the HL-A antigens of the donors several anomalous cytotoxicity reactions were noted (Bernoco et al., 1969; Ferrone et al., 1971; Dick et al., 1972; Lindblom and Nilsson, 1973; Pious et al., 1974). These "extra" HL-A reactivities have recently been found to be partly due to the presence in the HL-A alloantisera of antibodies against "Ia", expressed at the surface of lymphoid cell lines (Dick et al., 1975; Bodmer et al., 1975). The expression and turnover of the invariant smaller chain of HL-A, β_2-μ, has also been extensively studied in lymphoid cell lines (see Nilsson et al., 1974).

In lines of the BED type, HL-A antigens seem to be expressed in increased amounts on the surface as compared to normal lymphocytes (McCune et al., 1975; Welsh et al., 1977). The quantity of HL-A per BED cell is similar to (Welsh et al., 1977) or greater than (McCune et al., 1975) on mitogen-(PHA, PWM) stimulated lymphoblasts, and considerably greater (10–30 fold) than on peripheral B or T lymphocytes. All new BED lines tested have expressed HL-A in similar amounts except in two chromosomally altered, old lines (NC 37 and U-61 M) where a slightly higher number of HL-A determinants was found (Welsh et al., 1977). It is possible that not only the amount per cell but also the density of HL-A antigens is increased compared to normal lymphocytes, although estimations of the cell surface area are very uncertain (McCune et al., 1975).

The HL-A expression in BL lines is quantitatively similar to that in BED lines. However, here again heterogeneity is found. One cell line, Daudi, lacks the capacity to produce HL-A (Bodmer et al., 1975); P$_3$HR-1 expresses a lower amount than BED lines (Östberg et al., 1975), and the few other lines tested have had amounts similar to the BED lines (Welsh et al., 1977).

β_2-μ is expressed in a slight excess of HL-A (ratio $1:1 - 3:1$) at the surface of EBV-carrying cell lines and is subject to a very high turnover at the membrane or is possibly secreted via a separate pathway (Nilsson et al., 1974; Welsh et al., 1977). Cell surface β_2-μ has been quantitated by different methods in BL and BED lines (Nilsson et al., 1974; Östberg et al., 1975; Welsh et al., 1977), and taken together these studies indicate that the expression of β_2-μ is homogeneous in new BED lines, and variable in BL and old BED lines; the amount of surface β_2-μ ranges from zero (the Daudi line) to quantities similar to that on BED lines (the Raji line) (Nilsson et al., 1974). In most BL lines, however, there seems to be a reduction of surface β_2-μ density in comparison to normal lymphocytes and BED cells (Nilsson et al., 1974; Welsh et al., 1977). Since the amount of HL-A is not similarly reduced (Welsh et al., 1977) this reduction must involve free β_2-μ molecules or β_2-μ associated with other, not yet defined, antigenic structures. It is possible that decreased expression of surface β_2-μ is a general feature of malignant hematopoietic cells, since non-BL lymphoma, leukemia, and myeloma lines also have low amounts of surface β_2-μ (Nilsson et al., 1974).

The rate of accumulation of free β_2-μ chains in the medium (secretion) during logarithmic growth is similar in all new BED lines, but variable in the group of BL lines and two chromosomally altered BED lines (Nilsson et al., 1973; Evrin and Nilsson, 1974; Nilsson et al., 1974). In the BL group the rate of secretion has been found to be 0%–20% of that in BED lines (Nilsson et al., 1974).

All BED and BL lines (including the HL-A and β_2-μ-negative Daudi, but excluding the P$_3$HR-1) have been found to express "Ia" (Dick et al., 1975; Bodmer, 1975; Gahmberg et al., 1977; Trowbridge et al., 1977).

EBV-carrying cell lines have also been shown to express new, or altered, surface antigens that stimulate allogeneic and autochthonous lymphocytes in mixed leukocyte cultures (MLC) (Hardy et al., 1969; Flier et al., 1970; Green and Sell, 1970; Steel and Hardy, 1970; Han et al., 1971; Junge et al., 1971; Knight et al., 1971; Golub et al., 1972; Steel et al., 1973; Ling et al., 1974; Svedmyr et al., 1974). The stimulatory antigens in the MLC are unrelated to the presence of EBV (Steel et al., 1977) and are thought to be the "Ia" antigens (Wernet, 1976; Humphreys et al., 1976; Geier and Creswell, 1977). Recently Steel et al., (1978) reported that one BL line, EB1, which expresses "Ia" antigens nevertheless does not stimulate allogeneic lymphocytes in MLC. Using this line for absorption a rabbit anti-B cell serum could be rendered noncytotoxic to lymphocytes in complement-dependent cytotoxicity tests, although this serum was still inhibitory in MLC. The authors conclude that with this serum they had distinguished between "Ia" antigens detectable by complement-dependent cytotoxicity tests and very similar antigenic determinants responsible for stimulation in MLC.

3. Concanavalin A (Con A)-Induced Agglutinability and Mobility of Con A Receptors

The lectin Concanavalin A (Con A) has been extensively used as a probe in studies of cell surface changes related to malignancy. A high agglutinability in the presence of Con A has been found to be typical of malignant cells in many (Rapin and Burger, 1974), but not all (Glimelius et al., 1975; Berman, 1975), rodent and human cell systems. A reduced lateral mobility of Con A receptors has been another feature commonly associated with malignancy (Inbar et al., 1973 a, b; Ben-Bassat et al., 1974; Ben-Bassat and Goldblum, 1975).

All EBV-carrying cell lines have been found to agglutinate readily in the presence of Con A (De Salle et al., 1972; Glimelius et al., 1975; Ben-Bassat et al., 1976). Glimelius et al. (1975) found that a panel of newly established BED lines had closely similar agglutinability and that the degree of agglutination was higher than that of normal lymphocytes but similar to PHA-stimulated lymphocytes; two old lines showed a considerably higher agglutinability (Sect. G). All BL lines were significantly more agglutinable than BED lines, but a variability, unrelated to the age of the line, was noted. Ben-Bassat et al. (1976) have confirmed this high degree of Con A agglutinability in an extensive study on some old BL lines and fresh BL-tumor biopsy cells and the BL lines derived from them. The increased agglutinability may be unrelated to the neoplastic state per se, since in a large number of other types of EBV genome-negative malignant hematopoietic cell lines no consistently increased Con A agglutination was found (Glimelius et al., 1975). Interestingly, however, a positive correlation between EBV carrier state and high Con A agglutination was observed and this finding has been further substantiated by Yefenof et al. (1977), who demonstrated that conversion of EBV genome-negative lymphoma lines to an EBV carrier state was followed by an increased Con A agglutinability.

Compared to normal lymphocytes all BL lines, except the P_3HR1, have been found to have a reduced cap-forming ability when exposed to fluoresceinated Con A and incubated under capping conditions (Ben-Bassat et al., 1976). It is possible that this membrane change as well, although encountered in other malignant lymphoid cells (Ben-Bassat et al., 1974; Ben-Bassat and Goldblum, 1975), is directly related to the presence of EBV in BL cells rather than being a characteristic of the malignant phenotype, since studies on the EBV genome-negative lymphomas and their sublines infected with EBV have regularly shown that the ability to form caps is reduced in the sublines after staining with fluorescein-labeled anti-Ig or Con A (Yefenof and Klein, 1976; Yefenof et al., 1977b).

In conclusion, both BED and BL lines are more agglutinable by Con A than normal lymphocytes and a reduced lateral mobility has been demonstrated in BL lines, although BED lines have not been similarly examined. It is possible that these surface alterations are related to the presence of the EBV genomes.

4. Surface Glycoprotein Pattern

Recently some of the newly developed methods for specific radiolabeling of surface proteins (Gahmberg, 1977) have been employed to study the surface glycoprotein composition of cells in hematopoietic cell lines (Trowbridge et al., 1976; Andersson et al., 1977; Nilsson et al., 1977a; Gahmberg et al., 1978). With galactose-oxidase-catalyzed tritiated sodium borohydride-labeling it has been possible to show that the surface glycoprotein composition is different in the cells of BED and BL lines (Nilsson et al., 1977a; Gahmberg et al., 1978) (Fig. 8).

BED cells have a surface glycoprotein pattern similar to that of PWM-stimulated B lymphocytes, while in contrast, the basic surface glycoprotein pattern of BL cells resembles to some extent that of normal B lymphocytes. This difference provides further nonmorphologic distinguishing features for BED and BL cells. Moreover, it indicates that BL-tumor cells might originate from a lymphoid cell "frozen" at a differentiation stage close to that of the B lymphocyte, whereas B lymphocytes during development to BED cells after EBV infection not only become immortalized but also further differentiated to the B blast stage (Sect. E.V.1).

In addition to the surface glycoproteins detected on resting B lymphocytes, all six EBV-carrying BL lines examined, but none of six BED lines, had two characteristic pairs of glycoproteins of apparent molecular weights of 87,000/85,000 and 71,000/69,000 and some individually distinct bands. However, these pairs of glyco-proteins were also found on three EBV genome-negative lymphocytic lymphoma lines and are therefore not specific for BL, but rather perhaps for B lymphomas. The nature of the 87,000/85,000 and 71,000/69,000 glycoprotein is still unknown. It was speculated (Nilsson et al., 1977a) that they might represent markers for a certain stage of lymphoid differentiation or, but less likely, C-type oncornavirus-associated surface

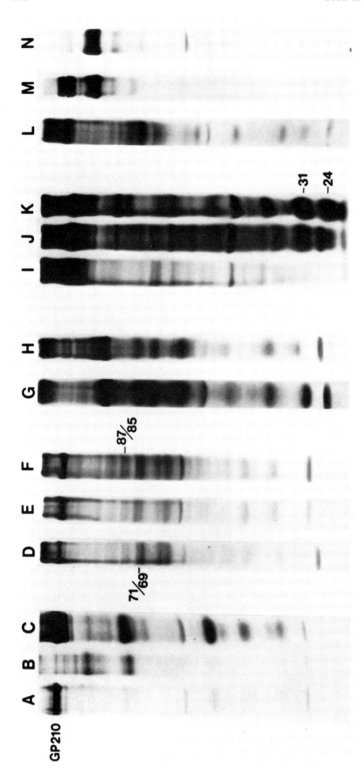

Fig. 8. Polyacrylamide gel electrophoresis patterns of surface glycoproteins of lymphoid cells labeled after treatment with neuraminidase and galactose oxidase. *A,* spleen B cells; *B,* blood B blasts; *C,* spleen B blasts; *D,* BL line Ramos; *E,* lymphocytic lymphoma line U-698; *F,* lymphocytic lymphoma line U-715; *G,* BED line U-61 M; *H,* BED line U-974; *I,* BL line P 3; *J,* BL line Daudi; *K,* BL line Raji; *L,* myeloma line RPMI 8226; *M,* blood T cells; *N,* acute lymphoblastic leukemia line Molt 4. The apparent molecular weights of some relevant glycoproteins are indicated. (Gahmberg et al., 1978)

glycoproteins analogous to the GP 70 found on murine leukemia virus-infected mouse thymocytes.

5. Hormone Receptors

A few lymphoid lines of the BED type have been examined for polypeptide hormone cell surface receptors. High affinity receptors have been found for insulin (Gavin et al., 1972 a, b), human growth hormone (Lesniak et al., 1973, 1974), and calcitonin (Marx et al., 1974). BL lines have only been included in the study of Marx et al. (1974) on calcitonin receptors and were found to have a significantly lower amount of receptor than the BED lines. However, since the lines tested were few and old no conclusion can be drawn about whether or not the difference observed might be general. Recently Carpenter et al. (1975) and Westermark (personal communication) have examined BED and BL lines for the presence of epidermal growth-factor receptors with negative results.

IV. GROWTH CHARACTERISTICS

All newly established BED lines have very similar requirements for growth in vitro (Nilsson and Pontén, 1975). In the absence of feeder cells they are dependent on a rich medium (e. g., Ham's F-10, F-12, and RPMI 1640) for maintenance and can grow in comparatively low concentrations of serum. However, growth is optimal with serum concentrations in the range of $5\%-10\%$ and newborn calf serum is usually as efficient as fetal calf serum in sustaining good growth. The cells grow in dense clumps without adherence to glass or plastic surfaces. The population doubling time in optimally fed, mycoplasma-free cultures is usually around 30 h giving a maximal cell density $1-1.2 \times 10^6$. At cell concentrations below 10^4 cells/ml, growth is very poor and the cells may eventually die. Growth is best in stationary suspension cultures; the use of spinner cultures will increase the frequency of dead cells. With feeder cells present BED cells will also grow in comparatively simple media (e. g., Eagle's MEM), although at a slower rate. Single cells and cell clumps will attach rapidly to feeder cells (Sect. E.II) leaving a minority of the cells floating free. BED lines have only a limited potential for growth in semisolid agar or agarose; the cloning efficiency is low and the colonies formed are microscopic (Moore, 1972; Nilsson and Pontén, 1975) (Sect. E. VII and G).

The growth characteristics of individual BL lines are variable (Nilsson and Pontén, 1975). Most lines grow easily in stationary suspension cultures but a few lines are strictly dependent on feeder cells for survival even after some months of continuous cultivation (Nilsson, unpublished). Many BL lines can grow in suspension without rich media, but the majority seem to proliferate more rapidly in such media; growth is usually slower in low concentrations of serum. As a group, BL lines tend to have a shorter population doubling time than BED lines and the maximum cell density described is 3×10^6 cells/ml (Pope et al., 1967), a density higher than that of any BED line. BL cells grow in suspension in loose clumps, single cells, or short chains; some attachment takes place when feeder cells are present, but the process of attachment is slow (days). Many BL lines grow in agar or agarose with a relatively high cloning efficiency and the formation of large colonies which are often macroscopically visible (Moore, 1972; Nilsson and Pontén, 1975).

V. FUNCTIONAL PROPERTIES

The extensive use of EBV-carrying lymphoid cell lines over the past 10 years has shown that they produce Ig, interferon, and a variety of biologically active products assumed to represent mediators of lymphoid cell functions during the delayed type of hypersensitivity reaction. Most of the non-Ig proteins produced are also synthesized both by mitogen-stimulated normal lymphocytes (e.g., interferon) and by non-lymphoid cells.

1. Immunoglobulin Production

The production of Ig has been studied extensively in both BED and BL cell lines. At the cell population level the synthesis of Ig has usually been recorded by immunochemical methods and the Ig has been identified either as secreted molecules in the spent supernatant or in cell lysates. At the single cell level immunofluorescence techniques or a combination of cloning and immunochemical methods have been used. Several qualitative and quantitative differences have been noted between the Ig production of BL and BED lines.

A fraction of the *BL lines* does not produce Ig (Finegold et al., 1967; Klein et al., 1967; Finegold et al., 1968; Klein et al., 1968; Osunkoya et al., 1969; Nadkarni et al., 1969; Scherr et al., 1971; van Furth et al., 1972; Béchet et al., 1974; Nilsson and Pontén, 1975); the most extensive studies show their frequency varying from 50% (Finegold et al., 1967) to 20% (van Furth et al., 1972). The synthesis in lines which do produce is monoclonal and identical to that synthesized by the tumor cells in vivo (Fahey et al., 1966; Tanigaki et al., 1966; Finegold et al., 1967; Klein et al., 1967; Wakefield et al., 1967; Finegold et al., 1968; Osunkoya et al., 1968; Takahashi et al., 1969 a; van Furth et al., 1972; Béchet et al., 1974; Evans et al., 1974; Klein et al., 1975; Nilsson and Pontén, 1975).

The predominant class of Ig synthesized by BL cells is IgM; three exceptional lines producing IgG have been reported (Fahey et al., 1967; Osunkoya et al., 1968; Klein et al., 1975), but of these only the line described by Klein et al. (1975) was positively identified as a BL line.

The BL lines usually produce Ig with normal antigenicity, electrophoretic mobility, and elution pattern on chromatography (Finegold et al., 1967). However, synthesis of incomplete Ig molecules (free heavy or light chains) has often been noted (Tanigaki et al., 1966; Wakefield et al., 1967; Finegold et al., 1968; Evans et al., 1974), and that other defects of the molecular structure may occur has been demonstrated by studies on Daudi IgM (Kennel, 1974).

The IgM manufactured by most BL lines is predominantly, or perhaps exclusively, destined for insertion in the plasma membrane (see Sherr et al., 1971) as suggested by recent observations on a limited number of cell lines (Nilsson and Pontén, 1975), and the release into the medium of a very few Ig molecules is probably due to membrane turnover. The quantity of S-IgM is variable but usually comparatively high, e.g., 8×10^4 molecules per Daudi cell (Klein et al., 1970; Sherr et al., 1972; Ghetie et al., 1974).

The rate of Ig synthesis has been examined in Daudi cells, where Ig represented 1%– 2% of all protein synthesized (Sherr et al., 1971) and accumulated in the membrane continuously during interphase (Killander et al., 1974), in contrast to the Ig production related to the cell cycle phase sometimes noted in myeloma and BED cells. Other BL lines have not been examined.

All *BED lines* synthesize Ig. The pattern of synthesis is polyclonal for $\sim 1-2$ years of continuous cultivation after establishment, and thereafter a gradual selection of one clone occurs (Glade and Chessin, 1968a; Nilsson, 1971b; Béchet et al., 1973, 1974) (Fig. 2).

In the early studies, the class of Ig most commonly synthesized was found to be IgG (Tanigaki et al., 1966; Finegold et al., 1967; Wakefield et al., 1967; Nilsson et al., 1968; Takahashi et al., 1969a; Nilsson, 1971b), but more recently IgM (Evans et al., 1974; Yount et al., 1976), IgM together with IgG (Litwin et al., 1973), or IgM together with IgD (Gordon et al., 1977) have been reported to be the predominant classes. A possible explanation for this discrepancy may be that the methods used in the early studies only identified secreted IgG and not IgM, which is largely membrane-associated (Premkumar et al., 1975). BED lines may synthesize complete molecules of Ig but a molar excess of light chains is often expressed at the surface and secreted (Tanigaki et al., 1966; Wakefield et al., 1967; McConahey et al., 1972; Litwin et al., 1974a; Nilsson and Pontén, 1975; Gordon et al., 1977). Exceptionally, old lines may lose the capacity to synthesize intact Ig and become converted to an exclusive production of either heavy or light chains (Tanigaki et al., 1966; Yount et al., 1976).

Cloning experiments and analysis of S-Ig by immunofluorescence (Hinuma and Grace, 1967; Takahashi et al., 1969b; Bloom et al., 1971; Nilsson et al., 1971a; Litwin and Lin, 1976) suggest that, almost without exception, all cells within a BED line have the capacity for Ig synthesis. Individual cells usually produce only one immunoglobulin, but in some lines the simultaneous synthesis of two heavy and one light chain has been detected.

The rate of Ig secretion in BED lines during the logarithmic growth phase has been reported to be of the order of $2.4-3$ $\mu g/10^6$ cells/day (Fahey and Finegold, 1967; Matsuoka et al., 1968; Nilsson and Pontén, 1975). Expression at the cell surface of 2×10^4 molecules per cell (McConahey et al., 1972) must be regarded as an approximation, since Litwin et al. (1974a), using a different methodology, detected $1-4.5 \times 10^5$ molecules per cell.

The synthesis of Ig has been thought to occur only during a limited part of the cell cycle in BED lines. Lerner and Hodgke (1971) and Buell et al. (1969) found a maximal rate of Ig synthesis in late G1 and early S phase while Watanabe et al. (1973) found an additional peak in G2 with intracellular accumulation occurring slightly later. The synthesis of secretory and membrane Ig at least in some BED lines has been suggested to be under separate control and to take place in separate cellular compartments with export perhaps along separate pathways (Lerner et al., 1972; Litwin et al., 1974b).

Immunoglobulins with antibody activity against available common antigens are not usually produced (Glade and Chessin, 1968a; Bloom et al., 1973). One BL line (P3-J) was claimed to make antibodies in response to exposure to coliphages (Kamei and Moore, 1967), but this observation was never confirmed (Krueger et al., 1974). However, Evans et al. (1974), Steel et al. (1974), and Joss et al. (1976) have reported that 4 out of 39 BED lines produced hemagglutinins with the characteristics of IgM.

Baskin et al. (1976a) found one BED line (PGL-33H) responsive to *Candida albicans* antigen (CaAg) using a migration-inhibition assay; loss of responsiveness to the CaAg was noted after exposure of the cells to anti-IgM-containing serum, but whether or not these findings indicate that surface IgM with antibody activity against CaAg is present on the PGLC-33HC cells has not been further elucidated.

Recently it was demonstrated that the simultaneous exposure of human B lymphocytes to EBV and an antigen (SRBC) resulted in the development of plaque-forming cells producing anti-SRBC (Luzzati et al., 1972). Thus it should be possible to establish permanent antibody-producing BED lines by this technique. However, only a minority of the multiple clones present shortly after EBV immortalization (Rosén et al., 1977) can be expected to produce the relevant antibody and selective methods have to be applied to isolate the antibody-producing cells from the other clones of Ig-secreting BED cells. With this in mind, Steinitz et al. (1977) have succeeded in establishing BED lines producing anti-hapten (anti-NNP) antibody from a population of surface anti-NNP antibody-carrying lymphocytes preselected from non-antibody expressing cells by rosetting with NNP-coated erythrocytes.

In conclusion, certain differences in the Ig production of BL and BED lines have usually been found and these seem to suggest that BL and BED cells represent different stages of lymphoid differentiation. The group of BL cells has been found to be heterogeneous with regard to the capacity to synthesize Ig. A minor fraction of the lines does not produce Ig but those which do usually do not secrete the Ig, but rather contain a comparatively high amount of it at the surface. The synthesis of Ig is not restricted to any particular phase of the cell cycle. The stage of differentiation shown by BL lines with regard to Ig production, is reminiscent of that of resting B cells. BED lines, in contrast, always synthesize and secrete Ig at a rate that is 1:5 – 1:3 of that observed in myeloma lines and only a minor amount of this Ig is retained at the cell surface; this stage of differentiation may roughly correspond to that of antigen-stimulated B blasts.

2. Synthesis of Putative Mediators of Cell-Mediated Immunity

Several extensive reviews have been written about the production and biologic properties of a number of different proteins that are putative mediators of cell-mediated immunity (Glade and Hirschhorn, 1970; Papageorgiou and Glade, 1972; Glade and Papageorgiou, 1973 a, b; Glade and Beratis, 1976).

All the studies on such mediators have employed BED lines and it is therefore impossible to judge whether or not a difference between BED lines and BL lines exists in this connection. Production of macrophage-inhibition factor (MIF) has been described by several laboratories (Glade et al., 1970; Granger et al., 1970; Papageorgiou et al., 1972; Tsuschimoto et al., 1972; Tubergen et al., 1972; Papageorgiou et al., 1974) and this MIF seems to have the same biochemical and biologic properties as that produced by sensitized guinea pig macrophages (Tubergen et al., 1972). The production by BED lines of two other, less well-characterized "factors" has also been reported; thus, Granger et al. (1970) have described the release by BED lines of a substance (lymphotoxin) with the capacity to kill fibroblast monolayers, and Smith et al. (1970), Hersh and Drewinko (1974), Hersh et al. (1974), and Han et al. (1975) have found a lymphoblastogenesis-inhibition factor.

3. Phagocytosis and Production of Interferon

Kammermeyer et al. (1968) and Sundström (1977) have established that EBV-carrying cell lines have a phagocytic capacity, a function generally attributed to granulocytes and monocytes. No consistent differences between the BL and BED types of lines were demonstrated.

Different laboratories have also shown that interferon (Deinhardt and Burnside, 1967; McCombs and Benyesh-Melnick, 1967; Kasel et al., 1968; Zajac et al., 1969; Haase et al., 1970; Minnefor, 1970; Adams et al., 1975) and a B_{1c}/B_{1a} globulin (C′3) (Glade and Chessin, 1968b) are produced by both BED and BL lines.

Since interferon is also synthesized spontaneously by macrophages (Smith and Wagner, 1967; Stecher and Thorbecke, 1967) BED cells seem to share at least five characteristics with macrophages – MIF, C′3, and interferon production, phagocytic activity, and the pattern of movement observed on allogeneic fibroblasts (Sect. E.II).

VI. CYTOCHEMICAL CHARACTERISTICS

Enzyme cytochemistry has been widely used by hematologists in the differential diagnosis of leukemia and lymphoma (Hayhoe and Cawley, 1972; Stuart et al., 1975).

Two extensive cytochemical studies on large panels of lymphoid cell lines have recently been published (Karpas et al., 1977; Sundström and Nilsson, 1977). The cell reactivity in the various enzyme-staining reactions, and especially the esterase reactions, is subject to considerable variation depending on differences in substrate, incubation time, pH, etc., and the amount of enzyme seems to be dependent on the culture conditions. It is therefore difficult to compare cytochemical results from different laboratories. However, some staining reactions are in good agreement, despite the variability that has been noted.

BED lines seem to have the following cytochemical characteristics: Staining is weakly to moderately positive with the periodic acid Schiff reaction, and for acid phosphatase, naphthol AS-D acetate esterase, naphthol AD chloroacetate esterase, α-naphthol acetate esterase, and β-glucoronidase. All lines are negative with peroxidase and stains for neutral fat (Sudan black B, Oil Red 0). Karpas et al. (1977) found staining for alkaline phosphatase, but this enzyme was not detected by Sundström and Nilsson (1977); the reason for this difference is probably methodologic.

BL lines have only been included in the study of Sundström and Nilsson (1977) and the only difference observed from the BED lines was a regular finding of neutral fat, a well-known constituent of the BL cell cytoplasm (Sect. E.I).

A new alkaline phosphatase with some unique properties has recently been described by Neumann et al. (1976) in lines of both BL and BED type.

VII. TUMORIGENICITY

BL lines have almost without exception been shown to originate from the malignant cell population in vivo (Sects. D and F). The nature of the BED lines has, however, long remained unclear. All BED lines certainly have one characteristic in common with truly malignant cells – the capacity for infinite growth in vitro. However, the lines are of polyclonal derivation (Sect. D), have normal diploid karyotypes (Sect. F), and share other features in common with mitogen-stimulated normal lymphocytes (e. g., morphology, motility, agglutinability by Con A, HL-A, and β-μ production, surface glycoprotein pattern, production of MIF, interferon, and Ig). It has therefore been suggested that BED lines are of non-neoplastic derivation (Nilsson, 1971 b; Belpomme et al., 1972; Béchet et al., 1973; Nilsson and Pontén, 1975) and that cells of BED lines could thus be regarded as only partly "transformed".

The direct test for malignancy – inoculation into an autologous host – cannot, for obvious reasons, be used to decide the nature of the BED lines. Other tests, which have been comparatively reliable in studies on animal tumors (i. e., colony formation in agar in vitro and heterologous transplantation), have therefore been used to judge the possible neoplastic state of EBV-carrying lymphoid cell lines. The early work by Imamura and Moore (1968), Southam et al. (1969 a), Southam et al. (1969 b), Huang et al. (1969), Levin et al. (1969), Christofinis (1969), Imamura et al. (1970), Adams et al. (1970), Adams et al. (1971), Deal et al. (1971), and Adams et al. (1973) indicated some difference between the lines from patients with BL and those originating from normal donors or patients with tumors other than BL. The BL-derived lines usually formed colonies in agar and produced tumors in newborn or immunosuppressed mice, rats, or hamsters, whereas with non-BL lines, a high cloning efficiency and growth in such animals were infrequently encountered. These results, based on studies with lines of various age, and probably therefore also heterogeneous with regard to chromosome constitution and clonality, did not allow any conclusion about possible consistent differences between the BL and BED type of EBV-carrying cell line.

A large number of EBV-carrying lines characterized as BL or BED by morphology and chromosome analysis, was studied recently for growth capacity in agarose (Nilsson et al., 1977 b) and tumorigenicity after transplantation subcutaneously into nude mice (Diehl et al., 1977; Nilsson et al., 1977 b). In agreement with earlier studies, the BL lines formed colonies in agarose, and most also grew subcutaneously in the nude mice; some exceptional lines were found both among old and new lines. In contrast, the BED lines did not form colonies in agar or grow in the nude mice unless they had an aneuploid karyotype. It is therefore possible that lines from healthy donors or patients with acute IM which have previously been reported to be transplantable (Christofinis, 1969; Imamura et al., 1970; Adams et al., 1970, 1973) were old and chromosomally altered, Alternatively, the use of different animals and/or inoculation routes could explain the successful growth.

The recent findings thus establish a clear difference in tumorigenicity between BL and BED lines inoculated subcutaneously in nude mice. They also suggest a non-neoplastic derivation of BED cells. Furthermore, they demonstrate that the spontaneous chromosomal alterations occurring in BED lines during prolonged cultivation in vitro (Sect. F.II) may sometimes be accompanied by the acquisition of "malignant" characteristics. EBV infection of B lymphocytes leads to immortality in vitro, but additional changes are apparently needed to render the cells capable of autonomous growth subcutaneously in nude mice. It has been hypothesized that unless EBV is different or has a different influence on the host-cell genome in BL than in BED cells, the evolution of a BL tumor-cell clone from an EBV infected B-cell(s) in vivo likewise is progressive and involves not only the immortalization by EBV, but also a sequence of chromosomal alterations and subsequent changes of the phenotype, which all interact and lead stepwise to independence from host control mechanisms (Nilsson et al., 1977 b).

F. CHROMOSOME STUDIES ON EBV-CARRYING LYMPHOID CELL LINES

The chromosomes of lymphoid cell lines have been extensively studied. Before the introduction of banding techniques only major abnormalities in chromosome structure and numerical aberrations could be detected and most of the reports concern BL-derived cell lines (Stewart et al., 1965; Chu et al., 1966; Cooper et al., 1966; Rabson et al., 1966; Bishun and Sutton, 1967; Kohn et al., 1967; Miles and O'Neill, 1967; Toshima et al., 1967; Hughes, 1968; Kurita et al., 1968; Tomkins, 1968; Tough et al., 1968; Huang et al., 1969; Nadkarni et al., 1969; Macek and Benyesh-Melnick, 1969; Zajac and Kohn, 1970; Rabson et al., 1970; Whang-Peng et al., 1970; Ikeuchi et al., 1971; Macek et al., 1971). Other studies were performed on newly established and old BED lines from normal donors (Kohn et al., 1968; Miles et al., 1968; Saksela and Pontén, 1968; Sandberg et al., 1968; Christophinis, 1969; Huang and Moore, 1969; Macek et al., 1971), from patients with IM (Kohn et al., 1968; Tomkins, 1968; Macek et al., 1971; Steel et al., 1971), and from donors with hematopoietic malignany other than BL (McCarthy et al., 1965; Lucas et al., 1966; Moore et al., 1966 a; Clarkson et al., 1967; zur Hausen, 1967; Ito et al., 1968; Miles et al., 1968; Saksela and Pontén, 1968; Sandberg et al., 1968; Tomkins, 1968; Huang et al., 1969; Macek et al., 1971; Steel et al., 1971).

All lines, regardless of origin, were found to have diploid or near-diploid chromosome numbers. Some structural abnormalities, such as marker chromosomes, have also been identified. One of these markers was a C-group chromosome characterized by a prominent subterminal construction on the long arms, which was found in BL lines (Kohn et al., 1967; Miles and O'Neill, 1967). A marker found in several BED lines including some that had been established by cocultivation with EBV-carrying BL cells or with lysates from BED lines (Henle et al., 1967; Kohn et al., 1968; Pope et al., 1968; Chessin et al., 1968; Miles et al., 1968; Macek and Benyesh-Melnick, 1969) was indistinguishable from the BL "C-marker" and this chromosome lesion was thought to have been induced by EBV (Kohn et al., 1968).

However, Tomkins (1968), Saksela and Pontén (1968), Steel et al. (1971), and Steel (1972) found no C-group marker chromosomes in BED lines and Macek and Benyesh-Melnick (1969) and Huang et al. (1970) detected the same abnormality in only a minority of the lines and at a very low frequency of the metaphases. Furthermore, Huang et al. (1970) and Whang-Peng et al. (1970) showed that there was no consistent relation between the presence of the C-group marker and EBV-related antigens.

I. STUDIES WITH BANDING TECHNIQUES IN NEWLY ESTABLISHED LINES

The new banding techniques (Caspersson et al., 1970; Dutrillaux and Lejeune, 1971; Sumner et al., 1971; Seabright, 1972) have made it possible to reveal several important cytogenic differences between BL and BED cells.

All newly established BED lines have been found to be normal diploid. The panel of lines analyzed includes BED lines established spontaneously from blood of patients with acute IM (Jarvis et al., 1974) and leukemia (Hellriegel et al., 1977), from lymph nodes of patients with Hodgkin's disease (Zech et al., 1976; Hellriegel et al., 1977), and lines established from cord and adult peripheral blood by exogeneous EBV or by

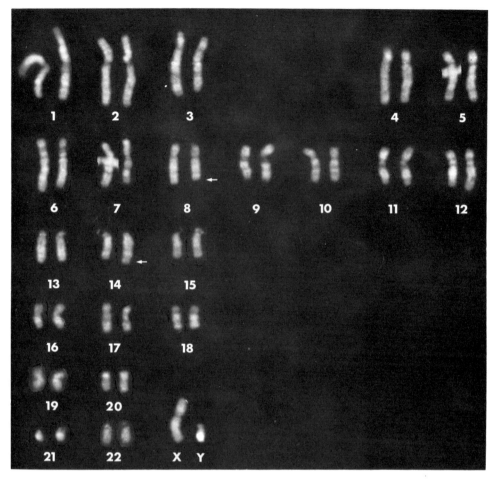

Fig. 9. Karyotype of a cell from a Burkitt lymphoma biopsy. *Arrows* indicate the 8q⁻; 14q⁺ translocation; Q-banding. (Zech et al., 1976)

cocultivation with X-irradiated EBV-producing cells (Jarvis et al., 1974; Zech et al., 1976; Hellriegel et al., 1977).

All BL lines have proved aneuploid. The chromosome 14 marker, first detected by Manolov and Manolova (1972) in BL biopsies and BL cell lines, has subsequently been identified in all BL lines examined with but few exceptions (Table 6) (Petit, 1972; Jarvis et al., 1974; Zech et al., 1976; Hellriegel et al., 1977; Kaiser-McCaw et al., 1977; Temple et al., 1977).

The chromosome 14 marker was originally described as an extra band located at the end of both long arms of one chromosome 14. Zech et al. (1976) found a translocation of a segment from the end of the long arms of one chromosome 8 to chromosome 14 (Fig. 9) (t [8q −; 14q +]) but in three other cases, the metaphases were of poor quality and did not allow detailed analysis of chromosome 8. It is not known if the extra band on the long arms of the chromosome 14 could be of some other origin. The 14q + marker was not found in the blood of BL patients (Zech et al., 1976), but it or similar chromosome 14 abnormalities have been identified in other malignant lymphomas besides BL (Reeves et al., 1973; Lawler, 1975; Mark, 1975; Prigogina and Fleischmann, 1975; Fukuhara et al., 1976; Zech et al., 1976) and in multiple myeloma (Wurster-Hill, 1973; Philip, 1975), but not in lymphocytic leukemias of 0 or T cell origin. It is therefore possible that the 14q + marker is associated with neoplasms of the B cell series although the frequency of the marker in lymphomas other than BL has not been determined.

Table 6. Frequency of 14q$^+$ marker in BL lines

References	Number of cell lines	
	With 14q$^+$	Without 14q$^+$
Manolov and Manolova, 1972	7	2
Petit et al., 1972	1	0
Jarvis et al., 1974	7	0
Zech et al., 1976	3	1
Hellriegel et al., 1977	5	0
Total	23	3

The role of the chromosome 14 in the development of lymphomas and myelomas is unknown, but it has been postulated that the rearrangement of the distal part of the long arm is advantageous for lymphoid cells during the suggested stepwise development of an autonomous BL clone (Zech et al., 1976) (Sect. E.VII). This assumption is supported by the finding of rearrangements of chromosome 14 in ataxia-telangiectasia, a hereditary disease known to be associated with an increased frequency of lymphoid neoplasia (Bochkov et al., 1974; Hayashi and Schmid, 1975; Oxford et al., 1975; McCaw et al., 1975).

In addition, other chromosomal abnormalities have been described in BL lines. Steel (1971) and Zech et al. (1976) reported a trisomy 7 which, like the chromosome 14 abnormality, seems also to be frequent in non-BL lymphomas (Zech et al., 1976), and minor numerical abnormalities were detected by Zech et al. in a limited number of BL lines. Finally, a region in the long arm of one chromosome 15 was lost or translocated in two cell lines, Daudi and Namalwa (Zech et al., 1976; Zeuthen et al., 1977); this deletion was associated with the complete absence of β_2-μ production in Daudi (Nilsson et al., 1973) and a reduced expression of β_2 in Namalwa (Zeuthen et al., 1977).

II. SPONTANEOUS CHROMOSOMAL ALTERATIONS DURING CONTINOUS CULTURE

In the prebanding era EBV-carrying lymphoid cell lines of both types were observed to be remarkably stable during prolonged cultivation and differed in this respect from cell lines established from nonhematopoietic tissue (Saksela and Pontén, 1968; Sandberg et al., 1968; Kurita et al., 1968; Huang and Moore, 1969; Huang et al., 1970; Krishan and Raychaudhari, 1970; Pontén, 1971). Signs of major rearrangements and changes in chromosome mode to hyper- or hypodiploidy, or occasionally near tetraploidy were, however, observed in some lines after 1–2 years in continous culture (Huang and Moore, 1969; Huang et al., 1969; Steel et al., 1971; Nilsson and Pontén, 1975).

Using banding techniques, Zech et al. (1976) found several changes of the karyotype in a few lines examined after prolonged in vitro culture. In a recent extensive study, Steel et al. (1977) examined the chromosomal evolution in 72 BED and 8 BL lines.

In BED lines examined within 1 year after establishment, the incidence of aneuploidy was 2 out of 25, while in old lines (> 1 year of continous cultivation) the corresponding figure was 25 out of 30. These secondarily altered lines usually remained diploid or near diploid with gains more frequent than losses, and these gains were not random. Trisomy was often found for chromosomes 3, 7, 8, 9, 12; the trisomy 7 is particularly interesting since it has been detected not only in BL but also in non-BL lymphoma lines (Zech et al., 1976; Steel et al., 1977).

Secondary chromosomal alterations in BED lines may sometimes be followed by changes in phenotypic characteristics (Sect. G) and a few lines have even acquired the capacity for growth subcutaneously in nude mice (Sect. E.VII). It is not yet known whether the development of any particular chromosomal alteration (e. g., trisomy 7) correlates with the acquisition of a more "malignant" phenotype in BED lines.

Little is yet known about chromosomal changes in BL lines. Three of the old lines included in the study of Steel et al. (1977) were near tetraploid; since the chromosome $14q^+$ marker is usually the only detectable deviation from normal in fresh BL biopsy cells the findings of Steel et al. (1977) indicate that changes also occur during the prolonged culture of BL lines. The number of BL lines examined repeatedly over a long period of time during continuous cultivation is, however, too limited to allow any conclusions about the rate and type of spontaneous chromosomal changes in BL as compared to BED lines.

G. PHENOTYPIC STABILITY DURING LONG-TERM CULTIVATION

There have been no systematic studies on phenotypic changes in BED and BL lines during prolonged cultivation in vitro except those on Ig production (Sect. E.V.1). However, in many reports on various phenotypic characteristics, deviations from the general pattern have been found in some old aneuploid BED lines. Although such lines were only rarely examined both at an early and a late stage in culture making direct comparisons impossible, one may assume that the inconsistencies observed were examples of secondary phenotypic alterations in vitro. Because of individuality among BL lines even at the time of establishment, a similar assumption about the nature of aberrant phenotypic characteristics found in old BL lines is more difficult to make. Only the changes in old BED lines will therefore be described.

The regular evolution of BED lines toward monoclonality (Sect. D) and aneuploidy (Sect. F.II) during the first 1 – 2 years of continous culture is only rarely correlated with any change in phenotypic characteristics, with the exception of growth properties (Nilsson, 1977). In fact, BED lines have a remarkable stability in the expression of isoenzymes such as phosphoglucomutase (PGM) and G-6-PD (Fialkow, personal communication), Ig and β_2-μ synthesis, and cell surface characteristics (Moore, 1972; Nilsson and Pontén, 1975; Nilsson, 1977).

The "abnormal" phenotypic expressions observed in old BED lines in our laboratory are summarized in Table 7. It should be noted that most old and monoclonal BED lines grow better in vitro than the polyclonal, newly established ones, as is to be expected, since the fastest growing cell clone will become selected during the gradual evolution toward monoclonality. The medium requirements are less stringent and the growth rate is usually higher in old lines.

It is also notable that some secondarily altered BED lines have acquired phenotypic characteristics which are commonly encountered among malignant EBV-carrying and EBV genome-negative hematopoietic cell lines, i. e., the capacity for colony formation in agarose and a potential for tumor formation subcutaneously in nude mice (Sect. E. VII). It is therefore possible that a full "malignant transformation" of BED cells can occur spontaneously during prolonged in vitro cultivation.

Table 7. Secondary phenotypic alterations in lymphoblastoid (BED) lines during long-term cultivation

Type of alteration	Reference
Shortened doubling time	Nilsson, 1977a
Growth in low serum concentrations	Nilsson, unpublished observations
Growth in Eagle's medium	Nilsson, unpublished observations
Increased frequency of surface-attached cells	Nilsson, unpublished observations
Growth in agarose	Nilsson et al., 1977b
Morphologic changes (e. g., Fig. 3b)	Nilsson and Pontén, 1975
Change in cytochemical profile (cytoplasmic fat)	Sundström and Nilsson, 1977
Increased expression of Fc receptors	Huber et al., 1976
Increased Con A-induced agglutinability	Glimelius et al., 1975
Increased expression of HL-A and β_2-μ	Welsh et al., 1977
Increased or decreased secretion of β^2-μ	Nilsson et al., 1974
In balance of Ig synthesis	
surface expression	see Sect. E.V.1
synthesis	see Sect. E.V.1
Tumorigenicity	Nilsson et al., 1977b

H. EBV GENOME-NEGATIVE HEMATOPOIETC CELL LINES

All EBV genome-negative hematopoietic cell lines seem to be representative of the malignant cell population of the donor as evidenced by such features as monoclonal derivation, production of Ig identical to that produced by the tumor in vivo, aneuploidy, and a potential for growth subcutaneously in nude mice. The frequency of establishment is low (Table 4), illustrating the unique ease by which EBV-carrying BL biopsy cells can be grown in vitro.

I. BURKITT'S LYMPHOMA LINES

Lymphomas with histopathologic features indistinguishable from those of the African BL occur at a low frequency in other parts of the world. In contrast to African BL, the cells of such lymphomas seem only rarely to carry EBV genomes, as studied by nucleic acid hybridization or EBNA tests (Pagano et al., 1973; Nonoyama et al., 1974; Klein et al., 1974, 1975; Andersson et al., 1976b; Bornkamm et al., 1976; Epstein et al., 1976; Gravell et al., 1976; Ben-Bassat et al., 1977; Goldblum et al., 1977), and respond poorly to therapy (Ziegler and Carbone, 1966). It has been suggested that EBV-negative BL, including the rare cases found in Africa (Lindahl et al., 1974; Klein et al., 1974), is a disease distinct from EBV-associated BL (zur Hausen, 1975) (Chap. 14).

In a few cases it has been possible to establish cell lines from EBV-negative BL (Tables 2 and 3). The lines have been derived from one African (Menezes et al., 1975), two American (Klein et al., 1975; Epstein et al., 1976), one Israeli (Ben-Bassat et al., 1977), and one Japanese BL (Miyoshi et al., 1977b).

The EBV-negative lines have many similarities to the two EBV-negative lymphocytic lymphoma lines of Nilsson and Sundström (1974) but also resemble EBV-positive BL lines. In contrast, they are all easily distinguishable from the BED type of EBV-carrying lines. Like all other malignant cell lines, they have individually unique features in addition to those common to other BL and lymphocytic lymphoma lines (Table 8).

All the EBV-negative BL lines seem to have been established with some difficulty; the BJAB (Menezes et al., 1975) only after almost 2 months of poor growth, the Ramos (Klein et al., 1975) after a lag of 3 weeks, the SU-AmB-1 (Epstein et al., 1976) with feeder cells, the DG-75 after 8 weeks, and the JBL after 6 weeks (Miyoshi et al., 1977b). Information about growth properties is only available for DG-75, BJAB, and Ramos. The two latter lines appear to be relatively difficult to grow and have a comparatively pronounced sensitivity to saturation density conditions and low concentrations of serum (Steinitz and Klein, 1975, 1976). However, DG-75 grows vigorously with a short doubling time (18–20 h) and an extremely high maximal cell density (5×10^6 cells/ml). All lines carry S-Ig of the IgM type while the expression of other B-lymphocyte surface markers varies. Three of the lines (Ramos, DG-75, SU-AmB-1) have the chromosome

Table 8. Characteristics of EBV genome-negative BL lines

Characteristic	Cell line				
	BJAB	RAMOS	SU-AmB-1	JBL	DG-75
Establishment	slow	like BL[EBV+]	feeder cells used	slow	slow
Growth in low serum concentration	poor	poor	n.t.[b]	n.t.	n.t.
Lymphocyte surface markers					
S-Ig	IgM κ	IgM λ	IgM	IgM λ	IgM κ
Fc receptor (Aggr. Ig)	n.t.	(+)	(+)	n.t.	−
Fc receptor	(+)	n.t.	−	+	n.t.
C receptor	+	+	−	+	−
EBV receptor	+	+	−	n.t.	−
SRBC receptor (E)	−	−	−	−	−
Tumorigenicity in nude mice	+	+	n.t.	+[a]	−
Chromosome 14 marker	−	+	+	−	+
BL[EBV+] surface glycoprotein pattern	−	+	n.t.	n.t.	+

[a] Tumorigenic in hamsters.   [b] Not tested.

14 marker (Sect. F.I). The surface glycoprotein pattern of DG-75 and Ramos was similar to that of EBV genome-containing BL lines (Nilsson et al., 1977a) while in the BJAB line some of the major glycoproteins had different molecular weights.

Since the number of lines examined is limited, the present results from studies on the phenotype of EBV-negative BL lines do not allow any general conclusions about possible biologic differences between EBV-negative and EBV-positive BL.

However, EBV-negative BL lines have been useful tools in studies on the biologic properties of EBV. Comparative studies from Klein's group have resulted in some interesting information on phenotypic changes in lymphocytes following EBV infection (Steinitz and Klein, 1975, 1976, 1977; Yefenof and Klein, 1976; Yefenof et al., 1977b). The EBV-converted BJAB and Ramos sublines were found to differ from the parental lines in being less dependent on serum and less sensitive to saturation-density conditions. Furthermore, the introduction of the EBV genome was correlated with impaired lateral diffusion of surface glycoproteins as evidenced by a reduced ability to form caps after staining with fluorescein labeled anti-IgM and Con A, and by an increased Con A-induced agglutinability. Recently, Yefenof et al. (1978) have also reported a reduced ability to shed S-Ig.

II. NON-BURKITT'S LYMPHOMA MALIGNANT HEMATOPOIETIC CELL LINES: COMPARATIVE ASPECTS

Lines derived from leukemia, myeloma, and non-BL lymphoma have not usually been found to carry EBV; the few exceptions are shown in Tables 2 and 3. It is not within the scope of this review to detail the characteristics of these lines. However, some important similarities and differences between the cells of BL lines and those of other lymphocytic lymphoma lines expressing B cell markers should be stressed.

The following similarities between BL and lymphocytic lymphoma lines (U-698 and U-715) are notable: (1) the morphologic homogeneity within each line, (2) the slow and loose attachment to feeder fibroblasts or glia cells, (3) the growth in suspension as single cells or loose clumps, (4) the synthesis of monoclonal Ig usually expressed at the cell surface but not secreted, (5) the aneuploid karyotype with a $14q^+$ marker, (6) the tumorigenicity subcutaneously in nude mice with only few exceptions, and (7) the identical pattern of major surface glycoproteins.

Other features of non-BL B lymphoma lines are dissimilar from those observed in BL lines: (1) the efficiency of establishment is low, (2) growth is only possible in rich media, (3) lines have been dependent on the presence of feeder cells for survival during the first few months in vitro, and (4) Con A-induced agglutinability is comparatively low while capping with Con A is more rapid than in BL lines.

In conclusion, the two lymphocytic lymphoma lines have many features in common with BL lines. Both types of tumor may therefore be derived from cells in closely similar stages of lymphoid differentiation.

I. CONCLUDING REMARKS

By comparative studies on functional characteristics and surface properties, chromo-somal analyses, and tests for tumorigenicity in nude mice, it has been possible to distinguish two distinct types of EBV-carrying human lymphoid cell lines – BL and BED lines (Nilsson and Pontén, 1975). The BL type of line has only been derived from BL tumor tissue and is charcterized by monoclonal derivation, morphologic ste-reotypia within each line, aneuploidy with a chromosome 14 marker almost always present, a potential for tumor formation subcutaneously in nude mice, and a characteristic surface glycoprotein pattern with some similarities to that of resting B lymphocytes. The BED type of EBV-carrying lymphoid cell line may be derived spontaneously from normal or neoplastic hematopoietic tissue from EBV-seropositive donors or by in vitro immortalization of human B lymphocytes by EBV. The most important features of the BED lines are polyclonal derivation, morphologic hetero-geneity within individual lines, diploidy, capacity for secretion of Ig, no capacity for growth subcutaneously in nude mice, and a basic surface glycoprotein pattern distinct from that of BL lines and similar to that of mitogen-stimulated B lymphoblasts. Individual BED lines are indistinguishable from each other, while in the group of BL lines each line has its own characteristic phenotypic profile.

All these differences are regularly found only when cell lines are characterized shortly after establishment. The BED lines will become monoclonal and aneuploid within 1–2 years of continous cultivation. The aneuploidy may be followed by changes of the phenotypic characteristics, sometimes in the direction of a more "malignant" phenotype. However, no secondarily altered BED line has proved impossible to distinguish from a BL line, since the acquisition of a chromosome 14 marker and a "lymphoma" major surface glycoprotein pattern has never been encountered.

The finding of two biologically distinct types of EBV-carrying cell lines, both apparently derived from EBV-carrying B lymphocytes, suggests that EBV infection per se will only make the B lymphocyte immortal in vitro and that additional changes are needed to give the immortal cell the potential for autonomous growth in vivo. The studies on BL and secondarily altered BED lines suggest that these other changes somehow involve chromosomal rearrangements and in particular the presence of a chromosome 14 alteration.

REFERENCES

Adams, A., Lidin, B., Strander, H., Cantell, K.: Spontaneous interferon production and Epstein-Barr virus antigen expression in human lymphoid cell lines. J. Gen. Virol. **28**, 219–223 (1975)

Adams, R. A., Flowers, A., Davis, B. J.: Direct implantation and serial transplantation of human lymphoblastic leukemia in hamsters, SB 2. Cancer Res. **28**, 1121–1125 (1968)

Adams, R. A., Foley, G. E., Farber, S., Flowers, A., Lazarus, H., Hellerstein, E. E.: Serial transplantation of Burkitt's tumor (EB 3) cells in newborn Syrian hamsters and its facilitation by antilymphocyte serum. Cancer Res. **30**, 338–345 (1970)

Adams, R. A., Hellerstein, E. E., Pothier, L., Foley, G. E., Lazarus, H., Stuart, A. B.: Malignant potential of a cell line isolated from the peripheral blood in infectious mononucleosis. Cancer **27**, 651–657 (1971)

Adams, R. A., Pothier, L., Hellerstein, E. E., Boileau, G.: Malignant immunoblastoma: immunoglobulin synthesis and the progression to leukemia in heterotransplanted acute lymphoblastic leukemia, chronic lymphatic leukemia, lymphoma, and infectious mononucleosis. Cancer **31**, 1397–1407 (1973)

Andersson, L. C., Wasastjerna, C., Gahmberg, C. G.: Different surface glycoprotein patterns on human T-, B- and leukemic lymphocytes. Int. J. Cancer **17**, 40–46 (1976 a)

Andersson, L. C., Gahmberg, C. G., Nilsson, K., Wigzell, H.: Surface glycoprotein patterns of normal and malignant human lymphoid cells. I. T cells, T blasts and leukemic T cell lines. Int. J. Cancer **20**, 702–707 (1977)

Andersson, M., Klein, G., Ziegler, J. L., Henle, W.: Association of Epstein-Barr viral genome with American Burkitt lymphoma. Nature **260**, 357–359 (1976b)

Armstrong, D.: Serial cultivation of human leukemic cells. Proc. Soc. Exp. Biol. Med. **122**, 475–481 (1966)

Baskin, B. L., Meltz, S. K., Glade, P.: Antigen responsiveness of an established human B-lymphoid cell line. I. Evidence for a surface receptor for Candida antigen detected by direct migration inhibition. Cellular Immunol. **26**, 264–273 (1976a)

Baskin, B. L., Meltz, S. K., Glade, P. R.: Antigen responsiveness of an established human B-lymphoid cell line. II. Loss of Candida antigen responsiveness following exposure of cells to specific anti-human immunoglobulin antisera. Cellular Immunol. **26**, 274–283 (1976b)

Béchet, J. M., Nilsson, K., Klein, G.: Polyclonal origin of lymphoblastoid cell lines established from normal and neoplastic human lymphoid tissue. In: Oncogenesis and herpesviruses. Biggs, P. M., de-Thé, G., Payne L. N. (eds.), pp. 249–252. Lyon: IARC 1972

Béchet, J. M., Nilsson, K., Pontén, J.: Establishment of multiple lymphoblastoid lines from single lymph nodes and study of their Ig synthesis. Int. J. Cancer **11**, 58–63 (1973)

Béchet, J. M., Fialkow, P., Nilsson, K., Klein, G.: Immunoglobulin synthesis and glucose-6-phosphate dehydrogenase as cell markers in human lymphoblastoid cell lines. Exp. Cell Res. **89**, 275–282 (1974)

Belpomme, D., Sewan, G., Doré, J.-F., Veanal, A.-M., Berumen, L., le Borgue de Kaouel, C., Mathé, G.: Established cell line (IcI 101) obtained from frozen human lymphoblastic leukemia cells: Morphologoical and immunological comparison with the patient's fresh cells. Eur. J. Canc. **5**, 55–59 (1969)

Belpomme, D., Minowada, J., Moore, G. E.: Are some human lymphoblastoid cell lines established from leukemic tissues actually derived from normal leukocytes? Cancer **30**, 282–287 (1972)

Ben-Bassat, H., Goldblum, N., Manny, N., Sachs, L.: Mobility of Concanavalin A receptors on the surface membrane of lymphocytes from normal persons and patients with chronic lymphocytic leukemia. Int. J. Cancer **14**, 367–371 (1974)

Ben-Bassat, H., Goldblum, N.: Concanavalin A receptors on the surface membrane of lymphocytes from patients with Hodgkin's disease and other malignant lymphomas. Proc. Natl. Acad. Sci. USA **72**, 1046–1049 (1975)

Ben-Bassat, H., Goldblum, N., Mitrani, S., Klein, G., Johansson, B.: Concanavalin A receptors on the surface membrane of lymphocytes from patients with African Burkitt's lymphoma and lymphoma cell lines. Int. J. Cancer **17**, 448–454 (1976)

Ben-Bassat, H., Goldblum, N., Mitrani, S., Goldblum, T., Yoffey, J. M., Cohen, M. M., Bentwich, Z., Ramot, B., Klein, E., Klein, G.: Establishment in continuous culture of a new type of lymphocyte from a "Burkitt-like" malignant lymphoma (Line D. G.-75). Int. J. Cancer **19**, 27–33 (1977)

Benyesh-Melnick, M., Fernbach, D. J., Lewis, R. T.: Studies on human leukemia. I. Spontaneous lymphoblastoid transformation of fibroblastic bone marrow cultures derived from leukemic and non-leukemic children. J. Natl. Cancer Inst. **31**, 1311–1325 (1963)

Benyesh-Melnick, M., Fernbach, D. J., Dessy, S., Lewis, R. T.: Studies on acute leukemia and infectious monoculeosis of childhood. III. Incidence of spontaneous lymphoblastoid transformation in bone marrow cultures. J. Natl. Canc. Inst. **40**, 111–122 (1968a)

Benyesh-Melnick, M., Phillips, C. F., Lewis, R. T., Seidel, E. H.: Studies on acute leukemia and infectious mononucleosis of childhood. IV. Continuous propagation of lymphoblastoid cells from spontaneously transformed bone marrow cultures. J. Natl. Canc. Inst. **40**, 123–134 (1968b)

Berman, L. D.: Lack of correlation between characteristics, agglutinability by plant lectins and the malignant phenotype. Int. J. Cancer **15**, 973–979 (1975)

Bernoco, D., Glade, P. R., Broder, S., Miggiano, V. C., Hirschhorn, K., Ceppellini, R.: Stability of HL-A and appearance of other antigens (LIVA) at the surface of lymphoblasts grown in vitro. Folia Hematol. **54**, 795–895 (1969)

Bichel, J.: Cultivation of leukemic cells in tissue culture. Acta Pathol. Microbiol. Scand. **31**, 410–419 (1952)

Bishun, N. P., Sutton, R.: Cytogenetic and other studies on the EB 4 line of Burkitt tumour cells. Br. J. Cancer **21**, 675–678 (1967)

Bloom, A. D., Choi, K. W., Lamb, B. J.: Immunoglobulin production by human lymphocytoid lines and clones: Absence of genic exclusion. Science **172**, 382–384 (1971)

Bloom, A. D., Wong, A., Tsuchimoto, T.: Bursa-dependent lymphocyte function in established cell lines: An in vitro model for the study of immunoglobulin and specific antibody synthesis. In: Birth defects.

Vol. IX: Long-term lymphocyte cultures in human genetics. Bergsma, D., Smith, G. F., Bloom, A. D. (eds.), pp. 62–72. New York: The National Foundation, March of Dimes 1973

Bochkov, N. P., Lopuchin, J. M., Kuleshow, N. P., Kovalchuk, L. V.: Cytogenetic study of patients with ataxia-telangiectasia. Humangenetik **24**, 115–128 (1974)

Bodmer, W. F., Jones, E. A., Young, D., Goodfellow, P. N., Bodmer, J. G., Dick, H. M., Steel, C. M.: Serology of human Ia type antigens detected in lymphoid lines: An analysis of the 6th Workshop sera. In: Histocompatibility Testing. Kiesmeyer-Nielsen, F. (ed.), pp. 677–684. Copenhagen: Munksgaard 1975

Bornkamm, G. W., Stein, H., Lennert, K., Ruggeberg, F., Bartels, H., zur Hausen, H.: Attempts to demonstrate virus-specific sequences in human tumors. IV. EB viral DNA in European Burkitt lymphoma and immunoblastic lymphadenopathy with excessive plasmacytosis. Int. J. Cancer **17**, 177–181 (1976)

Broder, S. W., Glade, P. R., Hirschhorn, K.: Establishment of long-term lines from small aliquots of normal lymphocytes. Blood **35**, 539–542 (1970)

Brodsky, A. L., Hurd, E. R.: Enhanced establishment of lymphoblastoid cell lines with the ficollhypaque density gradient. Proc. Soc. Exp. Biol. Med. **147**, 612–615 (1974)

Buell, D. N., Fahey, J. L.: Limited periods of gene expression in immunoglobulin-synthesizing cells. Science **164**, 1524–1525 (1969)

Carpenter, G., Lembach, K. J., Morrison, M. M., Cohen, W.: Characterization of the binding of ^{125}I-labeled epidermal growth factor to human fibroblasts. J. Biol. Chem. **250**, 4297–4304 (1975)

Caspersson, T., Zech, L., Johansson, C., Modest, E. J.: Identification of human chromosomes by DNA-binding fluorescing agents. Chromosoma **30**, 215–227 (1970)

Chandra, S., Moore, G. E., Brandt, P. M.: Similarity between leukocyte cultures from cancerous and noncancerous human subjects: An electron microscopic study. Cancer Res. **28**, 1982–1989 (1968)

Chang, R. S., Hsieh, M.-W., Blankenship, W.: Cell line initiation from cord blood leukocytes treated with viruses, chemicals and radiation. J. Natl. Cancer Inst. **47**, 479–483 (1971a)

Chang, R. S., Hsieh, M.-W., Blankenship, W.: Initiation and establishment of lymphoid cell lines from blood of healthy persons. J. Natl. Cancer Inst. **47**, 469–477 (1971b)

Chessin, L. N., Glade, P. P., Kasel, J. A., Moses, H. L., Heberman, R. B., Hirshaut, Y.: N. I. H. Clinical Staff Conference. The circulatory lymphocyte, its role in infectious mononucleosis. Ann. Intern. Med. **69**, 333–359 (1968)

Chu, E. W., Whang, J. J. K., Rabson, A. S.: Cytogenetic studies of lymphoma cells from an American patient with a tumor similar to Burkitt's tumors in African children. J. Natl. Cancer Inst. **37**, 885–891 (1966)

Clarkson, B.: Formal discussion: On the cellular origins and distinctive features of cultured cell lines derived from patients with leukemias and lymphomas. Cancer Res. **26**, 2483–2488 (1967)

Clarkson, B., Strife, A., de Harven, E.: Continuous culture of seven new cell lines (SK-L1 to 7) from patients with acute leukemia. Cancer **20**, 926–947 (1967)

Clements, G. B., Klein, G., Povey, S.: Production by EBV infection of an EBNA-positive subline from an EBNA-negative human lymphoma cell line without detectable EBV DNA. Int. J. Cancer **16**, 125–133 (1975)

Cooper, E. H., Hughes, D. T., Topping, N. E.: Kinetics and chromosome analysis of tissue culture lines derived from Burkitt lymphomata. Br. J. Cancer **20**, 102–113 (1966)

Christofinis, G. J.: Chromosome and transplantation results of a human leukocyte cell line derived from a healthy individual. Cancer **24**, 649–651 (1969)

Deal, D. R., Gerber, P., Chisari, F. V.: Heterotransplantation of two human lymphoid cell lines transformed *in vitro* by Epstein-Barr virus. J. Natl. Cancer Inst. **47**, 771–780 (1971)

Deinhardt, F., Burnside, J.: Spontaneous interferon production in cultures of a cell line from a human myeloblastic leukemia. J. Natl. Cancer Inst. **39**, 681–683 (1967)

de-Thé, G., Ho, H. C., Kwan, H. C., Desgranges, C., Favre, M. C.: Nasopharyngeal carcinoma (NPC). I. Types of cultures derived from tumour biopsies and non-tumour tissues of Chinese patients with special reference to lymphoblastoid transformation. Int. J. Cancer **6**, 189–206 (1970)

Dick, H. M., Steel, C. M., Crichton, W. B.: HL-A typing of cultured peripheral lymphoblastoid cells. Tissue Antigens **2**, 85–93 (1972)

Dick, H. M., Bodmer, W. F., Bodmer, J. G., Steel, C. M., Crichton, W. B., Evans, J.: HL-A typing of lymphoblastoid cell lines. In: Histocompatibility Testing. Kiessmeyer-Nielsen, F. (ed.), pp. 671–676. Copenhagen: Munksgaard 1975

Diehl, V., Henle, G., Henle, W., Kohn, G.: Demonstration of a herpes group virus in cultures of peripheral leucocytes from patients with infectious mononucleosis. J. Virol. **2**, 663–669 (1968)

Diehl, V., Henle, G., Henle, W., Kohn, G.: Effect of a herpes group virus (EBV) on growth of peripheral leucocyte cultures. In Vitro **4**, 92–99 (1969)

Diehl, V., Johansson, B.: Establishment of peripheral lymphoid cell cultures from patients with Hodgkin's disease depending on Epstein-Barr-Virus-reactivity and cellular immunity. Blut, **34**, 227–236 (1977 a)

Diehl, V., Krause, P., Hellriegel, K. P., Busche, M., Schedel, I., Laskewitz, E.: Lymphoid cell lines: *in vitro* cell markers in correlation to tumorigenicity in nude mice. In: Immunological diagnosis of leukemias and lymphomas. Thierfelder, T., Rodt, H., Thiel, E. (eds.), pp. 289–296. Berlin, Heidelberg, New York: Springer 1977b

Douglas, S. D., Fudenberg, H. H., Glade, P. R., Chessin, L. N., Moses, H. L.: Fince structure of leukocytes in infectious mononucleosis: In vivo and in vitro studies. Blood **34**, 42–51 (1969)

Dutrillaux, B., Lejeune, J.: Sur une nouvelle technique d'analyse du caryotype humain. C. R. Acad. Sci. (Paris) **272**, 2638–2640 (1971)

Epstein, A. L., Kaplan, H. S.: Biology of the human malignant lymphomas. I. Establishment in continuous cell culture and heterotransplantation of diffuse histiocytic lymphomas. Cancer **34**, 1851–1872 (1974)

Epstein, A. L., Henle, W., Henle, G., Hewetson, J. F., Kaplan, H. S.: Surface marker characteristics and Epstein-Barr virus studies of two established North American Burkitt's lymphoma cell lines. Proc. Natl. Acad. Sci. USA **73**, 228–232 (1976)

Epstein, A. L., Levy, R., Henle, W., Henle, G., Kaplan, H.: Biology of the human malignant lymphomas. IV. Functional characterization of ten diffuse histiocytic lymphoma cell lines. Cancer (in press) (1978)

Epstein, M. A.: Transformation in vivo – a review. In: Oncogenesis and herpesviruses II. de-Thé, G., Epstein, M. A., zur Hausen, H., (eds.), Part 2, pp. 141–151. Lyon: IARC 1975

Epstein, M. A., Achong, B. G.: Fine structural organization of human lymphoblasts of a tissue culture strain (EB1) from Burkitt's lymphoma. J. Natl. Cancer Inst. **34**, 241–253 (1965)

Epstein, M. A., Barr, Y. M.: Cultivation *in vitro* of human lymphoblasts from Burkitt's malignant lymphoma. Lancet **1964 I**, 252–253

Epstein, M. A., Barr, Y. M.: Characteristics and mode of growth of a tissue culture strain (EBl) of human lymphoblasts from Burkitt's lymphoma. J. Natl. Cancer Inst. **34**, 231–240 (1965)

Epstein, M. A., Achong, B. G., Barr, Y. M.: Virus particles in cultured lymphoblasts from Burkitt's lymphoma. Lancet **1964 a I**, 702–703

Epstein, M. A., Barr, Y. M., Achong, B. G.: A second virus-carrying tissue culture strain (EB2) of lymphoblasts from Burkitt's lymphoma. Pathol. Biol. (Paris) **12**, 1233–1234 (1964b)

Epstein, M. A., Barr, Y. M., Achong, B. G.: The behaviour and morphology of a second tissue culture strain (EB2) of lymphoblasts from Burkitt's lymphoma. Br. J. Cancer **19**, 108–115 (1965 a)

Epstein, M. A., Barr, Y. M., Achong, B. G.: Studies with Burkitt's lymphoma. Wistar Inst. Symp. Monogr. **4**, 69–82 (1965b)

Epstein, M. A., Henle, G., Achong, B. G., Barr, Y. M.: Morphological and biological studies on a virus in cultured lymphoblasts from Burkitt's lymphoma. J. Exp. Med. **121**, 761–770 (1965 c)

Epstein, M. A., Barr, Y. M., Achong, B. G.: Preliminary observations on new lymphoblast strains (EB4, EB5) from Burkitt tumours in a British and a Ugandan patient. Br. J. Cancer **20**, 475–479 (1966 a)

Epstein, M. A., Achong, B. G., Barr, Y. M., Zajac, B., Henle, G., Henle, W.: Morphological and virological investigations on cultured Burkitt tumor lymphoblasts (strain Raji). J. Natl. Cancer Inst. **37**, 547–559 (1966b)

Evans, J., Steel, M., Arthur, E.: A hemagglutination inhibition technique for detection of immunoglobulins in supernatants of human lymphoblastoid cell lines. Cell **3**, 153–158 (1974)

Evrin, P. E., Nilsson, K.: B_2-microglobulin production in vitro by hematopoietic, mesenchymal and epithelial cells. J. Immunol. **112**, 137–144 (1974)

Fagraeus, A., Nilsson, K., Lidman, K., Norberg, R.: Reactivity of smooth-muscle antibodies, surface ultrastructure, and mobility in cells of human hematopoietic cell lines. J. Natl. Cancer Inst. **55**, 783–789 (1975)

Fahey, J. L., Finegold, I., Rabson, A. S., Manaker, R. A.: Immunoglobulin synthesis in vitro by established human cell lines. Science **152**, 1259–1261 (1966)

Fahey, J. L., Finegold, I.: Synthesis of immunoglobulins in human cell lines. Cold Spring Harbor Symp. Quant. Biol. **32**, 283–289 (1967)

Ferrone, S., Pellegrino, M. A., Reisfeld, R. A.: A rapid method for direct HL-A typing of cultured lymphoid cells. J. Immunol. **107**, 613–615 (1971)

Fialkow, P. J.: Clonal origin of human tumors. Biochim. Biophys. Acta **458**, 283–321 (1976)

Fialkow, P. J.: Glucose-6-phosphate dehydrogenase (G-6-PD) markers in Burkitt lymphoma and other malignancies. In: Immunological diagnosis of leukemias and lymphomas. Thierfelder, S., Rodth, H., Thiel, E. (eds.), pp. 297–305. Berlin, Heidelberg, New York: Springer 1977

Fialkow, P. J., Klein, G., Gartler, S. M., Clifford, P.: Clonal origin for individual Burkitt tumours. Lancet 1970 I, 384–386

Fialkow, P. J., Klein, G., Giblett, R. E., Gothoskar, B., Clifford, P.: Foreign-cell contamination in Burkitt tumours. Lancet 1971 I, 883–886

Fialkow, P. J., Klein, E., Klein, G., Clifford, P., Singh, S.: Immunoglobulin and glucose-6-phosphate dehydrogenase as markers of cellular origin in Burkitt lymphoma. J. Exp. Med. 138, 89–102 (1973)

Finegold, I., Fahey, J. L., Granger, H.: Synthesis of immunoglobulins by human cell lines in tissue culture. J. Immunol. 99, 839–848 (1967)

Finegold, I., Fahey, J. L., Dutcher, T.: Immunofluorescent studies of immunoglobulins in human lymphoid cells in continuous culture. J. Immunol. 101, 366–373 (1968)

Flier, S. J., Glade, P. R., Broder, S. W., Hirschhorn, K.: Lymphocyte stimulation by allogeneic and autochthonous cultured lymphoid cells. Cell. Immunol. 1, 596–602 (1970)

Foley, G. E., Lazarus, H., Farber, S., Uszman, B. G., Boone, B. A., McCarthy, R. E.: Continuous culture of human lymphoblasts from peripheral blood of a child with acute leukemia. Cancer 18, 522–529 (1965)

Fresen, K. O., zur Hausen, H.: Establishment of EBNA-expressing cell lines by infection of Epstein-Barr virus (EBV) genome-negative human lymphoma cells with different EBV strains. Int. J. Cancer 17, 161–166 (1976)

Fukuhara, S., Shirakawa, S., Uchino, H.: Specific marker chromosome 14 in malignant lymphomas. Nature 259, 210–211 (1976)

Gahmberg, C. G.: Cell surface proteins: changes during cell growth and malignant transformation. In: Cell surface reviews, Poste, G., Nicolson, G. L. (eds.), pp. 371–421. ASP Biolog. and Medical Press B. B. 1977

Gahmberg, C. G., Andersson, L. C., Nilsson, K.: Surface glycoprotein patterns of human hematopoietic cell lines. In: Oncogenesis and herpesviruses III. de-Thé, G. Henle, W., Rapp, F. (eds.), pp. 649–654. Lyon: IARC 1978

Gavin, J. III, Buell, D. N., Roth, J.: Water-soluble insulin receptors from human lymphocytes. Science 178, 168–169 (1972 a)

Gavin, J. R., Roth, J., Jen, P., Freychet, P.: Insulin receptors in human circulating cells and fibroblasts. Proc. Natl. Acad. Sci. USA 69, 747–751 (1972 b)

Geier, S. G., Cresswell, P.: Rabbit antisera to human B cell alloantigens: Effects on the mixed lymphocyte response. Cell Immunol. 28, 341–354 (1977)

Gerber, P.: Occurence of Epstein-Barr virus in human leukocyte cultures. In Vitro 10, 247–252 (1974)

Gerber, P., Monroe, J. H.: Studies on leukocytes growing in continuous culture derived from normal human donors. J. Natl. Cancer Inst. 40, 855–866 (1968)

Gerber, P., Whang-Peng, J., Monroe, J. H.: Transformation and chromosome changes induced by Epstein-Barr virus in normal human leucocyte cultures. Proc. Natl. Acad. Sci. USA 63, 740–747 (1969)

Ghetie, V., Nilsson, K., Sjöquist, J.: Detection and quantitation of IgG on the surface of human lymphoid cells by rosette formation with protein A-coated sheep red blood cells. Eur. J. Immunol. 4, 500–505 (1974)

Giovanella, B. C., Stehlin, J. S.: Heterotransplantation of malignant tumors in "nude" thymusless mice. I. Breeding and maintenance of nude mice. J. Natl. Cancer Inst. 51, 615–619 (1973)

Giovanella, B. C., Yim, S. O., Stehlin, J. S., Williams, L. J.: Development of invasive tumors in the "nude" mouse after injection of cultured human melanoma cells. J. Natl. Cancer Inst. 48, 1531–1533 (1972)

Glade, P. R., Beratis, N. G.: Long-term lymphoid cell lines in the study of human genetics. Prog. Med. Gen. 1, 1–48 (1976)

Glade, P. R., Chessin, L. N.: Infectious mononucleosis: Immunoglobulin synthesis by cell lines. J. Clin. Invest. 47, 2391–2401 (1968 a)

Glade, P. R., Chessin, L. N.: Synthesis of B_{1c}/B_{1a}-globulin (C′3) by human lymphoid cells. Int. Arch. Allergy 34, 181–187 (1968 b)

Glade, P. R. Hirschhorn, K.: Products of lymphoid cells in continuous culture. Am. J. Pathol. 60, 483–492 (1970)

Glade, P. R., Grotsky, H., Broder, S. W., Hirschhorn, K.: Production of migration inhibitory factors by established lymphoid cell lines. Proceedings of 5th Leukocyte Culture Conference, pp. 607–617. New York: Academic Press 1970

Glade, P. R., Papageorgiou, P. S. Application of human long-term lymphocyte cultures to immunologic problems: Mediators of cellular immunity. In: Birth Defects. Vol. IX: Long-term lymphocyte cultures in human genetics. Bergsma, D., Smith, G. F., Bloom, A. D. (eds.), pp. 90–97. New York: The National Foundation, March of Dimes, 1973 a

Glade, P. R., Papageorgiou, P. S.: Human lymphoid cell lines: Models for immunological analysis. In Vitro **9**, 202–215 (1973 b)

Glade, P. R., Kare, J. A., Moses, H. L., Whang-Peng, J., Hoffman, P. F., Kammermeyer, J. K., Chessin, L. N.: Infectious mononucleosis continuous suspension culture of peripheral blood leukocytes. Nature **217**, 564–565 (1968 a)

Glade, P. R., Hirshaut, Y., Douglas, S. D., Hirschhorn, K.: Lymphoid suspension cultures from patients with viral hepatitis. Lancet **1968 b II**, 1273–1275

Glimelius, B., Nilsson, K., Pontén, J.: Lectin agglutinability of non-neoplastic and neoplastic human lymphoid cells in vitro. Int. J. Cancer **15**, 888–896 (1975)

Goldblum, N., Ben-Bassat, H., Mitrani, S., Andersson-Anvret, M., Goldblum, T., Aghai, E., Ramot, B., Klein, G.: A case of Epstein-Barr virus (EBV) genome-carrying lymphoma in an Isreali arab child. Eur. J. Cancer, **13**, 693–698 (1977)

Golub, S. H., Svedmyr, E. A. J. Hewetson, J. F., Klein, G.: Cellular reactions against Burkitt lymphoma cells. III. Effector cell activity of leukocytes stimulated *in vitro* with autochtonous cultured lymphoma cells. Int. J. Cancer **10**, 157–164 (1972)

Gordon, J., Hough, D., Karpas, A., Smith, J. L.: Immunoglobulin expression and synthesis by human haemic cell lines. Immunology **32**, 559–565 (1977)

Grace, J. T.: Formal discussion: hematopoietic cell cultures and associated herpes-type viruses. Cancer Res. **27**, 2494–2499 (1967)

Granger, G. A., Moore, G. E., White, J. G., Matzinger, P., Sundsmo, J. S., Shupe, S., Kolb, W. P., Kramer, J., Glade, P. R.: Production of lymphotoxin and migration inhibitory factor by established human lymphocytic cell lines. J. Immunol. **104**, 1476–1485 (1970)

Gravell, M., Levine, P. H., McIntyre, R. F., Land, V. J., Pagano, J. S.: Epstein-Barr virus in an American patient with Burkitt's lymphoma: Detection of viral genome in tumor tissue and establishment of a tumor-derived cell line (NAB). J. Natl. Cancer Inst. **56**, 701–704 (1976)

Greaves, M. F., Brown, G., Rickinson, A. B.: Epstein-Barr virus binding sites on lymphocyte subpopulations and the origin of lymphoblasts in cultured lymphoid cell lines and in the blood of patients with infectious mononucleosis. Clin. Immunol. Immunopathol. **3**, 514–524 (1975)

Greaves, M. F., Janossy, G., Roberts, M., Rapson, N. T., Ellis, R. B., Chessels, J., Lister, T. A., Catovsky, D.: Membrane phenotyping: Diagnosis, monitoring and classification of acute "lymphoid" leukaemias. In: Immunological diagnosis of leukemias and lymphomas. Thierfelder, S., Rodt, H., Thiel, E. (eds.), pp. 61–75. Berlin, Heidelberg, New York: Springer 1977

Green, S. S., Sell, K.W.: Mixed leukocyte stimulation of normal peripheral leukocytes by autologous lymphoblastoid cells. Science **170**, 989–999 (1970)

Gripenberg, U., Levan, A., Clifford, P.: Chromosome studies in Burkitt lymphomas. I. Serial studies in a case with bilateral tumors showing different chromosomal stemlines. Int. J. Cancer **4**, 334–349 (1969)

Haase, A. T., Johnson, J. S., Kasel, J. A., Margolis, S., Levy, H. B.: Induction of interferon in lymphoblastoid cell lines. Proc. Soc. Exp. Biol. Med. **133**, 1076–1083 (1970)

Hammond, E.: Ultrastructural characteristics of surface IgM reactive malignant lymphoid cells. Exp. Cell Res. **59**, 359–370 (1970)

Han, T., Moore, G. E., Sokal, J.: In vitro lymphocyte response to autologous cultured lymphoid cells. Proc. Soc. Exp. Biol. Med. **136**, 976–979 (1971)

Han, T., Pauly, J. L., Minowada, J.: Disparity in the production of lymphoblastogenesis inhibition factor by cultured human B and T lymphoid cell lines. Clin. Exp. Immunol. **20**, 73–81 (1975)

Hardy, E. A., Ling, N. R., Knight, S.: Exceptional lymphocyte stimulating capacity of cells from lymphoid cell lines. Nature **223**, 511–512 (1969)

Hayashi, K., Schmid, W.: Tandem duplication q14 by end to end chromosome fusions in ataxia-telangiectasia (AT). Clinical and cytogenetic findings in 5 patients. Humangenetik **30**, 135–141 (1975)

Hayhoe, F. G. J., Cawley, J. C.: Acute leukemia: cellular morphology, cytochemistry and fine structure. Clin. Haematol. **1**, 49–94 (1972)

Hellriegel, K. P., Diehl, V., Krause, P. H., Meier, S., Blankenstein, M., Busche, W.: The significance of chromosomal findings for the differentiation between lymphoma and lymphoblastoid cell lines. In: Haematology and blood transfusion. Immunological diagnosis of leukemias and lymphomas. Thierfelder, S., Rodt, H., Thiel, E. (eds.), pp. 307–313. Berlin, Heidelberg, New York: Springer 1977

Henle, G., Henle, W.: Immunofluorescence in cells derived from Burkitt's lymphoma. J. Bacteriol **91**, 1248–1256 (1966)

Henle, W., Diehl, V., Kohn, G., zur Hausen, H., Henle, G.: Herpes-type virus and chromosome marker in normal leukocytes after growth with irradiated Burkitt cells. Science **157**, 1064–1065 (1967)

Henle, G., Henle, W., Diehl, V.: Relation of Burkitt's tumor-associated herpes-type virus to infectious mononucleosis. Proc. Natl. Acad. Sci. USA **59**, 94–101 (1968)

Hersh, E. M., Drewinko, B.: Specific inhibition of lymphocyte blastogenic responses to mitogens by a factor produced by cultured human malignant lymphoma cells. Cancer Res. **34**, 215–220 (1974)

Hersh, E. M., McCredie, K. B., Freireich, E. J.: Inhibition of in vitro lymphocyte blastogenesis by inhibitor produced by cultured human lymphoblasts. Clin. Exp. Immunol. **17**, 463–473 (1974)

Heyden, H. W. v., Heyden, D. v.: Criteria for the differentiation of lymphoid cell lines. Blut **24**, 323–331 (1974)

Hinuma, Y., Grace, J. T.: Cloning of immunoglobulin-producing human leukemic and lymphoma cells in long term cultures. Proc. Soc. Exp. Biol. Med. **124**, 107–111 (1967)

Hiraki, S., Miyoshi, I., Msuji, H., Kubonishi, I., Matsuda, Y., Nakayama, T., Kishimoto, H., Chen, P., Kimura, I.: Establishment of an Epstein-Barr virus nuclear antigen-negative human B-cell line from an acute lymphoblastic leukemia: Brief communication. J. Natl. Cancer Inst. **59**, 93–94 (1977)

Huang, C. C., Moore, G. E.: Chromosomes of 14 hematopoietic cell lines derived from peripheral blood of persons with and without chromosome anomalies. J. Natl. Cancer Inst. **43**, 1119–1128 (1969)

Huang, C. C., Imamura, T., Moore, G. E.: Chromosomes and cloning efficiencies of hematopoietic cell lines derived from patients with leukemia, melanoma, myeloma and Burkitt lymphoma. J. Natl. Cancer Inst. **43**, 1129–1146 (1969)

Huang, C. C., Minowada, J., Smith, R. T., Osunkoya, B. O.: Reevaluation of relationship between C chromosome marker and Epstein-Barr virus: Chromosome and immunofluorescence analysis of 16 human hematopoietic cell lines. J. Natl. Cancer Inst. **45**, 815–829 (1970)

Huber, C., Sundström, C. C., Nilsson, K., Wigzell, H.: Surface receptors on human haematopoietic cell lines. Clin. Exp. Immunol. **25**, 367–376 (1976)

Hughes, D. T.: Cytogenetical polymorphism and evolution in mammalian somatic cell populations in vivo and vitro. Nature **217**, 518–523 (1968)

Humphreys, R. E., McCune, J. M., Chess, L., Herrman, H. C., Malenka, D. J., Mann, D. L., Parham, P., Schlossman, S. F., Strominger, J. L.: Isolation and immunologic characterization of a human, B-lymphocyte specific, cell surface antigen. J. Exp. Med. **144**, 98–112 (1976)

Ikeuchi, T., Minowada, J., Strandberg, A. A.: Chromosomal variability in ten cloned sublines of a newly established Burkitt's lymphoma cell line. Cancer **28**, 499–512 (1971)

Imamura, T., Moore, G. W.: Ability of human hematopoietic cell lines to form colonies in soft agar. Proc. Soc. Exp. Biol. **128**, 1179–1183 (1968)

Imamura, T., Huang, Ch. C., Minowada, J., Moore, G. E.: Heterologous transplantation of human hematopoietic cell lines. Cancer **25**, 1320–1331 (1970)

Inbar, M., Ben-Bassat, H., Fibach, E., Sachs, L.: Mobility of carbohydrate-containing structures on the surface membrane and the normal differentiation of myeloid leukemic cells to macrophages and granulocytes. Proc. Natl. Acad. Sci. USA **70**, 2577–2581 (1973 a)

Inbar, M., Ben-Bassat, H., Sachs, L.: Difference in the mobility of lectin sites on the surface membrane of normal lymphocytes and malignant lymphoma cells. Int. J. Cancer **12**, 93–99 (1973 b)

Ito, Y., Shiratori, O., Kurita, S., Takahashi, T., Kurita, Y., Ota, K.: Some chracterization of a human cell line (AICHI-4) established from tumorous lymphatic tissue of Hodgkin's disease. J. Natl. Cancer Inst. **41**, 1367–1375 (1968)

Iwakata, S., Grace, J. T.: Cultivation in vitro of myeloblasts from human leukemia. NY State J. Med. **64**, 2279–2282 (1964)

Jarvis, J. E., Ball, G., Rickinson, A. B., Epstein, M. A.: Cytogenetic studies on human lymphoblastoid cell lines from Burkitt's lymphomas and other sources. Int. J. Cancer **14**, 716–721 (1974)

Jensen, F. C., Gwatkin, R. B. L., Biggers, J. D.: A simple culture which allows simultaneous isolation of specific types of cells. Exp. Cell Res. **34**, 440–447 (1964)

Jensen, E. M., Korol, W., Dittmar, S. L., Medrek, T. J.: Virus containing lymphocyte cultures from cancer patients. J. Natl. Cancer Inst. **39**, 745–754 (1967)

Jondal, M.: Antibody-dependent cellular cytotoxicity (ADCC) against Epstein-Barr virus-determined membrane antigens. I. Reactivity in sera from normal persons and from patients with acute infectious mononucleosis. Clin. Exp. Immunol. **25**, 1–5 (1976)

Jondal, M., Klein, G.: Surface markers on human B and T lymphocytes. II. Presence of Epstein-Barr virus receptors on B lymphocytes. J. Exp. Med. **138**, 1365–1378 (1973)

Jondal, M., Klein, G., Oldstone, M. B. A., Bokish, V., Yefenof, E.: An association between complement and Epstein-Barr virus receptors on human lymphoid cells. Scand. J. Immunol. **5**, 401–410 (1976)

Joss, A. W. L., Evans, J., Veitch, D. T., Arthyr, E., Steel, C. M.: Haemagglutinins produced in vitro by human lymphoblastoid cells. J. Immunogen. **3**, 323–328 (1976)

Junge, U., Hoekstra, J., Deinhardt, R.: Stimulation of peripheral lymphocytes by allogeneic and autochthonous mononucleosis lymphocyte cell line. J. Immunol. **106**, 1306–1315 (1971)

Kaiser-McCaw, B., Epstein, A. L., Kaplan, H. S., Hecht, F.: Chromosome 14 translocation in African and North American Burkitt's lymphoma. Int. J. Cancer **19**, 482–486 (1977)

Kamei, H., Moore, G. E.: Antibody production stimulated in vitro in Burkitt lymphoma cells. J. Immunol. **101**, 587–593 (1968)

Kammermeyer, J. K., Root, R. K., Stites, D. P., Glade, P. R., Chessin, L. N.: The detection and characterization of phagocytic cells in established human cell lines synthesizing immunoglobulins. Proc. Soc. Exp. Biol. Med. **129**, 522–527 (1968)

Kaplan, J., Shope, T. C., Peterson (Jr.), W. D.: Epstein-Barr virus-negative human malignant T-cell lines. J. Exp. Med. **139**, 1070–1076 (1974)

Karpas, A., Hayhoe, F. G. J., Greenberger, J. S., Barker, C. R., Cawley, J. D., Lowenthal, L. M., Moloney, W. C.: The establishment and cytological cytochemical and immunological characterization of human haemic cell lines: evidence for heterogeneity. Leukaemia Res. **1**, 35–39 (1977)

Kasel, J. A., Haase, A. T., Glade, P. R., Chessin, L. N.: Interferon production in cell lines derived from patients with infectious mononucleosis. Proc. Soc. Exp. Biol. Med. **128**, 351–353 (1968)

Kennel, S. J.: The K-chains of the immunoglobulin from a continuous culture of human lymphocytes (Daudi) have an unusual molecular size. J. Exp. Med. **139**, 1031–1036 (1974)

Killander, D., Klein, E., Levin, A.: Expression of membrane-bound IgM and HL-A antigens on lymphoblastoid cells in different stages of the cell cycle. J. Immunol. **4**, 327–332 (1974)

Klein, E., Klein, G., Nadkarni, J. Nadkarni, J. J., Wigzell, H., Clifford, P.: Surface IgM specificity on cells derived from a Burkitt's lymphoma. Lancet **1967 II**, 1068–1070

Klein, E., Klein, G., Nadkarni, J. S., Nadkarni, J. J., Wigzell, H., Clifford, K.: Surface IgM-kappa specificity on a Burkitt lymphoma cell in vivo and in derived culture lines. Cancer Res. **28**, 1300–1310 (1968)

Klein, E., Eskeland, T., Inoue, M., Strom, R., Johansson, B.: Surface immunoglobulin-moieties on lymphoid cells. Exp. Cell Res. **62**, 133–148, (1970)

Klein, E., Nilsson, K., Yefenof, E.: An established Burkitt's lymphoma line with cell membrane IgG. Clin. Immunol. Immunopathol. **3**, 575–583 (1975)

Klein, E., Ben-Bassat, H., Neumann, H., Ralph, P., Zeuthen, J., Polliack, A., Vanky, F.: Properties of the K 562 cell lines, derived from a patient with chronic myeloid leukemia. Int. J. Cancer **18**, 421–431 (1976)

Klein, G.: Tumor immunology. Transplant. Proc. **5**, 31–41 (1973)

Klein, G.: Studies on the Epstein-Barr virus genome and the EBV-determined nuclear antigen in human malignant disease. Cold Spring Harbor Symp. Quant. Biol. **39**, 783–790 (1974)

Klein, G., Lindahl, T., Jondal, M., Leibold, W., Menézes, J., Nilsson, K., Sundström, C.: Continuous lymphoid cell lines with characteristics of B cells (bone marrow-derived), lacking the Epstein-Barr virus genome and derived from three human lymphomas. Proc. Natl. Acad. Sci. USA **71**, 3283–3286 (1974)

Klein, G., Giovanella, B., Westman, A., Stehlin, J., Mumford, D.: An EBV-genome-negative cell line established from an American Burkitt lymphoma: Receptor characteristics, EBV infectability and permanent conversion into EBV-positive sublines by in vitro infection. Intervirology **5**, 319–334 (1975)

Knight, S. C., Moore, G. E., Clarkson, B. D.: Stimulation of autochthonous lymphocytes by cells from normal and leukemic lines. Nature **229**, 185–187 (1971)

Kohn, G., Mellman, W. J., Moorhead, P. S., Loftus, J. Henle, G.: Involvement of C-group chromosomes in five Burkitt lymphoma cell lines. J. Natl. Cancer Inst. **38**, 209–222 (1967)

Kohn, G., Diehl, V., Mellman, W. J., Henle, W., Henle, G.: C-group chromosome marker in long-term leucocyte cultures. J. Natl. Cancer Inst. **41**, 795–804 (1968)

Kreuger, R. G., Watkins, A. C., Volkman, L. E.: Attempts to induce cultures of BALB/c myeloma and P3-J Burkitt's lymphoma cells to produce specific phage neutralizing antibody. J. Immunol. **112**, 1415–1419 (1974)

Krishan, A., Raychaudhuri, R., Flowers, A.: Karyotype studies on human leukemic lymphoblasts *in vitro* and serial transplantants in neonatal Syrian hamsters. J. Natl. Cancer Inst. **43**, 1203–1214 (1969)

Kurita, Y., Osato, T., Ito, Y.: Studies on chromosomes of three human cell lines harboring EB virus particles. J. Natl. Cancer Inst. **41**, 1355–1366 (1968)

Lawler, S. D., Reeves, B. R., Hamlin, J. M. E.: A comparison of cytogenetic and histopathology in the malignant lymphomata. Br. J. Cancer **31**, 162–167 (1975)

Lerner, R. A., Hodge, L. D.: Gene expression in synchronized lymphocytes: studies on the control of synthesis of immunoglobulin polypeptides. J. Cell Physiol. **77**, 265–276 (1971)

Lerner, R. A., McConahey, P. J., Jansen, I., Dixon, F.: Synthesis of plasma membrane-associated and secretory immunoglobulin in diploid lymphocytes. J. Exp. Med. **135**, 136–149 (1972)

Lesniak, M. A., Roth, J., Gorden, P., Gavin, III, J. R.: Human growth hormone radioreceptor assay using cultured human lymphocytes. Nature New Biol. **241**, 20–21 (1973)

Lesniak, M. A., Gorden, P., Roth, J., Gavin, III, J. R.: Binding of ^{125}I-human growth hormone to specific receptors in human cultured lymphocytes. J. Biol. Chem. **249**, 1661–1667 (1974)

Levin, A. G., Friberg, Jr. S., Klein, E.: Xenotransplantation of a Burkitt lymphoma culture line with surface immunoglobulin specificity. Nature **222**, 997–998 (1969)

Levy, J. A., Virolainen, M., Defendi, V.: Human lymphoblastoid lines from lymph node and spleen. Cancer **22**, 517–524 (1968)

Levy, J. A., Buell, N. D., Creech, C., Hirshaut, Y., Silverberg, H.: Further chracterization of the WI-L1 and WI-L2 lymphoblastoid lines. J. Natl. Cancer Inst. **46**, 647–652 (1971)

Lindblom, B., Nilsson, K.: HL-A antigens in established human cell lines. International Symposium on HL-A Reagents. Symposium Series on Immunological Standardization **18**, 124–128 (1972)

Lindahl, T., Klein, G., Reedman, B. M., Johansson, B., Singh, S.: Relationship between Epstein-Barr virus (EBV) DNA and the EBV-determined nuclear antigen (EBNA) in Burkitt lymphoma biopsies and other lymphoproliferative malignancies. Int. J. Cancer **13**, 764–772 (1974)

Ling, N. R., Hardy, D. A., Steel, C. M.: Human mixed cell reactions in relation to surveillance of lymphoid tissue. Proceedings of 8th Leukocyte Culture Conference Uppsala. Lindahl-Kiessling, K., Osoba, D. (eds.), pp. 235–241. London: Academic Press 1974

Litwin, S. D., Lin, P. K., Hütteroth, T. H., Cleve, H.: Multiple heavy chain classes and light chain types on surfaces of cultured human lymphoid cells. Nature **246**, 179–181 (1973)

Litwin, S. D., Hütteroth, T. H., Lin, P. K., Kennard, J., Cleve, H.: Immunoglobulin expression of cells from human lymphoblastoid lines. I. Heavy and light chain antigens of the cell surface. J. Immunol. **113**, 661–667 (1974 a)

Litwin, S. D., Hütteroth, T. H., Lin, P. K., Kennard, J., Cleve, H.: Immunoglobulin expression of cells from human lymphoblastoid lines. II. Interrelationship among surface, cellular, and secreted immunoglobulins. J. Immunol. **113**, 668–672 (1974 b)

Litwin, S. D., Lin, P. K.: Phenotypic heterogeneity for cells bearing surface immunoglobulin in human lymphoid lines. Cell. Immunol. **24**, 270–276 (1976)

Long, J. C., Zamecnik, P. C., Aisenberg, A. C., Atkins, L.: Tissue culture studies in Hodgkin's disease. Morphologic, cytogenetic, cell surface, and enzymatic properties of cultures derived from splenic tumors. J. Exp. Med. **145**, 1484–1500 (1977)

Lozzio, C. B., Lozzio, B. B.: Human chronic myelogeneous leukemia cell-line with positive Philadelphia chromosome. Blood **45**, 321–334 (1975)

Lucas, L. S., Whang, J. J. K., Thio, J. H., Manaker, R. A., Zeve, V. H.: Continuous cell culture from a patient with chronic myelogenous leukemia. I. Propagation and presence of Philadelphia chromosome. J. Natl. Cancer Inst. **37**, 753–759 (1966)

Luzatti, A. L., Hengartner, H., Schreier, M. H.: Induction of plaque-forming cells in cultured human lymphocytes by combined action of antigen and EB virus. Nature **269**, 419–420 (1977)

Macek, M., Benyesh-Melnick, M.: Cytogenetic comparison of lymphoblastoid cells containing or lacking EB herpesvirus. Bacteriol. Proc. **154**, (1969)

Macek, M., Seidel, E. H., Lewis, R. T., Brunschwig, J. P., Wimberly, I., Benyesh-Melnick, M.: Cytogenetic studies of EB virus-positive and EB virus-negative lymphoblastoid cell lines. Cancer Res. **31**, 308–321 (1971)

Manolov, G., Manolova, Y.: Marker band in one chromosome 14 from Burkitt lymphomas. Nature **237**, 33–34 (1972)

Mark, J.: Histiocytic lymphomas with the marker chromosome 14q+. Hereditas **81**, 289–292 (1975)

Matsouka, Y., Moore, G. E., Yagi, Y., Pressman, D.: Production of free light chains of immunoglobulin by a hematopoietic cell line derived from a patient with multiple myeloma. Proc. Soc. Exp. Biol. Med. **125**, 1246–1250 (1967)

Matsouka, Y., Takahashi, M., Yagi, Y., Moore, G. E., Pressman, D.: Synthesis and secretion of immunoglobulins by established cell lines of human hematopoietic origin. J. Immunol. **101**, 1111–1120 (1968)

Marx, S. J., Aurbach, G. D., Gavin, III, J. R., Buell, D. W.: Calcitonin receptors on cultured human lymphocytes. J. Biol. Chem. **249**, 6812–6816 (1974)

McCarthy, R. E., Junius, V., Farber, S., Lazarus, H., Foley, G. E.: Cytogenetic analysis of human lymphoblasts in continuous culture. Exp. Cell Res. **40**, 197–200 (1965)

McCaw, K. B., Hecht, F., Harnden, D. G., Teplitz, R. L.: Somatic rearrangement of chromosome 14 in human lymphocytes. Proc. Natl. Acad. Sci. USA **72**, 2071–2075 (1975)

McCombs, R. M., Benyesh-Melnick, M.: Studies on acute leukemia and infectious mononucleosis of childhood. I. Viral interference with lymphoblastoid cells of spontaneously transformed bone marrow cultures. J. Natl. Cancer Inst. **39**, 1187–1196 (1967)

McConahey, P. J., Lerner, R. A., Dixon, F. J.: Quantitation of plasma membrane and cytoplasmic Ig of human diploid lymphocyte clones. Fed. Proc. **30**, 588 (1971)

McCune, J. M., Humphreys, R. E., Yocum, R. R., Strominger, J. L.: Enhanced representation of HL-A antigens on human lymphocytes after mitogenesis induced by phytohemagglutinin or Epstein-Barr virus. Proc. Natl. Acad. Sci. USA **72**, 3206–3209 (1975)

Menezes, J., Leibold, W., Klein, G., Clements, G.: Establishment and characterization of an Epstein-Barr virus (EBV)-negative lymphoblastoid B cell line (BJA-B) from an exceptional, EBV-genome-negative African Burkitt's lymphoma. Biomedicine **22**, 276–284 (1975)

Miles, C. P., O'Neill, F.: Chromosome studies of 8 in vitro lines of Burkitt's lymphoma. Cancer Res. **27**, 392–402 (1967)

Miles, C. P., O'Neill, F., Armstrong, D., Clarkson, B., Keane, J.: Chromosome patterns of human leukocyte established cell lines. Cancer Res. **28**, 481–490 (1968)

Miller, G.: Human lymphoblastoid cell lines and Epstein-Barr virus: a review of their interrelationships and their relevance to the etiology of lymphoproliferative states in man. Yale J. Biol. Med. **43**, 358–384 (1971)

Miller, G.: The oncogenicity of Epstein-Barr virus. J. Infect. Dis. **130**, 187–205 (1974)

Miller, G., Enders, J. F., Lisco, H., Kohn, H. I.: Establishment of lines from normal human leucocytes by co-cultivation with a leucocyte line derived from a leukemic child. Proc. Soc. Exp. Biol. Med. **132**, 247–252, (1969)

Miller, G., Lipman, M.: Release of infectious Epstein-Barr virus by transformed marmoset leukocytes. Proc. Natl. Acad. Sci. USA **70**, 190–194 (1973)

Minnefor, A. B., Halsted, C. C., Seto, D. S. Y., Glade, P. R., Moore, G. E., Carver, D. H.: Interferon production by long term suspension cultures of leucocytes derived from patients with viral and non-viral diseases. J. Infect. Dis. **121**, 442–445 (1970)

Minowada, J., Moore, G. E.: T-lymphocyte cell lines derived from patients with acute lymphoblastic leukemia. In: Comparative leukemia research. Ito, Y., Dutcher, R. M. (eds.), pp. 251–261. Tokyo: University of Tokyo Press 1975

Minowada, J., Klein, G., Clifford, P., Klein, E., Moore, G. E.: Studies of Burkitt lymphoma cells. I. Establishment of a cell line (B35M) and its characteristics. Cancer **20**, 1430–1437 (1967)

Minowada, J., Ohnuma, T., Moore, G. E.: Brief communication: Rosette-forming human lymphoid cell lines. I. Establishment and evidence for origin of thymus-derived lymphocytes. J. Natl. Cancer Inst. **49**, 891–895 (1972)

Minowada, J., Oshimura, M., Tsubota, T., Higby, D. J., Sandberg, A. A.: Human leukemic B-cell lines: Presence of cytogenetic and immunoglobulin markers. Cancer Res. **37**, 3096–3099 (1977a)

Minowada, J., Tsubota, T., Nakazawa, S., Srivastava, B. I. S., Huang, C. C., Oshimura, M., Sonta, S., Han, T., Sinks, L. F., Sandberg, A. A.: Establishment and characterization of leukemic T-cell lines, B-cell lines, and null-cell line: a progress report on surface antigen study of fresh lymphocytic leukemias in man. In: Immunological diagnosis of leukemias and lymphomas. Thierfelder, T., Rodth, H., Thiel, E. (eds.), pp. 241–251. Berlin, Heidelberg, New York: Springer 1977b

Minowada, J., Tsubota, T., Greaves, M. F., Walters, T. R.: A non-T, non-B human leukemia cell line (Nalm-1): establishment of the cell line and presence of leukemia-associated antigens. J. Natl. Cancer Inst. **59**, 83–87 (1977c)

Miyoshi, I., Hiraki, S., Tsubota, T., Kubonishi, I., Matsuda, Y., Nakayama, T., Kishimoto, H., Kimura, I., Masuji, H.: Human B cell, T cell and null cell leukemic cell lines derived from acute lymphoblastic leukemias. Nature **267**, 843–844 (1977a)

Miyoshi, I., Hiraki, S., Kubonishi, I., Matsuda, Y., Kishimoto, H., Nakayama, T., Tanaka, T., Masuji, H., Kimura, I.: Establishment of an Epstein-Barr virus negative B-cell lymphoma line from a Japanese Burkitt lymphoma and its serial passage in hamsters. Cancer **40**, 2999–3003 (1977b)

Moore, G. E.: Cultured human lymphocytes. J. Surg. Oncol. **4**, 320–353 (1972)

Moore, G. E., Ito, E., Ulrich, K., Sandberg, A. A.: Culture of human leukemia cells. Cancer **19**, 713–723 (1966a)

Moore, G. E., Grace, Jr., J. T., Citron, P., Gerner, R. E., Burns, A.: Leukocyte cultures of patients with leukemia and lymphomas. NY State J. Med. **66**, 2757–2764 (1966b)

Moore, G. E., Gerner, R. E., Franklin, H. A.: Culture of normal leukocytes. J. Am. Med. Assoc. **199**, 519–524 (1967)

Moore, G. E., Kitamura, H., Toshima, S.: Morphology of cultured hematopoietic cells. Cancer **22**, 245–267 (1968)

Moore, G. E., Minowada, J.: Human hemapoietic cell lines: A progress report. In: Hemic cells in vitro. Farnes, P. (ed.), pp. 100–114. Baltimore: Williams & Wilkins 1969

Moses, H. L., Glade, P. R., Kasel, J. A., Rosenthal, A. S., Hirshaut, Y., Chessin, L. N.: Infectious mononucleosis: Detection of herpes-like virus and reticular aggregates of small cytoplasmic particles in continuous lymphoid cell lines derived from peripheral blood. Proc. Natl. Acad. Sci. USA **60**, 489–496 (1968)

Möller, G. (ed.): T and B lymphocytes in humans. Transplant. Rev. **16**, (1973)

Möller, G. (ed.): β_2-Microglobulin and HL-A antigens. Transplant. Rev. **21**, (1974)

Möller, G. (ed.): Biochemistry and biology of Ia antigens. Transplant. Rev. **30**, (1976)

Nadkarni, J. S., Nadkarni, J. J., Clifford, P., Manolov, G., Fenyö, E. M., Klein, E.: Characteristics of new cell lines derived from Burkitt lymphomas. Cancer **23**, 64–79 (1969)

Neumann, H., Klein, D., Hauck-Granoth, R., Yachnin, S., Ben-Bassat, H.: Comparative study of alkaline phosphatase acitivity in lymphocytes, mitogen-induced blasts, lymphoblastoid cell lines, acute myeloid leukemia, and chronic lymphatic leukemia cells. Proc. Natl. Acad. Sci. USA **73**, 1432–1436 (1976)

Niederman, J. C., McCollum, R. V., Henle, G., Henle, W.: Infectious mononucleosis: Clinical manifestations in relation to EB virus antibodies J. Am. Med. Assoc. **205**, 205–209 (1968)

Nilsson, K.: Human hematopoietic cells in continuous culture (diss.). Acta Univ. Upsaliensis **107**, (1971a)

Nilsson, K.: Histochemical changes in long term explants of human lymph nodes during lymphoblastoid transformation. Acta Pathol. Microbiol. Scand. A **79**, 243–248 (1971b)

Nilsson, K.: High frequency-establishment of human immunoglobulin producing lymphoblastoid lines from normal and malignant lymphoid tissue and peripheral blood. Int. J. Cancer **8**, 432–442 (1971c)

Nilsson, K.: Characteristics of established human myeloma and lymphoblastoid cell lines in long term culture. A comparative study. Int. J. Cancer **7**, 380–396 (1971d)

Nilsson, K.: Established cell lines as tools in the study of human lymphoma and myeloma cell characteristics. Hematology and blood transfusion. In: Immunological diagnosis of leukemias and lymphomas. Thierfelder, S., Rodt, H., Thiel, E. (eds.), pp. 253–264. Berlin, Heidelberg, New York: Springer 1977

Nilsson, K., Pontén, J.: Classification and biological nature of established human hematopoietic cell lines. Int. J. Cancer **15**, 321–341 (1975)

Nilsson, K., Sundström, C.: Establishment and characteristics of two unique cell lines from patients with lymphosarcoma. Int. J. Cancer **13**, 808–823 (1974)

Nilsson, K., Pontén, J., Philipson, L.: Development of immunocytes and immunoglobulin production in long term cultures from normal and malignant human lymph nodes. Int. J. Cancer **3**, 183–190 (1968)

Nilsson, K., Bennich, H., Johansson, S. G. O., Pontén, J.: Established immunoglobulin producing myeloma (IgE) and lymphoblastoid (IgG) cell lines from an IgE myeloma patient. Clin. Exp. Immunol. **7**, 477–489 (1970a)

Nilsson, K., Nilsson, L., Pontén, J.: Lymphocytes are mobile. (Film). 3rd International Conference on Lymphatic Tissue and Germinal Centers in Immune Reactions. Uppsala, 1970b

Nilsson, K., Klein, G., Henle, G., Henle, W.: The establishment of lymphoblastoid cell lines and its dependence on EBV. Int. J. Cancer **8**, 443–450 (1971)

Nilsson, K., Evrin, P. E., Berggård, L., Pontén, J.: β_2-microglobulin, a homologue of the constant domains of IgG, is produced by both lymphoid and non-lymphoid cells. Nature New Biol. **244**, 44–45 (1973)

Nilsson, K., Evrin, P. E., Welsh, K. I.: Production of β_2-microglobulin by normal and malignant human cell lines and peripheral lymphocytes. Transplant. Rev. **21**, 53–84 (1974)

Nilsson, K., Ghetie, V., Sjöquist, J.: A human lymphoid cell line with an IgG-like membrane component. Eur. J. Immunol. **5**, 518–526 (1975)

Nilsson, K., Andersson, L. C., Gahmberg, C. G., Wigzell, H.: Surface glycoprotein patterns of normal and malignant human lymphoid cells. II. B cells, B blasts and Epstein-Barr virus (EBV) positive and negative B-lymphoid cell lines. Int. J. Cancer **20**, 708–718 (1977a)

Nilsson, K., Giovanella, B. C., Stehlin, J. S., Klein, G.: Tumorigenicity of human hematopoietic cell lines in athymic nude mice. Int. J. Cancer **19**, 337–344 (1977b)

Nonoyama, M., Pagano, J. S.: Detection of Epstein-Barr viral genome in nonproductive cells. Nature New Biol. **233**, 103–106 (1971)

Nonoyama, M., Kawai, Y., Huang, C. H., Pagano, J. S., Hirshaut, Y., Levine, P.: Epstein-Barr virus DNA in Hodgkin's disease, American Burkitt's lymphoma and other human tumors. Cancer Res. **34**, 1228–1231 (1974)

Nowell, P. C.: Phytohemagglutinin: An initiator of mitosis in cultures of normal human leukocytes. Cancer Res. **20**, 462–466 (1960)

Oboshi, S.: Continous suspension culture of human neoplastic lymph nodes in cell culture. Identification and detection of Herpes-type EB-virus. Gann **7**, 191–199 (1969)

O'Conor, G. T., Rabson A. S.: Herpes-like particles in an American lymphoma: preliminary note. J. Natl. Cancer Inst. **35**, 899–903 (1965)

Östberg, L., Rask, L., Nilsson, K., Peterson, P. A.: Independent expression of the two HL-A antigen polypeptide chains. Eur. J. Immunol. **5**, 462–468 (1975)

Osgood, E. E.: Tissue culture in the study of leukocytic function. Ann. NY Acad. Sci. **59**, 806–814 (1958)

Osgood, E. E., Brooke, J. H.: Continous tissue culture of leukocytes from human leukemic blood by application of "gradient" principles. Blood **10**, 1010–1022 (1955)

Osunkoya, B. O.: Various aspects of the Burkitt tumor cell in tissue culture with reference to host defences. In: Treatment of Burkitt's tumor. Burchenal, J. H., Burkitt, D. (eds.), pp. 233–247. Berlin, Heidelberg New York: Springer 1967

Osunkoya, B. O., Mottram, F. C.: Formal discussion: Observations on the establishment of Burkitt's tumor lymphoblasts in serially propagated cultures. Cancer Res. **27**, 2500–2503 (1967)

Osunkoya, B. O., McFarlane, H., Luzatto, L., Udeozo, I. O. K., Mottram, F. C., Williams, A. I. O., Ngu, V. A.: Immunoglobulin synthesis by fresh cells and established cell lines from Burkitt's lymphoma. Immunology **14**, 851–860 (1968)

Oxford, J. M., Harnden, D. G., Parrington, J. M., Delhanty, J. D. A.: Specific chromosome aberrations in ataxia-telangiectasia. J. Med. Genetics **12**, 251–260 (1975)

Pagano, J., Huang, C. H., Levine, P.: Absence of Epstein-Barr viral DNA in American Burkitt's lymphoma. N. Engl. J. Med. **289**, 1395–1399 (1973)

Paltrowitz, I. M., Hirshaut, Y., Papenhausen, P., Henley, W., Hirschhorn, K., Glade, P. R.: Establishment of lymphoid cell lines in patients with common viral diseases. M. Sinai J. Med. NY **38**, 284–292 (1971)

Pantelouris, E. M.: Absence of thymus in a mouse mutant. Nature **217**, 370–371 (1968)

Papageorgiou, P. S., Glade, P. R.: Progress in lymphology. The cultured lymphocyte in clinical and experimental medicine. Lymphology **5**, 80–89 (1972)

Papageorgiou, P. S., Hemley, W. L., Glade, P. R.: Production and characterization of migration inhibitory factor(s) (MIF) of established lymphoid and non-lymphoid cell lines. J. Immunol. **108**, 494–504 (1972)

Papageorgiou, P. S., Sorokin, C. F., Glade, P. R.: Similarity of migration inhibitory factor(s) produced by human lymphoid cell line and phytohemagglutinin and tuberculin-stimulated human peripheral lymphocytes. J. Immunol. **112**, 675–682 (1974)

Papenhausen, P. S., Papageorgiou, P., Hirschhorn, K.: Complement receptor in synchronized cultures of human hematopoietic cell lines. J. Immunol. **114**, 519–521 (1975)

Papermaster, V. M., Papermaster, B. W., Moore, G. E.: Histocompatibility antigens of human lymphocytes in long term culture. Fed. Proc. **28**, 379 (1969)

Pattengale, P. K., Smith, R. W., Gerber, P.: Selective transformation of B lymphocytes by E. B. virus. Lancet **1973 II**, 93–94

Petit, P., Verhiest, A., LeCluse van der Bilt, F., Jongsma, A.: The chromosomes of the EB virus-positive Burkitt cell line P3JHR1K studied by the fluorescent staining technique. Pathol. Eur. **7**, 17–21 (1972)

Philip, P.: Marker chromosome 14q$^+$ in multiple myeloma. Hereditas **80**, 155–156 (1975)

Pious, D., Bodmer, J., Bodmer, W.: Antigenic expression and cross reactions in HL-A variants of lymphoid cell lines. Tissue Antigens **4**, 247–256 (1974)

Pontén, J.: Spontaneous lymphoblastoid transformation of long-term cell cultures from human malignant lymphoma. Int. J. Cancer **2**, 311–325 (1967)

Pontén, J.: Spontaneous and virus induced transformation in cell culture. In: Gard, S., Hallauer, C., Meyer, K. F. (eds.). Vienna, New York: Virology Monographs 8. Springer, 1971

Pontén, J.: Contact Inhibition. In: Cancer. Becker, F. F. (ed.), Vol. 4, pp. 55–100. New York: Plenum 1975

Pope, J. H.: Establishment of cell lines from peripheral leukocytes in infectious mononucleosis. Nature **216**, 810–811 (1967)

Pope, J. H.: Transformation in vitro by herpesviruses, a review. In: Oncogenesis and herpesviruses II. de-Thé, G., Epstein, M. A., zur Hausen, H., (eds.), Part 1, pp. 367–378. Lyon: IARC 1975

Pope, J. H., Achong, B. G., Epstein, M. A.: Burkitt lymphoma in New Guinea: Establishment of a line of lymphoblasts in vitro and description of their fine structure. J. Natl. Canc. Inst. **39**, 933–945 (1967)

Pope, J. H., Horne, M. K., Scott, W.: Transformation of foetal human leucocytes in vitro by filtrates of a human leukemic cell line containing herpes-like virus. Int. J. Cancer **3**, 857–866 (1968)

Povlsen, C. O., Rygaard, J.: Heterotransplantation of human adenocarcinomas of the colon and rectum to the mouse mutant nude. A study of nine consecutive transplantations. Acta Pathol. Microbiol. Scand. A **79**, 159–169 (1971)

Premkumar, E., Singer, P. A., Williamson, A. R.: A human lymphoid cell line secreting immunoglobulin G and retaining immunoglobulin M in the plasma membrane. Cell **5**, 87–92 (1975)

Prigogina, E. L., Fleischman, E. W.: Marker chromosome 14q$^+$ in two non-Burkitt lymphomas. Humangenetik **30**, 109–112 (1975)

Pulvertaft, R. J. V.: Cytology of Burkitt's tumour (African lymphoma). Lancet **1964 a I**, 238–240

Pulvertaft, R. J. V.: Phytohemagglutinin in relation to Burkitt's tumour (African lymphoma). Lancet **1964 b II**, 552–553

Pulvertaft, R. J. V.: A study of malignant tumours in Nigeria by short-term tissue culture. J. Clin. Pathol. **18**, 261–273 (1965)

Rabson, A. S., O'Conor, G. T., Baron, S., Whang, J. J., Legallais, F. Y.: Morphologic, cytogenetic and virologic studies in vitro of a malignant lymphoma from an African child. Int. J. Cancer **1**, 89–106 (1966)

Rabson, A. S., Chu, E. W., Berezesky, I. K., Legallais, F. Y., Grimley, P. M.: Morphological and cytogenetic studies in vitro of surface-adherent lymphoreticular cells derived from Burkitt lymphoma tissue. Int. J. Cancer **5**, 217–222 (1970)

Rapin, A. M. C., Burger, M. M.: Tumor cell surfaces: general alterations detected by agglutinins. Adv. Cancer Res. **20**, 1–92 (1974)

Rappaport, H.: Tumors of the hematopoietic system. Atlas of tumor pathology. Sect. III, Fasc. 8. Washington D. C.: Armed Forces Institute of Pathology 1966

Recher, L., Sinkovics, J. G., Sykes, J. A., Whitescarver, J.: Electron microscopic studies of suspension cultures derived from human leukemic and non leukemic sources. Cancer Res. **29**, 271–285 (1969)

Reedman, B. M., Klein, G.: Cellular localization of an Epstein-Barr virus (EBV) associated complement-fixing antigen in producer and non-producer lymphoblastoid cell lines. Int. J. Cancer **11**, 499–520 (1973)

Reeves, B. R.: Cytogenetics of malignant lymphomas. Studies utilising a Giemsa-banding technique. Humangenetik **20**, 231–250 (1973)

Reisner, E. H. (Jr.): Tissue culture of bone marrow. Ann. NY Acad. Sci. **77**, 487–500 (1959)

Rickinson, A. B., Jarvis, J. E., Crawford, D. H., Epstein, M. A.: Observations on the type of infection by Epstein-Barr virus in peripheral lymphoid cells of patients with infectious mononucleosis. Int. J. Cancer **14**, 704–715 (1974)

Rickinson, A. B., Epstein, M. A., Crawford, D. H.: Absence of infectious Epstein-Barr virus in blood in acute infectious mononucleosis. Nature **258**, 236–238 (1975)

Rickinson, A. B., Finerty, S., Epstein, M. A.: Comparative studies on adult donor lymphocytes infected by EB virus *in vivo* or *in vitro*: origin of transformed cells arising in cocultures with foetal lymphocytes. Int. J. Cancer **19**, 775–782 (1977)

Robinson, J. E., Andiman, W. A., Henderson, E., Miller, G.: Host-determined differences in expression of surface marker characteristics on human and simian lymphoblastoid cell lines transformed by Epstein-Barr virus. Proc. Natl. Acad. Sci. USA **74**, 749–753 (1977)

Rogentine, G. N., Gerber, P.: HL-A antigens of human lymphoid cells in long term tissue culture. Transplantation **8**, 28–37 (1969)

Rogentine, G. N., Gerber, P.: Qualitative and quantitative comparisons of HL-A antigens on different lymphoid cell types from the same individuals. In: Histocompatibility testing. Kiessmeyer-Nielsen, F. (ed.), pp. 333–338. Copenhagen: Munksgaard 1970

Rosén, A., Gergely, P., Jondal, M., Klein, G.: Polyclonal Ig production after Epstein-Barr virus infection of human lymphocytes in vitro. Nature **267**, 52–54 (1977)

Rosenfeld, C., Maciera-Coelho, A.: Mathematical analysis of the establishment of human peripheral blood cell lines. J. Natl. Canc. Inst. **43**, 597–602 (1969)

Rosenfeld, C., Gounter, A., Choquet, C., Venaut, A. M., Kayibinda, B., Pico, J. L., Greaves, M. F.: Phenotypic characterization of a unique non-T, non-B acute lymphoblastic leukaemia cell line. Nature **267**, 841–843 (1977)

Royston, I., Smith, R. W., Buell, D. N., Huang, E.-S., Pagano, J. S.: Autologous human B and T lymphoblastoid cell lines. Nature **251**, 745–746 (1974)

Rygaard, J.: Immunobiology of the mouse mutant "nude". Acta Pathol. Microbiol. Scand. **77**, 761–762 (1969)

Rygaard, J., Povlsen, C. O.: Heterotransplantation of a human malignant tumor to "nude" mice. Acta Pathol. Microbiol. Scand. **77**, 758–760 (1969)

Saksela, E., Pontén, J.: Chromosomal changes of immunoglobulin producing cell lines from human lymph nodes with and without lymphoma. J. Natl. Cancer Inst. **41**, 359–372 (1968)

Salle, L., De, Munakata, N., Pauli, R. M., Strauss, B. S.: Receptor sites for Concanavalin A on human peripheral lymphocytes and on lymphoblasts grown in long-term culture. Cancer Res. **32**, 2463–2468 (1972)

Sandberg, A. A., Takagi, N., Kato, H.: Cytogenetic studies of normal and neoplastic cells in vitro. In: The proliferation and spread of neoplastic cells pp. 99–136. Baltimore: Williams & Wilkins 1968

Schneider, U., Schwenk, H.-U., Bornkamm, G.: Characterization of EBV-genome negative "null" and "T" cell lines derived from children with acute lymphoblastic leukemia and leukemic transformed non-Hodgkin lymphoma. Int. J. Cancer **19**, 621–626 (1977)

Schwenk, H.-U., Schneider, U.: Cell cycle dependency of a T-cell marker on lymphoblasts. Blut **31**, 299–306 (1975)

Seabright, M.: The use of proteolytic enzymes for the mapping of structural rearrangements in the chromosomes of man. Chromosoma **36**, 204–210 (1972)

Sherr, C. J., Schenkein, I., Uhr, J. W.: Synthesis and intracellular transport of immunoglobulin in secretory and nonsecretory cells. Ann. NY Acad. Sci. **190**, 250–267 (1971)

Sherr, C. J., Baur, S., Grundgke, I., Zeligs, J., Zeligs, B., Uhr, J. W.: Cell surface immunoglobulin. III. Isolation and charcterization of immunoglobulin from nonsecretory human lymphoid cells. J. Exp. Med. **135**, 1392–1405 (1972)

Shevach, E. M., Herbermann, R., Frank, M. M., Green, I.: Receptors for complement and immunoglobulin on human leukemic cells and human lymphoblastoid cell lines. J. Clin. Invest. **51**, 1933–1938 (1972)

Shreffler, D. C., David, C. S.: The H-2 major histocompatibility complex and the I immune response region: Genetic variations, function, and organization. Adv. Immunol. **20**, 125–195 (1975)

Siegert, W., Moar, M. H., Bell, C., Klein, G.: Demonstration of complement receptors on lymphoblastoid cells by radiolabeled antibodies and *in situ* autoradiography. Cell. Immunol. **31**, 234–241 (1977)

Sinkovics, J. G.: Lymphoid cells in long term cultures. Med. Rec. (Houston) **61**, 50–56 (1968)

Sinkovics, J. G., Sykes, J. A., Schullenberger, C. C., Howe, C. D.: Patterns of growth in cultures deriving from human leukemic sources. Tex. Rep. Biol. Med. **25**, 466–467 (1967)

Smith, T. J., Wagner, R. R.: Rabbit macrophage interferons. I. Conditions for biosynthesis by virus-infected and uninfected cells. J. Exp. Med. **125**, 559–577 (1967)

Smith, R. T., Bauscher, J. A., Adler, W. H.: Studies of an inhibitor of DNA synthesis and a non-specific mitogen elaborated by human lymphoblasts. Am. J. Pathol. **60**, 495–504 (1970)

Southam, C. M., Burchenal, J. H., Clarkson, B., Tanzi, A., Mackey, R., McComb, V.: Heterotransplantation of human cell lines from Burkitt's tumors and acute leukemia into newborn rats. Cancer **23**, 281–299 (1969a)

Southam, C. M., Burchenal, J. H., Clarkson, B., Tanzi, A., Mackey, R., McComb, V.: Heterotransplantability of human cell lines derived from leukemia and lymphomas into immunologically tolerant rats. Cancer **24**, 211–222 (1969b)

Stecher, V. J., Thorbecke, G. J.: Sites of synthesis of serum proteins. I. Serum proteins produced by macrophages in vitro. J. Immunol. **99**, 643–652 (1967)

Steel, C. M.: Non-identy of apparently similar chromosome aberrations in human lymphoblastoid cell lines. Nature. **233**, 555–556 (1971)

Steel, C. M.: Human lymphoblastoid cell lines. III. Cocultivation technique for establishment of new lines. J. Natl. Cancer Inst. **48**, 623–628 (1972)

Steel, C. M., Hardy, D. A.: Evidence of altered antigenicity in cultured lymphoid cells from patients with infectious mononucleosis. Lancet **1970 I**, 1322–1323

Steel, C. M., Edmond, E.: Human lymphoblastoid cell lines. I. Culture methods and examination for Epstein-Barr virus. J. Natl. Cancer Inst. **47**, 1193–1201 (1971)

Steel, C. M., McBeath, S., O'Riordan, M. L.: Human lymphoblastoid cell lines. II. Cytogenetic studies. J. Natl. Cancer Inst. **47**, 1203–1214 (1971)

Steel, C. M., Hardy, D. A., Ling, N. R., Dick, H. M., Macintosh, P., Crichton, W. B.: The interaction of normal lymphocytes and cells from lymphoid cell lines. III. Studies on activation in an autochthonous system. Immunology **24**, 177–189 (1973)

Steel, C. M., Evans, J., Joss, A. W. L., Arthur, M. E.: Antibody activity associated with immunoglobulins secreted by human lymphoblastoid cell lines. Nature **252**, 604–605 (1974)

Steel, C. M., Deane, D. L., Philipson, J. Dick H. M., Crichton, W. B.: Characterization of altered surface antigens on human B lymphoblastoid cells. In: Proceedings 25th Annual Colloquium Protides of Biological Fluids. 25th Colloquium 1977. Peeters, H. (ed.), pp. 697–702. London: Pergamon Press 1978

Steel, C. M., Woodward, M. A., Davidson, C., Philipson, J., Arthur, E.: Non random chromosome gains in human lymphoblastoid cell lines. Nature **270**, 349–351 (1977)

Steinitz, M., Klein, G.: Comparison between growth characteristics of an Epstein-Barr virus (EBV)-genome-negative lymphoma line and its converted subline in vitro. Proc. Natl. Acad. Sci. USA **72**, 3518–3520 (1975)

Steinitz, M., Klein, G.: Epstein-Barr virus (EBV)-induced change in the saturation sensitivity and serum dependence of established EBV-negative lymphoma lines in vitro. Virology **70**, 570–573 (1976)

Steinitz, M., Klein, G.: Further studies on the differences in serum dependence in EBV negative lymphoma lines and their in vitro EBV converted virus-genome carrying sublines. Eur. J. Cancer. **13**, 1269–1275 (1977)

Steinitz, M., Klein, G., Koskimies, S., Mäkelä, O.: EB virus-induced B lymphocyte cell lines producing specific antibody. Nature **269**, 420–422 (1977)

Stevens, D. P., Barker, L. F., Fike, R., Hopps, H. E., Meyer, H. M.: Lymphoblastoid cell cultures from patients with infectious hepatitis. Proc. Soc. Exp. Biol. Med. **132**, 1042–1046 (1969)

Stewart, S. E., Lovelace, E., Whang, J. J., Ngu, V. A.: Burkitt tumor: tissue culture, cytogenetic and virus studies. J. Natl. Cancer Inst. **34**, 319–327 (1965)

Stuart, J., Gordon, P. A., Lee, T. R.: Enzyme cytochemistry of blood and bone marrow cells. Histochem. J. **7**, 471–487 (1975)

Sumner, A. T., Evans, H. J., Buckland, R. A.: New techniques for distinguishing between human chromosomes. Nature New Biol. **232**, 31–32 (1971)

Sundström, C.: Biology of human malignant lymphomas in vitro: Characterization of biopsy cells and established cell lines. Acta Univ. Upsaliensis **261**, 1–57 (1977)

Sundström, C., Nilsson, K.: Establishment and characterization of a human histiocytic lymphoma cell line (U-937). Int. J. Cancer **17**, 565–577 (1976)

Sundström, C., Nilsson, K.: Cytochemical profile of human haematopoietic biopsy cells and derived cell lines. Br. J. Haematol. **37**, 489–501 (1977)

Svedmyr, E. D., Deinhardt, F., Gatti, R. A., Golub, S., Gunvén, P., Hoekstra, K., Klein, G., Leibold, W., Menezes, J., Wigzell, H.: Sensitization of human lymphocytes with autologous lymphoblastoid cell line. In: Lymphocyte recognition and effector mechanisms. Lindahl-Kiessling, K., Osoba, O. (eds.), pp. 217–222. New York: Academic Press 1974

Takahashi, M., Yagi, Y., Moore, G. E., Pressman, D.: Pattern of immunoglobulin production in individual cells of human hematopoietic origin in established culture. J. Immunol. **102**, 1274–1283 (1969 a)

Takahashi, M., Tanigaki, N., Yagi, Y., Moore, G. E., Pressman, D.: Immunoglobulin production in cloned sublines of a human lymphocytoid cell line. J. Immunol. **102**, 1388–1393 (1969 b)

Tanigaki, N., Yagi, Y., Moore, G. E., Pressman, D.: Immunoglobulin production in human leukemia cell lines. J. Immunol. **97**, 634–646 (1966)

Temple, M. J., Baumiller, R. C., Feller, W. C.: Chromosomal aberrations in EBV-positive and EBV-negative human lymphoid cell lines. In: Oncogenesis and herpesviruses III. de-Thé, G., Henle, W., Rapp, F. (eds.). Lyon: IARC (in press) 1978

Theofilopoulos, A. N., Dixon, F. J., Bokisch, V. A.: Binding of soluble immune complexes to human lymphoblastoid cells. 1. Characterization of receptors for IgG Fc and complement and description of the binding mechanism. J. Exp. Med. **140**, 887–894 (1974)

Tomkins, G. A.: Chromosome studies on cultured lymphoblastoid cells from cases of New Guinea Burkitt lymphoma, myeloblastic and lymphoblastic leukemia and infectious mononucleosis. Int. J. Cancer **3**, 644–653 (1968)

Toshima, S., Takagi, N., Minowada, J., Moore, G. E., Sandberg, A. A.: Electron microscopic and cytogenetic studies of cells derived from Burkitt's lymphoma. Cancer Res. **27**, 753–759 (1967)

Tough, I. M., Harnden, D. G., Epstein, M. A.: Chromosome markers in cultured cells from Burkitt's lymphoma. Eur. J. Cancer **4**, 637–646 (1968)

Trowbridge, I. S., Ralph, P., Bevan, M. J.: Differences in the surface proteins of mouse T and B cells. Proc. Natl. Acad. Sci. USA **72**, 157–161 (1975)

Trowbridge, I. S., Hyman, R., Mazauskas, C.: Surface molecules of cultured human lymphoid cells. Eur. J. Immunol. **6**, 777–782 (1976)

Trowbridge, I. S., Hyman, R., Klein, G.: Human B cell line deficient in the expression of B cell-specific glycoproteins (GP 27, 35). Eur. J. Immunol. **7**, 640–645 (1977)

Trowell, O. A.: Lymphocytes. In: Cells and tissues in culture, Vol. 2. Willmer, E. N. (ed.), pp. 96–172. London: Academic Press 1965

Trujillo, J. M., List-Young, B., Butler, J. J., Schullenberger, C. C., Gott, C.: Long term culture of lymph node tissue from a patient with lymphocytic lymphoma. Nature **209**, 310–311 (1966)

Tsuchimoto, T., Tubergen, D. G., Bloom, A. D.: Synthesis of macrophage migration inhibition factor (MIF) by immunoglobulin-producing lymphocyte lines and their clones. J. Immunol. **109**, 884–886 (1972)

Tubergen, D. G., Feldman, J. D., Pollock, E. M., Lerner, R. A.: Production of macrophage migration inhibition factor by continous cell lines. J. Exp. Med. **135**, 255–266 (1972)

Uzman, B. G., Foley, G. E., Farber, S., Lazarus, H.: Morphologic variations in human leukemic lymphoblasts (CCRF-CEM cells) after long-term culture and exposure to chemotherapeutic agents. Cancer **19**, 1725–1742 (1966)

van Furth, R., Gorter, H., Nadkarni, J. S., Klein, E., Clifford, P.: Synthesis of immunoglobulins by biopsied tissues and cell lines from Burkitt's lymphoma. Immunology **22**, 847–857 (1972)

Wakefield, J. D., Thorbecke, G. J., Old, L. J., Boyse, E. A.: Production of immunoglobulins and their subunits by human tissue culture cell lines. J. Immunol. **99**, 308–319 (1967)

Watanabe, S., Yagi, Y., Pressman, D.: Immunoglobulin production in synchronized cultures of human hematopoietic cell lines. II. Variation of synthetic and secretion activities during the cell cycle. J. Immunol. **111**, 797–804 (1973)

Welsh, K. I., Dorval, G., Nilsson, K., Clements, G., Wigzell, H.: Quantitation of β_2-microglobulin and HLA on the surface of human cells. II. In vitro cell lines and their hybrids. Scand. J. Immunol. **6**, 265–271 (1977)

Wernet, P.: Human Ia-type alloantigens: Methods of detection, aspects of chemistry and biology, markers for disease states. Transplant. Rev. **30**, 271–298 (1976)

Whang-Peng, J., Gerber, P., Knutsen, T.: So called C marker chromosome and Epstein-Barr virus. J. Natl. Cancer Inst. **45**, 831–839 (1970)

Wurster-Hill, D. H., McIntyre, O. R., Cornwell, G. G., Maurer, L. H.: Marker-chromosome 14 in multiple myeloma and plasma-cell leukaemia. Lancet **1973 II**, 1031

Yefenof, E., Klein, G.: Difference in antibody induced redistribution of membrane IgM in EBV-genome free and EBV-positive human lymphoid cells. Exp. Cell Res. **99**, 175–178 (1976)

Yefenof, E., Klein, G., Jondal, M., Oldstone, M. B. A.: Surface markers on human B- and T-lymphocytes. IX. Two-color immunofluorescence studies on the association between EBV receptors and complement receptors on the surface of lymphoid cell lines. Int. J. Cancer **17**, 693–700 (1976)

Yefenof, E., Klein, G.: Membrane receptor stripping confirms the association between EBV receptors and complement receptors on the surface of human B lymphoma lines. Int. J. Cancer **20**, 347–352 (1977)

Yefenof, E., Klein, G., Kvarnung, K.: Relationships between complement activation, complement binding, and EBV absorption by human hematopoietic cell lines. Cell. Immunol. **31**, 225–233 (1977a)

Yefenof, E., Klein, G., Ben-Bassat, H., Lundin, L.: Difference in the Con A induced redistribution and agglutination patterns of EBV genome free and EBV carrying human lymphoma lines. Exp. Cell Res. **108**, 185–190 (1977b)

Yefenof, E., Lundin, L., Klein, G.: Shedding of anti-IgM from antibody coated human lymphoma lines: differences between EBV negative lines and their virus converted sublines. Europ. J. Immunol. **8**, 190–193 (1978)

Yount, W. J., Utsinger, P. D., Hutt, L. M., Buchanan, P. D., Korn, J. H., Fuller, C. R., Logue, M., Pagano, J. S.: Subpopulations of human lymphoblastoid cell lines. Scand. J. Immunol. **5**, 795–810 (1976)

Zajac, B. A., Henle, W., Henle, G.: Autogenous and virus-induced interferons from lines of lymphoblastoid cells. Cancer Res. **29**, 1467–1475 (1969)

Zajac, B. A., Kohn, G.: Epstein-Barr virus antigens, marker chromosome and interferon production in clones derived from cultured Burkitt tumor cells. J. Natl. Cancer Inst. **45**, 399–406 (1970)

Zech, L., Haglund, U., Nilsson, K., Klein, G.: Characteristic chromosomal abnormalities in biopsies and lymphoid-cell lines from patients with Burkitt and non-Burkitt lymphomas. Int. J. Cancer **17**, 47–56 (1976)

Zeuthen, J., Friedrich, U., Rosén, A., Klein, E.: Structural abnormalities in chromosome 15 in cell lines with reduced expression of Beta-2-microglobulin. Immunogenetics **4**, 567–580 (1977)

Ziegler, J. L., Carbone, P. P.: Burkitt tumor in the United States: Diagnosis, treatment and prognosis. Blood **28**, 982–983 (1966)

zur Hausen, H.: Chromosomal changes of similar nature in seven established cell lines derived from the peripheral blood of patients with leukemia. J. Natl. Cancer Inst. **38**, 683–696 (1967)

zur Hausen, H.: Oncogenic herpes viruses. Biochem. Biophys. Acta **417**, 25–53 (1975)

zur Hausen, H., Schulte-Holthausen, H., Klein, G., Henle, W., Henle, G., Clifford, P., Sanesson, L.: EBV DNA in biopsies of Burkitt tumours and anaplastic carcinomas of the nasopharynx. Nature **228**, 1056–1058 (1970)

zur Hausen, H., Diehl, V., Wolf, H., Schulte-Holthause, H., Schneider, U.: Occurrence of Epstein-Barr virus genomes in human lymphoblastoid cell lines. Nature New Biol. **237**, 189–190 (1972)

12 Activation of the Viral Genome In Vitro

B. Hampar

Laboratory of Molecular Virology, National Cancer Institute, National Institutes of Health, Building 560, Frederick Cancer Research Center, Frederick, Bethesda, MD 20014 (USA)

A. INTRODUCTION

The Epstein-Barr virus (EBV) occupies a unique position among human herpesviruses in that it is the only one which has been shown to be capable of forming a true latent infection whereby complete copies of the virus genome persist in replicating cells (reviewed by Epstein and Achong, 1977). Two human cell types have been demonstrated to harbor latent EBV genomes, B lymphocytes (bone marrow-derived lymphocyte) (Jondal et al., 1973; Pattengale et al., 1973), and epithelial tumor cells in nasopharyngeal carcinomas (NPC) (Wolf et al., 1973).

Latency by EBV has been confirmed by several methods. First, clonal isolates of EBV-harboring lymphoblastoid cells contain the virus genome (Hinuma et al., 1967; Zajac and Kohn, 1970; Sugawara et al., 1972). Second, when lymphoblastoid cells harboring EBV are made resistant to the halogenated pyrimidine, 5-bromode-oxyuridine (BUDR), spontaneous virus activation is accompanied by the appearance of thymidine kinase (dTK), while the enzyme remains suppressed in cells carrying repressed virus genomes (Hampar et al., 1971a). Third, treatment of lymphoblastoid cells with BUDR results in activation of repressed virus genomes (Gerber, 1972; Hampar et al., 1972a). Finally, lymphoblastoid cells showing no evidence of productive EBV infection express EBV nuclear antigen (EBNA) (Reedman and Klein, 1973).

This chapter is concerned with events accompanying activation of latent EBV genomes, irrespective of whether activation occurs spontaneously or is induced by a specific agent. The term "activation" as used here refers to any condition which allows the virus genome to enter a productive cycle, notwithstanding the possibility that the cycle may be aborted prior to formation of infectious virions.

B. PROPERTIES OF HUMAN LYMPHOBLASTOID CELL LINES[1]

Lymphoblastoid cell lines harboring EBV are classified with respect to virus production into two broad categories. Producer lines are those in which spontaneous activation occurs in a varying percentage of the cells, usually resulting in synthesis of virus particles characteristic of a productive cycle. Nonproducer lines are those in which spontaneous virus activation occurs only rarely with the virus productive cycle being aborted prior to completion.

Immunofluorescence (IF) has been employed most extensively for detecting intracellular antigens associated with productive EBV infection following spontaneous or induced activation (Chap. 3). EBNA, detected by anticomplement IF (Reedman and Klein, 1973), shows many analogies to the nuclear T antigens expressed in cells latently infected with small DNA tumor viruses. Expression of EBNA is evident in latently infected cells and does not require activation of the EBV genome. The EBNA binds to cellular DNA and is associated with methaphase-arrested chromosomes. The first antigen to appear in cells in which the genome is activated to a productive cycle is the early antigen (EA), consisting of a restricted (R) and a diffuse (D) component differentiated by IF (Henle et al., 1970). The EA complex is presumably composed of nonstructural antigens and is synthesized prior to replication

---

[1] In this chapter "lymphoblastoid" is applied to cell lines of both lymphoma and nonmalignant origin – c.f. Chap. 11.

of "free" virus DNA (vDNA) in productively infected cells (Gergely et al., 1971 a). The EA complex appears first in the nucleus and later is also found in the cytoplasm (Gergely et al., 1971 b). The virus productive cycle in activated nonproducer cells is aborted subsequent to the synthesis of EA (Gerber and Lucas, 1972) and prior to the synthesis of "free" vDNA. Synthesis of EA is sufficient to ensure cell death (Diehl et al., 1972), although the activated cells may progress through the cell cycle to reach mitosis where EA can be found associated with chromosomes during metaphase (Hampar et al., 1974 c) or telophase (Glaser et al., 1977). The virus productive cycle in activated producer cells progresses beyond EA to the synthesis of "free" vDNA and the second antigen complex, viral capsid antigen (VCA) (Henle and Henle, 1966), consisting of virus structural proteins.

C. STATE OF THE VIRUS GENOME IN LYMPHOBLASTOID CELLS

Human lymphoblastoid cells may harbor up to 50 or more copies of the EBV genome in a repressed state (zur Hausen and Schulte-Holthausen, 1970; Nonoyama and Pagano, 1971; zur Hausen et al., 1972). The number of vDNA copies increases dramatically during productive infection in producer cells, while activated nonproducer cells show no increase in vDNA copies since the productive cycle is aborted prior to synthesis of "free" vDNA (Glaser and Nonoyama, 1974; Hampar et al., 1974 c).

Most EBV genome copies persist in lymphoblastoid cells in a nonintegrated state, although there is some physical association with the cellular DNA (Nonoyama and Pagano, 1972). At least some cells also contain circularized vDNA (Lindahl et al., 1976) characteristic of episomes (Adams and Lindahl, 1975). Additional evidence suggests that some vDNA may actually be integrated into the cell DNA by covalent linkage (Adams et al., 1973) (Chap. 8).

At present it is not known whether activation (spontaneous or induced) occurs via the nonintegrated vDNA or the putative integrated copy(s). Recent findings indicate that treatment of producer P_3HR-1 cells with cycloheximide can reduce the amount of vDNA (Tanaka et al., 1976), and at least one clone (Cl. 9) of drug-treated cells has been shown to contain only one vDNA copy. Clone 9 is EBNA-positive, but shows no evidence of spontaneous virus activation or sensitivity to activation by 5-iododeoxyuridine (IUDR) in contrast to the parent P_3HR-1 cells. Studies presently underway on the state of the vDNA in Cl. 9 cells may allow definitive conclusions concerning integration of EBV DNA in human cells.

Autoradiographic evidence suggests that the multiple copies of EBV DNA in lymphoblastoid cells are not associated with specific chromosomes (zur Hausen and Schulte-Holthausen, 1972). Despite this apparently random distribution, the vDNA is closely associated with the cellular DNA. First, vDNA can be isolated together with metaphase chromosomes (Nonoyama and Pagano, 1971). Second, replication of repressed vDNA occurs synchronously during the early part of the cell's S phase (S-1 period) (Hampar et al., 1974 b). Finally, replication of repressed vDNA but not "free" vDNA is under control of the host cell; hydroxyurea (HU), which inhibits replication of cellular DNA, also inhibits replication of repressed vDNA, whereas replication of "free" vDNA made during productive infection is not inhibited by HU (Hampar et al., 1972 b; Mele et al., 1974) as a result of the appearance in cells of a new ribonucleotide reductase resistant to the action of the drug (Henry et al., 1978). In contrast to the effects of HU on vDNA replication, phosphonoacetic acid (PAA) inhibits replication of "free" vDNA at concentrations which do not inhibit replication of cellular or repressed vDNA (Summers and Klein, 1976; Nyormoi et al., 1976). This effect of PAA has been ascribed to the appearance in productively infected cells of a virus-coded DNA polymerase sensitive to the action of the drug.

D. SPONTANEOUS ACTIVATION

Spontaneous activation of EBV is seen in producer cells although the percentage of cells undergoing activation may vary considerably with time in an unpredictable fashion. Procedures reported to enhance EBV production include single-cell cloning to obtain high producer populations (Hinuma et al., 1967b), incubation at suboptimal temperatures (Hinuma et al., 1967b), temperature cycling (Maurer et al., 1970), aging of stationary phase cultures (Hinuma et al., 1967a), incubation in medium deficient in arginine (Henle and Henle, 1968), cocultivation or fusion with nonlymphoid cells (Hampar et al., 1971b; Matsuo et al., 1976), colcemid treatment to block cell division (Sairenji and Hinuma, 1971), ultraviolet- (Lai et al., 1973) or X-irradiation (Yata et al., 1970), infection with adenovirus type 5 (Faucon et al., 1974), and treatment with hydrocortisone (Joncas et al., 1973).

As already mentioned, the programming of the virus productive cycle following spontaneous activation has been shown to consist, in order of appearance, of EA, "free" vDNA, and VCA, and additional information has been derived from studies employing producer P_3HR-1 cells made resistant to BUDR (Hampar et al., 1974a, 1975). Such cells (P_3HR-1 [BU]) are characterized by the absence of a functional dTK when they harbor repressed virus genomes, and by the appearance of dTK when these genomes are activated. Studies with these cells indicate that during any one cell cycle only a limited number of cells are capable of undergoing virus activation spontaneously (Hampar et al., 1972b). A critical period for initiating virus activation has been localized at the beginning of the cells' S phase (S-1 period) (Hampar et al., 1973). Following initiation of the activation sequence, the P_3HR-1(BU) cells continue through the S phase in the absence of a functional dTK pathway. The EA complex is synthesized and the cells initiate a new cycle of DNA synthesis characterized by the presence of dTK. The dTK-positive cells synthesize both cell DNA and "free" vDNA (Derge et al., 1975), and this synthesis of DNA in dTK-positive P_3HR-1(BU) cells is resistant to normally inhibitory concentrations of HU, although it remains sensitive to other DNA inhibitors (Hampar et al., 1972b).

Maintenance of P_3HR-1(BU) cells on high concentrations of BUDR (≥ 20 µg/ml) does not prevent synthesis of EA, but VCA and virus particles are not produced. Removal of the BUDR allows the EA-positive cells to resume synthesis of "free" vDNA and ultimately VCA and virus particles (Hampar et al., 1971a).

Studies of DNA synthesis in P_3HR-1(BU) cells support the generally accepted conclusion that productive infection with EBV results ultimately in cell death (Hampar et al., 1975). When P_3HR-1 cells, which express dTK, are grown for several generations in the presence of BUDR, the DNA following isopyknic centrifugation shows three peaks corresponding to light-light (absence of BUDR), light-heavy (presence of BUDR in only one DNA strand), and heavy-heavy (presence of BUDR in both DNA strands) DNA. The presence of a heavy-heavy DNA band indicates that the cells can progress through two or more cycles of DNA synthesis in the presence of BUDR. When P$_3$HR-1(BU) cells are grown for several generations in the presence of BUDR, only two DNA peaks are evident corresponding to light-light and light-heavy DNA. The absence of a heavy-heavy DNA band indicates that P$_3$HR-1(BU) cells which have undergone virus activation and are dTK-positive do not undergo more than one cycle of DNA synthesis.

Finally, the question of whether EBV induces a new virus-coded dTK is still unresolved. Studies to date have failed to reveal differences in the properties of the dTK that appears in EBV-infected cells, including P$_3$HR-1(BU) cells, compared to those of the normal human enzyme. The possible absence of an EBV-coded dTK indicates that the enzyme which appears in EA-positive P$_3$HR-1(BU) cells may be a human enzyme which is derepressed during productive infection.

E. ACTIVATION INDUCED BY CHEMICALS

Several chemicals possess an ability to induce EBV in human cells. In the case of producer cells, activation by chemicals may lead to the synthesis of EA, "free" vDNA, and VCA, while nonproducer cells treated with chemicals only synthesize EA. The only reported exceptions occur when nonproducer cells are treated for prolonged periods (several weeks or more) with BUDR (Hampar et al., 1972 a) or when hybrids of nonproducer cells and human epithelial cells are treated for short periods with IUDR (Glaser and Nonoyama, 1972) (see Sect. F).

Only a few of the various agents which induce EBV cause significant levels of activation, and on an empirical basis, it is probable that inducing agents merely enhance the levels of spontaneous virus activation. It is unlikely that activation of EBV could be induced in cells which were incapable of undergoing any spontaneous activation, although the detection of spontaneous activation may be below observable levels. Latency probably depends upon an equilibrium between the cell and the virus that maintains the EBV genome in a repressed state in a majority of the cells, while in a few cells the equilibrium may shift in favor of the virus. The latter condition would allow activation with resultant productive or abortive infection and cell death. Agents which induce EBV probably function by shifting the equilibrium in favor of the virus in a higher than normal percentage of the cells.

I. HALOGENATED PYRIMIDINES (IUDR AND BUDR)

Activation of EBV was first achieved with BUDR in human lymphoblastoid cells (Gerber, 1972; Hampar et al., 1972 a) and NPC cells (Trumper et al., 1976), but IUDR has proven more efficient and is used in most studies today (Sugawara et al., 1972; Klein and Dombos, 1973; Glaser et al., 1976 a). Halogenated pyrimidines have also been employed for activation of SV40 (Rothschild and Black, 1970) and oncorna-viruses (Lowy et al., 1971).

Incorporation into cells of IUDR and BUDR occurs via the thymidine salvage pathway utilizing dTK for phosphorylation. Virus activation by these analogues requires their incorporation into the cell DNA and consequently is dependent on the cells being in the S phase. As expected, activation by IUDR or BUDR can be prevented by blocking cell DNA synthesis (Klein and Dombos, 1973) or by adding an excess of thymidine, which is preferentially incorporated by the cells (Gerber and Lucas, 1972). Producer cells in the presence of high concentrations ($> 20 \,\mu g/ml$) of IUDR or BUDR synthesize EA, but "free" vDNA and VCA are not synthesized unless the drug is removed, and even then VCA may not appear in all cells (Hampar et al., 1971a; Glaser et al., 1973). In contrast, activation of nonproducer cells by IUDR or BUDR results only in EA synthesis regardless of whether or not the drug is removed (Gerber and Lucas, 1972; Hampar et al., 1974c). Some EBV-positive lymphoblastoid cells cannot be activated by either IUDR or BUDR (Klein and Dombos, 1973), although the reason for their resistance is not readily apparent. One possibility may be related to the wide variations observed in the levels of thymidine incorporated by different lymphoblastoid cells lines (Lazarus et al., 1974).

Synchronization has been employed for studying the events associated with EBV activation by IUDR. The double-thymidine blocking technique has proven effective for synchronizing some, but not all, producer and nonproducer lymphoblastoid cell lines (Hampar et al., 1973, 1974c). The synchronization procedure itself, which employs excess thymidine for blocking cells at the G-1/S border, results in low levels of activation. This is not unexpected since DNA inhibitors when added at the proper time in the cell cycle also induce low levels of virus activation (Hampar et al., 1974a; Long et al., 1974).

Although synchronization is not required for EBV activation by IUDR, it does allow localization within the cell cycle of specific events associated with the initiation and progression of the virus productive cycle (Fig. 1) (Hampar et al., 1975). When synchronized producer or nonproducer cells are treated for short periods (30–60 min) with IUDR ($20 \,\mu g/ml$), maximum levels of virus activation are observed when the drug is added $\sim$ 60 min after the cells enter the S phase (S-1 period). The critical S-1 period

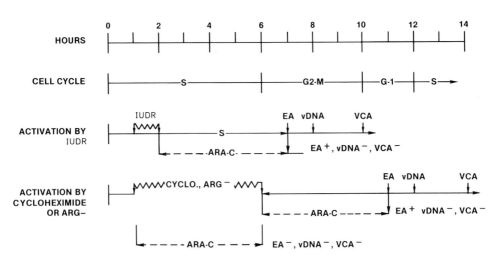

Fig. 1. Temporal sequence of events associated with virus activation by IUDR or cycloheximide and Arg-. The sequence in each case is for activated producer cells where EA, "free" vDNA, and VCA are synthesized. Additional details are given in the text

for IUDR incorporation to induce EBV does not coincide with the period of maximum drug incorporation into cell DNA, which occurs during the mid-S phase (S-2 period) (Hampar et al., 1974c). The S-1 period is also the time when the repressed vDNA replicates (Hampar et al., 1974b), suggesting a temporal if not a causal relationship between activation and vDNA replication. Cell DNA synthesis during the 30–60 min period of IUDR incorporation is inhibited by $\sim 80\%$, but removal of the drug allows resumption of DNA synthesis and completion of the S phase. The time of completion of the S phase is delayed by approximately the same time interval as is needed for IUDR incorporation. Toxicity due to the incorporated IUDR occurs either during the G-2 or M period, and is evident at mitosis where $\sim 50\%$ of the cells fail to complete division and enter a new S phase.

Synthesis of EA occurs ~ 5 h after removal of the IUDR at a time corresponding to the S/G-2 border of the cell cycle. Inhibition of cell DNA synthesis following removal of the IUDR during the S-1 period does not inhibit subsequent EA synthesis, which occurs at the same time (5 h) as in cells in which DNA synthesis is not inhibited. Consequently, while synthesis of EA coincides temporally with entry of the cell into G-2, it is not dependent upon the cell completing the S phase. As expected, however, inhibition of cell DNA synthesis following IUDR treatment does preclude synthesis of "free" vDNA and VCA in producer cells (Gergely et al., 1971a). It would appear that EA is transcribed either from preexisting DNA or DNA synthesized during the period of IUDR incorporation. Further, the temporal sequence of transcriptional and translation events associated with EA appear to be predetermined and may include synthesis of as yet undetected antigens.

Synthesis of EA in IUDR-activated producer cells is followed by a new cycle of DNA synthesis during which "free" vDNA is made and VCA appears after ~ 3 h. The addition of DNA inhibitors during the first hour following the appearance of EA will prevent synthesis of VCA, but the inhibitors will not prevent VCA synthesis if added at later times.

The situation with nonproducer cells is quite different in that the virus productive cycle is aborted subsequent to EA synthesis and prior to synthesis of "free" vDNA and VCA. The EA-positive nonproducer cells do show very low levels of DNA synthesis after the appearance of EA, which suggests an abortive attempt to enter a new cycle of DNA synthesis (Hampar et al., 1974c). The inability of IUDR-activated nonproducer cells to undergo a complete productive cycle may be ascribed to a post-transcriptional block as evidenced by the finding that whereas $\sim 50\%$ of the virus genome is transcribed in nonactivated Raji cells (Hayward and Kieff, 1976), essentially the entire virus genome is transcribed following IUDR treatment (Tanaka et al., 1977).

Approximately 50% of producer cells activated by IUDR during the S-1 period fail to synthesize "free" vDNA and VCA (Hampar et al., 1974c). This percentage is comparable to the observed toxic effects of the incorporated IUDR and suggests a causal relationship between IUDR-induced toxicity and abortive infection in producer cells.

II. INHIBITORS OF PROTEIN SYNTHESIS OR ARGININE DEFICIENCY (ARG-)

Inhibitors of protein synthesis or media deficient in specific amino acids have been employed for activating latent DNA (Kaplan et al., 1972) and RNA (Aaronson and

Dunn, 1974) viruses. In the case of EBV, medium deficient in arginine (Arg-) enhances the levels of spontaneous activation in producer cells (Henle and Henle, 1968).

The events associated with activation of EBV by the protein inhibitor cycloheximide or Arg- medium have been studied using synchronized producer and nonproducer cells (Fig. 1) (Hampar et al., 1976). In contrast to IUDR, which does not require synchronized cells for activation, cycloheximide shows no activating potential in nonsynchronized cells. Activation by cycloheximide or Arg- medium in synchronized cultures occurs when treatment is initiated during the S-1 period of the cell cycle and is terminated after 5 h. The times for initiating and terminating the treatment appear critical and are not amenable to variation. As already discussed (see Sect. E.I), the S-1 period is also critical for initiating activation by IUDR.

During the 5-h treatment with cycloheximide or Arg- medium, DNA synthesis is inhibited by 80%–85%. Surprisingly, the remaining low levels of DNA synthesis are required for antigen expression and presumably virus activation. The addition of DNA inhibitors (ara-C or HU) during the 5-h period of treatment prevents subsequent expression of EA or VCA even if DNA synthesis is allowed to resume following termination of the treatment with cycloheximide or Arg- medium. This differs from what is observed with IUDR, where inhibition of cell DNA synthesis following 60-min treatment with the analogue does not prevent subsequent expression of EA.

Synthesis of EA occurs $\sim$ 5 h after termination of treatment with cycloheximide or Arg- medium and is followed in $\sim$ 3 h by synthesis of VCA. Producer cells activated by cycloheximide or Arg- medium synthesize both EA and VCA, while only EA is made in nonproducer cells. In this respect, cycloheximide and Arg- medium are similar to IUDR.

F. VIRUS EXPRESSION IN HYBRID CELLS

Somatic cell hybrids have been employed for studying control of EBV expression. These hybrids have furnished information not readily obtained with lymphoblastoid cells alone (Glaser and Rapp, 1975). The most extensively studied hybrids between EBV-harboring lymphoblastoid cells and human nonlymphoid cells (Glaser and O'Neil, 1972; Glaser and Rapp, 1972; Glaser et al., 1973) were produced by fusion of producer P_3HR-1 cells and epithelial-like D98 cells (D98/HR-1), and nonproducer Raji cells and D98 cells (D98/Raji). Both D98/HR-1 and D98/Raji hybrids contain multiple copies of the EBV genome, express EBNA, and show no evidence of spontaneous virus activation. Since producer P_3HR-1 cells do show spontaneous virus activation, often at relatively high levels, the lack of spontaneous activation in D98/HR-1 cells suggest the presence in these hybrids of a factor(s) that maintains the virus genome in a repressed state.

Treatment of D98/HR-1 hybrids with IUDR results in virus activation similar to that which occurs when P_3HR-1 cells are treated with the drug. The IUDR-activated hybrid cells synthesize EA in the presence of the analogue and "free" vDNA, VCA, and virus particles following removal of the drug (Glaser et al., 1973) The levels of virus activation in IUDR-treated hybrid cells may be higher than those observed in drug-treated P_3HR-1 cells. Further, dibutyryl cyclic AMP (cAMP), known to affect cellular regulation, can induce low levels of virus activation in D98/HR-1 hybrid cells and may enhance the levels of virus activation induced by IUDR (Zimmermann et al., 1973). A similar effect of cAMP on lymphoblastoid cells has not been observed.

When Raji cells are treated for short periods with IUDR, only EA is synthesized, indicating an abortive infection (Gerber and Lucas, 1972). Treatment of D98/Raji hybrid cells with IUDR results in a complete productive cycle similar to that observed with D98/HR-1 hybrid cells (Glaser et al., 1973). It would appear that factors present in Raji cells which preclude a complete virus productive cycle are circumvented or neutralized in D98/Raji hybrid cells.

Hybrid cells have also been produced by fusion of lymphoblastoid cells themselves. When two nonproducer cells differing in their sensitivity to IUDR-induced activation were fused, the resultant hybrid cells showed such levels of IUDR-induced EA synthesis as to indicate that sensitivity to IUDR activation was dominant over resistance (Nyormoi et al., 1973). In contrast, when producer Daudi cells were fused with nonproducer Raji cells (Raji/Daudi), the IUDR inducibility of the hybrid cells occurred at levels comparable to those of the less sensitive Raji cells, suggesting a negative control mechanism (Klein et al., 1976). The Raji-Daudi hybrid cells also showed spontaneous expression of EA and VCA, suggesting that the producer status of the Daudi cells dominated over the nonproducer status of the Raji cells. This differs considerably from D98/HR-1 hybrid cells where the producer status of the P_3HR-1 cells is abolished by fusion with nonlymphoid D98 cells.

Hybrids prepared by fusion of nonproducer Raji cells and EBV-negative lymphoblastoid BJAB cells (Raji/BJAB) showed levels of IUDR inducibility significantly higher than observed with Raji cells alone (Klein et al., 1976), suggesting some type of complementation. It has been suggested that similar control mechanisms are involved in the response of lymphoblastoid cells to superinfection with EBV and inducibility by IUDR with respect to EA synthesis (Klein and Dombos, 1973; Klein et al., 1976). Results consistent with this suggestion have been obtained recently by comparing the inducibility of EA by superinfection and IUDR using Raji cells and tetraploid Raji cells obtained by colcemid treatment (Shapiro et al., 1978). The levels of EA synthesis following superinfection or IUDR treatment were significantly lower in the tetraploid cells than in diploid Raji cells. Further, tetraploidization of Raji cells did not result in the expected doubling in number of EBV DNA copies. These observations are consistent with the reported correlation between IUDR inducibility and number of vDNA copies (Pritchett et al., 1976; Tanaka et al., 1976).

Hybrids have also been prepared by fusion of EBV-harboring lymphoblastoid cells and virus-negative mouse cells (Klein et al., 1974). The mouse/human hybrid cells contain vDNA and express EBNA. With one reported exception (Glaser et al., 1976b), all mouse/human hybrids thus far studied are noninducible by IUDR for EA or VCA expression. In most cases, the virus is eliminated from the hybrid cells as human chromosomes are segregated out. Exceptions occur, however, as evidenced by the isolation of hybrid clones that contain vDNA and EBNA in the absence of recognizable human chromosomes (Glaser et al., 1978; Steplewski et al., 1978) These hybrids still contain human enzymes, which raises the possibility that some human DNA has been translocated to mouse chromosomes. The vDNA may be carried along with the human DNA in an integrated state or may persist in an episomal state independent of the retained human DNA.

G. CONCLUDING REMARKS

EBV is similar to other latent mammalian DNA (Kaplan et al., 1975) and RNA (Greenberger and Aaronson, 1975; Schwartz et al., 1975) viruses in its dependence on the stage of the cell cycle for activation by various agents. Latent herpesviruses, other than EBV, which are sensitive to activation by IUDR include those from subhuman primates (Neubauer et al., 1974; Neubauer und Rabin, 1978) and the Marek's disease virus of chickens (Nazerian, 1975; Dunn and Nazerian, 1977). The mechanism of EBV activation has yet to be determined, and in each instance where one mechanism of cell control appears operative, a different and often opposite mechanism is deduced from additional studies (Sect. F). If EBV activation occurs via integrated vDNA, it may involve an excision step such as that proposed for SV40 (Rakusanova et al., 1976). Alternatively, if activation occurs via nonintegrated vDNA, it may depend upon faulty reassociation of the cell and vDNA following their replication during the S-1 period (Hampar et al., 1976). The final resolution of the problem of EBV activation must await more definitive studies.

REFERENCES

Aaronson, S. A., Dunn, C. Y.: High frequency C-type virus induction by inhibitors of protein synthesis. Science **183**, 422–424 (1974)

Adams, A., Lindahl, T., Klein, G.: Linear association between cellular DNA and Epstein-Barr virus in a human lymphoblastoid cell line. Proc. Natl. Acad. Sci., USA **70**, 2888–2892 (1973).

Adams, A., Lindahl, T.: Intracellular forms of Epstein-Barr virus DNA in Raji cells. In: Oncogenesis and herpesviruses II. de-Thé, G., Epstein, M. A., zur Hausen, H. (eds.), Part 1, pp. 125–132. Lyon: IARC 1975

Derge, J. G., Birkhead, S. L., Hemmaplardh, T., Hampar, B.: DNA synthesis in cells activated for the Epstein-Barr virus. In: Oncogenesis and herpesviruses II. de-Thé, G., Epstein, M. A., zur Hausen, H. (eds), Part 1, pp. 467–474. Lyon: IARC 1975

Diehl, V., Wolf, H., Schulte-Holthausen, H., zur Hausen, H.: Re-exposure of human lymphoblastoid cell lines to Epstein-Barr virus. Int. J. Cancer **10**, 641–651 (1972)

Dunn, K., Nazerian, K.: Induction of Marek's disease virus by IdUrd in a chicken lymphoblastoid cell line. J. Gen. Virol. **34**, 413–419 (1977).

Epstein, M. A., Achong, B. G.: Recent progress in Epstein-Barr virus research. Annu. Rev. Microbiol. **31**, 421–445 (1977).

Faucon, N., Chardonnet, Y., Perrinet, M. C., Sohier, R.: Superinfection with adenovirus of Burkitt lymphoma cell lines. J. Natl. Cancer Inst. **53**, 305–308 (1974).

Gerber, P.: Activation of Epstein-Barr virus by 5-bromodeoxyuridine in "virus-free" human cells. Proc. Natl. Acad. Sci. USA **69**, 83–85 (1972)

Gerber, P., Lucas, S.: Epstein-Barr virus-associated antigens activated in human cells by 5-bromodeoxyuridine. Proc. Soc. Exp. Biol. Med. **141**, 431–435 (1972)

Gergely, L., Klein, G., Ernberg, I.: The action of DNA antagonists on Epstein-Barr virus (EBV)-associated early antigen (EA) in Burkitt lymphoma lines. Int. J. Cancer **7**, 293–302 (1971a)

Gergely, L., Klein, G., Ernberg, I.: Appearance of Epstein-Barr virus-associated antigens in infected Raji cells. Virology **45**, 10–21 (1971b)

Glaser, R., O'Neil, F. J.: Hybridization of Burkitt lymphoblastoid cells. Science **176**, 1245–1247 (1972)

Glaser, R., Rapp, F.: Rescue of Epstein-Barr virus from somatic cell hybrids of Burkitt lymphoblastoid cells. J. Virol. **10**, 288–296 (1972)

Glaser, R., Nonoyama, M., Becker, B., Rapp, F.: Synthesis of Epstein-Barr virus antigens and DNA in activated somatic cell hybrids. Virology **55**, 62–69 (1973)

Glaser, R., Nonoyama, M.: Host cell regulation of induction of Epstein-Barr virus. J. Virol. **14**, 174–176 (1974)

Glaser, R., Rapp, F.: Biological properties of the Epstein-Barr virus and its possible role in human malignancy. Prog. Med. Virol. **21**, 43–57 (1975)

Glaser, R., de-Thé, G., Lenoir, G., Ho, J. H. C.: Superinfection of epithelial nasopharyngeal carcinoma cells with Epstein-Barr virus. Proc. Natl. Acad. Sci. USA **73**, 960–963 (1976 a)

Glaser, R., Farrugia, R., Brown, N.: Effect of the host cell on the maintenance and replication of Epstein-Barr virus. Virology **69**, 132–142 (1976 b)

Glaser, R., Lenoir, G., Ferrone, S., Pellegrino, M. A., de-Thé, G.: Cell surface markers on epithelial-Burkitt hybrid cells superinfected with Epstein-Barr virus. Cancer Res. **37**, 2291–2296 (1977)

Glaser, R., Nonoyama, M., Hampar, B., Croce, C. M.: Studies on the association of the Epstein-Barr virus genome and human chromosomes. (submitted) (1978)

Greenberger, J. S., Aaronson, S. A.: Cycloheximide induction of xenotropic type-C virus from synchronized mouse cells: Metabolic requirement for virus activation. J. Virol. **15**, 64–70 (1975)

Hampar, B., Derge, J. G., Martos, L. M., Walker, J. L.: Persistence of a repressed Epstein-Barr virus genome in Burkitt lymphoma cells made resistant to 5-bromodeoxyuridine. Proc. Natl. Acad. Sci. USA **68**, 3185–3189 (1971a)

Hampar, B., Martos, L. M., Walker, J. L.: Epstein-Barr virus in human lymphoblastoid cells: Enhancing the percentage of virus-positive cells by co-cultivation with African Green monkey (VERO) cells. J. Natl. Cancer Inst. **47**, 535–537 (1971b)

Hampar, B., Derge, J. G., Martos, L. M., Walker, J. L.: Synthesis of Epstein-Barr virus after activation of the viral genome in a "virus negative" human lymphoblastoid cell (RAJI) made resistant to 5-bromodeoxyuridine. Proc. Natl. Acad. Sci. USA **69**, 72–82 (1972 a)

Hampar, B., Derge, J. G., Martos, L. M., Tagamets, M. A., Burroughs, M. A.: Sequence of spontaneous Epstein-Barr virus activation and selective DNA synthesis in activated cells in the presence of hydroxyurea. Proc. Natl. Acad. Sci. USA **69**, 2589–2593 (1972b)

Hampar, B., Derge, J. G., Martos, L. M., Tagamets, M. A., Chang, S-Y, Chakrabarty, M.: Identification of a critical period during the S Phase for activation of the Epstein-Barr virus by 5-iododeoxyuridine. Nature (New Biol.) **244**, 214–217 (1973)

Hampar, B., Derge, J. G., Showalter, S. D.: Enhanced activation of the repressed Epstein-Barr viral genome by inhibitors of DNA synthesis. Virology **58**, 298–301 (1974a)

Hampar, B., Tanaka, A., Nonoyama, M., Derge, J. G.: Replication of the resident repressed Epstein-Barr virus genome during the early S phase (S-1 period) of non-producing RAJI cells. Proc. Natl. Acad. Sci. USA **71**, 631–633 (1974b)

Hampar, B., Derge, J. G., Nonoyama, M., Chang, S-Y, Tagamets, M. A., Showalter, S. D.: Programming of events in Epstein-Barr virus-activated cells induced by 5-iododeoxyuridine. Virology **62**, 71–89 (1974 c)

Hampar, B., Derge, J. G., Tanaka, A., Nonoyama, M.: Sequence of Epstein-Barr virus productive cycle in human lymphoblastoid cells. Cold Spring Harbor Symp. Quant. Biol. **39**, 811–815 (1975)

Hampar, B., Lenoir, G., Nonoyama, M., Derge, J. G., Chang, S-Y.: Cell cycle dependence for activation of Epstein-Barr virus by inhibitors of protein synthesis or medium deficient in arginine. Virology **69**, 660–668 (1976)

Hayward, S. D., Kieff, E. D.: Epstein-Barr virus specific RNA. I. Analysis of viral RNA in cellular extracts and in the polyribosomal fraction of permissive and non-permissive lymphoblastoid cell lines. J. Virol. **18**, 518–525 (1976)

Henle, G., Henle, W.: Immunofluorescence in cells derived from Burkitt's Lymphoma. J. Bacteriol. **91**, 1248–1256 (1966)

Henle, W., Henle, G.: Effect of arginine-deficient media on the herpes-type virus associated with cultured Burkitt tumor cells. J. Virol. **2**, 182–191 (1968)

Henle, W., Henle, G., Zajac, B. A., Pearson, G., Waubke, R., Scriba, M.: Differential reactivity of human serums with early antigens induced by Epstein-Barr virus. Science **169**, 188–190 (1970)

Henry, B. E., Glaser, R., Hewetson, J., O'Callaghan, D. J.: Expression of altered ribonucleotide reductase activity associated with the replication of the Epstein-Barr virus (in press) (1978)

Hinuma, Y., Konn, M., Yamaguchi, J., Wudarski, D. J., Blakeslee, J. R.: Immunofluorescence and herpes-type particles in P$_3$HR-1 Burkitt lymphoma cell line. J. Virol. **1**, 1045–1051 (1967a)

Hinuma, Y., Konn, M., Yamaguchi, J., Grace, J. T., Jr.: Replication of herpes-type virus in a Burkitt lymphoma cell line. J. Virol. **1**, 1203–1206 (1967b)

Joncas, J., Boucher, J., Boudreault, A., Granger-Julien, M.: Effect of hydrocortisone on cell viability, Epstein-Barr virus genome expression, and interferon synthesis in human lymphoblastoid cell lines. Cancer Res. **33**, 2142–2148 (1973)

Jondal, M., Klein, G.: Surface markers on human B and T lymphocytes. II. Presence of Epstein-Barr virus receptors on B lymphocytes. J. Exp. Med. **138**, 1365–1368 (1973)

Kaplan, J. C., Wilbert, S. M., Black, P. H.: Analysis of simian virus 40-induced transformation of hamster kidney cells in vitro. VIII. Induction of infectious simian virus 40 from virogenic transformed hamster cells by amino acid deprivation or cycloheximide treatment. J. Virol. **9**, 448–453 (1972)

Kaplan, J. C., Kleinman, L. F., Black, P. H.: Cell cycle dependence of SV40 virus induction from transformed hamster cells by UV-irradiation. Virology **68**, 215–220 (1975)

Klein, G., Dombos, L.: Relationship between the sensitivity of EBV-carrying lymphoblastoid lines to superinfection and the inducibility of the resident viral genome. Int. J. Cancer **11**, 327–337 (1973)

Klein, G., Wiener, F., Zech, L., zur Hausen, H., Reedman, B.: Segregation of the EBV-determined nuclear antigen (EBNA) in somatic cell hybrids derived from the fusion of a mouse fibroblast and human Burkitt lymphoma line. Int. J. Cancer **14**, 54–64 (1974)

Klein, G., Clements, G., Zeuthen, J., Westman, A.: Somatic cell hybrids between human lymphoma lines. II. Spontaneous and induced patterns of Epstein-Barr virus (EBV) cycle. Int. J. Cancer **17**, 715–724 (1976)

Lai, P. K., Mackay-Scollay, E. M., Alpers, M. P.: Synthesis of virus-capsid antigen (VCA) enhanced by ultraviolet irradiation of a lymphoblastoid cell line carrying Epstein-Barr virus. J. Gen. Virol. **21**, 135–143 (1973)

Lazarus, H., Barell, E. F., Oppenheim, S., Krishan, A.: Divergent properties of two human lymphocytic cell lines isolated from a single specimen of peripheral blood. In Vitro **9**, 303–310 (1974)

Lindahl, T., Adams, A., Bjursell, G., Bornkamm, G. W., Kaschka-Dierich, C., John, U.: Covalently closed circular duplex DNA of Epstein-Barr virus in Raji cells. J. Mol. Biol. **102**, 511–530 (1976)

Long, C., Derge, J. G., Hampar, B.: Procedure for activating Epstein-Barr virus early antigen in non-producer cells by 5-iododeoxyuridine. J. Natl. Cancer Inst. **52**, 1355–1357 (1974)

Lowy, D. R., Rowe, W. P., Teich, N., Hartley, J. W.: Murine leukemia virus: High frequency activation in vitro by 5-iododeoxyuridine and 5-bromodeoxyuridine. Science **174**, 155–156 (1971)

Matsuo, T., Yamamoto, K., Osato, T.: Differential induction of Epstein-Barr virus-related antigens in human lymphoblastoid cells by virus-mediated cell-to-cell contact. Int. J. Cancer **17**, 423–428 (1976)

Maurer, B. A., Glick, J. L., Minowada, J.: DNA synthesis in EB virus-containing Burkitt lymphoma cultures during a temperature cycling procedure. Proc. Soc. Exp. Biol. Med. **133**, 1226–1030 (1970)

Mele, J., Glaser, R., Nonoyama, M., Zimmerman, J., Rapp, F.: Observations on the resistance of Epstein-Barr virus DNA synthesis to hydroxyurea. Virology **62**, 101–111 (1974)

Nazerian, K.: Induction of an early antigen of Marek's disease virus in a lymphoblastoid cell line. In: Oncogenesis and herpesviruses II. de-Thé, G., Epstein, M. A., zur Hausen, H. (eds.), Part 1, pp. 345–350. Lyon: IARC 1975

Neubauer, R. H., Wallen, W. C., Rabin, H.: Stimulation of herpesvirus saimiri expression in the absence of evidence for Type C virus activation in a marmoset lymphoid cell line. J. Virol. **14**, 745–750 (1974)

Neubauer, R. H., Rabin, H.: Selective stimulation and differentiation of early antigens in a baboon lymphoblastoid cell line producing transforming Epstein-Barr like virus J. Gen. Virol. **48**, 295–301 (1978)

Nonoyama, M., Pagano, J. S.: Detection of Epstein-Barr viral genome in nonproductive cells. Nature (New Biol.) **233**, 103–106 (1971)

Nonoyama, M., Pagano, J. S.: Separation of Epstein-Barr virus DNA from large chromosomal DNA in non-virus-producing cells. Nature (New Biol.) **238**, 169–171 (1972)

Nyormoi, O., Klein, G., Adams, A., Dombos, L.: Sensitivity to EBV superinfection and IUDR inducibility of hybrid cells formed between a sensitive and a relatively resistant Burkitt lymphoma cell line. Int. J. Cancer **12**, 396–408 (1973)

Nyormoi, O., Thorley-Lawson, D. A., Elkington, J., Strominger, J. L.: Differential effect of phosphonoacetic acid on the expression of Epstein-Barr viral antigens and virus production. Proc. Natl. Acad. Sci. USA **73**, 1745–1748 (1976)

Pattengale, P. K., Smith, R. W., Gerber, P.: Selective transformation of B lymphocytes by EB virus. Lancet **1973 II**, 93–94

Pritchett, R., Pedersen, M., Kieff, E.: Complexity of EBV homologous DNA in continuous lymphoblastoid cell lines. Virology **74**, 227–231 (1976)

Rakusanova, T., Kaplan, J. C., Smales, W. P., Black, P. H.: Excision of viral DNA from host cell DNA after induction of Simian Virus 40-transformed hamster cells. J. Virol. **19**, 279–285 (1976)

Reedman, B., Klein, G.: Cellular localization of an Epstein-Barr virus (EBV)-associated complement-fixing antigen in producer and non-producer lymphoblastoid cell lines. Int. J. Cancer **11**, 499–520 (1973)

Rothschild, H., Black, P. H.: Analysis of SV40-induced transformation of hamster kidney tissue in vitro. VII.Induction of SV40 virus from transformed hamster cell clones by various agents. Virology **42**, 251–256 (1970)

Sairenji, T., Hinuma, Y.: Relationship between the synthesis of Epstein-Barr virus and growth of host cells in a Burkitt lymphoma cell line, P₃HR-1. Gann Monogr. **10**, 113–122 (1971)

Schwartz, S. A., Panem, S., Kirsten, W. H.: Distribution and virogenic effects of 5-bromodeoxyuridine in synchronized rat embryo cells. Proc. Natl. Acad. Sci. USA **72**, 1829–1833 (1975)

Shapiro, I., Andersson-Anvret, Klein, G.: Polyploidization of EBV-carrying lymphoma lines decreases the inducibility of EBV-determined early antigen following P₃HR-1 virus superinfection or iododeoxyuridine treatment. Intervirology **10**, 94–101 (1978)

Steplewski, Z., Koprowski, H., Andersson-Anvet, M., Klein, G.: Epstein-Barr virus in somatic cell hybrids between mouse cells and human nasopharyngeal carcinoma cells. J. Cell. Phys. **97**, 1–8 (1978)

Sugawara, K., Mizuno, F., Osato, T.: Epstein-Barr virus-associated antigens in non-producing clones of human lymphoblastoid cell lines. Nature (New Biol.) **239**, 242–243 (1972)

Summers, W. C., Klein, G.: Inhibition of Epstein-Barr virus DNA synthesis and late gene expression by phosphonoacetic acid. J. Virol. **18**, 151–155 (1976)

Tanaka, A., Nonoyama, M., Hampar, B.: Partial elimination of latent Epstein-Barr virus genomes from virus producing cells by cycloheximide. Virology **70**, 164–170 (1976)

Tanaka, A., Nonoyama, M., Glaser, R.: Transcription of latent Epstein-Barr virus genomes in human epithelial/Burkitt hybrid cells. Virology **82**, 63–68 (1977)

Trumper, P. A., Epstein, M. A., Giovanella, B. C.: Activation in vitro by BUDR of a productive EB virus infection in the epithelial cells of nasopharyngeal carcinoma. Int. J. Cancer **17**, 578–587 (1976)

Wolf, H., zur Hausen, H., Becker, V.: EB viral genome in epithelial nasopharyngeal carcinoma cells. Nature (New Biol.) **244**, 245–247 (1973)

Yata, J., Klein, G., Hewetson, J., Gergely, L.: Effect of metabolic inhibitors on membrane immunofluorescence reactivity of established Burkitt lymphoma cell lines. Int. J. Cancer **5**, 394–403 (1970)

Zajac, B. A., Kohn, G.: Epstein-Barr virus antigen, marker chromosome and interferon production in clones derived from cultured Burkitt tumour cells. J. Natl. Cancer Inst. **45**, 399–406 (1970)

Zimmerman, J. E. (Jr.), Glaser, R., Rapp, F.: Effect of dibutyryl cyclic AMP on the induction of Epstein-Barr virus in hybrid cells. J. Virol. **12**, 1442–1445 (1973)

zur Hausen, H., Schulte-Holthausen, H.: Presence of EB virus nucleic acid homology in a "virus-free" line of Burkitt tumor cells. Nature **227**, 245–248 (1970)

zur Hausen, H., Schulte-Holthausen, H.: Detection of Epstein-Barr viral genomes in human tumour cells by nucleic acid hybridization. In: Oncogenesis and herpesviruses. Biggs, P. M., de-Thé, G., Payne, L. N. (eds.), pp. 321–325. Lyon: IARC (1972)

zur Hausen, H., Diehl, V., Wolf, H., Schulte-Holthausen, H., Schneider, U.: Epstein-Barr virus genomes in human lymphoblastoid cell lines. Nature (New Biol.) **237**, 189–190 (1972)

13 The Virus as the Etiologic Agent of Infectious Mononucleosis[1]

G. Henle and W. Henle[2]

Division of Virology, The Joseph Stokes, Jr. Research Institute at The Children's Hospital of Philadelphia, School of Medicine, University of Pennsylvania, 34th Street & Civic Center Boulevard, Philadelphia, PA 19104 (USA)

[1] Work by the authors was supported by research grant CA-04568 and contract NO1-CP-33272 from the National Cancer Institute, U. S. Public Health Service.
[2] W. H. is the recipient of Career Award 5-K6-AI-22683 from the National Institutes of Health, Public Health Service.

The world-wide distribution and high incidence of antibodies to the Epstein-Barr virus (EBV) (see Chap. 4) strongly suggested that the virus might be the unsuspected cause of a common disease, besides its association with two rare malignancies i. e., Burkitt's lymphoma (BL) and nasopharyngeal carcinoma (NPC). Consequently, numerous paired acute-phase and convalescent sera from patients with unidentifiable infections of presumably viral origin were examined for an emergence or increase in titer of antibodies to EBV. While these efforts in search of a disease caused by the virus were initially unrewarding, they prepared the stage for what appeared to be a fortuitous observation and led to the identification of EBV as the long-sought cause of infectious mononucleosis (IM).

A. EVIDENCE FOR THE ETIOLOGIC ROLE OF EBV IN INFECTIOUS MONONUCLEOSIS

I. INITIAL OBSERVATIONS

The first suggestion that EBV might be etiologically related to IM was obtained when a laboratory technician who previously had no antibodies to the virus, as determined by indirect immunofluorescence (G. Henle and W. Henle, 1966), seroconverted in the course of this disease (G. Henle et al., 1968). It was of some significance, too, that cultures of her leukocytes initiated during the acute phase and early convalescence readily developed into permanently growing lymphoid cell lines (LCL), whereas cultures set up prior to her illness or in late convalescence failed to survive (G. Henle et al., 1968). A small proportion of cells in the established cultures was found to synthesize EBV as shown by immunofluorescence and electron microscopy. Comparable observations were made a few months later when another antibody-negative technician developed IM (Diehl et al., 1968). It was quickly found that sera from IM patients uniformly showed elevated titers of antibodies to EBV, which actually were directed against EB viral capsid antigen (VCA) (W. Henle et al., 1966; zur Hausen et al., 1967; Mayyasi et al., 1967). Of particular significance were results obtained with serial sera from students collected in a prospective study of IM at Yale University and kindly provided under code by Drs. McCollum and Niederman; all the pre-illness sera were correctly identified, having no antibodies to VCA, whereas consecutive acute-phase and convalescent sera from the same students showed high and, in part, still rising anti-VCA titers (G. Henle et al., 1968; Niederman et al., 1968). In addition, LCL showing small proportions of VCA-positive cells, were readily established from leukocytes of nearly every IM patient tested; they were obtained at a reduced frequency from leukocytes of donors with past histories of IM but not from leukocytes of individuals without antibodies to EBV (Diehl et al., 1968). These observations strongly indicated that EBV is the cause of IM, a conclusion subsequently confirmed by similar observations and extended by additional evidence (W. Henle and G. Henle, 1972, 1973a; Miller, 1975).

Identification of EBV as the cause of IM was in retrospect not particularly surprising. It was already known that EBV was an essentially lymphocytotropic virus since it was found to replicate only in cells of the lymphoid series. All attempts to transmit it to other types of cells had been unsuccessful (Epstein et al., 1965), a fact holding to the present date. EBV thus should have been suspected of causing an essentially lymphoproliferative disease, such as IM. It had also been shown prior to the discovery of the role of EBV in IM that cultures of leukocytes from IM patients developed more readily into continuous LCL than leukocyte cultures from other donors (Pope, 1967; Glade et al., 1968). Furthermore, there were already indications of the capacity of EBV to transform normal lymphocytes in vitro into LCL containing small numbers of VCA-positive cells (W. Henle et al., 1967); and finally, the seroepidemiology of EBV had revealed features which were compatible with the epidemiology of IM. It was known that in populations living under conditions of crowding or poor hygiene, among which IM is essentially unknown, antibodies to VCA are acquired at high frequencies in early childhood (Levy and G. Henle, 1966; Tischendorf et al., 1970), whereas under high socioeconomic conditions acquisition of this antibody is often delayed to adolescence and later (G. Henle and W. Henle, 1966, 1967, 1970); IM is most frequently observed in this social class and age range.

The indirect immunofluorescence test for the titration of anti-VCA was found to have limitations since (a) the lowest titers observed in IM overlapped with the highest titers seen in healthy individuals after long-past primary infections; and (b) diagnostically significant increments in titers from the acute to convalescent phases were observed in no more than 10%–20% of the patients. Other more discerning serologic tests were needed.

Two different complement fixation (CF) tests were introduced. Gerber et al. (1968) used virus suspensions derived from the HR-1 subculture of the P_3J line of BL cells (Hinuma et al., 1967) as antigen and found that pre-illness sera gave negative reactions, whereas high antibody titers were recorded in the acute-phase sera of IM patients; but again significant increases in titers between the acute and convalescent phases were observed in only some of the patients. Difficulties in obtaining virus suspensions in sufficient concentration and quantities have limited the use of this test to a few studies (Gerber and Deal, 1970; Vonka et al., 1970).

Extracts of cells from virus-producing LCL were found to contain a soluble (S) antigen reactive in CF tests with many human sera (Armstrong et al., 1966). The antigen was not thought to be EBV-related at that time because the same sera also reacted with extracts of cells from nonproducer LCL. It was subsequently shown (Pope et al., 1969 a) that only anti-VCA positive sera fixed C′ in the presence of S antigen, thus linking it with EBV. This relationship was substantiated later by the demonstration of EBV genomes in nonproducer LCL by nucleic acid hybridization techniques (zur Hausen and Schulte-Holthausen, 1970; Nonoyama and Pagano, 1971; zur Hausen et al., 1972). It was further noted that anti-S was usually absent in acute-phase IM sera but appeared regularly weeks or even months after onset of illness (Vonka et al., 1972). The regular anti-S seroconversion following IM lent additional support to the etiologic role of EBV in this disease, but the late development of this antibody limited its serodiagnostic value.

II. ADDITIONAL SEROLOGIC TESTS

1. Antibodies to EBV-Determined Membrane Antigens

It was shown by Klein and his associates (1967) that biopsy and cultured BL cells had antigens on their membranes which were detectable on live cells by indirect immunofluorescence, using sera from BL patients as well as from many other donors. These antigens were subsequently found to be EBV-determined (Klein et al., 1968a) and were also observed on the membranes of cultured lymphoblasts derived from leukocytes of IM patients (Klein et al., 1968b). Correspondingly, IM patients were shown to develop antibodies to these membrane antigens (MA) in the course of the disease. The indirect immunofluorescence test for detection of anti-MA was later replaced by a blocking procedure to avoid interaction of antibodies to membrane antigens unrelated to EBV. Live cells were first exposed to test serum and then, after washing, to fluorescein isothiocyanate (FITC)-conjugated antibodies to EBV-specific MA from a donor without detectable iso- or other nonspecific antibodies to cell membrane components (Klein et al., 1969). MA proved to be a complex of several components, some being synthesized before (early MA) and others only after (late MA) viral DNA replication (Ernberg et al., 1974; Silvestre et al., 1974). Due to their complexities, tests for antibodies to MA components have not been widely applied in IM.

2. Antibodies to the EBV-Induced Early Antigen Complex

Superinfection of lymphoblasts from nonproducer LCL with EBV derived from P_3HR-1 cultures was found to reduce or abolish their growth in vitro, yet few or none of the exposed cells stained in the indirect immunofluorescence test for VCA when positive sera from healthy donors were employed (W. Henle, et al., 1970a). This paradox was resolved when sera from patients with IM, BL, or NPC were used in the assay. The reactive antibodies appeared to be largely disease-associated and with sera from such patients, up to 90% of the cells stained brilliantly 1–3 days after exposure to EBV and the percentages of positive cells were proportional to the dose of virus used. The antigen(s) appeared in the cells within a few hours after exposure, often being the only component(s) synthesized. In 10% or less of the infected cells VCA also ultimately developed. Antibodies to these "early antigen(s)" (EA) were observed in 70%–85% of patients during the acute phase of IM (W. Henle et al., 1971). They arose transiently and returned to nondetectable levels usually within a few weeks after onset of illness.

In the course of examining numerous sera for antibodies to EA, two patterns of immunofluorescence became evident, showing that EA is a complex of at least two components (G. Henle et al., 1971). One, causing diffuse staining of the nucleus and cytoplasm of infected cells and resistant to methanol fixation, has been called D; the other, staining a restricted antigenic mass in the cytoplasm and denatured by methanol, has been designated R. Antibodies to the EA complex in the acute phase of IM are invariably directed against the D component (G. Henle et al., 1971; W. Henle et al., 1974a), but in prolonged cases of the disease anti-R may occasionally arise and replace anti-D (Horwitz et al., 1975). In NPC, anti-D is usually the dominant antibody, whereas in BL anti-R is often the sole antibody to the EA complex. As anti-EA is observed infrequently in healthy individuals and then only at low titers, the anti-D response in IM turned out to be of considerable diagnostic value (W. Henle et al., 1974a).

3. EBV-Specific IgM Antibodies

Early attempts by the authors to detect VCA-specific IgM antibodies by indirect immunofluorescence in sera of IM patients failed due to the fact that most commercially available antihuman IgM conjugates are unsatisfactory for this purpose. However, after separation of the IgM fractions from IM sera, positive results were recorded (Hampar et al., 1971; Banatvala et al., 1972). Schmitz and Scherer (1972) demonstrated VCA-specific IgM antibodies by using a triple-layer technique; i. e., fixed cell smears from producer LCL were successively exposed to test serum dilution, antihuman IgM rabbit serum, and FITC-conjugated goat antibodies to rabbit globulins. While the demonstration of VCA-specific IgM antibodies confirmed that IM represents a primary EBV infection, the test procedures were as yet too inconvenient for routine serodiagnosis. It was shown subsequently that VCA-specific IgM antibodies can be readily determined by indirect immunofluorescence provided the anti-human IgM conjugate is satisfactory (Nikoskelainen and Hänninen, 1973; Edwards and McSwiggan, 1974; Nikoskelainen et al., 1975; Horwitz et al., 1976 a). With the proper reagent, the IgM antibody test has become a readily applicable and the most essential serodiagnostic procedure for identification of primary EBV infections. Peak titers are usually reached in the early acute phase and the antibodies subsequently decline to lower levels and disappear within one or more months.

4. Antibodies to EBV Nuclear Antigen

In attempts to localize the soluble (S) complement-fixing antigen in cells from nonproducer LCL, Reedman and Klein (1973) applied the sensitive anti-complement immunofluorescence reaction. By this technique brilliant fluorescence is elicited in every nucleus of cells from nonproducer as well as producer LCL. Antibodies to this EBV nuclear antigen (EBNA) are present in practically all anti-VCA positive sera. For accurate antibody determinations it is essential to use a three-step procedure, i. e., cell smears from nonproducer LCL are exposed successively to test serum dilution, appropriately diluted serum of an anti-VCA negative donor as source of C', and the anti-human $\beta_1 C/\beta_1 A$ conjugate as the admixture of C' to an anti-complementary test serum in a two-step test may yield false negative or prozone reactions (W. Henle et al., 1974b). Application of the anti-EBNA test to sera from IM patients has shown that this antibody, with few exceptions, arises only weeks or months after onset of illness (G. Henle et al., 1974). As mentioned earlier, antibodies to the soluble (S) CF antigen also arise late in the course of IM (Vonka et al., 1972). This parallel behavior and the fact that generally anti-EBNA titers closely match anti-S titers (Klein and Vonka, 1974) suggest that the antigens involved in the two tests are identical (Chap. 3).

5. Virus Neutralization Tests

Several neutralization tests have been developed which are based on either (a) the induction of abortive EBV superinfections in nonproducer LCL or (b) the in vitro transformation of lymphocytes by EBV. In the case of (a), neutralization of the virus is detected by prevention of EA synthesis in the exposed cells (Pearson et al., 1970) or by survival of the cells so that they form colonies in wells of microtiter plates (Rocchi and

Hewetson, 1973). In the case of (b), evidence of neutralization is provided by failure to establish LCL (Pope et al., 1969 b; Gerber et al., 1969 a; Miller et al., 1971, 1972), by undiminished incorporation of ^{3}H-thymidine into the exposed cells (Robinson and Miller, 1975), or by emergence of EBNA-positive cells in the test cultures (Aya et al., 1974; Leibold et al., 1975; Moss and Pope, 1975). Using these techniques, especially the microtest based on colony formation and most suitable for large-scale assays, it became evident that EBV-neutralizing antibodies were already present in early acute-phase sera from IM patients and that they increased in titer subsequently to higher persistent levels (Hewetson et al., 1973). There is some evidence that neutralizing antibodies are possibly identical with antibodies to some of the MA components (Pearson et al., 1970; De Schryver et al., 1974).

III. EBV IN THE OROPHARYNX OF INFECTIOUS MONONUCLEOSIS PATIENTS

Demonstration of the virus was initially unsuccessful when lymphoblasts from nonproducer LCL were exposed to throat washings or swabs collected during the acute phase of IM. No EA synthesis became apparent because there was either too little or no "lytic" virus or because the virus was of the "transforming" type (Miller et al., 1974). Indeed, exposure of peripheral or umbilical-cord blood lymphocytes to oropharyngeal excretions of IM patients leads readily to the establishment of LCL (Chang and Golden, 1971; Pereira et al., 1972; Gerber et al., 1972; Miller et al., 1973). Virus is demonstrable by this technique in the oropharynx of nearly every IM patient. Excretion of the virus may persist for as long as 18 months after onset of IM (Miller et al., 1973; Niederman et al., 1976) and virus is also detectable in throat washings of an appreciable percentage (12%–18%) of healthy donors long after primary EBV infection (Gerber et al., 1972; Chang et al., 1973; Miller, 1975). The fact that EBV-positive lymphoblast lines can be established at a moderate frequency from peripheral leukocytes of anti-VCA positive donors (Moore et al., 1967; Diehl et al., 1968; Gerber et al., 1968 a; Miller et al., 1971) and uniformly from lymph nodes (Nilsson et al., 1971) already showed that, like other herpesviruses, EBV establishes a persistent viral-carrier state after the primary infection, in this specific instance in the lymphoreticular system. The persistent EBV infection may become activated sporadically, especially under immunosuppressive conditions, and lead to renewed, presumably intermittent excretion of virus into the oropharynx (Strauch et al., 1974; Miller, 1975). Whether the virus is derived from the lymphoid tissues or from other organs in the oropharynx, possibly salivary glands (Niederman et al., 1976), has not been established.

IV. ATTEMPTS TO INDUCE INFECTIOUS MONONUCLEOSIS IN VOLUNTEERS OR NONHUMAN PRIMATES

A number of attempts to transmit IM experimentally were made prior to the discovery of EBV by injection of volunteers with blood, throat washings, or stool suspensions from patients in the acute phase of illness, but the results were inconclusive or outright negative (Sohier et al., 1940; Evans, 1947, 1950; Evans et al., 1953; Taylor, 1953;

Niederman and Scott, 1965). However, Wising (1942) transmitted the disease to a volunteer by transfusion of blood from an IM patient, a result later confirmed several times accidentally (Gerber et al., 1969 b; Blacklow et al., 1971; Turner et al., 1972). Preinoculation sera from some of the volunteers had been frozen and, when tested later, were found to have antibodies to VCA, i. e., all the volunteers were immune prior to inoculation (Niederman, personal communication). Since the majority of sera from old-world nonhuman primate species are now known to have antibodies reacting with EBV VCA and some also with D (Gerber and Deal, 1970; Dunkel et al., 1972; Kalter et al., 1972; Gerber et al., 1976), it is likely that the animals used in early transmission attempts were also immune. The potential oncogenicity of EBV has prevented experimental inoculation of volunteers with the virus. However, injection of EBV into antibody-negative gibbons has led to seroconversion after an incubation period of 5 weeks. At that time the two animals that had been injected into the tonsils with either P_3HR-1 virus or autochthonous lymphocytes, exposed in vitro for 18 h to the virus, developed a mild exudative tonsillitis (Werner et al., 1972). Following injection of EBV into cotton-top marmosets, some responded with silent seroconversion, others with a self-limited lymphoproliferative disease, and the remainder developed disseminated fatal lymphomas within 6–14 weeks (Shope et al., 1973; Deinhardt et al., 1975; Chap.16). These results come close to fulfilling the third Henle-Koch postulate.

B. IMPLICATIONS OF THE SEROLOGIC AND VIROLOGIC OBSERVATIONS IN INFECTIOUS MONONUCLEOSIS

From the observations presented in the preceding section, the serologic and virologic events occurring in the course of IM can be summarized schematically as shown in Fig. 1. A number of conclusions can be drawn.

I. SUSCEPTIBILITY OR IMMUNITY TO INFECTIOUS MONONUCLEOSIS

IM only occurs in individuals without antibodies to EBV. All pre-illness sera available by chance or by design from prospective studies of IM proved to be uniformly devoid of all antibodies to EBV (G. Henle et al., 1968; Niederman et al., 1968, 1970; Evans et al., 1968; Hirshaut et al., 1969; Tischendorf et al., 1970; Wahren et al., 1970; Sawyer et al., 1971; University Health Physicians and PHLS Laboratories, 1971; Hallee et al., 1974). Absence of anti-VCA thus denotes susceptibility and its presence, immunity to IM. Although anti-VCA is not a virus-neutralizing antibody, sera containing anti-VCA with rare exceptions also reveal neutralizing antibodies (Rocchi et al., 1973; Hewetson et al., 1973). The anti-VCA test serves therefore as a convenient and dependable indicator of the immune status.

II. EBV-SPECIFIC SERODIAGNOSIS

Primary EBV infections, whether or not accompanied by classic signs of IM, can be dependably diagnosed by criteria derived from the antibody patterns presented in

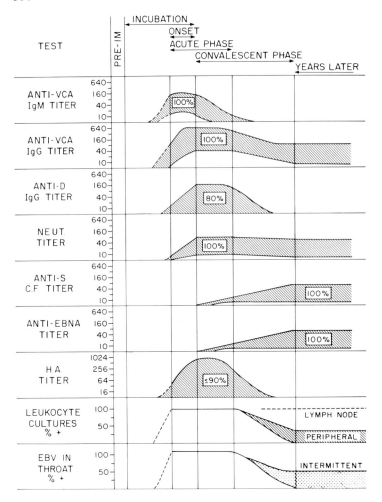

Fig. 1. Antibody responses and other observations in the course of IM. From Henle, W., Henle, G.: The seroepidemiology of Epstein-Barr virus. Adv. Pathol. (1975): Courtesy of the editor and publisher

Fig. 1. A *current primary EBV infection* is identified by (a) the early demonstration of high titers of VCA-specific IgM antibodies and their later decline to lower, ultimately nondetectable levels; (b) high and in 10%–20% of the patients still rising VCA-specific IgG antibody titers and their subsequent decline to lower but then persistent levels; (c) a transient anti-D response, observed in over 80% of IM patients; and (d) the early absence and later emergence of anti-EBNA and of the probably identical antibodies to S antigen. Anti-R may occasionally arise and replace anti-D late in the course of IM in patients showing persistent signs of illness (Horwitz et al., 1975). While these criteria were derived mainly from studies of adolescent or adult IM patients, they hold equally for primary EBV infections with typical signs of IM in children (Ginsburg et al., 1977 a) and in adults above 40 years of age (Horwitz et al., 1976 a), and also in silent infections uncovered by chance (Horwitz et al., 1976 b). Antibodies to MA components or EBV-neutralizing antibodies are usually not determined for routine purposes because of the time required, the complexities of the tests, and the limited additional information they may provide.

A *long-past primary EBV infection* is identified by (a) absence of VCA-specific IgM antibodies; (b) usually moderate, unchanging titers of VCA-specific IgG antibodies; (c) absence of anti-EA, as a rule, although low levels of anti-R, rarely anti-D, may occasionally be found in sera from some of those individuals who maintain relatively high VCA-specific IgG antibody titers; and (d) detection of anti-EBNA or anti-S at unchanging, moderate titers. Consecutively negative results in all tests denote, of course, that the illness under study is not caused by EBV and that the donors have not as yet been infected by the virus.

To perform four separate immunofluorescence tests for the serodiagnosis of primary EBV infections may appear unusually demanding. Yet, for evaluation of serodiagnostic results on patients with an IM-like illness who may have additional, unrelated clinical problems, all tests are needed. For example, reactivation of persistent EBV infections by immunosuppressive malignant or nonmalignant diseases such as Hodgkin's disease, other lymphomas, leukemias, sarcoidosis, systemic lupus erythematosus, etc., may lead to elevated anti-VCA titers and occasionally re-emergence of anti-D (W. Henle and G. Henle, 1973b) and conceivably also re-emergence of VCA-specific IgM antibodies at low to moderate titers. In such cases, elevated anti-EBNA titers would exclude a primary EBV infection. In some cases of prolonged severe immunosuppression, e. g., in renal transplant patients or individuals with genetic T cell (thymus-dependent lymphocyte) defects, anti-EBNA may be undetectable even though VCA-specific IgG antibodies are maintained at moderate or even high titers. In such instances, the absence of VCA-specific IgM antibodies would exclude a primary EBV infection. Thus, only the complete serologic pattern may permit interpretation of the results in such situations. As will be discussed below, the detection of heterophil antibody responses would, of course, readily identify primary EBV infections.

III. DETECTION OF HETEROPHIL ANTIBODY RESPONSES IN INFECTIOUS MONONUCLEOSIS

A considerable number of heterophil antibodies, mostly of the IgM class, develop transiently in the course of IM. These antibodies are directed against sheep, horse, and bovine erythrocytes, the I/i blood groups, Ig, nuclear factors, Proteus OX_{19} and other antigens evidently unrelated to EBV (Carter, 1966; Lee and Davidsohn, 1972), and although such antibody responses are presently unexplained they provide an important diagnostic tool. It has been suggested, among other things, that already committed B lymphocytes (bone marrow-derived lymphocyte) are stimulated by EBV or a byproduct of the disease process to synthesize enhanced amounts of antibody. This hypothesis has the advantage that it would explain the great variety of heterophil antibody responses, whereas the sharing, uncovering, or derepression of antigens by the virus, another hypothesis, seems unlikely because of the multitude of antigens involved.

The most frequent and most extensively studied heterophil antibodies in IM are the agglutinins for sheep or horse erythrocytes and the hemolysins for bovine red blood cells (RBC). The development of high titers of sheep RBC agglutinins in IM was first described by Paul and Bunnell (1932). It was subsequently shown that these antibodies have to be differentiated from other types of sheep and horse RBC agglutinins. In the differential absorption test, the agglutinins arising in IM are not absorbed by guinea pig kidney suspensions (Forssman antigen), but are removed from the sera by bovine erythrocytes (Davidsohn and Nelson, 1969). The heterophil agglutinins of the Paul-Bunnell-Davidsohn (PBD) type are, with very rare exceptions, specific for IM, as are the ox cell hemolysins, which are determined directly without requiring absorption procedures (Mason, 1951; Leyton, 1952; Davidsohn and Lee, 1964). Rapid differential slide agglutination tests have been developed (Lee et al., 1968; Galloway, 1969) for which the required reagents are provided commercially in tests kits. While these tests, too, are generally specific for IM, false negative results may be observed when the heterophil antibody titers are low, and false positive results may also be occasionally recorded.

Heterophil agglutinins of the PBD type or ox cell hemolysins are usually already detectable during the 1st week of illness but occasionally arise later or not at all in a small proportion of the patients. It has been estimated that $\sim 10\%$ of adolescent or young adult patients and a larger percentage of children fail to show heterophil antibodies when their sera are tested against sheep RBC. With the more sensitive horse RBC test (Lee and Davidsohn, 1972), the percentage of nonresponders is smaller, yet EBV-associated IM without PBD antibody responses has remained a reality (Evans et al., 1968; Klemola et al., 1970; Nikoskelainen et al., 1974; Ginsburg et al., 1977; Horwitz et al., 1977). The heterophil antibodies may persist at gradually diminishing titers for many months or even over a year after onset of IM (Evans et al., 1975; Horwitz et al., 1976b), with the ox cell hemolysins disappearing first and the horse RBC agglutinins, last.

The high degree of specificity of the PBD agglutinins and ox cell hemolysins for IM denotes that EBV-specific serodiagnostic tests are not usually needed in classic cases of the disease. They are required, however, for heterophil antibody-negative cases of IM-like illnesses that in part are due to EBV but more frequently to cytomegalovirus (CMV), and occasionally to adenovirus or other viruses, or *Toxoplasma gondii* (Klemola et al., 1967, 1970; Evans et al., 1968; Wahren et al., 1969; Nikoskelainen et al., 1974; Evans; 1975, Horwitz et al., 1977). Furthermore, primary EBV infections show a wide range of clinical responses and severity, and a remarkable variety of complications involving various organs which may follow, accompany, or even precede typical signs of IM or represent at times the only clinical features. Thus, in spite of detection of heterophil antibodies, physicians may often want confirmation of the diagnosis by EBV-specific serology.

IV. DEMONSTRATION OF EBV IN INFECTIOUS MONONUCLEOSIS PATIENTS

Isolation of the virus has proved to be of limited diagnostic value. The nearly uniform establishment of LCLs from peripheral leukocytes and the almost regular demonstration of EBV in oropharyngeal secretions (Fig. 1) provide supporting evidence of primary EBV infections, but do not prove it. As already discussed, a persistent viral-carrier state regularly ensues after overt or silent EBV infections. EBV carriers may intermittently excrete virus into the oropharynx and LCL can be established from their circulating leukocytes at moderate frequencies and almost uniformly from lymph nodes. This persistent viral infection is undoubtedly responsible for the life-long maintenance of various virus-related antibodies.

C. FACTS AND SPECULATIONS REGARDING PATHOGENESIS

I. THE SOURCE OF INFECTION

This can rarely be identified, since, as a rule, no chains of cases of IM are observed. Indeed, the incidence of IM among roommates of patients at colleges or other schools has been comparable to that seen among the students at large (Sawyer et al., 1971; University Health Physicians and PHLS Laboratories, 1971; Hallee et al., 1974). In families, secondary cases may occasionally be observed (Wahren et al., 1970; Joncas and Mitnyan, 1970). For every overt case of IM, one silent primary EBV infection can be identified on the average by seroconversion. The ratio between overt cases and primary infections which remain silent or are accompanied by such mild symptoms as not to be registered has ranged between > 2:1 and 1:2 (Niederman et al., 1970; Sawyer et al., 1971; University Health Physicians and PHLS Laboratories, 1971; Hallee et al., 1974). Such silent cases can undoubtedly transmit infections. Furthermore, since anti-VCA positive individuals are permanent carriers of EBV and intermittent excreters of the virus (Gerber et al., 1972; Miller et al., 1973; Chang et al., 1973; Miller, 1975), they provide ample sources of infection.

II. THE ROUTE OF TRANSMISSION

As a rule, close salivary contact (Hoagland, 1955) or contaminated eating and drinking utensils provide the route of infection. Air-borne dissemination of the virus may possibly occur occasionally (Ginsburg et al., 1976), although multicase outbreaks of IM are most uncommon. Infections are transmitted most likely by extracellular virus, but perhaps occasionally also by infected cells. IM has been transmitted on rare occasions to antibody negative recipients by blood transfusions (Gerber et al., 1969b; Blacklow et al., 1971; Turner et al., 1972). In two of these instances, the donors turned out to be in the incubation period of IM and thus were probably viremic although their blood could also have contained virus-infected lymphocytes. Such cells must be expected to be regularly transmitted by blood transfusions from anti-VCA positive donors, but they usually do not cause illness in susceptible recipients because antibodies are also transfused simultaneously. Thus, only silent seroconversions are generally observed under these conditions (W. Henle et al., 1970b).

III. THE INCUBATION PERIOD

This has been estimated to be 5–7 weeks in young adults, but it is possibly somewhat shorter in children, although there are no solid data for this suggestion. The events occurring between exposure to the virus and the development of the disease are essentially unknown, but have been the subject of speculations which will be presented later.

IV. CLINICAL FEATURES

IM is essentially a self-limited lymphoproliferative disease with a usually benign course, but is occasionally accompanied by severe though rarely fatal complications. After vague prodromal symptoms, the disease presents in its typical form with a triad of fever, sore throat, and extensive cervical lymphadenopathy. The spleen is often enlarged and liver involvement, leading to abnormal liver-function tests, is frequent. The uncomplicated illness usually lasts 2–4 weeks, but may be prolonged occasionally for several months. Complications involving the central nervous system, such as the Guillain-Barré syndrome, Bell's palsy, transverse myelitis, and meningoencephalitis, were known to occur in heterophil antibody-positive IM prior to the discovery of EBV. It has been shown now by EBV-specific serodiagnostic tests that they may also develop in the absence of heterophil antibody responses and in patients who may show minimal or no other signs of IM (Grose et al., 1975; Lange et al., 1976). Complications involving other organs are pneumonitis, myo- or pericarditis, nephritis, rupture of the spleen, acquired hemolytic anemia, thrombocytopenic purpura, agranulocytosis, etc. Here again, EBV-specific serology may identify unsuspected cases of IM.

V. THE WHITE BLOOD CELL PICTURE

Early after onset of IM, leukocyte counts may be normal or show a leukopenia due to a decrease in granulocytes. By the 2nd or 3rd week, the counts are elevated to between 10,000 and 20,000 WBC mm^3, rarely higher. Blood smears obtained during the 1st or 2nd week of illness characteristically show more than 50%, usually 60%–80% mononuclear cells (lymphocytes and monocytes) with at least 10, and generally more than 25 atypical lymphocytes/100 WBCs and considerable pleomorphism. These abnormalities persist for at least 2 weeks and occasionally for several months.

The atypical lymphocytes have been reported to have T cell characteristics (Sheldon et al., 1973; Pattengale et al., 1974 a), but other studies have shown that B cells also contribute to the pool of atypical cells (Enberg et al., 1974; Giulano et al., 1974). In fact, the absolute number of atypical lymphocytes may often exceed the total number of T cells (Mangi et al., 1974). It is conceivable that not only T cells, but also B lymphocytes producing heterophil IgM antibodies might form rosettes with sheep RBC, although this has not been clearly demonstrated. Increases in the relative proportion of T cells (Sheldon et al., 1973; Virolainen et al., 1974) or of B cells (Piessens et al., 1973) have been reported. These discrepant observations have been resolved by determination of the absolute numbers of B and T cells (Mangi et al., 1974). The B lymphocytes, including presumably atypical cells, are increased and present in peak numbers during the 1st week of IM and then decline to normal levels within 3 weeks. In contrast, T lymphocytes, many of them atypical, increase to peak levels in the 2nd week after onset of illness and remain elevated for ∼ 5 weeks. While the atypical B lymphocytes may include nonlytically EBV-infected cells, they would at most account for a small fraction (Klein et al., 1976), as will be discussed later. The atypical T cells are thought to be activated, at least in part, by EBV-infected B cells expressing virus-determined antigens on their surfaces.

During the period of lymphocytosis and presence of numerous atypical lymphocytes, a decline in cell-mediated immunity is apparent. There is a transient depression in responses to skin test antigens, perhaps due to antigenic competition, as well as hyporesponsiveness of lymphocytes in vitro to phytohemagglutinin, allogeneic lymphocytes, or certain specific antigens (Bentzon, 1955; Haider et al., 1973; Sheldon et al., 1973; Mangi et al., 1974). The nature of this immunosuppressive effect is not clear, but may be similar for other viral diseases.

VI. PATHOLOGY

There is extensive hyperplasia of lymphoreticular tissues, but the lymph nodes usually retain their follicular structure, although the sinuses are partially obliterated and distended by macrophages, atypical lymphocytes, and pyroninophilic immunoblasts. Variable numbers of plasma cells, occasional Reed-Sternberg cells, and focal necrosis are also present (Dorfman and Warnke, 1974). Focal and perivascular infiltration of mononuclear cells, which are largely atypical, may be seen in nearly every organ. In the liver, patchy mononuclear cell infiltrates are observed in the portal tracts and lobular sinusoids as well as around parenchymal cells. These infiltrates may be the cause of functional disturbances. The bone marrow may often reveal ill-defined granulomas.

VII. EVENTS DURING THE INCUBATION PERIOD

The host-virus interactions can only be surmised on the basis of in vitro studies and observations made during the acute phase of IM. One can merely raise questions and suggest possible answers.

To begin with, it is unknown whether *the infecting virus* has to be of the "lytic," or whether it can also be of the "transforming" type (Miller et al., 1974). EBV present in the oropharynx of IM patients or viral carriers has invariably been detectable only by its capacity to transform B lymphocytes in vitro into permanently growing lymphoblasts; it has failed to induce EA synthesis (lytic cycles) in cells of nonproducer LCL. Most virus populations are, however, likely to be mixtures of the two viral variants, the dominant one determining the demonstrable activity.

The *initial target cells* remain to be identified. It has been suggested that as yet unknown cells, possibly of epithelial nature, may be highly permissive for EBV and serve as initial targets. This suggestion is based, among other considerations, on the intimate association of EBV genomes with NPC cells, which are of epithelial derivation (Wolf et al., 1973, 1975; Klein et al., 1974; Huang et al., 1974). On the basis of results obtained by in situ nucleic acid hybridization tests with exfoliated oropharyngeal epithelial cells from IM patients, Lemon et al. (1977) have claimed that these cells support replication of EBV. Additional evidence is needed to substantiate this conclusion. If correct, the question remains why, with the accessibility of the oropharyngeal epithelium, clinical signs of IM do not develop sooner than observed.

With the evident tropism of EBV for B lymphocytes (Jondal and Klein, 1973; Pattengale et al., 1974b) the lymphoid tissues of the oropharynx may not only be the later, but also the initial sites of infection. B lymphocytes, however, cannot be considered more than partially permissive for EBV according to observations made in vitro. In LCL derived from leukocytes of IM patients or viral carriers, or established by exposure of lymphocytes from antibody negative children or adults to transforming EBV, only a small proportion of the cells support at any given time lytic cycles of viral replication, although all cells express EBNA and thus harbor viral genomes. The percentages of spontaneously induced lymphoblasts depend on the cell line and on the period of maintenance in vitro, since on prolonged cultivation, most LCL gradually become nonproducers. Synthesis of viral antigen and viral particles can be induced in some of the cells by exposure of the LCL to 5-bromodeoxyuridine (BUDR) or 5-iododeoxyuridine (IUDR) (Hampar et al., 1972; Gerber, 1972; Chap. 12), or by super-infection with lytic EBV (P_3HR-1 virus) (W. Henle et al., 1970 a; G. Henle et al., 1971). Recent observations indicate that the viral progeny obtained after superinfection is derived largely from the indigenous viral genomes rather than the superinfecting virus (Nonoyama; zur Hausen, personal communications). However, some lymphoid cell lines devoid of EBV genomes have been found now to be remarkably susceptible to P_3HR-1 virus, leading to EA synthesis in all of the cells and VCA in a high percentage of them (A. L. Epstein et al., 1978).

According to these various observations, if they were applicable to in vivo conditions, B lymphocytes could be primary targets for EBV. If so, virus production and the spread of the infection by viremia or dissemination of infected B cells would probably be relatively slow, thus possibly accounting for the long incubation period of IM.

As to *EBV-specific antibody responses,* considerable numbers of target cells, whatever their nature, must gradually become lytically infected during the incubation period to produce and release sufficient EA, MA, VCA, and virus particles to evoke peak titers, as a rule, of VCA-specific IgM and IgG antibodies by the time of onset of illness as well as substantial levels of anti-MA and neutralizing antibodies (Fig. 1). While viral replication in all probability is preceded by EBNA synthesis, too little of this antigen becomes available or EBNA is too weak an antigen to induce detectable antibody responses during the incubation period. There remains, however, another possible explanation for the late emergence of anti-EBNA.

Since antibodies to EBNA become detectable usually only weeks or even months after onset of IM when viral replication has undoubtedly long since subsided to very low levels, the suggestion has been made (G. Henle et al., 1974) that EBNA for antibody stimulation is derived mainly from nonlytically infected, EBV-transformed B lymphocytes. The virus detectable in the oropharynx during the acute phase, and presumably earlier, is mainly of the transforming type. It is likely therefore that transformation of B lymphocytes occurs not only in vitro, but also in vivo in lymphoid organs *before* significant development of EBV-neutralizing antibodies. Such nonlyti-cally infected, EBNA-positive cells would be expected to survive and divide, as they do in vitro and exhibit new antigens in their membranes, thereby becoming targets for T lymphocytes and possibly other host defenses and releasing EBNA in the process of their destruction. Such a course of events could well explain the delayed anti-EBNA responses. Indeed, T cells specifically attacking EBV-transformed cells in vitro have been demonstrated in the acute phase of IM but no longer in convalescence (Svedmyr and Jondal, 1975; Royston et al., 1975; Hutt et al., 1975).

The *demonstration of EBV-infected lymphocytes* in support of the various specu-lations presented above may no longer be achieved convincingly during the acute phase of IM. First of all, the lytic and nonlytic infections of B lymphocytes might have passed their peaks by the time of onset of illness which, in fact, might be due to immune responses to the infected cells. Secondly, lytically or nonlytically infected cells may not be spilled in substantial numbers into the blood, the only type of specimen readily available for examination. They may be concentrated in affected lymphoid organs or lymph nodes, which very rarely become available for study. Lytically infected cells, whether producing virus or solely EAs, may generally not survive for long because they are doomed to degenerate spontaneously (W. Henle et al., 1970 a; Gergely et al., 1971 a, b) and are possibly destroyed and removed even faster by developing host defenses. Lytically infected, i. e., EA, VCA, and virus particle positive cells have never been observed among circulating leukocytes obtained during the acute phase of IM. Cells with virus particles have been demonstrated, however, by electron microscopy within a lymph node of a patient who died from an overwhelming primary EBV infection, having shown high heterophil antibody titers but not as yet antibodies to EBV (Bar et al., 1974). Nonlytically infected, EBNA-positive cells have been observed in small numbers among B lymphocyte populations separated from the blood of IM patients in the early acute phase by Klein et al. (1976), in a lymph node from a child with a prolonged course of IM by Lenoir et al. (1977), and in lymphoid organs of a fatal case of IM by Britton et al. (1977). Others have failed to detect EBNA-positive cells in the circulation of IM patients (Rickinson et al., 1977; Crawford et al., 1978). Since their numbers are small it may be technically difficult to identify them by the anti-C′ immunofluorescence technique among the numerous other lymphocytes, often nonspecifically stained due to C′ receptors or other reasons. EBNA is also known to escape from the nucleus under adverse conditions such as those involved in the separation of lymphocyte subpopulations and preparation of cell smears. It has been proposed, however, that nonlytic infections of B lymphocytes may occur in which the EBV genome is perpetuated without expression of EBNA (Rickinson et al., 1974, 1977). Both forms of nonlytic infections are not mutually exclusive and both might be involved in the establishment of LCL but in a different manner.

Two mechanisms for the in vitro emergence of LCL are being considered: (a) the cell lines arise from lymphoblasts already transformed in vivo, as observed when cells of BL biopsies are cultured (Epstein et al., 1964; Pulvertaft, 1964; Nadkarni et al., 1968). In fact, Epstein and his associates established the first BL lines in a medium containing human serum which in all probability contained EBV neutralizing antibodies; and (b) on cultivation in vitro, the EBV genomes become derepressed in some of the nonlytically infected cells, whether EBNA-positive or not, so that viral replication ensues and the viral progeny then procedes to transform other B lymphocytes present in the cultured population into permanently growing, EBNA-positive lymphoblasts (Rickinson et al., 1974). This interpretation is supported by the fact that addition of cord blood lymphocytes from infants of one sex to leukocytes of IM patients of the opposite sex leads to polyclonal LCL with representation of cells from both donors as determined by chromosomal analysis. Induction of viral synthesis is observed also with BL cells, which are uniformly EBNA-positive, in that VCA- and/or EA-positive cells are generally not detectable in cell smears from fresh biopsies, but they appear regularly within 24–72 h when placed in culture, amounting to up to 10% of the population (Nadkarni et al., 1970). Virus released from the BL cells also transforms added cord blood lymphocytes (Dalens et al., 1975). Since the establishment of LCL from leukocytes of IM patients is almost completely inhibited when the cells are cultured in the presence of EBV-neutralizing antibodies (Rickinson et al., 1974), or when the cells are treated with phosphonoacetic acid (PAA), which blocks transformation but does not affect already transformed cells (Summers and Klein, 1976; Rickinson et al., 1978), there is no doubt that the great majority of LCL from IM patients are established by the 'two-step' mechanism. The question remains whether the occasional LCL obtained in the presence of neutralizing antibodies or after PAA treatment arose because the inhibitiors failed to neutralize all viral progeny or to prevent virus production completely, or whether they developed directly from the few EBNA-positive large B lymphocytes observed in the blood (Klein et al., 1976). Consideration must be given also to the fact that activated T cells are undoubtedly present in the cultures and attack already transformed cells, but T cells might not remain alive and active sufficiently long to affect the growth of all the cells transformed by the 'two step' mechanism.

The numbers of *circulating EBV-infected lymphocytes* in the course of IM have been estimated by determining the numbers of mononuclear cells required to establish LCL on cocultivation with a constant number of cord blood leukocytes (Rocchi et al., 1977). Maximally 1 in 2000 mononuclear cells was found to carry EBV during the 1st week of illness. This ratio declined by 3 weeks to 1 in 70,000 and by 3 months to 1 in about 10^7 mononuclear cells, with a range of 1 in 10^6 to 1 in $>10^7$, which held also for healthy donors long after past primary infections. In the absence of cord blood lymphocytes LCL were established at a 100 times lower frequency. The actual numbers of EBV-infected lymphocytes could be somewhat larger since not all of them may be induced in vitro to synthesize virus. Nevertheless, these results indicate that circulating EBNA-positive cells should be detectabale at most during the 1st week of illness, but not later. In fact their peak numbers may well precede the onset of illness. The results also denote that EBV-infected cells do not contribute significantly to the pool of atypical lymphocytes.

The *immune responses to EBV-infected cells* have been mentioned repeatedly in the foregoing discussions. These are expected to be evoked by lytically as well as nonlytically infected B lymphoid cells due to EBV-determined membrane antigens. The appearance and increasing concentrations of EBV-neutralizing antibodies will gradually prevent further exogenous infections of cells so that the targets ultimately should be limited to nonlytically infected cells per se or after spontaneous induction of viral replication. The immune responses include the emergence of activated T cells specifically primed against EBV-transformed lymphoblastoid cells and possibly also antibody-dependent cellular cytotoxicity (ADCC) (Pearson and Orr, 1976). They would obviously trail EBV-infected cells as to the time of appearance, attainment of peak concentration, and duration of detectability.

T cells which specifically destroy EBNA-positive cells from EBV-transformed LCL in vitro have been demonstrated by the ^{51}Cr-release technique among circulating lymphocytes of IM patients during the acute phase of illness, but no longer in late convalescence (Svedmyr and Jondal, 1975; Royston et al., 1975; Hutt et al., 1975). There are, however, T cell populations that nonspecifically attack cultured lymphoblasts from EBNA-positive as well as negative LCL. Demonstration of the EBV-specific activity depends therefore to a large extent on successful separation of subpopulations of T cells (Svedmyr and Jondal, 1975; Svedmyr et al., unpublished). EBV-specific killer T cells have not been found among lymphocytes from patients whose IM-like illness was unrelated to EBV as judged by serodiagnostic tests although nonspecific killer cells were readily demonstrable. The nonspecifically active T cell fraction could also be effective, of course, in the control of EBV-infected cells, but the possibility has not been excluded that this in vitro activity might be due to a laboratory artifact, i. e., the incorporation of bovine serum components into the membranes of the cultured target cells (Irie et al., 1974; Sulit et al., 1976) to which T lymphocyte donors may have become sensitized in the course of time through ingestion of bovine food products. It would seem essential to use target cells maintained on media containing human anti-VCA negative serum or perhaps sera of other species to reduce the possibility of such nonspecific interactions.

Cells from a nonproducer LCL, such as the Raji line of BL origin, are labeled with ^{51}Cr for the ADCC test 48–72 h after superinfection with P_3HR-1 virus. The labeled target cells are exposed to serial dilutions of heat-inactivated test sera and then to lymphocytes from unselected donors. The resulting cytotoxicity is mediated by antibodies to cell membrane components, presumably late MA (Pearson and Orr, 1976). While several types of effector cells have been implicated, lymphocytes with Fc receptors appear to be the most active (Pearson, 1977). High titers of antibodies reactive in the ADCC test have been noted among sera from BL, NPC, and IM patients (Jondal, 1976; Pearson and Orr, 1976; Pearson, 1977). In IM, peak antibody titers are reached only several weeks after onset of illness (Hewetson et al., unpublished). Although not proven, it is likely that ADCC reactions occur not only in vitro but also in vivo (Pearson, 1977).

These immune responses, and possibly others directed against EBV-infected cells could well account for part of the symptomatology of IM, especially the tonsillitis and extensive lymphadenopathy. Thus, IM would have features resembling an autoimmune disease not only with regard to some of the heterophil antibody responses, such as anti-i, which may be the cause of the hemolytic anemia seen as a complication of IM. The action of T lymphocytes could also account for the late development of anti-EBNA, as discussed earlier. There is additional indirect evidence that an efficient T cell system is required for the emergence and/or maintenance of anti-EBNA.

Uremic conditions are known to be immunosuppressive (Wilson et al., 1965), a fact which might explain why hemodialysis or renal transplant patients with past EBV infections have moderate to high anti-VCA titers and occasionally low levels of anti-EA, but often no or only barely detectable levels of anti-EBNA (unpublished). A primary EBV infection observed in two such patients, who were siblings, remained silent in one and resulted in only mild signs of IM in the other (Grose et al., 1977). The VCA-specific IgM and IgG antibody responses were of the usual order, but anti-EBNA emerged only after more than 8 and 11 months, respectively, and never exceeded barely detectable levels. Immunologically compromised patients, e. g., patients with inherited T cell defects or ataxia-telangiectasia, may show high anti-VCA titers as well as anti-D, but no or very low levels of anti-EBNA (Rocchi, personal communication; Berkel et al., unpublished). In BL, absence or low levels of anti-EBNA were found to correlate with anergy to dermal recall antigens (Olweny et al., unpublished). While these and other observations support a relation between T cell function and anti-EBNA production further studies are needed for substantiation.

As mentioned earlier, *after recovery from IM*, EBV-infected lymphoid cells, whether EBNA positive or not, persist in lymph nodes and lymphoid organs in presumably small numbers, with a few being spilled into the circulation. In some of these cells lytic cycles of viral replication must be induced occasionally to provide sufficient antigen and virus to maintain anti-VCA and neutralizing antibodies at detectable levels for life. The nonlytically infected cells are generally held in check presumably by T cells or other immune reactions. They are weeded out but never completely eliminated, and EBNA-positive cells when destroyed would release enough of the antigen for continuing production of the corresponding antibody. While EBV-specific killer T cells can no longer be demonstrated in the circulation after recovery from IM, they might still persist at subdetectable levels. These interactions must be in a stable equilibrium, as a rule, judging by the nearly constant titers of the detectable antibodies over many years, if not for life. This equilibrium may be upset, however, by immunosuppressive diseases or immunosuppressive therapy leading to a reactivation of the persistent viral carrier state and with it to enhanced titers of anti-VCA and, less frequently, re-emergence of anti-EA. Anti-EBNA usually remains stationary under these conditions or may even decline to low or nondetectable levels.

Obviously numerous questions regarding the pathogenesis of IM remain which require answers, as well as suggested answers that must be confirmed. One of the key problems has been the inability to assess the actual events occurring during the incubation period of the disease. No animal model is available in which typical IM can be reproduced. Further advances in understanding the pathogenesis of IM must rest therefore on intensive study of unusual cases of IM, e. g., patients requiring lymph node biopsies for diagnosis or removal of a ruptured spleen, patients with fatal complications, or immunologically compromised patients who may succumb rapidly to the disease. Since all these conditions are fortunately rare, progress is not expected to be rapid.

REFERENCES

Armstrong, D., Henle, G., Henle, W.: Complement fixation tests with cell lines derived from Burkitt's lymphoma and acute leukemias. J. Bacteriol. **91**, 1257–1262 (1966)

Aya, T., Osato, T.: Early events in transformation of human cord leukocytes by Epstein-Barr virus; Induction of DNA synthesis and virus-associated nuclear antigen. Int. J. Cancer **13**, 341–347 (1974)

Banatvala, J. E., Best, J. M., Waller, D. K.: Epstein-Barr virus-specific IgM in infectious mononucleosis, Burkitt's lymphoma, and nasopharyngeal carcinoma. Lancet **1972 I**, 1205–1208

Bar, R., DeLor, C. L., Clausen, K. P., Hurtubise, P., Henle, W., Hewetson, J.: Fatal infectious mononucleosis in a family. N. Engl. J. Med. **290**, 363–367 (1974)

Bentzon, J. W.: The effect of certain infectious diseases on tuberculin allergy. Tubercle **34**, 34–41 (1955)

Blacklow, N. R., Watson, B. K., Miller, G., Jacobson, B. M.: Mononucleosis with heterophil antibodies and EB virus infection. Acquisition by an elderly patient in hospital. Am. J. Med. **51**, 549–552 (1971)

Britton, S., Andersson-Anvret, M., Gergely, P., Henle, W., Jondal, M., Klein, G., Sandstedt, B., Svedmyr, G.: EB virus immunity and tissue distribution in a fatal case of infectious mononucleosis. N. Engl. J. Med. **298**, 89–92 (1978)

Carter, R. L.: Antibody formation in infectious mononucleosis. II. Other 19S antibodies and false-positive serology. Br. J. Hematol. **12**, 268–275 (1966)

Chang, R. S., Golden, H. D.: Transformation of human leukocytes by throat washing from infectious mononucleosis patients. Nature **234**, 359–360 (1971)

Chang, R. S., Lewis, J. P., Abildgaard, C. F.: Prevalance of oropharyngeal excretors of leukocyte-transforming agents among a human population. N. Engl. J. Med. **289**, 1325–1329 (1973)

Crawford, D. H., Rickinson, A. B., Finerty S., Epstein, M. A.: Epstein-Barr (EB) virus genome-containing, EB nuclear antigen-negative B-lymphocyte populations in blood in acute infectious mononucleosis. J. Gen. Virol. **38**, 449–460 (1978)

Davidsohn, I., Lee, C. L.: Serologic diagnosis of infectious mononucleosis. A comparative study of five tests. Am. J. Clin. Pathol. **41**, 115–125 (1964)

Dalens, M., Zech, L., Klein, G.: Origin of lymphoid lines established from mixed cultures of cord blood lymphocytes and explants from infectious mononucleosis, Burkitt lymphoma and healthy donors. Int. J. Cancer **16**, 1008–1014 (1975)

Davidsohn, I., Nelson, D. A.: The blood. In: Todd-Sanford's clinical diagnosis by laboratory methods, 14th ed. Davidsohn, I., Henry, J. B. (eds.), Chap. 5. Philadelphia: Saunders 1969

De Schryver, A., Klein, G., Hewetson, J., Rocchi, G., Henle, W., Henle, G., Pope, J.: Comparison of EBV neutralization tests based on abortive infection or transformation of lymphoid cells and their relation to membrane reactive antibodies (anti-MA). Int. J. Cancer **13**, 353–362 (1974)

Deinhardt, F., Falk, L., Wolfe, L. G., Paciga, J., Johnson, D.: Response of marmosets to experimental infection with Epstein-Barr virus. In: Oncogenesis and herpesviruses II. de-Thé, G., Epstein, M. A., zur Hausen, H. (eds.), Part 2, pp. 161–168. Lyon: IARC 1975

Diehl, V., Henle, G., Henle, W., Kohn, G.: Demonstration of a herpes group virus in cultures of peripheral leukocytes from patients with infectious mononucleosis. J. Virol. **2**, 663–669 (1968)

Dorfman, R. F., Warnke, R.: Lymphadenopathy simulating the malignant lymphomas. Human Pathol. **5**, 519 (1974)

Dunkel, V., Pry, T., Henle, G., Henle, W.: Immunofluorescence tests for antibodies to Epstein-Barr virus with sera of lower primates. J. Nat. Cancer Inst. **49**, 435–440 (1972)

Edwards, J. M. B., McSwiggan, D. A.: Studies on the diagnostic value of an immunofluorescence test for EB virus-specific IgM. J. Clin. Pathol. **27**, 647–651 (1974)

Enberg, R. N., Eberle, B. J., Williams, C. R. (Jr.): T- and B-cells in peripheral blood during infectious mononucleosis. J. Infect. Dis. **130**, 104–111 (1974)

Epstein, A. L., Levy, R., Henle, W., Henle, G., Kaplan, H. S.: Biology of the human malignant lymphomas: IV. Functional characterization of 10 diffuse histiocytic lymphoma cell lines. Cancer **42**, 2379–2391 (1978)

Epstein, M. A., Achong, B. G., Barr, Y. M.: Virus particles in cultured lymphoblasts from Burkitt's lymphoma. Lancet **1964 I**, 702–703

Epstein, M. A., Henle, G., Achong, B. G., Barr, Y. M.: Morphological and biological studies on a virus in cultured lymphoblasts from Burkitt's lymphoma. J. Exp. Med. **121**, 761–770 (1965)

Ernberg, I., Klein, G., Kourilsky, F. M., Silvestre, D.: Differentiation between early and late membrane antigen on human lymphoblastoid cell lines infected with Epstein-Barr virus. I. Immunofluorescence. J. Natl., Cancer Inst. **53**, 61–65 (1974)

Evans, A. S.: Experimental attempts to transmit infectious mononucleosis to man. Yale J. Biol. Med. **20**, 19–26 (1947)

Evans, A. S.: Further experimental attempts to transmit infectious mononucleosis to man. J. Clin. Invest. **29**, 508–512 (1950)

Evans, A. S., Evans, B. K., Sturtz, V.: Standards for hepatic and hematologic tests in monkeys: Observations during experiments with hepatitis and mononucleosis. Proc. Soc. Exp. Biol. Med. **82**, 437–440 (1953)

Evans, A. S., Niederman, J. C., McCollum, R. W.: Seroepidemiologic studies of infectious mononucleosis with EB virus. N. Engl. J. Med. **279**, 1121–1127 (1968)

Evans, A. S., Niederman, J. C., Canabre, L. C., West, B., Richards, V. A.: A prospective evaluation of heterophile and Epstein-Barr virus-specific IgM antibody tests in clinical and subclinical infectious mononucleosis: Specificity of and sensitivity of the tests and persistance of antibody. J. Infect. Dis. **132**, 546–554 (1975)

Galloway, E.: Comparison of three slide tests for infectious mononucleosis with Davidsohn's presumptive and differential heterophil test. Canad. J. Med. Technol. **31**, 197–206 (1969)

Gerber, P.: Activation of Epstein-Barr virus by 5-bromodeoxyuridine in "virus-free" human cells. Proc. Natl. Acad. Sci. USA **69**, 83–85 (1972)

Gerber, P., Deal, D. R.: Epstein-Barr virus-induced viral and soluble complement-fixing antigens in Burkitt's lymphoma cell cultures. Proc. Soc. Exp. Biol. Med. **134**, 748–751 (1970)

Gerber, P., Hamre, D., Moy, R. A., Rosenblum, E. N.: Infectious mononucleosis: Complement-fixing antibodies to herpes-like virus associated with Burkitt's lymphoma. Science **161**, 173–175 (1968)

Gerber, P., Whang-Peng, J., Monroe, J. H.: Transformation and chromosome changes induced by Epstein-Barr virus in normal human leukocyte cultures. Proc. Nat. Acad. Sci. USA **63**, 740–747 (1969 a)

Gerber, P., Walsh, J. H., Rosenblum, E. N., Purcell, R. H.: Association of EB virus infection with the post-perfusion syndrome. Lancet **1969 b I**, 593–596

Gerber, P., Nonoyama, M., Lucas, S., Perlin, E., Goldstein, L. I.: Oral excretion of Epstein-Barr virus by healthy subjects and patients with infectious mononucleosis. Lancet **1972 II**, 988–989

Gerber, P., Pritchett, R. F., Kieff, E. D.: Antigens and DNA of a chimpanzee agent related to Epstein-Barr virus. J. Virol. **19**, 1090–1099 (1976)

Gergely, L., Klein, G., Ernberg, I.: The action of DNA antagonists on Epstein-Barr virus (EBV)-associated early antigens (EA) in Burkitt lymphoma lines. Int. J. Cancer **7**, 293–302 (1971 a)

Gergely, L., Klein, G., Ernberg, I.: Effect of EBV-induced early antigens on host macromolecular synthesis, studied by combined immunofluorescence and radioautography. Virology **45**, 22–29 (1971 b)

Ginsburg, C. M., Henle, G., Henle, W.: An outbreak of infectious mononucleosis among the personnel of an outpatient clinic. Am. J. Epidemiol. **104**, 571–575 (1976)

Ginsburg, C. M., Henle, W., Henle, G., Horwitz, C. A.: Infectious mononucleosis in children: evaluation of the Epstein-Barr virus-specific serology. J. Am. Med. Assoc. **237**, 781–785 (1977)

Giulano, V. J., Jasin, H. A., Ziff, M.: The nature of the atypical lymphocyte in infectious mononucleosis. Clin. Immunol. Immunopathol. **3**, 90–98 (1974)

Glade, P. R., Karel, J. A., Morse, H. L., Whang-Peng, J., Hoffman, P. E., Kammermeyer, J. K., Chessin, L. N.: Infectious mononucleosis continuous suspension cultures of peripheral leukocytes. Nature **217**, 564–565 (1968)

Grose, C., Henle, W., Henle, G., Feorino, P. M.: Primary Epstein-Barr virus infections in acute neurologic diseases. N. Engl. J. Med. **292**, 392–395 (1975)

Grose, C., Henle, W., Horwitz, M. S.: Primary Epstein-Barr virus infection in a renal transplant recipient. South. Med. J. **70**, 1276–1278 (1978)

Haider, S., Coutino, M. D., Emond, R. T. D.: Tuberculin anergy and infectious mononucleosis. Lancet **1973 II**, 74

Hallee, T. J., Evans, A. S., Niederman, J. C.: Infectious mononucleosis at the United States Military Academy. A prospective study of a single class over 4 years. Yale J. Biol. Med. **47**, 182–192 (1974)

Hampar, B., Hsu, K. C., Martos, L. M., Walker, J. L.: Serologic evidence that a herpes-type virus is the etiologic agent of heterophile-positive infectious mononucleosis. Proc. Natl. Acad. Sci. USA **68**, 1407–1411 (1971)

Hampar, B., Derge, J. G., Martos, L. M., Walker, J. L.: Synthesis of Epstein-Barr virus after activation of the viral genome in a "virus-negative" human lymphoblastoid cell (Raji) made resistant to 5-bromodeoxyuridine. Proc. Natl. Acad. Sci. USA **69**, 78–82 (1972)

Henle, G., Henle, W.: Immunofluorescence in cells derived from Burkitt's lymphoma. J. Bacteriol. **91**, 1248–1256 (1966)

Henle, G., Henle, W.: Immunofluorescence, interference and complement fixation techniques in the detection of the herpes-type virus in Burkitt tumor cell lines. Cancer Res. **27**, 2442–2446 (1967)

Henle, G., Henle, W.: Observations on childhood infections with the Epstein-Barr virus. J. Infect. Dis. **121**, 303–310 (1970)

Henle, G., Henle, W., Diehl, V.: Relation of Burkitt tumor associated herpes-type virus to infectious mononucleosis. Proc. Natl. Acad. Sci. USA **59**, 94–101 (1968)

Henle, G., Henle, W., Klein, G.: Demonstration of two distinct components in the early antigen complex of Epstein-Barr virus infected cells. Int. J. Cancer **8**, 272–282 (1971)

Henle, G., Henle, W., Horwitz, C. A.: Antibodies to Epstein-Barr virus-associated nuclear antigen in infectious mononucleosis. J. Infect. Dis. **130**, 231–239 (1974)

Henle, W., Henle, G.: Epstein-Barr virus: The cause of infectious mononucleosis. In: Oncogenesis and herpesviruses. Biggs, P. M., de-Thé, G., Payne, L. N. (eds.), pp. 269–274. Lyon: IARC

Henle, W., Henle, G.: Epstein-Barr virus and infectious mononucleosis. N. Engl. J. Med. **288**, 263–264 (1973a)

Henle, W., Henle, G.: Epstein-Barr virus (EBV)-related serology in Hodgkin's disease. Natl. Cancer Inst. Monogr. **36**, 79–84 (1973b)

Henle, W., Hummeler, K., Henle, G.: Antibody coating and agglutination of virus particles separated from the EB3 line of Burkitt lymphoma cells. J. Bacteriol. **92**, 269–271 (1966)

Henle, W., Diehl, V., Kohn, G., zur Hausen, H., Henle, G.: Herpes-type virus and chromosome marker in normal leukocytes after growth with irradiated Burkitt cells. Science **157**, 1064–1065 (1967)

Henle, W., Henle, G., Zajac, B., Pearson, G., Waubke, R., Scriba, M.: Differential reactivity of human sera with EBV-induced "early antigens". Science **169**, 188–190 (1970a)

Henle, W., Henle, G., Scriba, M., Joyner, C. R., Harrison, F. (Jr.), von Essen, R., Paloheimo, J., Klemola, E.: Antibody responses to the Epstein-Barr virus and cytomegaloviruses after open-heart and other surgery. N. Engl. J. Med. **282**, 1068–1074 (1970b)

Henle, W., Henle, G., Niederman, J. C., Klemola, E., Haltia, K.: Antibodies to early antigens induced by Epstein-Barr virus in infectious mononucleosis. J. Infect. Dis. **124**, 58–67 (1971)

Henle, W., Henle, G., Horwitz, C. A.: Epstein-Barr virus-specific diagnostic tests in infectious mononucleosis. Human Pathol. **5**, 551–565 (1974a)

Henle, W., Guerra, A., Henle, G.: False negative and prozone reactions in tests for antibodies to Epstein-Barr virus-associated nuclear antigen. Int. J. Cancer **13**, 751–754 (1974b)

Hewetson, J. F., Rocchi, G., Henle, W., Henle, G.: Neutralizing antibodies against Epstein-Barr virus in healthy populations and patients with infectious mononucleosis. J. Infect. Dis. **128**, 283–289 (1973)

Hinuma, Y., Kohn, M., Yamaguchi, J., Wudarski, D. J., Blakesee, J. R. (Jr), Grace, J. T. (Jr.): Immunofluorescence and herpes-type virus particles in the P3HR-1 Burkitt lymphoma cell line. J. Virol. **1**, 1045–1051 (1967)

Hirshaut, Y., Christenson, W. N., Perlmutter, J. C.: Prospective study of herpes-like virus role in infectious mononucleosis. Clin. Res. **19**, 459–463 (1971)

Hoagland, R. J.: The transmission of infectious mononucleosis. Am. J. Med. Sci. **229**, 262–272 (1955)

Horwitz, C. A., Henle, W., Henle, G., Schmitz, H.: Clinical evaluation of patients with infectious mononucleosis and development of antibodies to the R component of the Epstein-Barr virus-induced early antigen complex. Am. J. Med. **58**, 330–338 (1975)

Horwitz, C. A., Henle, W., Henle, G., Segal, M., Arnold, T., Lewis, F. B., Zanick, D., Ward, P. C. J.: Clinical and laboratory evaluation of elderly patients with heterophil-antibody positive infectious mononucleosis; report of seven patients, ages 40–78. Am. J. Med. **61**, 333–339 (1976a)

Horwitz, C., Henle, W., Henle, G., Polesky, H., Wexler, H., Ward, P.: The specificity of heterophil antibodies and healthy donors with no or minimal signs of infectious mononucleosis. Blood **47**, 91–98 (1976b)

Horwitz, C. A., Henle, W., Henle, G., Polesky, H., Balfour, H. H. (Jr.), Siem, R. A., Borken, S., Ward, P. C. J.: Heterophil-negative infectious mononucleosis and mononucleosis-like illnesses: laboratory confirmation of 43 cases. Am. J. Med. **63**, 947–956 (1977)

Huang, D. P., Ho, J. H. C., Henle, W., Henle, G.: Demonstration of EBV-associated nuclear antigen in NPC cells from fresh biopsies. Int. J. Cancer **14**, 580–588 (1974)

Hutt, L. M., Huang, Y. T., Dascomb, H. E., Pagano, J. S.: Enhanced destruction of lymphoid cell lines by peripheral blood leukocytes taken from patients with acute infectious mononucleosis. J. Immunol. **115**, 243–248 (1975)

Irie, R. F., Irie, K., Morton, D.: Natural antibody in human serum to a neoantigen in human cultured cells grown in fetal calf serum. J. Natl. Cancer Inst. **52**; 1051–1057 (1974)

Joncas, J., Mitnyan, C.: Serologic response of the EBV antibodies in pediatric cases of infectious mononucleosis and their contacts. Can. Med. Assoc. J. **102**, 1260–1263 (1970)

Jondal, M., Klein, G.: Surface markers on human B and T lymphocytes. II. Presence of Epstein-Barr virus receptors on B lymphocytes. J. Exp. Med. **138**, 1365–1378 (1973)

Jondal, M.: Antibody-dependent cellular cytotoxicity (ADCC) against Epstein-Barr virus-determined antigens. I. Reactivity in sera from normal persons and from patients with acute infectious mononucleosis. Clin. Exp., Immunol. **25**, 1–10 (1976)

Kalter, S. S., Heberling, R. L., Ratner, J. J.: EBV antibody in sera of non-human primates. Nature **238**, 353–354 (1972)

Klein, G., Vonka, V.: Relationship between the Epstein-Barr virus (EBV) determined complement-fixing antigen and the nuclear antigen (EBNA) detected by anti-complement fluorescence. J. Nat. Cancer Inst. **53**, 1645–1646 (1974)

Klein, G., Clifford, P., Klein, E., South, R. T., Minowada, J., Kourilsky, F., Burchenal, J. H.: Membrane immunofluorescence reactions of Burkitt lymphoma cells from biopsy specimens and tissue cultures. J. Natl., Cancer Inst. **39**, 1027–1044 (1967)

Klein, G., Pearson, G., Nadkarni, J. S., Nadkarni, J. J., Klein, E., Henle, G., Henle, W., Clifford, P.: Relation between Epstein-Barr viral and cell membrane immunofluorescence of Burkitt tumor cells. I. Dependence of cell membrane immunofluorescence on presence of EB virus. J. Exp. Med. **128**, 1011–1020 (1968a)

Klein, G., Pearson, G., Henle, G., Henle, W., Diehl, V., Niederman, J. C.: Relation between Epstein-Barr viral and cell membrane immunofluorescence in Burkitt tumor cells. II. Comparison of cells and sera from patients with Burkitt's lymphoma and infectious mononucleosis. J. Exp. Med. **128**, 1021–1030 (1968b)

Klein, G., Pearson, G., Henle, G., Henle, W., Goldstein, G., Clifford, P.: Relation between Epstein-Barr viral and cell membrane immunofluorescence in Burkitt tumor cells. III. Comparison of blocking and direct membrane immunofluorescence and anti-EBV reactivities of different sera. J. Exp. Med. **129**, 697–705 (1969)

Klein, G., Giovanella, B. C., Lindahl, T., Fialkow, P. J., Singh, S., Stehlin, J. S.: Direct evidence for the presence of Epstein-Barr virus DNA and nuclear antigen in malignant epithelial cells from patients with poorly differentiated carcinoma of the nasopharynx. Proc. Natl. Acad. Sci. USA **71**, 4737–4741 (1974)

Klein, G., Svedmyr, E., Jondal, M., Persson, P. O.: EBV-determined nuclear antigen (EBNA)-positive cells in the peripheral blood of infectious mononucleosis patients. Int. J. Cancer **17**, 21–26 (1976)

Klemola, E., Kääriäinen, L., von Essen, R., Haltia, K., Koivuniemi, A., von Bonsdorff, C-H.: Further studies on cytomegalovirus mononucleosis in previously healthy individuals. Acta Med. Scand. **182**, 311–322 (1967)

Klemola, E., von Essen, R., Henle, G., Henle, W.: Infectious mononucleosis-like disease with negative heterophil agglutination test. Clinical features in relation to Epstein-Barr virus and cytomegalovirus antibodies. J. Infect. Dis. **121**, 608–614 (1970)

Lange, B. J., Berman, P. H., Bender, J., Henle, W., Hewetson, J. F.: Encephalitis in infectious mononucleosis: diagnostic considerations. Pediatrics **58**, 877–880 (1976)

Lee, C. L., Davidsohn, I.: Serologic test for infectious mononucleosis. Chicago: American Society of Clinical Pathologists Commission on Continuing Education 1972

Lee, C. L., Davidsohn, I., Panczyszyn, O.: Horse agglutinins in infectious mononucleosis. II. The spot test. Am. J. Clin. Pathol. **49**, 12–18 (1968)

Leibold, W., Flanagan, T. D., Menezes, J., Klein, G.: Induction of Epstein-Barr virus (EBV)-associated nuclear antigen (EBNA) during *in vitro* transformation of human lymphoid cells. J. Natl. Cancer Inst. **54**, 65–68 (1975)

Lemon, S. M., Hutt, L. M., Shaw, J. E., Li, J-L., Pagano, J. S.: Replication of EBV in epithelial cells during infectious mononucleosis. Nature **268**, 268–270 (1977)

Lenoir, J. L., de-Thé, G., Virelizier, J. L., Griscelli, C.: Epstein-Barr virus nuclear antigen (EBNA) positive cells in a lymph node of a child with severe primary EBV infection. In: Oncogenesis and herpesviruses III. de-Thé, G., Henle, W., Rapp, F. (eds.), pp. 733–738. Lyon: IARC 1978

Levy, J. A., Henle, G.: Indirect immunofluorescence tests with sera from African children and cultured Burkitt lymphoma cells. J. Bacteriol. **92**, 275–276 (1966)

Leyton, G. B.: Ox-cell hemolysins in human serum. J. Clin. Pathol. **5**, 324–328 (1952)

Mangi, R. J., Niederman, J. C., Kelleher, J. E. (Jr.), Dwyer, J. M., Evans, A. S., Kantor, F. S.: Depression of cell mediated immunity during acute infectious mononucleosis. N. Eng. J. Med. **291**, 1149–1153 (1974)

Mason, J. K.: An ox cell haemolysin test for the diagnosis of infectious mononucleosis. J. Hyg. (Camb.) **49**, 471–481 (1951)

Mayyasi, S. A., Schidlovsky, G., Bulfone, L. M., Buscheck, F. T.: The coating reaction of the herpes-type virus isolated from malignant tissues with an antibody present in sera. Cancer Res. **27**, 2020–2024 (1967)

Miller, G.: Epstein-Barr herpesvirus and infectious mononucleosis. Progr. Med. Virol. **20**, 84-112 (1975)

Miller, G., Lisco, H., Kohn, H. I., Stitt, D.: Establishment of cell lines from normal adult human blood leukocytes by exposure to Epstein-Barr virus and neutralization by human sera with Epstein-Barr virus antibody. Proc. Soc. Exp. Biol. Med. **137**, 1459–1465 (1971)

Miller, G., Niederman, J. C., Stitt, D. L.: Infectious mononucleosis: appearance of neutralizing antibody to Epstein-Barr virus measured by inhibition of formation of lymphoblastoid cell lines. J. Infect. Dis. **125**, 403–406 (1972)

Miller, G., Niederman, J. C., Andrews, L.: Prolonged oropharyngeal excretion of EB virus following infectious mononucleosis. N. Engl. J. Med. **137**, 140–147 (1973)

Miller, G., Robinson, J., Heston, L., Lipman, M.: Differences between laboratory strains of Epstein-Barr virus based on immortalization, abortive infection and interference. Proc. Natl. Acad. Sci. USA **71**, 4006–4010 (1974)

Moore, G. E., Gerner, R. E., Franklin, H. A.: Culture of normal human leukocytes. J. Am. Med. Assoc. **199**, 519–524 (1967)

Moss, D. J., Pope, J. H.: EB virus-associated nuclear antigen production and cell proliferation in adult peripheral leukocytes inoculated with the QIMR-WIL strain of EB virus. Int. J. Cancer **15**, 503–511 (1975)

Nadkarni, J. S., Nadkarni, J. J., Clifford, P., Manolov, G., Fenyö, E. N., Klein, E.: Characteristics of new cell lines derived from Burkitt's lymphomas. Cancer **23**, 64–79 (1968)

Nadkarni, J. S., Nadkarni, J. J., Klein, G., Henle, W., Henle, G., Clifford, P.: EB viral antigens in Burkitt tumor biopsies and early cultures. Int. J. Cancer **6**, 10–17 (1970)

Niederman, J. C., Scott, R. B.: Studies on infectious mononucleosis: Attempts to transmit the disease to human volunteers. Yale J. Biol. Med. **38**, 1–10 (1965)

Niederman, J. C., McCollum, R. W., Henle, G., Henle, W.: Infectious mononucleosis. J. Am. Med. Assoc. **203**, 139–143 (1968)

Niederman, J. C., Evans, A. S., Subramanyan, M. S., McCollum, R. W.: Prevalence incidence and persistence of EB virus antibody in young adults. N. Eng. J. Med. **282**, 361–365 (1970)

Niederman, J. C., Miller, G., Pearson, H. A., Pagano, J. S., Dowalibi, J. M.: Infectious mononucleosis. Epstein-Barr virus shedding in saliva and the oropharynx. N. Engl. J. Med. **294**, 1355–1359 (1976)

Nikoskelainen, J., Hänninen, P.: Antibody responses to Epstein-Barr virus in infectious mononucleosis. Infect. Immun. **11**, 42–51 (1975)

Nikoskelainen, J., Leikola, J., Klemola, E.: IgM antibodies specific for Epstein-Barr virus in infectious mononucleosis, without heterophil antibodies. Br. Med. J. **1974 IV,** 72–75

Nilsson, K., Klein, G., Henle, W., Henle, G.: The establishment of lymphoblastoid lines from adult and fetal human lymphoid tissue and its dependence on EBV. Int. J. Cancer **8**, 443–450 (1971)

Nonoyama, M., Pagano, J. S.: Detection of Epstein-Barr viral genome in non-productive cells. Nature **233**, 103–106 (1971)

Pattengale, P. K., Smith, R. W., Perlin, E.: Atypical lymphocytes in acute infectious mononucleosis. Identification by multiple T and B lymphocyte markers. N. Engl. J. Med. **291**, 1145–1148 (1974a)

Pattengale, P. K., Gerber, P., Smith, R. W.: B-cell characteristics of human peripheral and cord blood lymphocytes transformed by Epstein-Barr virus. J. Natl. Cancer Inst. **52**, 1081–1086 (1974b)

Paul, J. R., Bunnell, W. W.: The presence of heterophile antibodies in infectious mononucleosis. Am. J. Med. Sci. **183**, 80–104 (1932)

Pearson, G.: *In vitro* and *in vivo* investigations on antibody-dependent cellular cytotoxity. Curr. Top. Microbiol. Immunol. **80**, 65–96 (1978)

Pearson, G. R., Orr, T. W.: Antibody-dependent lymphocyte cytotoxicity against cells expressing Epstein-Barr virus antigens. J. Natl. Cancer Inst. **56**, 485–488 (1976)

Pearson, G., Dewey, F., Klein, G., Henle, G., Henle, W.: Relation between neutralization of Epstein-Barr virus and antibodies to cell membrane antigens induced by the virus. J. Natl. Cancer Inst **45**, 989–995 (1970)

Pereira, M. S., Field, A. M., Blake, J. M., Rodgers, F. G., Bailey, L. A., Davies, J. R.: Evidence for oral excretion of EB virus in infectious mononucleosis. Lancet **1972 I,** 710–711

Piessens, W. F., Schur, P. H., Moloney, W. C., Churchill, W. H.: Lymphocyte surface immunoglobulins. Distribution and frequency in lymphoproliferative diseases. N. Engl. J. Med. **288**, 176–180 (1973)

Pope, J. H.: Establishment of cell lines from peripheral leukocytes in infectious mononucleosis. Nature **216**, 810–811 (1967)

Pope, J. H., Horne, M. K., Wetters, E. J.: Significance of a complement-fixing antigen associated with herpes-like virus and detected in the Raji cell line. Nature **222**, 166–167 (1969a)

Pope, J. H., Horne, M. K., Scott, W.: Identification of the filtrable leukocyte-transforming factor of QIMR-WIL cells as herpes-like virus. Int. J. Cancer **4**, 255–260 (1969b)

Pulvertaft, R. J. V.: Cytology of Burkitt's tumor (African lymphoma). Lancet **1964 I,** 238–240

Reedman, B. M., Klein, G.: Cellular localization of an Epstein-Barr virus (EBV)-associated complement-fixing antigen in producer and non-producer lymphoblastoid cell lines. Int. J. Cancer **11**, 499–520 (1973)

Rickinson, A. B., Jarvis, J. E., Crawford, D. H., Epstein, M. A.: Observations on the type of infection by Epstein-Barr virus in peripheral lymphoid cells of patients with infectious mononucleosis. Int. J. Cancer **14**, 704–715 (1974)

Rickinson, A. B., Finerty, S., Epstein, M. A.: Comparative studies on adult donor lymphocytes infected by EB virus *in vivo* and *in vitro*. Origin of transformed cells arising in co-cultures with foetal lymphocytes. Int. J. Cancer **19**, 775–782 (1977)

Rickinson, A. B., Finerty, S., Epstein, M. A.: Inhibition by phosphonoacetate of the *in vitro* outgrowth of Epstein-Barr virus genome-containing cell lines from the blood of infectious mononucleosis patients. In: Oncogenesis and herpesviruses III. de-Thé, G., Henle, W., Rapp. F. (eds.), pp. 721–728. Lyon: IARC 1978

Robinson, J., Miller, G.: Assay for Epstein-Barr virus based on stimulation of DNA synthesis in mixed leukocytes from umbilical cord blood. J. Virol. **15**, 1065–1072 (1975)

Rocchi, G., Hewetson, J. F.: A practical and quantitative micro test for determination of neutralizing antibodies against Epstein-Barr virus. J. Gen. Virol. **18**, 385–391 (1973)

Rocchi, G., Hewetson, J., Henle, W.: Specific neutralizing antibodies in Epstein-Barr virus associated diseases. Int. J. Cancer **11**, 637–647 (1973)

Rocchi, G., de Felici, A., Ragona, G., Heinz, A.: Quantitative evaluation of Epstein-Barr-Virus-infected mononuclear peripheral blood leukocytes in infectious mononucleosis. N. Engl. J. Med. **296**, 132–134 (1977)

Royston, I., Sullivan, J. L., Perlman, P. O., Perlin, E.: Cell-mediated immunity to Epstein-Barr virus-transformed lymphoblastoid cells in acute infectious mononucleosis. N. Eng. J. Med. **293**, 1159–1163 (1975)

Sawyer, R. N., Evans, A. S., Niederman, J. C., McCollum, R. W.: Prospective studies of a group of Yale University freshmen. I. Occurence of infectious mononucleosis. J. Infect. Dis. **123**, 263–270 (1971)

Schmitz, H., Scherer, M.: IgM antibodies to Epstein-Barr virus in infectious mononucleosis. Arch. Ges. Virusforsch. **37,** 332–339 (1972)

Sheldon, P. J., Papamichael, M., Hemsted, E. H., Holborow, E. J.: Thymic origin of atypical lymphoid cells in infectious mononucleosis. Lancet **1973 I,** 1153–115

Shope, T., Dechairo, D., Miller, G.: Malignant lymphoma in cotton-top marmosets following inoculation of Epstein-Barr virus. Proc. Natl. Acad. Sci. USA **70,** 2487–2491 (1973)

Silvestre, D., Ernberg, I., Neauport-Sautes, C., Kourilsky, F. M., Klein, G.: Differentiation between early and late membrane antigen on human lymphoid cell lines infected with Epstein-Barr virus. II. Immunoelectron microscopy. J. Natl. Cancer Inst. **53,** 67–74 (1974)

Sohier, R., Lepine, P., Sautter, V.: Recherches sur la transmission experimentale de la mononucleose au singe et à l'homme. Ann. Inst. Pasteur **65,** 50–62 (1940)

Strauch, B., Andrews, L., Siegel, N., Miller, G.: Oropharyngeal excretion of Epstein-Barr virus by renal transplant recipients and other patients treated with immunosuppressive drugs. Lancet **1974 I,** 234–237

Sulit, H. L., Golub, S. H., Irie, R. F., Gupta, R. K., Grooms, G. A., Morton, D. L.: Human tumor cells grown in fetal calf serum and human serum: Influences on the tests for lymphocyte cycotoxicity, serum blocking and serum arming effects. Int. J. Cancer **17,** 461–468 (1976)

Summers, W. C., Klein, G.: Inhibition of EBV DNA synthesis and late gene expression by phosphonoacetic acid. J. Virol. **18,** 151–155 (1976)

Svedmyr, E., Jondal, M.: Cytotoxic effector cells specific for B cell lines transformed by Epstein-Barr virus are present within patients with infectious mononucleosis. Proc. Natl. Acad. Sci. USA **72,** 1622–1626 (1975)

Taylor, A. W.: Effects of glandular fever in acute leukemia. Br. Med. J. **1953 I,** 589–593

Tischendorf, P., Shramek, G. J., Balagtas, R. C., Deinhardt, F., Knospe, W. H., Noble, G. R., Maynard, J. E.: Development and persistence of immunity to Epstein-Barr virus in man. J. Infect. Dis. **122,** 401–409 (1970)

Turner, A. R., MacDonald, R. N., Cooper, B. A.: Transmission of infectious mononucleosis by transfusion of pre-illness plasma. Ann. Intern. Med. **77,** 751–753 (1972)

University Health Physicians and P.H.L.S. Laboratories: Infectious mononucleosis and its relation to EB virus antibody. Br. Med. J. **1971 IV,** 643–646

Virolainen, M., Andersson, L. C., Lalia, M., Van Essen, R.: T-lymphocyte proliferation in mononucleosis. Clin. Immunol. Immunopathol. **2,** 114–120 (1973)

Vonka, V., Benyesh-Melnick, M., McCombs, R. M.: Antibodies in human sera to soluble and viral antigens found in Burkitt's lymphoma and other lymphoblastoid cell lines. J. Natl., Cancer Inst. **44,** 865–872 (1970)

Vonka, V., Vlckova, I., Zavadova, H., Kouba, K., Lazonska, Y., Duben, J.: Antibodies to EB virus capsid antigen and soluble antigen of lymphoblastoid cells in infectious mononucleosis. Int. J. Cancer **9,** 529–535 (1972)

Wahren, B., Espmark, A., Waldén, G.: Serologic studies on cytomegalovirus infection in relation to infectious mononucleosis and similar conditions. Scand. J. Infect. Dis. **1,** 145–151 (1969)

Wahren, B., Espmark, A., Lantorp, K., Sterner, G.: EBV antibodies in family contacts of patients with infectious mononucleosis. Proc. Soc. Exp. Biol. Med. **133,** 934–939 (1970)

Werner, J., Pinto, C. A., Haff, R. F., Henle, W., Henle, G.: Responses of gibbons (Hylobates Lar) to inoculation of Epstein-Barr virus (EBV). J. Infect. Dis. **126,** 678–681 (1972)

Wilson, W. E. C., Kirkpatrick, C. H., Talmadge, D. W.: Suppression of immunologic responsiveness in uremia. Ann. Intern. Med. **62,** 1–14 (1965)

Wising, P. J.: A study of infectious mononucleosis (Pfeiffer's disease) from the etiological point of view. Acta Med. Scand. Suppl. **133,** 1–102 (1942)

Wolf, H., zur Hausen, H., Becker, V.: EB viral genomes in epithelial nasopharyngeal carcinoma cells. Nature **244,** 245–247 (1973)

Wolf, H., zur Hausen, H., Klein, G., Becker, V., Henle, G., Henle, W.: Attempts to detect virus-specific DNA sequences in human tumors. III. Epstein-Barr viral DNA in non-lymphoid nasopharyngeal carcinoma cells. Med. Microbiol. Immunol. **161,** 15–21 (1975)

zur Hausen, H., Schulte-Holthausen, H.: Presence of EB virus nucleic acid homology in a "virus-free" line of Burkitt tumor cells. Nature **227,** 245–248 (1970)

zur Hausen, H., Henle, W., Hummeler, K., Diehl, V., Henle, G.: Comparative study of cultured Burkitt tumor cells by immunofluorescence, autoradiography and electron microscopy. J. Virol. **1,** 830–837 (1967)

zur Hausen, H., Diehl, V., Wolf, H., Schulte-Holthausen, H., Schneider, U.: Occurence of Epstein-Barr virus genomes in human lymphoblastoid cell lines. Nature New Biol. **237,** 189–190 (1972)

14 The Relationship of the Virus to Burkitt's Lymphoma

M. A. Epstein and B. G. Achong

Department of Pathology, The Medical School, University of Bristol, University Walk, Bristol BS8 1TD (England)

A. INTRODUCTION

Burkitt's lymphoma (BL) (Burkitt, 1958) is a highly unusual tumor; as has been pointed out in Chap. 1, its unique and peculiar features first prompted the search for a causative agent, which led to the discovery of the Epstein-Barr virus (EBV) (Epstein et al., 1964). Although much was known at the time about BL (Burkitt, 1963), certain characteristics have come to assume special significance as its association with EBV has emerged and new information relevant to this has also been obtained. Before considering the relationship of the tumor to EBV, these special aspects call for comment.

B. BURKITT'S LYMPHOMA

I. DEFINITION

BL first came to be understood as a distinct entity when it was realized that a variety of lymphoid tumors seen frequently in children in Africa were all manifestations of a single malignant lymphoma syndrome (Burkitt, 1958) which had not been recognized before. In those parts of Africa where the tumor is common, it has been found to be commoner than all other malignant tumors of children added together, with a peak incidence at about 6–7 years of age (Burkitt, 1963). Clinically, the tumor is always multifocal with a bizarre organ distribution quite unlike that of any other lymphoma (Burkitt, 1963), and in terms of histology all examples have been characterized as poorly differentiated lymphocytic lymphomas containing variable numbers of non-malignant histiocytes, the presence of which is responsible for the well-known "starry sky" appearance (O'Conor and Davies, 1960; Wright, 1963 a). Cytologic and histochemical studies have fully confirmed this conclusion (Wright, 1963 b) and strict internationally recognized criteria for the diagnosis of BL have been drawn up (Berard et al., 1969). Subsequently, another area where BL is extremely common in children has been recognized in New Guinea (Ten Seldam et al., 1966).

Almost all the work on BL from the high incidence areas has been done with African rather than New Guinean material and the term African BL will therefore be used here in relation to the endemic form of the tumor. In addition, cases of lymphoma closely similar to African BL occur very rarely outside the endemic zones everywhere in the world where search has been made (Burkitt, 1967a) and although this sporadic tumor resembles endemic BL histologically and cytologically, it shows certain clear-cut differences. Thus, the organ distribution is somewhat different, the age peak is later, and the long-term response to therapy appears to be more favorable (Cohen et al., 1969; Aresenau et al., 1975; Mann et al., 1976; Ziegler, 1977).

Both endemic (African) and sporadic BL are B-cell (bone marrow-derived lymphocyte) tumors, and the former has been shown to be monoclonal in origin (Fialkow et al., 1970, 1973).

II. EPIDEMIOLOGY INDICATING AN INFECTIOUS CAUSE

Both the dependence of high incidence areas of African BL on certain conditions of temperature and rainfall and the implication this carries for a virus being involved in the etiology (Burkitt, 1962a, b) have already been pointed out in relation to the discovery of EBV (Chap. 1). The original observations on this temperature and rainfall dependence of African BL have stood the test of time (Burkitt, 1970) and have been extended to the other endemic area of the tumor, namely New Guinea (Booth et al., 1967).

Further evidence for the existence of an infectious cause of African BL has been provided by studies showing time-space clustering of the disease with the epidemic characteristic of "drift" (Pike et al., 1967; Williams et al., 1978) and a curious seasonal variation in onset (Williams et al., 1974). Two arresting new epidemiologic findings strongly indicating an infectious element in the etiology of BL have recently been reported; these concern a striking risk factor and case clustering – they are discussed in Sect. C.II and D below.

III. CLINICAL BEHAVIOR SUGGESTING HOST RESPONSES TO ANTIGENICITY

It has been recognized from the outset that African BL is a highly malignant tumor; without therapy the majority of affected children die within 4 months of clinical onset (Burkitt, 1962c). However, the occurrence of rare spontaneous remissions (Burkitt and Kyalwazi, 1967), remissions after nonspecific therapy (David and Burkitt, 1968), temporary remissions after transfusion of serum from successfully treated patients (Burkitt, 1967b; Ngu, 1967), and frequent striking long-term survivals following single dose chemotherapy (Burkitt, 1967c), all indicate that the tumor must be highly antigenic and capable of eliciting a potent host immunologic response.

IV. CYTOGENETICS

Early cytogenetic investigations on African BL biopsies showed abnormalities in the No. 2 and No. 4 chromosomes of the cells of some tumors, which it was thought at the time might be characteristic for the disease (Jacobs et al., 1963; Stewart et al., 1965; Rabson et al., 1966). Subsequently, a No. 10 chromosome marker abnormality was reported in cultured BL-derived and other EBV-carrying lymphoid cell lines by some investigators, but could not be found by others (Epstein and Achong, 1973). It would appear that none of these early reports of chromosonal abnormalities relates to changes specific either for BL or for EBV-infected cells.

More recently, the application of chromosome-banding techniques has revealed a consistent abnormality in one No. 14 chromosome in African BL biopsy cells and in lymphoid cell lines of African BL origin (Manolov and Manolova, 1972; Jarvis et al., 1974; Zech et al., 1976). This No. 14 chromosome change has been identified as a translocation from one No. 8 chromosome to give an extra band on both long arms of the No. 14 and is designated t(8q−; 14q+) (Zech et al., 1976). However, the t(8q−; 14q+) alteration has likewise failed to prove a marker specific either for BL or for EBV-infected cells — the same abnormality has been reported in several non-Burkitt lymphomas and a chronic lymphatic leukemia (Zech et al., 1976; Fleischman and Prigogina, 1977; Fukuhara and Rowley, 1978) and a seemingly identical translocation has been found in other lymphosarcomas, non-Burkitt lymphomas, multiple myeloma, and acute lymphatic leukemia (Reeves, 1973; Mark, 1975; Prigogina and Fleischman, 1975; Zech et al., 1976; Minowada et al., 1977; Catovsky et al., 1977; Liang and Rowley, 1978). Again, although the marker is present in all EBV genome-containing BLs and in the lymphoma cell lines derived from them, it has never been reported in EBV-positive nonmalignant lymphoblastoid lines (Jarvis et al., 1974; Chap. 11). Hence, although not a marker for BL or EBV (Kaiser-McCaw et al., 1977), the t(8q−; 14q+) translocation nevertheless seems to be related to malignant change in lymphoid cells in a more general way.

In any event, the No. 14 chromosome is perculiarly unstable since many other changes affecting it have been detected in such various conditions as ataxia telangiectasia (McCaw et al., 1975; Oxford et al., 1975), assorted malignant tumors (Wurster-Hill et al., 1973; Lawler et al., 1975; Philip, 1975; Fukuhara et al., 1976; Pickthall, 1976; Yamada et al., 1977; Hossfeld, 1978; Liang and Rowley, 1978; Fukuhara and Rowley, 1978), and even in normal lymphocytes after brief culture in vitro (Welch and Lee, 1975; Beatty-De Sana et al., 1975; Hecht et al., 1975).

Even though cytogenetic studies have failed to detect changes specific for BL or EBV, they have provided an important line of evidence showing that when BL biopsies are cultured it is the malignant tumor cells which grow out directly, since random chromosome changes in the biopsy cells are also found in the resulting cell lines (Gripenberg et al., 1969; Manolov and Manolova, 1972).

C. THE VIRUS AND AFRICAN BURKITT'S LYMPHOMA

I. SPECIFIC RESPONSES OF BURKITT'S LYMPHOMA PATIENTS TO EBV

The EBV-determined antigens identified so far are described in detail in Chap. 3. It is noteworthy that 100% of patients with African BL have antibodies to the viral capsid antigen (VCA) (Chap. 4), indicating that all individuals with the tumor have been infected by the virus.

The response of any EBV-infected host to the viral antigens varies considerably depending on the circumstances; thus, the levels of antibody to each antigen show quite different and characteristic patterns in normal seropositive individuals, in primary infection accompanied by infectious mononucleosis (IM), in patients with nasopharyngeal carcinoma, and in patients with African BL (Chaps. 4, 13, and 15).

Apart from the usual antibody responses to EBV antigens seen in all infected individuals (Chap. 4), the special features of the response mounted by patients with African BL are:

1. An unusually high level of antibodies to VCA with the geometric mean titer 8–10 times greater than that of control sera from African children or patients with other malignancies of the lymphoreticular system (Levy and Henle, 1966; Henle et al., 1969; Kafuko et al., 1972).
2. Uniquely high titers of antibodies to early antigen (EA) of the restricted (R) type; these predominante over antibodies directed against the other component of the EA

complex, frequently occur in the absence of the latter, and sometimes even reach a titer 8 times higher than antibodies to VCA (Henle et al., 1971; Henle and Henle, 1977).

3. Changes in antibody levels showing a close and peculiar association with certain clinical events in the course of African BL. A drop in, or low, anti-EA(R) titer relates to a good prognosis, whereas a rise in this antibody usually heralds a fatal relapse (Henle et al., 1973); in addition, a sudden drop in antibodies to membrane antigen (MA) often precedes tumor recurrence by several months (Gunvén et al., 1974). Further details of these various responses are given in Chap. 4.

II. RISK FACTOR

Even more striking evidence that EBV is in some way actually causally related to African BL has recently been reported. A 7-year prospective seroepidemiologic survey in Uganda has followed 42,000 children and found among them 12 cases of BL from whom predisease serum samples were available for study. This uniquely valuable material has shown that individuals who develop African BL already have remarkably raised titers of antibodies to VCA months or years before clinical onset of the tumor, and the data on this have made it possible to calculate the risk factor attached to such unusually marked responses to this EBV antigen so long before the disease. Thus, the risk of developing African BL was approximately 30 times higher for those with a VCA antibody titer of two doubling dilutions or more above the normal control population (de-Thé et al., 1978; Chap. 18), a risk appreciably greater than that for heavy cigarette smoking and bronchogenic carcinoma (Doll and Peto, 1976; Royal College of Physicians, London, 1977).

III. EBV IN TUMOR CELLS

EBV particles have never been observed directly in African BL biopsy material despite careful searching of nearly 150 tumors by experienced researchers in several laboratories (Epstein and Herdson, 1963; Dourmashkin, 1964; Achong and Epstein, 1966; Rabson et al., 1966; Bernhard, 1970). However, it was obvious from the outset that at least some of the cells harbored the virus genome, since a productive cycle of virus replication was activated by the in vitro environment when the cells were placed in culture (Epstein et al., 1965); indeed, it was this activation which allowed EBV to be discovered in the first place, when such cultured cells were examined by electron microscopy (Epstein et al., 1964; Chap. 1). Confirmation for the presence of the EBV genome in African BL cells was obtained by showing that live cells fresh from tumors expressed the EBV-determined MA (Klein et al., 1966, 1967, 1968 a, b, 1969).

It has now been established beyond doubt by nucleic acid hybridization experiments that every tumor cell does in fact contain multiple copies of EBV DNA (zur Hausen et al., 1970; zur Hausen and Schulte-Holthausen, 1972; Nonoyama and Pagano, 1973; Nonyama et al., 1973; Kawai et al., 1973; Chaps. 6 and 7) which are responsible for the expression of the EBV nuclear antigen (EBNA) demonstrable by anticomplement immunofluorescence (Reedman and Klein, 1973; Lindahl et al., 1974; Chap. 3) and the lymphocyte-detected membrane antigen (LYDMA) shown by in vitro T-cell (thymus-dependent lymphocyte) cytotoxicity tests (Svedmyr and Jondal, 1975; Jondal et al., 1975; Klein et al., 1976). The expression of these various neoantigens in African BL cells, particularly those in the cell membrane, provides the explanation of the strong antigenicity of the tumor observed in early clinical work (Sect. B.III).

IV. INFORMATION FROM LYMPHOID CELL LINES

Further confirmation of the special and significant relationship of EBV to the malignant cells of African BL is provided by findings on the mode of origin of lymphoid cell lines from the tumors, as compared to the origin of those from other types of EBV-carrying B cells. As has been pointed out in Chap. 1, EBV-containing lymphoid lines arise by the direct outgrowth of the tumor cells when African BL biopsies are cultured (Gripenberg et al., 1969; Nadkarni et al., 1969; Fialkow et al., 1970; Manolov and Manolova, 1972); in contrast, EBV-containing nonmalignant peripheral lymphocytes from seropositive individuals, which have a different relationship to the virus, namely latency (Chap. 1), give cell lines in vitro by a two-step mechanism unconnected with direct outgrowth (Rickinson et al., 1974, 1975, 1977a, b; Rocchi et al., 1977; Crawford et al., 1978).

It is of interest that these two modes of origin give rise to two different types of cell line with qualitatively different properties (Chap. 11).

V. COFACTORS

If, as now seems almost certain (Sect. F), EBV plays some sort of causative role in endemic BL, it clearly cannot do so alone. For, the virus is widespread throughout the world (Chaps. 1 and 4), whereas the high incidence endemic areas of the tumor are restricted to certain parts of Africa and New Guinea showing specific features of temperature and rainfall (Burkitt, 1962 a, b; Booth et al., 1967). Quite apart from the ubiquity of the virus, it has long been recognized that the original hypothesis that an oncogenic virus carried by a vector affected by climate was responsible for the temperature and rainfall dependence of the tumor (Burkitt, 1962, b) cannot be true, since even in regions with the highest incidence of African BL, vector mediated case-to-case infection is not possible (Haddow, 1964).

1. Hyperendemic Malaria

With the foregoing excluded, it follows that a climate-dependent cofactor is most likely to be involved; Burkitt has argued persuasively that hyperendemic malaria fits the requirements for such a cofactor (Burkitt, 1969) and a considerable body of evidence supports this notion:

1. Both malaria and African BL are limited by the same temperature and rainfall barriers (Burkitt, 1969).
2. There are only two areas in the world where malaria is hyperendemic, tropical Africa and New Guinea, and these are precisely where the tumor is endemic (Burkitt, 1969).

3. In other tropical areas where malaria is not hyperendemic the tumor is rare (Burkitt, 1969).
4. There are many areas where malaria and the tumor were both common, but since eradication of the former, tumor incidence has been drastically reduced (Burkitt, 1969).
5. Sickle cell trait confers partial protection against malaria and children with the trait have half the incidence of the tumor (Williams, 1966; Pike et al., 1970).
6. Severe malaria is not only important in the development of African BL, but seems to precipitate its onset (Morrow et al., 1976).

The exact mechanisms whereby hyperendemic malaria might interact with EBV infection to bring about a transformation event in vivo are currently ill-defined, but important pointers have begun to emerge. It has been known for some time that only B lymphocytes have receptors for EBV (Pattengale et al., 1973; Jondal and Klein, 1973) and also that malaria is both immunosuppressive and a stimulator of B cell proliferation (Salaman et al., 1969; O'Conor, 1970; Greenwood et al., 1972). Persistent malaria might therefore act as a cofactor by stimulating and maintaining a continuing large supply of lymphoid cells especially liable to undergo malignant change in response to infection by the virus. Such readily transformable cells could be a particular type of B cell, B cells with a particular chromosomal change, or B cells in the early stages of differentiation. There is indeed evidence now that at least in vitro certain subclasses of B lymphocytes constitute a special target for transformation by EBV (Katsuki et al., 1977; Steel et al., 1977) and recent observations on the lack of differentiation shown by cells from many acute leukemias (Greaves et al., 1977; Janossy et al., 1978) suggest that the cells transformed to malignancy to give African BL tumors might similarly be in the early regions of the differentiation pathway.

2. Genetic Predisposition

However important the role of hyperendemic malaria as a cofactor with EBV for the induction of African BL, the tumor must have a multifactorial causation with other influences playing a significant part. For, where BL is endemic, almost the entire population is infected by EBV at an early age (Henle and Henle, 1969) and hyperendemic malaria by definition affects over 50% of young children, yet only small numbers of these doubly infected individuals develop the tumor. It seems likely that a genetic predisposition to African BL must also be involved analogous to that seen with Marek's disease before the days of vaccines when only a minority of birds infected actually manifested the malignant disease (Chap. 17). Marek's disease is of particular interest in this context since it provides an example of a herpesvirus ubiquitous in its chicken host with a variety of well-defined cofactors influencing its oncogenicity (Payne, 1973).

An indication for the presence of a peculiar individual response to EBV infection in African BL patients which might well predispose to the tumor, has emerged from the long-term prospective study of a large group of children in a high incidence area for African BL. Those individuals destined to have BL showed unusually high antibody levels to EB VCA as compared to controls, over considerable periods before the onset of the tumors and, as discussed in Sect. C.II above, this individual characteristic constituted a major risk factor (de-Thé et al., 1978; Chap. 18).

VI. EBV ISOLATES FROM AFRICAN BURKITT'S LYMPHOMA

The question has naturally arisen as to whether EBV isolated from the tumor cells of African BL differs in its properties from that carried by normal seropositive individuals or patients with IM. With the exception of a single unusual mutant laboratory strain, all EBV isolates of whatever origin show such biologic, biochemical, and antigenic similarities as not to suggest major strain differences (Chaps. 1, 6, and 8) and any minor variations detected certainly cannot be specifically related to virus from malignant or nonmalignant sources.

D. SPORADIC BURKITT'S LYMPHOMA

The lymphoma somewhat similar to African BL which occurs sporadically but rarely outside the endemic areas of Africa and New Guinea (Burkitt, 1967a) has long presented a problem regarding its relationship to EBV. It will be remembered that this tumor resembles endemic BL histologically and cytologically and is likewise a B cell tumor (Mann et al., 1976) but shows a somewhat different age peak, organ distribution, and response to therapy (Sect. B.I).

Recent studies have provided some understanding of the question of EBV-relatedness; it is now clear that a small but significant minority of sporadic BL patients (about 12%) shows exactly the same close association with EBV as do African BL cases in having similar characteristic antibody responses to the virus and both virus DNA and virus-determined neoantigens in all the tumor cells (Andersson et al., 1976; Ziegler et al., 1976; Judson et al., 1977). In contrast, individuals with those sporadic BL whose tumor cells do not carry EBV DNA, show either no antibodies to EBV antigens or merely low titer antibodies without the characteristic pattern (Pagano et al., 1973; Epstein et al., 1976; Ziegler et al., 1976).

It is now being suggested that the condition we currently define as BL on clinical, histologic and cytologic criteria (Berard et al., 1969) may in fact be two distinct diseases (zur Hausen, 1975; Andersson et al., 1976; de-Thé et al., 1978) – on the one hand, endemic BL and the minority of sporadic BL cases, which are all EBV genome-positive; on the other hand, the majority of sporadic BL cases which do not have EBV DNA in the tumor cells. Since sporadic BL can seemingly occur anywhere in the world, the finding of a rare EBV genome-negative case of BL even in endemic areas (Lindahl et al., 1974) would fit well with this view of the dual nature of the disease. Furthermore, that endemic BL is relatively frequent, yet similarly genome-positive sporadic BL extremely rare clearly reflects the effect, additional to that of the virus, of such a climate-dependent cofactor as hyperendemic malaria (Sect. C.VI), whose distribution seems to determine the high indidence areas of the tumor. A recent account of a time-space cluster of the rare EBV-associated form of sporadic BL (Judson et al., 1977) provides another analogy relating this form of the disease to African BL, as well as further indications of an infectious origin.

E. ONCORNAVIRUSES AND BURKITT'S LYMPHOMA

A claim has been made that African BL biopsies have shown evidence for the presence of oncornavirus material in the tumor cells (Kufe et al., 1973 a, b). This material is said to consist of particles encapsulating a 70S RNA and a reverse transcriptase, both characteristic of oncornavirus and found in suspensions of disrupted tumors by means of a simultaneous detection test (Kufe et al., 1973 b). However, the results have only been positive in $\sim 80\%$ of African BL, similar positive results have been obtained with each of a wide assortment of other human tumors (Kufe et al., 1973 c; Cuatico et al., 1973, 1974; Balda et al., 1975; Witkin et al., 1975), and there has been no confirmatory morphologic evidence for the presence of the particles either in the original biopsies or in the positive fractions of the suspensions.

Apart from the foregoing it has been found possible to activate true, morphologically authenticated, oncornaviruses in the cells of certain EBV lines (Kotler et al., 1975) and the intermittent production of an oncornavirus by 1 out ot 11 such lines has been confirmed (Klucis et al., 1976). In addition, oncornaviruses have frequently been found in normal human placental and fetal tissue (Chandra et al., 1970; Kalter et al., 1973; Vernon et al., 1974; Panem et al., 1975; Imamura et al., 1976) and appear to be widespread in the normal cells of many mammalian species (Lieber et al., 1973).

Although the origin and significance of oncornaviruses actually detected in human malignant cells are at present unclear, it seems most probable that they are examples of the well-recognized, endogenous (class I) oncornaviruses which are likewise widely present but which, unlike the exogenous (class II) oncornaviruses, have never been shown to be carcinogenic (Gillespie and Gallo, 1975; Berard et al., 1976). In any event, there is certainly no evidence for any oncornaviruses playing a part in the etiology of BL.

F. DISCUSSION

With any putative human tumor virus there are obviously great difficulties in obtaining definitive proof that the agent is indeed carcinogenic in man. It is for this reason that more and more basic information has been sought on the role of EBV in BL; as a result enough is now known to draw meaningful conclusions if the facts are considered in an appropriate framework. Henle (1971) has proposed certain criteria which any human tumor virus should meet:
1. Virus, virus-determined neoantigens, or virus nucleic acid must be present in all the tumor cells.
2. Antibodies to virus-determined antigens must occur at higher frequency and/or titers with given malignancies than in controls.
3. The virus must be capable of transforming normal cells in vitro.
4. The virus must be capable of tumor induction in subhuman primates.

After 15 years intensive work since the discovery of EBV (Epstein et al., 1964), it is crystal clear that this agent, unlike any other virus suspected of oncogenicity in man, has fully satisfied the foregoing requirements and indeed gone far beyond them.

Several different techniques have established beyond doubt that EBV DNA and virus antigens are present in the cells of almost every African BL and a minority of sporadic BL (Chaps. 3, 6, 7, and 8). African BL has long been recognized as a monoclonal disease (Fialkow et al., 1970, 1973) and the presence of the virus DNA in every tumor cell indicates that the original cell undergoing malignant transformation must in each case have been infected at the outset – EBV does not at a later stage simply infect some of the tumor cells which happen to provide a suitable and accessible environment. Furthermore, that such a casual passenger event is not responsible for BL cell infection is demonstrated by the occurrence in seropositive patients of many other kinds of B cell tumors which are always EBV genome-negative, including now the majority of cases of sporadic BL (Ziegler et al., 1976). The significance of EBV genomes in African BL cells is heightened by the fact that at least one or two copies appear to be linearly covalently integrated into the host cell DNA (Kaschka-Dierich et al., 1976; Chap. 8) in a manner analogous to that of known DNA oncogenic animal viruses in the cells of the tumors they cause (Tooze, 1973).

Antibody responses to EBV in African BL and genome-positive cases of sporadic BL likewise fulfill Henle's requirements; indeed, not only are they always present and greatly raised in titer in the tumor patients as compared to controls, but in addition BL patients display a characteristic response pattern that varies specifically during the clinical course of the disease (Sect. C.I; Chap. 4). It seems clear that neither of these curious features of antibody response to EBV in BL patients can be explained merely on the basis of a passenger role for the virus.

That EBV is extraordinarily efficient at transforming normal primate B lymphocytes in vitro into continuously growing cell lines has been discussed fully in Chaps. 1, 10, and 11. The reasons for believing that these cell lines are malignantly transformed have likewise been discussed (Chap. 1). Although the malignant nature of such transformed human cells has not yet been fully resolved and the necessary experiments obviously cannot be performed with human cell lines, marmoset lymphocytes transformed by EBV in culture (Miller et al., 1972) give malignant tumors when inoculated back into these animals (Shope et al., 1973). EBV is thus clearly capable of the malignant transformation of such normal cells in vitro, even without considering its powerful effects on human B lymphocytes. To complete the picture, the virus is also experimentally oncogenic in vivo (Chap. 16) and in this respect matches the behavior of known oncogenic herpesviruses of animals (Chap. 17).

Added to all this, the unusual antibody response to EB VCA shown for long periods by individuals destined to have African BL (de-Thé et al., 1978) has now provided further epidemiologic evidence for a causal relationship between EBV and the tumor. This finding has permitted the calculation of a highly significant risk factor for tumor development in those showing this unusual response to infection by the virus (Sect. C.II; Chap. 18) which can only be explained on the basis of special interactions of EBV with its likely cofactors (Sect. C.V). Such interactions might involve an individual genetic predisposition to African BL when exposed to both EBV and malaria, or tumor development as a result of an especially early infection with these two agents, or again, some special sequence in the timing of the two infections in relation to one another. The possible role of persistent malaria in stimulating lymphoid target cells especially liable to EBV-induced malignant transformation has already been discussed (Sect. C.VI).

In the light of everything considered so far, EBV unquestionably brings about a transformation event in subhuman primate lymphocytes when it infects such cells in vitro and during experimental tumor induction in vivo; it is also not unreasonable to conclude now that it almost certainly brings about such an event under natural conditions in man during the genesis of EBV-related BL. The nature of the transformation event is not yet fully understood; however, in vitro it may be related either to amplification of the EBV DNA load or to integration of some viral DNA molecules into the genome of the newly infected cell (Thorley-Lawson and Strominger, 1976; Chap. 9) and similar phenomena might operate in malignant change in vivo.

There are at least some indications now regarding the series of steps into which such a transformation event in vivo might fit during the induction of African BL by EBV. The t(8q − ; 14q +) chromosome abnormality clearly predisposes to malignant change in lymphoid cells (Klein, 1975); it could well be that B cells carrying this spontaneous mutation increase in number during the lymphoid stimulation of chronic malaria (Sect. C.V.1) and that infection of a cell of this kind by EBV brings about the transformation event leading to the production of a malignant clone expressing EBV-determined cell membrane antigens. The additional immunosuppressive effect of the malaria (Sect. C.V.1) might result in failure to eliminate such clones with consequent development of African BL. The production of nonmalignant B cells with the 14q + abnormality is genetically determined in ataxia telangiectasia (Harnden, 1974; McCaw et al., 1975; Oxford et al., 1975), which is an autosomal recessive disease, and this suggests that the emergence of such cells before the onset of African BL may also have a genetic basis which would thus explain a genetic predisposition to the tumor (Sect. C.V.2).

Whether or not this should ultimately prove to be the case, definition of the EBV-induced transformation event will provide much needed insights at the molecular level regarding the way in which the virus exerts its carcinogenic function. Absolute proof that EBV actually plays a part in nature in the causation of those BL tumors with which it is associated will only be obtainable at the biologic level if the prevention of infection with a vaccine gives a consequent decrease in the number of tumors. A program of intervention of this kind in a high incidence area for African BL is no longer beyond the bounds of practical realization (Epstein, 1975, 1976); the factors involved are discussed in Chap. 19.

REFERENCES

Achong, B. G., Epstein, M. A.: Fine structure of the Burkitt tumor. J. Natl. Cancer Inst. **36**, 877–897 (1966)

Andersson, M., Klein, G., Ziegler, J. L., Henle, W.: Association of Epstein-Barr viral genomes with American Burkitt lymphoma. Nature **260**, 357–359 (1976)

Arsenau, J. C., Canellos, G. P., Banks, P. M., Berard, C. W., Gralnick, H. R., Devita, V. T.: American Burkitt's lymphoma: a clinicopathologic study of 30 cases. Am. J. Med. **58**, 314–321 (1975)

Balda, B-R., Hehlmann, R., Cho, J-R., Spiegelman, S.: Oncornavirus-like particles in human skin cancers. Proc. Natl. Acad. Sci. USA **72**, 3697–3700 (1975)

Beatty-DeSana, J. W., Hoggard, M. J., Cooledge, J. W.: Non-random occurrence of 7–14 translocations in human lymphocyte cultures. Nature **255**, 242–243 (1975)

Berard, C., O'Conor, G. T., Thomas, L. B., Torloni, H.: Histopathological definition of Burkitt's tumour. Bull. W. H. O. **40**, 601–607 (1969)

Berard, C. W., Gallo, R. C., Jaffe, E. S., Green, I., Devita, V. T.: Current concepts of leukemia and lymphoma: etiology, pathogenesis, and therapy. Ann. Intern. Med. **85**, 351–366 (1976)

Bernhard, W.: Fine structure of Burkitt's lymphoma. In: Burkitt's lymphoma. Burkitt, D. P., Wright, D. H. (eds.), pp. 103–117. Edinburgh, London: Livingstone 1970

Booth, K., Burkitt, D. P., Bassett, D. J., Cooke, R. A., Biddulph, J.: Burkitt lymphoma in Papua-New Guinea. Br. J. Cancer **21**, 657–664 (1967)

Burkitt, D.: A sarcoma involving the jaws in African children. Br. J. Surg. **46**, 218–223 (1958)

Burkitt, D.: A children's cancer dependent on climatic factors. Nature **194**, 232–234 (1962a)

Burkitt, D.: Determining the climatic limitations of a children's cancer common in Africa. Br. Med. J. **1962b II**, 1019–1023

Burkitt, D.: A tumour syndrome affecting children in tropical Africa. Postgrad. Med. J. **38**, 71–79 (1962c)

Burkitt, D.: A lymphoma syndrome in tropical Africa. Int. Rev. Exp. Pathol. **2**, 67–138 (1963)

Burkitt, D.: Burkitt's lymphoma outside the known endemic areas of Africa and New Guinea. Int. J. Cancer **2**, 562–565 (1967a)

Burkitt, D.: Clinical evidence suggesting an immunological response against African lymphoma. U.I.C.C. Monogr. **8**, 197–203 (1967b)

Burkitt, D.: Long-term remissions following one and two-dose chemotherapy for African lymphoma. Cancer **20**, 756–759 (1967c)

Burkitt, D. P.: Etiology of Burkitt's lymphoma – an alternative hypothesis to a vectored virus. J. Natl. Cancer Inst. **42**, 19–28 (1969)

Burkitt, D. P.: Geographical Distribution. In: Burkitt's lymphoma. Burkitt, D. P., Wright, D. H. (eds.), pp. 186–197. Edinburgh, London: Livingstone 1970

Burkitt, D. P., Kyalwazi, S. K.: Spontaneous remission of African lymphoma. Br. J. Cancer **21**, 14–16 (1967)

Catovsky, D., Pittman, S., Lewis, D., Pearse, E.: Marker chromosome 14q+ in follicular lymphoma in transformation. Lancet **1977 II**, 934

Chandra, S., Liszczak, T., Korol, W., Jensen, E. M.: Type-C particles in human tissues. I. Electron microscopic study of embryonic tissues *in vivo* and *in vitro*. Int. J. Cancer **6**, 40–45 (1970)

Cohen, M. H., Bennett, J. M., Berard, C. W., Ziegler, J. L., Vogel, C. L., Sheagren, J. N., Carbone, P. P.: Burkitt's tumor in the United States. Cancer **23**, 1259–1272 (1969)

Crawford, D. H., Rickinson, A. B., Finerty, S., Epstein, M. A.: Epstein-Barr (EB) virus genome-containing EB nuclear antigen-negative B-lymphocyte populations in blood in acute infectious mononucleosis. J. Gen. Virol. **38**, 449–460 (1978)

Cuatico, W., Cho, J-R., Spiegelman, S.: Particles with RNA of high molecular weight and RNA-directed DNA polymerase in human brain tumors. Proc. Natl. Acad. Sci. USA **70**, 2789–2793 (1973)

Cuatico, W., Cho, J-R., Spiegelman, S.: Evidence of particle associated RNA-directed DNA polymerase and high molecular weight RNA in human gastro-intestinal and lung malignancies. Proc. Natl. Acad. Sci. USA **71**, 3304–3308 (1974)

David, J., Burkitt, D.: Burkitt's lymphoma: remissions following seemingly non-specific therapy. Br. Med. J. **1968 IV**, 288–291

de-Thé, G., Geser, A., Day, N. E., Tukei, P. M., Williams, E. H., Beri, D. P., Smith, P. G., Dean, A. G., Bornkamm, G. W., Feorino, P., Henle, W.: Epidemiological evidence for causal relationship between Epstein-Barr virus and Burkitt's lymphoma: results of the Ugandan prospective study. Nature **274**, 756–761 (1978)

Doll, R., Peto, R.: Mortality in relation to smoking: 20 years' observation on male British doctors. Br. Med. J. **1976 II**, 1525–1536

Dourmashkin, R.: An electron microscope study of Burkitt tumour biopsies. Eur. J. Cancer **1**, 309–312 (1965)

Epstein, A. L., Henle, W., Henle, G., Hewetson, J. F., Kaplan, H. S.: Surface marker characteristics and Epstein-Barr virus studies of two established North American Burkitt's lymphoma cell lines. Proc. Natl. Acad. Sci. USA **73**, 228–232 (1976)

Epstein, M. A.: Towards an anti-viral vaccine for a human cancer. Nature **253**, 6 (1975)

Epstein, M. A.: Epstein-Barr virus – is it time to develop a vaccine program? J. Natl. Cancer Inst. **56**, 697–700 (1976)

Epstein, M. A., Achong, B. G.: The EB virus. Annu. Rev. Microbiol. **27**, 413–436 (1973)

Epstein, M. A., Achong, B. G., Barr, Y. M.: Virus particles in cultured lymphoblasts from Burkitt's lymphoma. Lancet **1964 I**, 702–703

Epstein, M. A., Henle, G., Achong, B. G., Barr, Y. M.: Morphological and biological studies on a virus in cultured lymphoblasts from Burkitt's lymphoma. J. Exp. Med. **121**, 761–770 (1965)

Epstein, M. A., Herdson, P. B.: Cellular degeneration associated with characteristic nuclear fine structural changes in the cells from two cases of Burkitt's malignant lymphoma syndrome. Br. J. Cancer **17**, 56–58 (1963)

Fialkow, P. J., Klein, G., Gartler, S. M., Clifford, P.: Clonal origin for individual Burkitt tumours. Lancet **1970 I**, 384–386

Fialkow, P. J., Klein, E., Klein, G., Clifford, P., Singh, S.: Immunoglobulin and glucose-6-phosphate dehydrogenase as markers of cellular origin in Burkitt lymphoma. J. Exp. Med. **138**, 89–102 (1973)

Fleischman, E. W., Prigogina, E. L.: Karyotype peculiarities of malignant lymphomas. Hum. Genet. **35**, 269–279 (1977)

Fukuhara, S., Rowley, J. D.: Chromosome 14 translocations in non-Burkitt lymphomas. Int. J. Cancer **22**, 14–21 (1978)

Fukuhara, S., Shirakawa, S., Uchino, H.: Specific marker chromosome 14 in malignant lymphomas. Nature **259**, 210–211 (1976)

Gillespie, D., Gallo, R. C.: RNA processing and RNA tumor virus origin and evolution. Science **188**, 802–811 (1975)

Greaves, M. F., Janossy, G., Roberts, M., Rapson, N. T., Ellis, R. B., Chassells, J., Lister, T. A., Catovsky, D.: Membrane phenotyping: diagnosis, monitoring and classification of acute 'lymphoid'leukaemias. In: Immunodiagnosis of leukaemias and lymphomas. Thierfelder, S., Rodt, H., Thiel, E. (eds.), pp. 61–75. Munich: Lehmans 1977

Greenwood, B. M., Bradley-Moore, A. M., Palit, A., Bryceson, A. D. M.: Immunosuppression in children with malaria. Lancet **1972 I**, 169–172

Gripenberg, U., Levan, A., Clifford, P.: Chromosomes in Burkitt lymphomas. I. Serial studies in a case with bilateral tumors showing different chromosomal stemlines. Int. J. Cancer **4**, 334–349 (1969)

Gunvén, P., Klein, G., Clifford, P., Singh, S.: Epstein-Barr virus-associated membrane-reactive antibodies during long term survival after Burkitt's lymphoma. Proc. Natl. Acad. Sci. USA **71**, 1422–1426 (1974)

Haddow, A. J.: Age incidence in Burkitt's lymphoma syndrome. East. Afr. Med. J. **41**, 1–6 (1964)

Harnden, D. G.: Ataxia telangiectasia syndrome: cytogenetic and cancer aspects. In: Chromosomes and cancer. German, J. (ed.), pp. 619–636. New York: Wiley 1974

Hecht, F., McCaw, B. K., Peakman, D., Robinson, A.: Non-random occurrence of 7–14 translocations in human lymphocyte cultures. Nature **255**, 243–244 (1975)

Henle, G., Henle, W., Clifford, V., Diehl, V., Kafuko, G., Kirya, B. G., Klein, G., Morrow, R. H., Munube, G. M. R., Pike, P., Tukei, P. M., Ziegler, J. L.: Antibodies to Epstein-Barr virus in Burkitt's lymphoma and control groups. J. Natl. Cancer Inst. **43**, 1147–1157 (1969)

Henle, G., Henle, W., Klein, G.: Demonstration of two distinct components in the early antigen complex of Epstein-Barr virus-infected cells. Int. J. Cancer **8**, 272–282 (1971)

Henle, W.: Evidence for a relation of the Epstein-Barr virus to Burkitt's lymphoma and nasopharyngeal carcinoma. In: Proceedings of the 1st International Symposium of the Princess Takamatsu Cancer Research Fund: Recent advances in human tumor virology and immunology. Nakahara, W., Nishioka, K., Hirayama, T., Ito, Y. (eds.), pp. 361–367. Tokyo: University of Tokyo Press 1971

Henle, W., Henle, G.: The relation between the Epstein-Barr virus and infectious mononucleosis, Burkitt's lymphoma and cancer of the postnasal space. East Afr. Med. J. **46**, 402–406 (1969)

Henle, W., Henle, G.: Antibodies to the R component of Epstein-Barr virus-induced early antigens in Burkitt's lymphoma exceeding in titer antibodies to Epstein-Barr viral capsid antigen. J. Natl. Cancer Inst. **58**, 785–786 (1977)

Henle, W., Henle, G., Gunvén, P., Klein, G., Clifford, P., Singh, S.: Patterns of antibodies to Epstein-Barr virus-induced early antigens in fatal cases of Burkitt's lymphoma and long term survivors. J. Natl. Cancer Inst. **50**, 1163–1173 (1973)

Hossfeld, D. K.: Chromosome 14q+ in a retinoblastoma. Int. J. Cancer **21**, 720–723 (1978)

Imamura, M., Phillips, P. E., Mellors, R. C.: The occurrence and frequency of type C virus-like particles in placentas from patients with systemic lupus erythematosus and from normal subjects. Am. J. Pathol. **83**, 383–394 (1976)

Jacobs, P. A., Tough, I. M., Wright, D. H.: Cytogenetic studies in Burkitt lymphoma. Lancet **1963 II**, 1144–1146

Janossy, G., Greaves, M. F., Sutherland, R., Durant, J., Lewis, C.: Membrane phenotypes of acute 'lymphoid' and undifferentiated leukaemias: relationship to target cells and differentiation pathways. Leukaemia Res. **1**, 289 (1977)

Jarvis, J. E., Ball, G., Rickinson, A. B., Epstein, M. A.: Cytogenetic studies on human lymphoblastoid cell lines from Burkitt's lymphomas and other sources. Int. J. Cancer **14**, 716–721 (1974)

Jondal, M., Klein, G.: Surface markers on human B and T lymphocytes. II. Presence of Epstein-Barr virus receptors on B lymphocytes. J. Exp. Med. **138**, 1365–1378 (1973)

Jondal, M., Svedmyr, E., Klein, E., Singh, S.: Killer T cells in a Burkitt's lymphoma biopsy. Nature **255**, 405–407 (1975)

Judson, S. C., Henle, W., Henle, G.: A cluster of Epstein-Barr-virus-associated American Burkitt's lymphoma. N. Engl. J. Med. **297**, 464–468 (1977)

Kafuko, G. W., Henderson, B. E., Kirya, B. G., Munube, G. M. R., Tukei, P. M., Day, N. E., Henle, G., Henle, W., Morrow, R. H., Pike, M. C., Smith, P. G., Williams, E. H.: Epstein-Barr virus antibody levels in children from the West Nile district of Uganda. Report of a field study. Lancet **1972 I**, 706–709

Kaiser-McCaw, B., Epstein, A. L., Kaplan, H. S., Hecht, F.: Chromosome 14 translocation in African and North American Burkitt's lymphoma. Int. J. Cancer **19**, 482–486 (1977)

Kalter, S. S., Helmke, R. J., Heberling, R. L., Panigel, M., Fowler, A. K., Strickland, J. E., Hellman, A.: Brief communication: C-type particles in normal human placentas. J. Natl. Cancer Inst. **50**, 1081–1084 (1973)

Kaschka-Dierich, C., Adams, A., Lindahl, T., Bornkamm, G. W., Bjursell, G., Klein, G., Giovanella, B. C., Singh, S.: Intracellular forms of Epstein-Barr virus DNA in human tumour cells *in vivo*. Nature **260**, 302–306 (1976)

Katsuki, T., Hinuma, Y., Yamamoto, N., Abo, T., Kumagai, K.: Identification of the target cells in human B lymphocytes for transformation by Epstein-Barr virus. Virology **83**, 287–294 (1977)

Kawai, Y., Nonoyama, M., Pagano, J. S.: Reassociation kinetics for Epstein-Barr virus DNA: nonhomology to mammalian DNA and homology of viral DNA in various diseases. J. Virol. **12**, 1006–1012 (1973)

Klein, G.: The Epstein-Barr virus and neoplasia . New Engl. J. Med. **293**, 1353–1357 (1975)

Klein, E., Klein, G., Levine, P. H.: Immunological control of human lymphoma: discussion. Cancer Res. **36**, 724–727 (1976)

Klein, G., Clifford, P., Klein, E., Stjernswärd, J.: Search for tumor-specific immune reactions in Burkitt lymphoma patients by the membrane immunofluorescence reaction. Proc. Natl. Acad. Sci. USA **55**, 1628–1635 (1966)

Klein, G., Klein, E., Clifford, P.: Search for host defences in Burkitt lymphoma: membrane immunofluorescence tests on biopsies and tissue culture lines. Cancer Res. **27**, 2510–2520 (1967)

Klein, G., Pearson, G., Nadkarni, J. S., Nadkarni, J. J., Klein, E., Henle, G., Henle, W., Clifford, P.: Relation between Epstein-Barr viral and cell membrane immunofluorescence of Burkitt tumor cells. I. Dependence of cell membrane immunofluorescence on presence of EB virus. J. Exp. Med. **128**, 1011–1020 (1968 a)

Klein, G., Pearson, G., Henle, G., Henle, W., Diehl, V., Niederman, J. C.: Relation between Epstein-Barr viral and cell membrane immunofluorescence in Burkitt tumor cells. II. Comparison of cells and sera from patients with Burkitt's lymphoma and infectious mononucleosis. J. Exp. Med. **128**, 1021–1030 (1968 b)

Klein, G., Pearson, G., Henle, G., Henle, W., Goldstein, G., Clifford, P.: Relation between Epstein-Barr viral and cell membrane immunofluorescence in Burkitt tumor cells. III. Comparison of blocking of direct membrane immunofluorescence and anti-EBV reactivities of different sera. J. Exp. Med. **129**, 697–705 (1969)

Klucis, E., Jackson, L., Parsons, P. G.: Survey of human lymphoblastoid cell lines and primary cultures of normal and leukaemic leukocytes for oncornavirus production. Int. J. Cancer **18**, 413–420 (1976)

Kotler, M., Balabanova, H., Weinberg, E., Friedmann, A., Becker, Y.: Oncornavirus-like particles released from arginine-deprived human lymphoblastoid cell lines. Proc. Natl. Acad. Sci. USA **72**, 4592–4596 (1975)

Kufe, D., Hehlmann, R., Spiegelman, S.: RNA related to that of a murine leukemia virus in Burkitt's tumors and nasopharyngeal carcinomas. Proc. Natl. Acad. Sci. USA **70**, 5–9 (1973 a)

Kufe, D., Magrath, I. T., Ziegler, J. L., Spiegelman, S.: Burkitt's tumors contain particles encapsulating RNA-instructed DNA polymerase and high molecular weight virus-related RNA. Proc. Natl. Acad. Sci. USA **70**, 737–741 (1973 b)

Kufe, D. W., Peters, W. P., Spiegelman, S.: Unique nuclear DNA sequences in the involved tissues of Hodgkin's and Burkitt's lymphomas. Proc. Natl. Acad. Sci. USA **70**, 3810–3814 (1973 c)

Lawler, S. D., Reeves, B. R., Hamlin, I. M. E.: A comparison of cytogenetics and histopathology in the malignant lymphomata. Br. J. Cancer **31** [Suppl. II], 162–167 (1975)

Levy, J. A., Henle, G.: Indirect immunofluorescence tests with sera from African children and cultured Burkitt lymphoma cells. J. Bacteriol. **92**, 275–276 (1966)

Liang, W., Rowley, J. D.: 14q+ marker chromosome in multiple myeloma and plasma-cell leukaemia. Lancet **1978 I**, 96

Lieber, M. M., Benveniste, R. E., Livingston, D. M., Todaro, G. J.: Mammalian cells in culture frequently release type C viruses. Science **182**, 56–59 (1973)

Lindahl, T., Klein, G., Reedman, B. M., Johansson, B., Singh, S.: Relationship between Epstein-Barr virus (EBV) DNA and the EBV-determined nuclear antigen (EBNA) in Burkitt lymphoma biopsies and other lymphoproliferative malignancies. Int. J. Cancer **13**, 764–772 (1974)

Mann, R. B., Jaffe, E. S., Braylan, R. C., Nanba, K., Frank, M. M., Ziegler, J. L., Berard, C. W.: Non-endemic Burkitt's lymphoma. A B-cell tumor related to germinal centers. N. Engl. J. Med. **295**, 685–691 (1976)

Manolov, G., Manolova, Y.: Marker band in one chromosome 14 from Burkitt lymphomas. Nature **237**, 33–34 (1972)

Mark, J.: Histiocytic lymphomas with the marker chromosome 14q+. Hereditas **81**, 289–292 (1975)

McCaw, B. K., Hecht, F., Harnden, D. G., Teplitz, R. L.: Somatic rearrangement of chromosome 14 in human lymphocytes. Proc. Natl. Acad. Sci. USA **72**, 2071–2075 (1975)

Miller, G., Shope, T., Lisco, H., Stitt, D., Lipman, M.: Epstein-Barr virus: transformation, cytopathic changes, and viral antigens in squirrel monkey and marmoset leukocytes. Proc. Natl. Acad. Sci. USA **69**, 383–387 (1972)

Minowada, J., Oshimura, M., Tsubota, T., Higby, D. J., Sandberg, A. A.: Cytogenetic and immunoglobulin markers of human leukemia B-cell lines. Cancer Res. **37**, 3096–3099 (1977)

Morrow, R. H., Kisuule, A., Pike, M. C., Smith, P. G.: Burkitt's lymphoma in the Mengo district of Uganda: epidemiologic features and their relationship to malaria. J. Natl. Cancer Inst. **56**, 479–483 (1976)

Nadkarni, J. S., Nadkarni, J. J., Clifford, P., Manolov, G., Fenyö, E. M., Klein, E.: Characteristics of new cell lines derived from Burkitt lymphomas. Cancer **23**, 64–79 (1969)

Ngu, V. A.: Host defences to Burkitt tumour, Br. Med. J. **1967 I**, 345–347

Nonoyama, M., Huang, C. H., Pagano, J. S., Klein, G., Singh, S.: DNA of Epstein-Barr virus detected in tissue of Burkitt's lymphoma and nasopharyngeal carcinoma. Proc. Natl. Acad. Sci. USA **70**, 3265–3268 (1973)

Nonoyama, M., Pagano, J. S.: Homology between Epstein-Barr virus DNA and viral DNA from Burkitt's lymphoma and nasopharyngeal carcinoma determined by DNA-DNA reassociation kinetics. Nature **242**, 44–47 (1973)

O'Conor, G. T.: Persistent immunologic stimulation as a factor in oncogenesis with special reference to Burkitt's tumor. Am. J. Med. **48**, 279–285 (1970)

O'Conor, G. T., Davies, J. N. P.: Malignant tumors in African children. J. Pediatrics **56**, 526–535 (1960)

Oxford, J. M., Harnden, D. G., Parrington, J. M., Delhanty, J. D. A.: Specific chromosome aberrations in ataxia telangiectasia. J. Med. Genetics **12**, 251–262 (1975)

Pagano, J. S., Huang, C. H., Levine, P. H.: Absence of Epstein-Barr viral DNA in American Burkitt's lymphoma. N. Engl. J. Med. **289**, 1395–1399 (1973)

Panem, S., Prochownik, E. V., Reale, F. R., Kirsten, W. H.: Isolation of type C virions from a normal human fibroblast strain. Science **189**, 297–299 (1975)

Pattengale, P. K., Smith, R. W., Gerber, P.: Selective transformation of B lymphocytes by EB virus. Lancet **1973 II**, 93

Payne, L. N.: Marek's disease: a possible model for herpesvirus-induced neoplasms in man. In: Proceedings of the 3rd International Symposium of the Princess Takamatsu Cancer Research Fund: Analytic and experimental epidemiology of cancer. Nakahara, W., Hirayama, T., Nishioka, K., Sugano, H. (eds.), pp. 235–257. Tokyo: University of Tokyo Press 1973

Philip, P.: Marker chromosome 14q+ in multiple myeloma. Hereditas **80**, 155–156 (1975)

Pickthall, V. J.: Detailed cytogenetic study of a metastatic bronchial carcinoma. Br. J. Cancer **34**, 272–278 (1976)

Pike, M. C., Morrow, R. H., Kisuule, A., Mafigiri, J.: Burkitt's lymphoma and sickle cell trait. Br. J. Prev. Soc. Med. **24**, 39–41 (1970)

Pike, M. C., Williams, E. H., Wright, B.: Burkitt's tumor in the West Nile District of Uganda 1961–5. Br. Med. J. **1967 II**, 395–399

Prigogina, E. L., Fleischman, E. W.: Marker chromosome 14q+ in two non-Burkitt lymphomas. Humangenetik **30**, 109–112 (1975)

Rabson, A. S., O'Conor, G. T., Baron, S., Whang, J. J., Legallais, F. Y.: Morphologic, cytogenetic and virologic studies *in vitro* of a malignant lymphoma from an African child. Int. J. Cancer **1**, 89–106 (1966)

Reedman, B. M., Klein, G.: Cellular localization of an Epstein-Barr virus (EBV)-associated complement-fixing antigen in producer and nonproducer lymphoblastoid cell lines. Int. J. Cancer **11**, 499–520 (1973)

Reeves, B. R.: Cytogenetics of malignant lymphomas. Studies utilising a Giemsa-banding technique. Humangenetik **20**, 231–250 (1973)

Rickinson, A. B., Epstein, M. A., Crawford, D. H.: Absence of infectious Epstein-Barr virus in blood in acute infectious mononucleosis. Nature **258**, 236–238 (1975)

Rickinson, A. B., Finerty, S., Epstein, M. A.: Comparative studies on adult donor lymphocytes infected by EB virus *in vivo* or *in vitro:* origin of transformed cells arising in co-cultures with foetal lymphocytes. Int. J. Cancer **19**, 775–782 (1977a)

Rickinson, A. B., Finerty, S., Epstein, M. A.: Mechanism of the establishment of Epstein-Barr virus genome-containing lymphoid cell lines from infectious mononucleosis patients: studies with phosphonoacetate. Int. J. Cancer **20**, 861–868 (1977b)

Rickinson, A. B., Jarvis, J. E., Crawford, D. H., Epstein, M. A.: Observations on the type of infection by Epstein-Barr virus in peripheral lymphoid cells of patients with infectious mononucleosis. Int. J. Cancer **14**, 704–715 (1974)

Rocchi, G., de Felici, A., Ragona, G., Heinz, A.: Quantitative evaluation of Epstein-Barr-virus-infected mononuclear peripheral blood leukocytes in infectious mononucleosis. N. Engl. J. Med. **296**, 132–134 (1977)

Royal College of Physicians, London: 3rd Report: Smoking or health. p. 54. London: Pitman Medical 1977

Salaman, M. H., Wedderburn, N., Bruce-Chwatt, L. J.: The immunodepressive effect of a murine plasmodium and its interaction with murine oncogenic viruses. J. Gen. Microbiol. **59**, 383–391 (1969)

Shope, T., Dechairo, D., Miller, G.: Malignant lymphoma in cottontop marmosets after inoculation with Epstein-Barr virus. Proc. Natl. Acad. Sci. USA **70**, 2487–2491 (1973)

Steel, C. M., Philipson, J., Arthur, E., Gardiner, S. E., Newton, M. S., McIntosh, R. V.: Possibility of EB virus preferentially transforming a subpopulation of human B lymphocytes. Nature **270**, 729–731 (1977)

Stewart, S. E., Lovelace, E., Whang, J. J., Ngu, V. A.: Burkitt tumor: tissue culture, cytogenetic and virus studies. J. Natl. Cancer Inst. **34**, 319–327 (1965)

Svedmyr, E., Jondal, M.: Cytotoxic effector cells specific for B cell lines transformed by Epstein-Barr virus are present in patients with infectious mononucleosis. Proc. Natl. Acad. Sci. USA **72**, 1622–1626 (1975)

Ten Seldam, R. E. J., Cooke, R., Atkinson, L.: Childhood lymphoma in the territories of Papua and New Guinea. Cancer **19**, 437–446 (1966)

Thorley-Lawson, D., Strominger, J. L.: Transformation of human lymphocytes by Epstein-Barr virus is inhibited by phosphonoacetic acid. Nature **263**, 332–334 (1976)

Tooze, J.: The molecular biology of tumour viruses. Cold Spring Harbor Laboratory 1973

Vernon, M. L., McMahon, J. M., Hackett, J. J.: Brief communication: additional evidence of type-C particles in human placentas. J. Natl. Cancer Inst. **52**, 987–989 (1974)

Welch, J. P., Lee, C. L. Y.: Non-random occurrence of 7–14 translocations in human lymphocyte cultures. Nature **255**, 241–242 (1975)

Williams, A. O.: Haemoglobin genotypes, ABO blood groups, and Burkitt's tumour. J. Med. Genet. **3**, 177–179 (1966)

Williams, E. H., Day, N. E., Geser, A. G.: Seasonal variation in onset of Burkitt's lymphoma in the West Nile District of Uganda. Lancet **1974 II**, 19–22

Williams, E. H., Smith, P. G., Day, N. E., Geser, A., Ellice, J., Tukei, P.: Space-time clustering of Burkitt's lymphoma in the West Nile District of Uganda: 1961–1975. Br. J. Cancer **37**, 109–122 (1978)

Witkin, S. S., Ohno, T., Spiegelman, S.: Purification of RNA-instructed DNA polymerase from human leukemic spleens. Proc. Natl. Acad. Sci. USA **72**, 4133–4136 (1975)

Wright, D. H.: A lymphoma syndrome in tropical Africa. Note on histology, cytology and histochemistry. Int. Rev. Exp. Pathol. **2**, 97–102 (1963a)

Wright, D. H.: Cytology and histochemistry of the Burkitt lymphoma. Br. J. Cancer **17**, 50–55 (1963b)

Wurster-Hill, D. H., McIntyre, O. R., Cornwell, G. G., Maurer, L. H.: Marker chromosome 14 in multiple myeloma and plasma cell leukaemia. Lancet **1973 II**, 1031

Yamada, K., Yoshioka, M., Oami, H.: A 14q + marker and a late replicating chromosome #22 in a brain tumor: brief communication. J. Natl. Cancer Inst. **59**, 1193–1195 (1977)

Zech, L., Haglund, U., Nilsson, K., Klein, G.: Characteristic chromosomal abnormalities in biopsies and lymphoid cell lines from patients with Burkitt and non-Burkitt lymphomas. Int. J. Cancer **17**, 47–56 (1976)

Ziegler, J. L.: Treatment results of 54 American patients with Burkitt's lymphoma are similar to the African experience. N. Engl. J. Med. **297**, 75–80 (1977)

Ziegler, J. L., Andersson, M., Klein, G., Henle, W.: Detection of Epstein-Barr virus DNA in American Burkitt's lymphoma. Int. J. Cancer **17**, 701–706 (1976)

zur Hausen, H.: Oncogenic herpes viruses. Biochim. Biophys. Acta **417**, 25–53 (1975) zur Hausen, H., Schulte-Holthausen, H., Klein, G., Henle, W., Henle, G., Clifford, P., Santesson, L.: EBV DNA in biopsies of Burkitt tumours and anaplastic carcinomas of the nasopharynx. Nature **228**, 1056–1058 (1970)

zur Hausen, H., Schulte-Holthausen, H.: Detection of Epstein-Barr viral genomes in human tumour cells by nucleic acid hybridization. In: Oncogenesis and herpesviruses. Biggs, P. M., de-Thé, G., Payne, L. N. (eds.), pp. 321–325. Lyon: IARC 1972

15 The Relationship of the Virus to Nasopharyngeal Carcinoma

G. Klein[1]

Department of Tumor Biology, Karolinska Institutet, S-104 01 Stockholm 60 (Sweden)

---

[1] This article is largely based on a previous chapter, written by Maria Andersson-Anvret, Nils Forsby, and George Klein (in: Progr. Exp. Tumor Res., 21: 100–116. Ed. Karger, Basel, 1978).

A. INTRODUCTION

Nasopharyngeal carcinoma (NPC) shows great ethnic variations between different human populations (see Muir, 1971, 1972, 1975; Ho, 1972, 1975; Muir and Shanmugaratnam, 1967; Clifford, 1970; Shanmugaratnam, 1971). It has been suggested that both genetic and environmental factors contribute to its etiology. Its frequency is remarkably high in certain areas of southern China, the Kwang-tung Province in particular. First generation immigrants of southern Chinese origin maintain a high frequency of NPC (Barr, 1974; Ho, 1975). In Singapore, different Chinese dialect groups show frequencies that correspond to their points of origin in China (Shanmugaratnam and Muir, 1967). Later generations of Chinese Americans show a decline in NPC mortality, but it is not clear whether this is due to their changed environment or to the intermarriage of different Chinese ehtnic subgroups with differing incidences of NPC.

Caucasians have a low incidence of NPC. Offspring of mixed marriages between southern Chinese and non-Chinese groups show an intermediate frequency (Shanmugaratnam and Muir, 1967; Muir, 1971). This further stresses that genetic factors must play an important role. Since the disease is rare in northern China and in Japan, there is obviously no association between high risk and the mongoloid race as such. Several reports speak of familial aggregation of NPC (Nevo et al., 1971; Shanmugaratnam, 1971; Ho, 1972; Williams and de-Thé, 1974). Males have a higher frequency of NPC than females, irrespective of race and geography.

While in Burkitt's lymphoma (BL) there is a clear environmental cofactor acting with Epstein-Barr virus (EBV) (Chap. 14), the epidemiology of NPC speaks more strongly in favor of intrinsic, probably genetic, cofactors.

B. HISTOPATHOLOGY

The normal nasopharynx is coated with different types of epithelia. The surface and the crypts are lined by stratified squamous or ciliated columnar epithelium. In addition to these two types of surface epithelium, there is a third type, designated transitional or intermediate epithelium (Ali, 1967). The walls also contain connective, glandular, and much lymphoid tissue.

Different types of nasopharyngeal cancers originate from various components of the walls. Carcinomas that arise from the surface epithelium are by far the most common and the term NPC is generally reserved for them. Only undifferentiated or anaplastic NPC are associated with EBV, as discussed below (Sect. D).

A variety of histopathologic classifications has been proposed for NPC (Liang et al., 1962; Yeh, 1962; Lin et al., 1969; Perez et al., 1969; Shanmugaratnam, 1972; Svoboda, 1972; Micheau, 1975) and the nomenclature is therefore rather confusing. The differentiated squamous-cell carcinomas with "intercellular bridges" and keratinization do not offer any problems. Undifferentiated NPC without squamous differentiation, the most common tumor of the region, presents a more controversial classification problem, however. A wide variety of subtypes has been suggested. Moreover, different pathologists may use different histologic criteria for subtype classification even if they use the same nomenclature. It is therefore difficult to compare the publications of different authors. It is also doubtful whether the subclassification of undifferentiated carcinomas into different subtypes that may actually coexist within the same tumor has any biologic significance.

Two subtypes of undifferentiated NPC distinguished in the past were "lymphoepithelioma" (Regaud, 1921; Schmincke, 1921; Ewing, 1929; Capell, 1938) and "transitional cell carcinoma" (Quick and Cutler, 1927; Capell, 1938), the main difference lying in the extensive and intimate admixture of lymphocytes with the tumor cells in the former. The lymphocytes are not neoplastic, however (Tech, 1957; Yeh, 1962; Klein et al., 1974a), but consist mainly of T cells (thymus-dependent lymphocytes) (Jondal and Klein, 1975) that may be remnants of the abundant lymphoid tissue in the nasopharyngeal walls. Since they appear to inflict no damage on the tumor cells and have a small, inactive appearance, it is unlikely that they represent an immunologic reaction.

Even undifferentiated NPC often contain small foci with a tendency to squamous differentiation. Some tumors may show a spindle-cell, clear-cell, basaloid, or pleomorphic appearance (Yeh, 1962; Shanmugaratnam, 1972). Since NPC is a uniclonal tumor (Fialkow et al., 1972), different cell types that occur in the same tumor may merely reflect different modulations of the original tumor cell type.

Light microscope studies have led to the view that all NPCs should be regarded as squamous cell carcinomas (New and Kirch, 1928; Hauser and Brownell, 1938; Tech, 1957; Yeh, 1962; Shanmugaratnam and Muir, 1967) and this has been further supported by electron microscope studies (Svoboda et al., 1965, 1967; Lin et al., 1969; Gazzolo et al., 1972; Shanmugaratnam, 1972; Prasad, 1974) which showed the presence of desmosomes between adjacent tumor cells, and tonofibrils and keratin-like structures within the cytoplasm of tumor cells from different types of NPC. In addition to squamous cell-derived NPC, other histologic types of carcinoma may arise from columnar and transitional cell epithelia (Liang et al., 1962; Ho, 1972; Klein et al., 1974), possibly without preceding squamous metaplasia.

It appears most straightforward to classify NPCs as squamous cell carcinomas with various degrees of differentiation and with the EBV association essentially restricted to the undifferentiated group, as discussed below (Sect. D).

C. EBV-RELATED SEROLOGY IN NASOPHARYNGEAL CARCINOMA

The association between EBV and NPC was first suggested by the demonstration of precipitating antibodies to EBV-related antigens in the sera of American NPC patients (Old et al., 1966). Subsequent studies confirmed the association and extended it to the EBV antigens demonstrated by immunofluorescense (De Schryver et al., 1969; W. Henle et al., 1970; de-Thé, 1972; Klein, 1972; Chap. 3). W. Henle et al. (1970) have shown that Chinese, African, and Caucasian NPC sera had an approximately tenfold elevated titer against viral capsid antigen (VCA) on the average, only parallelled by BL sera. These titers were clearly much higher than the anti-VCA titers of patients with other tumors of the head and the neck region. Antibodies to membrane antigen (MA) were also significantly elevated in NPC sera, comparable to BL sera (De Schryver et al., 1969).

Antibodies to the early antigen (EA) complex are regularly present in NPC sera. Antibodies against the diffuse (D) component are more frequent, although low levels of antibody against the restricted (R) component are frequently detectable as well. This is in contrast to the BL sera, in which most anti-EA antibodies are directed against the R component. W. Henle et al. (1973) have shown that the anti-D antibody titers of NPC patients increase with the progression of the disease from stage I to IV, as discussed in Sect. F below.

NPC sera also showed elevated titers against the complement fixing (CF) soluble antigen (S) (Sohier and de-Thé, 1971, 1972). This contrasted with BL patients' sera where CF antibody titers were usually lower than in NPC and also fluctuated during the clinical course of the disease. In NPC they were usually high and stable, regardless of the stage of the disease.

Among the different EBV-associated antibody titers, VCA and EA were correlated with each other as were anti-EBV nuclear antigen (EBNA) and CF/S titers (de-Thé et al., 1975). Anti-VCA titers were relatively stable over a lifetime. In contrast, the presence of anti-EA antibodies was related to the course of the disease. Association between EBNA and CF/S is not surprising, since they represent the same antigen (Ohno et al., 1977).

Only anaplastic NPC were characterized by regularly elevated anti-EBV titers (De Schryver et al., 1969; Henle et al., 1970) in contrast to other nasopharyngeal tumors and head and neck carcinomas.

NPC patients were found to have increased IgA levels (Wara et al., 1975); Henle and Henle (1976) showed the appearance of a specific IgA anti-VCA antibody, which is more or less completely absent from both BL patients and patients with head and neck carcinomas other than BL or NPC. Following successful treatment of the tumor, IgA anti-VCA and anti-EA(D) antibodies regularly decline to nondetectable levels (Henle and Henle, 1976). IgA anti-VCA appears therefore to have a diagnostic and also a certain prognostic value for NPC.

D. EBV GENOMES IN NASOPHARYNGEAL CARCINOMA

Zur Hausen et al. first demonstrated the presence of EBV DNA in NPC biopsies by DNA-DNA hybridization (zur Hausen et al., 1970; Nonoyama et al., 1973). Up to then, EBV had only been found to infect B lymphocytes (bone marrow-derived lymphocytes) in vitro. All known in vitro established EBV-carrying lines have B lymphocyte characteristics. The only other EBV-carrying tumor, BL, is a uniclonal malignancy of the B lymphocyte. For these reasons, it was first thought that the EBV DNA positivity of NPC was due to the abundant, infiltrating lymphocytes. This notion turned out to be incorrect, however, when it was clearly shown that EBV DNA was located in the epithelial carcinoma cells. Wolf et al. (1973) first demonstrated the presence of EBV DNA in the carcinoma cells of NPC by in situ cRNA/DNA hybridization on frozen sections. In a later paper, Wolf et al. found (1975) an inverse relationship between the number of EBV genome equivalents and the approximate amount of infiltrating lymphocytes. This was also consistent with the association of the viral genome with the carcinoma cells. The finding (Jondal and Klein, 1975) that most infiltrating lymphocytes of the NPC biopsies are EBV-negative T cells also supported this notion.

Conclusive evidence for the localization of the EBV DNA in the epithelial cells was obtained when NPC cells were serially passaged in athymic (nude) mice (Klein et al., 1974 a). During such passage, the human lymphocytes are eliminated and the human stroma is replaced by mouse stroma. The amount of mouse cell admixture was estimated by an enzyme marker, glucose-6-phosphate dehydrogenase. After two passages in nude mice, EBV DNA-negative human carcinoma cells remained negative, while EBV DNA-positive undifferentiated carcinomas retained their virus DNA, as determined by nucleic acid hybridization. They were also shown to contain EBNA and to carry it in the large carcinoma cells. EBNA was also demonstrated directly in the carcinoma cells of human NPC biopsy samples (Huang et al., 1974).

EBV DNA has been found in undifferentiated NPC specimens from different parts of the world, including Tunisia, Singapore, Kenya, and Taiwan (Pagano et al., 1975). We have recently investigated eight Swedish biopsies from tumors in the nasopharynx. Among these only two were found to be undifferentiated NPCs. EBV DNA was detected in these two tumors by nucleic acid hybridization. The other six tumors, including differentiated squamous cell carcinomas and malignant lymphomas, did not contain EBV DNA (M. Andersson-Anvret, N. Forsby, and G. Klein to be published).

The DNA-DNA renaturation kinetics studies of Nonoyama and Pagano (1973) have shown that the EBV DNA sequences carried by BL and NPC tumors are very similar, with more than 90% homology (Kawai et al., 1973). However, there appeared to be small but significant differences in the EBV-DNA sequences present in Tunisian *vs* Singapore derived NPC biopsies. These differences were reflected in the final extent of renaturation and were estimated to involve ∼ 10% of the sequences (Pagano, 1974b). The DNA of the Singapore NPC specimens accelerated the reannealing of a radioactive EBV DNA probe, derived from the EBV of a virus-producer African BL line, only to ∼ 85%. In contrast, the EBV DNA derived from a Tunisian NPC showed more than 95% homology with the same EBV DNA probe. These results suggested up to 15% lack of homology in the nucleotide sequences between the Singapore specimens and the BL-derived probe (Pagano, 1974 a). Although both disease labels, such as NPC and BL, and geographic designations of origin are used when speaking of these results, these differences may merely represent more-or-less random variations between different viral isolates that have no meaningful disease-related or epidemiologic association.

The resident EBV DNA in NPC tumor cells occurs partly in the form of integrated DNA sequences and partly as free episomes (Kaschka-Dierich et al., 1976; Lindahl et al., 1976). The latter represent the majority of the viral DNA molecules and appear as covalently closed circles. There is thus no difference, in principle, between the way in which the viral genome associates with the DNA of a BL or an NPC cell.

Kaschka-Dierich et al. (1976) observed a small size difference between the covalently closed DNA circles from BL and NPC tumors in sedimentation velocity experiments and by measuring the contour length by electron microscopy. While interesting, these experiments are open to the same questions with regard to random strain variations *vs* possible disease-related differences as the DNA sequence studies discussed in the preceding paragraph.

While earlier studies strongly suggested a regular association between EBV DNA and the anaplastic form of NPC (Klein et al., 1974 a; zur Hausen et al., 1974; Pagano et al., 1975), they suffered from the lack of parallel histopathologic examination of the specimens used for nucleic acid hybridization. This may lead to both false negative and false positive results. False negative results may be due to wrong histologic diagnosis, absence of tumor cells from the specimen, and necrosis of the tumor cells. False positive results can be due to the misdiagnosis of the EBV-carrying BL or NPC at the histologic level.

In a recent study, we critically examined 76 African tumor biopsies by a simultaneous nucleic acid hybridization and histopathologic scrutiny on parallel samples taken from the same biopsy (Andersson-Anvret et al., 1977): 51 were undifferentiated NPC, 4 were NPC with some signs of squamous differentiation, 7 turned out to be nasopharyngeal tumors of other histologic types, and 14 were head-and-neck carcinomas located outside the nasopharynx. All 51 undifferentiated NPCs contained significant numbers of EBV-genome copies per cell. Two of the somewhat differentiated NPCs were also EBV DNA-positive, whereas 2 were negative. Of the 7 other nasopharyngeal tumors, 1 was EBV DNA positive. Histologic examination, however, showed that this was a typical BL. The other 6 tumors were all EBV DNA-negative lymphoproliferative malignancies. All 14 head-and-neck carcinomas located outside the nasopharynx were EBV DNA negative. The sera of undifferentiated NPC patients had elevated antibody titers against the EBV-determined antigens, the EA (D) component in particular.

These results clearly confirmed that there is a unique and regular association of EBV with undifferentiated NPC. The association appears to be even more strictly regular than the relationship between EBV and African BL. So far there is no report of any histologically proven undifferentiated NPC that is shown to contain viable tumor tissue and to lack the EBV genome. This contrasts with the 3% EBV-negative African BL that have been described.

E. BIOLOGIC ACTIVITY OF NASOPHARYNGEAL CARCINOMA – ASSOCIATED EBV

NPC cells in vivo are virus nonproducers (i. e., EA- and VCA-negative). Considerable difficulties were encountered in trying to culture NPC-derived epithelial cells. For these reasons. the biologic activity of NPC-associated EBV could not be tested until recently. Previously lymphoblastoid cell lines (LCL) were derived from NPC and were shown to release transforming EBV (de-Thé et al., 1970). However, these experiments gave no assurance that the LCL-associated virus was representative for the virus associated with the epithelial tumor cells. It was therefore of considerable interest when Trumper et al. (1977) showed that two out of six NPC passaged through nude mice produced EBV which was competent to transform cord blood cells. Since nude mouse passage purifies the tumor from contaminating, non-neoplastic human stroma, including lymphocytes, this virus must have originated from the epithelial cells themselves. This opens the possibility of studying the epithelial cell-associated virus in more detail, perhaps after introduction into a marmoset lymphocyte that can be expected not only to proliferate but also to produce the virus.

Like the EBV associated with infectious mononucleosis (IM) and BL, the NPC-associated virus has thus also been identified as a transforming virus, further strengthening the impression that transformation (immortalization) is the natural property of different wild-type EBV substrains (Chap. 1).

F. DISEASE-RELATED SEROLOGIC STUDIES

EBV-related antibody patterns were found to change in the course of the disease and during therapy (Henle et al., 1973, 1977). It was found that the geometric mean titer (GMT) of VCA-specific IgG antibodies increases stepwise from stage I (slightly above that of healthy controls) to an ultimately eight or ten times higher level as compared to patients in stage I or healthy controls, respectively (Henle et al., 1973; de-Thé et al., 1975; Henle and Henle, 1976). The same was found for the GMT of anti-EBNA (de-Thé et al., 1975).

Since the anti-EBV antibody titers increased with the tumor burden, Henle et al. postulated that both should decline again after reduction or elimination of the tumor by effective therapy. A comparison of patients before initiation of therapy and treated patients who had survived 5 or more years, has shown that the GMT of VCA-specific IgG antibodies was substantially lower in the long-term survivors than in the untreated patients (Henle et al., 1973). Moreover, the incidence and GMT of IgG antibodies to EA(D) were distinctly reduced in the long-term survivors as compared to the untreated patients (Henle et al., 1973). Decreases in VCA-specific IgG and anti-EBNA titers have been noted among patients who were followed for a 2-year period after therapy (de-Thé et al., 1973).

In a subsequent study (Henle et al., 1977) more than 100 patients were examined periodically for their EBV-antibody spectra before therapy and until death, during a 4–5 year period. The sera were titrated for IgG, IgA, and IgM antibodies to VCA, for IgG and IgA antibodies to EA(D) and EA(R), and for antibodies to EBNA. In patients before treatment the incidences and titers of most of the antibodies increased with the stage of the disease, i. e., essentially with the total tumor burden. Such increases were observed in individual patients with an ultimately fatal disease at times well in advance of the recognition of relapses or metastases. Increases were not noted or were only minor and delayed in some fatal cases if the tumor extended to the cranial cavity in the absence of significant involvement of cervical lymph nodes. In contrast, patients who responded well to therapy and remained clinically free of disease during the 4–5 year observation period after – at the most – early minor relapses, showed gradual, steady declines in the titers of all antibodies except anti-EBNA. Thus, VCA-specific IgA and EA (D)-specific IgA and IgG became in time undetectable in many of the patients. In several long-term survivors the declines were arrested at given levels or a reversal to increasing titer was noted which was followed in time by detection of a recurrent tumor or metastases in some cases, but not in others. These findings showed that the serologic monitoring of NPC patients may be useful as a signal for recurrent tumor activity. The studies so far mentioned focused on anti-EA and anti-VCA antibodies. Since both EA and VCA are associated with the viral cycle and are not expressed on growing cells, these antibodies can obviously play no role in protection against residual tumor cells. A recent study of Pearson, Johansson, and Klein (1978) dealt with another type of antibody.

Antibody-dependent cellular cytotoxicity (ADCC) tests were performed with African NPC patient sera against EBV-superinfected, MA-positive Raji target cells. The serum donors were divided into two groups: (1) those individuals who died within 2 years following diagnosis of NPC; and (2) individuals who responded well to therapy and survived longer than 2 years following diagnosis. The ADCC GMT for the survivor group was significantly higher than the GMT for nonsurvivors (5410 vs 615).

Interestingly a number of discordant sera were found in the nonsurvivor group with very low ADCC titers (< 240) at diagnosis in the presence of high VCA titers. When ADCC titers were compared with anti-EA or IgA antibody titers to VCA, a statistically significant inverse correlation was noted.

These findings were interpreted to indicate that ADCC titers might be of prognostic value in patients with NPC. In contrast to the anti-EA and IgA anti-VCA titers discussed above, high ADCC titers appear to be indicators of a good prognosis, while low titers point to a poor prognosis. It is conceivable that antibody to MA may play an active role in immunity against this virus-associated tumor. For this to be proven, however, it will be necessary to demonstrate the presence of MA on carcinoma cells.

G. CONCLUDING REMARKS

EBV DNA is found in the undifferentiated form of NPC, but not in more differentiated types. In addition to the biologic difference in transforming *vs* nontransforming activity between different EBV strains (Klein et al., 1974b; Miller et al., 1975), the genetic constitution of the host may be responsible for the different virus-target cell interactions. A strong hereditary influence is probably involved in NPC (Ho, 1972). A possible association of NPC with the HL-A system has been reported among the Chinese in Singapore (Simons et al., 1975). Thus, an increase in the frequency of HL-A2 and a deficit of detectable antigens in the second locus appeared to be associated with a high risk of NPC. The study in Singapore was an attempt to identify specific genetic factors which could explain the high incidence of the disease in the Chinese population. An association with the HL-A system could not be discovered among Tunisians with NPC (Betuel et al., 1975).

The association of EBV with the carcinoma cells in NPC raises the question of the mode of infection. Do epithelial cells have EBV receptors or are they infected by transfer of viral information from lymphoid cells? Is there a virus variant with specific affinity and potential oncogenicity for the nasopharyngeal epithelium? As proposed by zur Hausen (1975), it may be speculated that the transformation of the epithelial cells takes place within the vicinity of permissive (EBV-synthesizing) cells. The shedding of EBV in the saliva of patients with acute IM points to the existence of virus-producing cells within the pharynx (Chang and Golden, 1971; Gerber et al., 1972; Miller et al., 1973).

The distinction between a secondary (passenger) and a causative virus-tumor cell association is a notoriously difficult task, even in experimental cancer research. As developed elsewhere in more detail (Klein 1971), consistency and regularity of association, irrespective of geography, are the few criteria that can be used. "Association" means the regular presence of the viral genome and certain viral products (not necessarily the productive viral cycle itself) in *all* tumor cells.

These expectations are fullfilled, to a surprising degree, as regards the association between EBV and NPC. The viral genome has been found, virtually without exception, in all undifferentiated NPCs, irrespective of geography. The few apparent exceptions in the literature were not subjected to critical, parallel histologic study and it cannot be excluded that the histologic diagnoses were wrong or the tumor pieces were devoid of viable tumor tissue. It is particularly remarkable that the association of EBV with NPC is not dependent on the frequency of the disease – tumors of the high-incidence Chinese ethnic groups, the moderate-incidence North African cases, and the sporadic Western cases, all show the same association as long as they belong to the proper histologic type. On the other hand, differentiated squamous cell carcinomas of the nasopharyngeal region and other tumors localized in the nasopharynx (including malignant lymphomas) lack the viral genome. None of these observations can be reconciled with a simple passenger hypothesis.

Another series of observations that has great bearing on the interpretation of the relationship of EBV to NPC concerns the localization of the viral genome in the tumor. EBV-carrying LCL have been readily established from NPC biopsies (de-Thé et al., 1970). For this reason, the B lymphocyte was seen as the only conceivable host for the virus. It was therefore natural to believe that the presence of the EBV genomes in NPC was merely a reflection of lymphocytic infiltration. The first doubt came (Wolf et al., 1973) when an inverse relationship was found between the average number of EBV genomes per cell and the degree of lymphocytic infiltration. In situ cytohybridization (Wolf et al., 1975) and nude mouse passage (Klein et al., 1974a) later conclusively proved that the viral genome and EBNA are associated with the carcinoma cells themselves.

The significance of these puzzling observations is not yet fully resolved. On the one hand, they are fully compatible with the possibility that EBV plays some etiologic role in NPC. In the experimental field, virus-induced transformation is regularly followed by the maintenance of the viral genome in the neoplastic cells and "hit-and-run" mechanisms have not been conclusively demonstrated in any system.

On the other hand, the association between EBV and epithelial cells is quite obscure. No informative in vitro studies have been carried out, probably due to the difficulties involved in the cultivation of the normal epithelial cells in vitro. It is often suspected that the normal epithelial cell may support the replication of EBV, but this is based on indirect hints rather than on experimental evidence. In the one EBV-carrying epithelial cell now known, the NPC cell, the association is strictly nonproductive, although it can be activated in short-term in vitro cultures. This does not necessarily exclude that normal epithelial cells may also be productive in vivo. It may be recalled that two other oncogenic DNA viruses, Shope papilloma virus and Marek's disease virus, are carried latently in the multiplying, basal epithelium and virus production starts in the differentiated, keratinized epithelium, i.e., cells beginning to die. If this should be the case for EBV, virus replication would have been missed in epithelial cells in the studies conducted so far.

If EBV does play an etiologic role in NPC, the same dilemma arises as in BL: How can one reconcile the ubiquitous presence of the virus with the relative rarity of the tumor? Hypothetical explanations include the possible existence of specific, oncogenic virus variants, and/or the interplay of the virus with environmental or genetic cofactors. Unlike BL, where the evidence of time-space clustering points toward environmental cofactors, the ethnic features of NPC stress the importance of host genetics.

REFERENCES

Andersson-Anvret, M., Forsby, N., Klein, G.: Nasopharyngeal carcinoma. Prog. Exp. Tumor Res. **21,** 100–116 (1978)

Andersson-Anvret, M., Forsby, N., Klein, G., Henle, W.: Relationship between the Epstein-Barr virus and undifferentiated nasopharyngeal carcinoma: Correlated nucleic acid hybridization and histopathological examination. Int. J. Cancer **20,** 486–494 (1977)

Ali, M. Y.: Distribution and character of the squamous epithelium in the human nasopharynx. In: Cancer of the nasopharynx. Muir, C. S., Shanmugaratnam, K. (eds.). pp. 138–146 Copenhagen: Munksgaad 1967

Betuel, H., Camoun, M., Colombin, J., Day, N. E., Ellouz, R., de-Thé, G.: The relationship between nasopharyngeal carcinoma and HL-A system among Tunisians. Int. J. Cancer **16,** 249–254 (1975)

Buell, P.: The effect of migration on the risk of nasopharyngeal cancer among Chinese. Cancer Res. **34,** 1189–1191 (1974)

Capell, D. F.: Pathology of nasopharyngeal tumours. J. Laryngol. Otol. **53,** 558–580 (1938)

Chang, R. S., Golden, H. D.: Transformation of human leukocytes by throat washing from infectious mononucleosis patients. Nature **234,** 359–360 (1971)

Clifford, P.: On the epidemiology of nasopharyngeal carcinoma. Int. J. Cancer **5,** 287–309 (1970)

De Schryver, A., Friberg, S. Jr., Klein, G., Henle, G., Henle W., de-Thé, G., Clifford, P., Ho, H. C.: Epstein-Barr virus-associated antibody patterns in carcinoma of the post-nasal space. Clin. Exp. Immunol. **5,** 443–459 (1969)

de-Thé, G.: The etiology of nasopharyngeal carcinoma. Pathobiol. Annu. **2,** 235–254 (1972)

de-Thé, G., Ho, H. C., Ablashi, D. V., Day, N. E., Macario, A. J. L., Martin-Berthelon, M. C., Sohier, R.: Nasopharyngeal carcinoma. IX. Antibodies to EBNA and correlation with response to other EBV antigens in Chinese patients. Int. J. Cancer **16,** 713–721 (1975)

de-Thé, G., Ho, H. C., Kwan, H. C., Desgranges, C., Favre, M. C.: Nasopharyngeal carcinoma (NPC). I. Types of cultures derived from tumor biopsies and non-tumorous tissues of Chinese patients with special reference to lymphoblastoid transformation. Int. J. Cancer **6,** 189–206 (1970)

de-Thé, G., Schier, R., Ho, J. H., Freund, R.: Nasopharyngeal carcinoma. IV. Evolution of complement-fixing antibodies during the course of the disease. Int. J. Cancer **12,** 368–377 (1973)

Ewing, J.: Lymphoepithelioma. Am. J. Pathol. **5,** 99–107 (1929)

Fialkow, P. J., Martin, G. M., Klein, G., Clifford, P., Singh, S.: Evidence for a clonal origin of head and neck tumors. Int. J. Cancer **9,** 133–142 (1972)

Gazzolo, L., de-Thé, G., Vuillaume, M., Ho, H. C.: Nasopharyngeal carcinoma. II. Ultrastructure of normal mucosa, tumor biopsies, and subsequent epithelial growth in vitro. J. Natl. Cancer Inst. **48,** 73–86 (1972)

Gerber, P., Nonoyama, M., Lucas, S., Perlin, E., Goldstein, L. J.: Oral excretion of Epstein-Barr virus by healthy subjects and patients with infectious mononucleosis. Lancet **1972 II,** 988–989

Hauser, I. J., Brownell, D. H.: Malignant neoplasm of the nasopharynx. J. Am. Med. Assoc. **111,** 2467–2473 (1938)

Henle, G., Henle, W.: Epstein-Barr virus-specific IgA serum antibodies as an outstanding feature of nasopharyngeal carcinoma. Int. J. Cancer **17,** 1–7 (1976)

Henle, W., Henle, G., Ho, H. C., Burtin, P., Cachin, Y., Clifford, P., De Schryver, A., de-Thé, G., Diehl, V., Klein, G.: Antibodies to Epstein-Barr virus in nasopharyngeal carcinoma, other head and neck neoplasms and control groups. J. Natl. Cancer Inst. **44,** 225–231 (1970)

Henle, W., Ho., J. H. C., Henle, G., Chau, J. C. W., Kwan, H. C.: Nasopharyngeal carcinoma: Significance of changes in Epstein-Barr virus related antibody patterns following therapy. Int. J. Cancer **20,** 663–672 (1977)

Henle, W., Ho, H. C., Henle, G., Kwan, H. C.: Antibodies to Epstein-Barr virus-related antigens in nasopharyngeal carcinoma. Comparison of active cases with long term survivors. J. Natl. Cancer Inst. **51,** 361–369 (1973)

Ho, J. H. C.: Nasopharyngeal carcinoma (NPC). Adv. Cancer Res. **15,** 57–92 (1972)

Ho, H. C.: Epidemiology of nasopharyngeal carcinoma. J. R. Coll. Surg. Edinb. **20,** 223–235 (1975)

Huang, D. P., Ho, J. H. C., Henle, G.: Demonstration of Epstein-Barr virus-associated nuclear antigen in nasopharyngeal carcinoma cells from fresh biopsies. Int. J. Cancer **14,** 580–588 (1974)

Jondal, M., Klein, G.: Classification of lymphocytes in nasopharyngeal carcinoma (NPC) biopsies. Biomedicine **23,** 163–165 (1975)

Kaschka-Dierich, C., Adams, A., Lindahl, T., Bornkamm, G. W., Bjursell, G., Klein, G.: Intracellular forms of Epstein-Barr virus DNA in human tumour cells in vivo. Nature **260,** 302–306 (1976)

Kawai, Y., Nonoyama, M., Pagano, J. S.: Reassociation kinetics for Epstein-Barr virus DNA: Nonhomology to mammalian DNA and homology of viral DNA in various diseases. J. Virol. **12**, 1066–1012 (1973)

Klein, G.: Immunological studies on a human tumor. Dilemmas of the experimentalist. Isr. J. Med. Sci. **7**, 111–131 (1971)

Klein, G.: Herpesviruses and oncogenesis. Proc. Natl. Acad. Sci. USA **69**, 1056–1064 (1972)

Klein, G., Giovanella, B. C., Lindahl, T., Fialkow, P. J., Singh, S., Stehlin, J.: Direct evidence for the presence of Epstein-Barr virus DNA and nuclear antigen in malignant epithelial cells from patients with anaplastic carcinoma of the nasopharynx. Proc. Natl. Acad. Sci. USA **71**, 4737–4741 (1974a)

Klein, G., Sugden, B., Leibold, W., Menezes, J.: Infection of EBV-genome negative and positive human lymphoblastoid lines with biologically different preparations of EBV. Intervirology **3**, 232–244 (1974b)

Liang, P. C., Ch'en, C. C., Chu, C. C., Hu, Y. F., Chu, K. M., Tsung, Y. S.: The histopathologic classification, biologic characteristics and histogenesis of nasopharyngeal carcinoma. Clin. Med. J. **81**, 629–658 (1962)

Lin, H. S., Lin, C. S., Yeh, S., Tu, S. M.: Fine structure of nasopharyngeal carcinoma with special reference to the anaplastic type. Cancer **23**; 390–405 (1969)

Lindahl, T., Adams, A., Bjursell, G., Bornkamm, G. W., Kaschka-Dierich, C., Jehn, U.: Covalently closed circular duplex DNA of Epstein-Barr virus in a human lymphoid cell line. J. Mol. Biol. **102**, 511–530 (1976)

Micheau, C.: Anatomie pathologique et essai de classification des epitheliomas du naso-pharynx. Bull. Cancer **62**, 277–286 (1975)

Miller, G., Niederman, J. C., Andrews, L.: Prolonged oropharyngeal excretion of Epstein-Barr virus after infectious mononucleosis. N. Engl. J. Med. **288**, 229–232 (1973)

Miller, G., Robinson, J., Heston, L., Lipman, M.: Differences between laboratory strains of Epstein-Barr virus based on immortalization, abortive infection and interference. In: Oncogenesis and herpesviruses II. de-Thé, G., Epstein, M. A.,zur Hausen, H. (eds.),Part 1, pp. 395–408, Lyon: IARC 1975

Muir, C. S.: Nasopharyngeal carcinoma in non-Chinese populations with special reference to South-East Asia and Africa. Int. J. Cancer **8**, 351–363 (1971)

Muir, C. S.: Epidemiology and etiology. J. Am. Med. Assoc. **220**, 393 (1972)

Muir, C. S.: L'épidemiologie du cancer du cavum. Bull. Cancer **62**, 261–264 (1975)

Muir, C. S., Shanmugaratnam, K. (eds.): Cancer of the nasopharynx. Copenhagen: Munksgaard 1967

Nevo, S., Meyer, W., Altman, M.: Carcinoma of nasopharynx in twins. Cancer **28**, 807–809 (1971)

New, G. B., Kirch, W.: Tumors of nose and throat: A review of literature. Arch. Otolaryngol. **8**, 600–607 (1928)

Nonoyama, M., Huang, C. H., Pagano, J. S., Klein, G., Singh, S.: DNA of Epstein-Barr virus detected in tissue of Burkitt's lymphoma and nasopharyngeal carcinoma. Proc. Natl., Acad. Sci. USA **70**, 3265–3268 (1973)

Nonoyama, M., Pagano, J. S.: Homology between Epstein-Barr virus DNA and viral DNA from Burkitt's lymphoma and nasopharyngeal carcinoma determined by DNA-DNA reassociation kinetics. Nature **242**, 44–47 (1973)

Ohno, S., Luka, J., Lindahl, T., Klein, G.: Identification of a purified complement-fixing antigen as Epstein-Barr-virus determined nuclear antigen (EBNA) by its binding to metaphase chromosomes. Proc. Natl. Acad. Sci. USA **74**, 1605–1609 (1977)

Old, L. J., Boyse, E. A., Oettgen, H. F., de Harven, E., Geering, G., Williamson, B., Clifford, P.: Precipitating antibody in human serum to an antigen present in cultured Burkitt's lymphoma cells. Proc. Natl. Acad. Sci. USA **56**, 1699–1704 (1966)

Pagano, J. S.: The Epstein-Barr virus and malignancy: Molecular evidence. Cold Spring Harbor Symp. Quant. Biol. **39**, 797–805 (1974a)

Pagano, J. S.: The Epstein-Barr viral genome and its interactions with human lymphoblastoid cells and chromosomes. In: Viruses, evolution and cancer. Kurstak, E., Maramorosch (eds.), pp. 79–116. New York: Academic Press 1974b

Pagano, J. S., Huang, C. H., Klein, G., de-Thé, G., Shanmugaratnam, K., Yang, C. S.: Homology of Epstein-Barr virus DNA in nasopharyngeal carcinomas from Kenya, Taiwan, Singapore and Tunisia. In: Oncogenesis and herpesviruses II. de-Thé, G., Epstein, M. A. zur Hausen, H. (eds.), Part 2, pp. 179–190. Lyon: IARC 1975

Pearson, G. R., Johansson, B., Klein, G.: Antibody-dependent cellular cytotoxicity against Epstein-Barr virus-associated antigens in African patients with nasopharyngeal carcinoma. Int. f. Cancer **22**, 120–125 (1978)

Perez, C. A., Ackerman, L. V., Mill, W. B., Ogura, J. H., Powers, W. E.: Cancer of the nasopharynx: Factors influencing prognosis. Cancer **24**, 1–17 (1969)

Prasad, U.: Cells of origin of nasopharyngeal carcinoma; an electron microscopic study. J. Laryngol. Otol. **88**, 1087–1094 (1974)

Quick, D., Cutler, M.: Transitional cell epidermoid carcinoma; radiosensitive type of intra-oral tumor. Surg. Gynecol. Obstet **45**, 320–331 (1927)

Regaud, C.: Discussion of: Lymphoépithéliome de l'hypopharynx traité par la roentgentherapie. Reverchon, L. Coutard, H.: Bull. Soc. Franc. Otorhinolaryngol. **34**, 209–214 (1921)

Schmincke, A.: Über lymphoepitheliale Geschwülste. Beitr. Pathol. **68**, 161–170 (1921)

Shanmugaratnam, K.: Studies on the etiology of nasopharyngeal carcinoma. Int. Rev. Exp. Pathol. **10**, 361–413 (1971)

Shanmugaratnam, K.: The pathology of nasopharyngeal carcinoma. A review. In: Oncogenesis and herpesviruses II. Biggs. P. M., de-Thé, G., Payne, L. N. (eds.), pp. 239–248. Lyon: IARC 1972

Shanmugaratnam, K., Muir, C. S.: The incidence of nasopharyngeal cancer in Singapore. In: Cancer of the nasopharynx Muir, C. S., Shanmugaratnam, K. (eds.), pp. 47–53 Copenhagen: Munksgaard 1967

Shanmugaratnam, K., Muir, C. S.: Nasopharyngeal carcinoma: origin and structure In: Cancer of the nasopharynx. Muir, C. S., Shanmugaratnam, K. (eds.), pp. 153–162 Copenhagen: Munksgaard 1967

Simons, M. J., Wee, G. B., Chan, S. H., Shanmugaratnam, K., Day, N.E., de-Thé, G. B.: Probable identification of an HL-A second-locus antigen associated with a high risk of a nasopharyngeal carcinoma. Lancet **1975 I**, 142–143

Sohier, R., de-Thé, G.: Fixation du complément avec un antigene soluble: Différences d'activité importantes entre les serums de lymphome de Burkitt, de cancer du rhinopharynx et de mononucleose infectieuse. C. R. Acad. Sci. (D) Paris **273**, 121–124 (1971)

Sohier, R., de-Thé, G.: Evolution of complement-fixing antibody titres with the development of Burkitt's lymphoma. Int. J. Cancer **9**, 524–528 (1972)

Svoboda, D. J.: Pathologic classification and fine structure. J. Am. Med. Assoc. **220**, 394–396 (1972)

Svoboda, D. J., Kirchner, F. R., Shanmugaratnam, K.: Ultrastructure of nasopharyngeal carcinomas in American and Chinese patients: an application of electron microscopy to geographic pathology. Exp. Mol. Pathol. **4**, 184–204 (1965)

Svoboda, D. J., Kirchner, F.R., Shanmugaratnam, K.: The fine structure of nasopharyngeal carcinomas. In: Cancer of the nasopharynx. Muir, C. S., Shanmugaratnam, K. (eds.), pp. 163–171 Copenhagen: Munksgaard 1967

Teoh, T. B.: Epidermoid carcinoma of the nasopharynx among Chinese: a study of 31 necropsies. J. Pathol. Bacteriol. **78**, 451–465 (1957)

Trumper, P. A., Epstein, M. A., Giovanella, B. C., Finerty, S.: Isolation of infectious EB virus from the epithelial tumour cells of nasopharyngeal carcinoma. Int. J. Cancer **20**, 655–662 (1977)

Wara, W. M., Wara, D. W., Philips, T. L., Ammann, A. J.: Elevated IgA in carcinoma of the nasopharynx. Cancer **35**, 1313–1315 (1975)

Williams, E. H., de-Thé, G.: Familial aggregation in nasopharyngeal carcinoma. Lancet **1974 II**, 295–296

Wolf, H., zur Hausen, H., Becker, V.: EB-viral genomes in epithelial nasopharyngeal carcinoma cells. Nature New Biol. **244**, 245–247 (1973)

Wolf, H., zur Hausen, H., Klein, G., Becker, V., Henle, G., Henle, W.: Attempts to detect virus-specific DNA sequences in human tumours. III. Epstein-Barr viral DNA in non-lymphoid nasopharyngeal carcinoma cells. Med. Microbiol. Immunol. **161**, 15–21 (1975)

Yeh, S.: A histological classification of carcinomas of the nasopharynx with a critical review as to the existence of lymphoepitheliomas. Cancer **15**, 895–920 (1962)

zur Hausen, H.: Oncogenic herpesviruses. Biochim. Biophys. Acta **417**, 25–53 (1975)

zur Hausen, H., Schulte-Holthausen, H., Klein, G., Henle, W., Henle, G., Clifford, P., Santesson, L.: EBV DNA in biopsies of Burkitt tumours and anaplastic carcinomas of the nasopharynx. Nature **228**, 1056–1058 (1970)

zur Hausen, H., Schulte-Holthausen, H., Wolf, H., Dörries, K., Egger, H.: Attempts to detect virus-specific DNA in human tumors. II. Nucleic acid hybridizations with complementary RNA of human herpes group viruses. Int. J. Cancer **13**, 657–664 (1974)

16 Experimental Carcinogenicity by the Virus In Vivo

G. Miller[1]

Department of Pediatrics, School of Medicine, Yale University, 333 Cedar Street, New Haven, CT 06510 (USA)

[1] The experiments described in this chapter which were carried out in the author's laboratory could not have been possible without the collaboration of T. C. Shope, J. Robinson, E. Henderson, and W. A. Andiman. Levin Waters provided patient and conservative guidance in interpretation of the pathology. W. Webb and D. Coope were expert in care of marmosets and handling their tissues and cells. Work on experimental tumorigenicity by EBV was supported by grants VC-107 from the American Cancer Society and grants CA-12055 and CA-16038 from the National Cancer Institute. G. M. is an investigator of the Howard Hughes Medical Institute.

A. INTRODUCTION

Epstein-Barr virus (EBV) induces lymphoid neoplasms in marmosets and owl monkeys (Shope et al., 1973; Epstein et al., 1973 a, b, 1975). The tumors caused experimentally resemble Burkitt's lymphomas (BL) in several ways: they arise in the germinal centers of lymphoid follicles, they contain many EBV DNA copies per cell, and they express the EBV nuclear antigen (EBNA). Not all individuals of susceptible species infected in the laboratory manifest malignant disease. Some seem to contract a benign lymphoproliferative syndrome while others remain healthy. Thus a spectrum of responses, such as is seen in human EBV infections, also occurs after infection of new-world primates in the laboratory.

For 20 years before the discovery of EBV efforts to transmit the etiologic agent of infectious mononucleosis (IM) to primates had failed (Frank et al., 1976). Several reasons for failure are now apparent. Some trials were carried out with specimens, such as acute phase sera, in which the virus was not likely to be present. Most experimentors used *Macaca mulatta* as the laboratory host. This choice seemed logical since the rhesus monkey is susceptible to a variety of human viruses such as those which cause poliomyelitis, mumps, and measles. However, most old-world monkeys and great apes have antibodies to EBV due to infection with related agents (Chap. 17). Even juvenile rhesus monkeys, which are EBV-seronegative, do not seem susceptible to the virus. Without the aid of serologic tests to monitor experimental infection there was no way to identify a successful but clinically inapparent transmission.

Even after the discovery of EBV initial efforts to transfer the infection to primates were also unsuccessful. Failure in retrospect can be partly attributed to reliance on African and Indian primates and to the use of certain new-world species which are not susceptible. In many early trials of experimental infection the P_3HR-1 virus strain was used. Most stocks of this strain had lost their ability to transform cells and were unable to initiate infection.

A series of findings in different laboratories made it possible to show eventually that EBV can cause tumors in primates. The method for distinguishing virus-producer from nonproducer cell lines by examining them with immunofluorescence for virus capsid antigen (VCA) was seminal, as was the delineation of the two major biologic activities of transformation and superinfection (Henle and Henle, 1966; Henle et al., 1967, 1970; Miller et al., 1974; Menezes et al., 1975). Conversion in vitro of marmoset lymphocytes into cell lines provided a regular source of high titered EBV capable of transforming in vitro (Miller et al., 1972; Miller and Lipman, 1973) (Chaps. 1 and 10). The methods developed to recognize EBV genomes in human tumors, nucleic acid hybridization for detection of the DNA and anti-complement immunofluorescence for demonstration of EBNA, were also crucial in showing the presence of the genome in the experimentally induced tumors (zur Hausen et al., 1970; Nonoyama et al., 1973; Reedman and Klein, 1973; Klein, 1975).

Perhaps most important in the history of the development of a laboratory model for EBV was the fortuitous selection of certain species of new-world primates as hosts. The impetus for this choice was the finding by Meléndez that cotton-top marmosets and owl monkeys were highly susceptible to tumor induction by herpesvirus saimiri (HVS) (Meléndez et al., 1969). As a group, new-world monkeys lack antibodies to EBV (Frank et al., 1976). Apparently they do not naturally carry a virus that is antigenically similar to human EBV nor are they easily infected in captivity by casual contact with man. Yet lymphoid cells from a number of species of new-world primates can be established as cell lines following exposure in culture to human EBV (Miller et al., 1972; Falk et al., 1974).

New-world monkey species differ in their sensitivity to infection, in their clinical and pathologic responses, and in various properties of cells that have been transformed. More understanding of the mechanisms of this variation in host response among different primate species might provide clues to the reasons for the highly variable outcome of EBV infections of man.

B. VIRUS FACTORS IN TUMORIGENESIS

I. SOURCE OF VIRUS (STRAIN)

One still unresolved hypothesis is that the diversity of EBV-associated disease in man results in part from heterogeneity of the virus. Such virus variation might arise by genetic interaction among strains of human EBV, by genetic interaction between EBV of man and related viruses of nonhuman primates, or by the acquisition of certain cellular genes or the genes of endogenous viruses by EBV. New-world primates may ultimately be the testing ground to determine whether some virus variants are oncogenic and others are not. In vitro transformation will not be a way to distinguish oncogenic from nononcogenic strains, because tumor formation and immortalization in culture are different phenomena. There are but a few high-titered EBV strains available for comparison of their tumorigenic capacities. The results at hand indicate that at least three EBV strains can induce malignant lymphoma (Shope et al., 1973; Epstein et al., 1973a; Werner et al., 1975). Two of the three, B95-8 and Kaplan, were originally obtained from patients with IM. The third, EB3, was derived from a child with BL. B95-8 and Kaplan release virus that has been shown to transform human lymphocytes in vitro. The transforming activity of EB3 has, thus far, only been detected by tumor formation.

The B95-8 strain, which has been most widely used for experimental tumorigenesis, is released from transformed marmoset cells (Miller and Lipman, 1973). Initially there was concern that B95-8 was not the same as human EBV or that the virus was contaminated with other agents. The DNA of B95-8 virus has now been shown, by nucleic acid hybridization and by the analysis of the size of DNA fragments generated by the restriction endonuclease E_{CO} RI, to be more than 90% homologous with the DNA of the P_3HR-1 EBV strain (Pritchett et al., 1975; Sugden et al., 1976) (Chap. 8). Furthermore, all the E_{CO}RI fragments of B95-8 DNA are also found directly in the DNA of BL biopsies (Sugden, 1977). No other viral agents have been detected in the B95-8 virus stocks by a variety of approaches employing biologic, antigenic, and physicochemical methods.

Although it is now clear that B95-8 is a human EBV, there nonetheless remain questions as to whether it is a "typical" EBV strain. The strain originated from the peripheral blood leukocytes of an elderly lady with IM following transfusion of fresh blood (Blacklow et al., 1971). There is evidence that human cells transformed by the B95-8 strain carry episomal genomes that are 10% smaller in size than those found in cell lines from BL or from normals (Adams et al., 1977; Chap. 8). However, since several EBV strains can cause tumors in marmosets there can be no contention that this is a property unique to B95-8 EBV. Furthermore, two of the tumorigenic strains, EB3 and Kaplan, have only been carried in human lymphoid lines.

In one experiment throat washing obtained from an immunosuppressed renal transplant recipient was used for inoculation of marmosets without further in vitro passage (Lipman et al., 1975). Typical herpes virions were found when this specimen was examined by electron microscopy. On the basis of biologic tests the throat washing contained only EBV. It immortalized leukocytes and did not cause cytopathic effects characteristic of the other human herpesviruses. One of two marmosets developed abdominal lymph node enlargement about 5 weeks after inoculation. A lymph node biopsy made 2 months after inoculation showed marked hyperplasia. The animal developed antibodies to EB VCA. An autopsy performed 9 months after initiation of the experiment showed normal lymph nodes. Thus EBV, which has never been carried in vitro is infectious for marmosets and can induce lymph node disease though such virus has not yet been shown to be tumorigenic.

Although P_3HR-1 virus stocks contain as many particles as B95-8 stocks and although the DNA of the two strains is more than 90% homologous, the non-transforming P_3HR-1 virus is not capable of causing tumors (Falk et al., 1974; Miller et al., 1977). Animals inoculated once with P_3HR-1 virus do not even develop antibodies to EBV. The P_3HR-1 variant probably does not replicate in the monkeys. This finding makes it unlikely that P_3HR-1 represents the lytic "wild" biotype of EBV. Instead the processes of experimental infection and in vitro transformation seem to be linked. The simplest model to account for this linkage is that the primary event in experimental infection is transformation of lymphoid cells. The transformed cells contain the whole genome, which is periodically activated and released. At this point antibodies are then produced to viral components. This model for experimental infection may not be true for infection of man in whom there may indeed be a lytic phase of the infection in the oropharynx apart from transformation.

II. AMOUNT OF VIRUS

The minimal tumorigenic dose of B95-8 EBV is in the range of 1000 transforming units as assayed on human umbilical cord leukocytes (Deinhardt et al., 1975). About 1 in 50 B95-8 DNA molecules is a transforming unit for human cells (Sugden et al., 1977). In order to transform marmoset cells in vitro between 100 to 1000 times more active virus is required than to transform human cells (Henderson et al., 1977). Therefore approximately 50,000 EBV genomes is the minimal tumorigenic dose in marmosets (1000 transforming units as measured on human cells × 50 genomes per transforming unit). It is likely that the minimal tumorigenic dose of EBV in marmosets is that amount of virus required to initiate one transformation event.

Some inferences about the mode of tumorigenesis may be drawn from the tumorigenic dose. The tumorigenic dose of HVS is one plaque-forming unit. This low tumorigenic dose in the intact animal suggests that HVS has an active site of replication. Indeed HVS is recovered from the kidneys of experimentally infected animals. Viral replication may precede transformation of lymphocytes by HVS. To cite another example, young Syrian hamsters develop malignant lymphoma and osteosarcoma following intravenous inoculation of Simian virus 40, but only if they are given

10^7–10^8 plaque-forming units (Diamondopoulos and McLane, 1975). The low ratio of tumor-forming units to plaque-forming units indicates that in this instance transformation is inefficient and suggests that there is probably not an additional site where virus is amplified. The data for EBV fall in between these two extremes. In the animal, EBV probably does not replicate widely. The tumorigenic dose and the transforming dose in vitro are nearly identical.

C. HOST FACTORS IN EXPERIMENTAL CARCINOGENICITY

I. SPECIES

Results of in vitro transformation experiments and in vivo inoculations of a number of different primate species are summarized in Table 1 (for more detailed information from which this summary was compiled see Frank et al., 1976). It can be seen that EBV-reactive antibodies and spontaneous formation of lymphoid cell lines occur in great apes and old-world monkeys but not in new-world species. EBV is carcinogenic in some species of new-world monkeys and not in others. For example, in our laboratory we have transformed lymphoid cells from squirrel monkeys *(Saimiri)*, woolly monkeys *(Lagothrix)*, common marmosets *(Callothrix)*, and cotton-top marmosets *(Saguinus)*. For all experiments we used the same EBV strain, B95-8. We have tested for oncogenicity in two ways: by returning large numbers of cells that had been transformed in vitro to the autologous host and by injecting biologically active virus. We have obtained clear-cut evidence of infection and tumor formation in only one species, the cotton-top marmoset.

Squirrel monkeys developed antibodies to EBV and heterophil antibodies when they were hyperimmunized with transformed cells (Shope and Miller, 1973). Both types of immune responses were transient and no tumors occurred. Neither antibodies to EBV nor disease was produced when young squirrel monkeys were given cell-free virus of high titer (L. Meléndez and G. Miller, unpublished). Woolly monkeys were given autologous transformed cells in an "immunologically privileged" site, namely into the cerebrospinal fluid via the cisterna magnum (Andiman and Miller, 1978). Transformed cells were cultured from the peripheral blood of one of two monkeys injected in this fashion. These transformed cells were retrieved 1 week after inoculation but not thereafter. They were probably survivors of the inoculum. Neither animal developed persistent antibodies nor tumors. Four woolly monkeys given virus did not become infected or show signs of disease. Similarly *Callothrix* marmosets inoculated with autologous transformed cells did not develop tumors.

Thus, the cells of three species can be immortalized in vitro but neither autologous cell lines nor the virus initiate tumor formation. It is therefore necessary to distinguish between transformation of cells in culture, i.e., imparting to them the ability to proliferate indefinitely, and the ability to induce tumors in the intact animal. Human cells that have been transformed in culture are not oncogenic in the nude mouse, whereas BL tumor cells are (Nilsson et al., 1977). Clearly host factors contribute to the oncogenicity of the virus and the species of experimental animal is of great importance.

At least two properties distinguish transformed cells of those species in which the virus is not oncogenic from those of the cotton-top marmoset in which the virus is carcinogenic. One is virus production – cotton-top marmoset cells shed considerably more virus. *Lagothrix* cells yield only minute amounts of virus following transformation and in this way they resemble human cells. Squirrel monkey and *Callothrix* cells produce small amounts of virus, but not as much as marmoset cells. The production of extracellular virus might permit spread and increase the number of transformation events within the intact host. The more transformed cells, the greater likelihood of escape from host surveillance mechanisms. A second property setting cotton-top marmoset transformants apart from those of other species is the loss of one normal B lymphocyte (bone marrow-derived lymphocyte) surface characteristic. Cotton-top marmoset cells lose the ability to form rosettes with complement-coated erythrocytes following transformation. This is discussed in greater detail later.

Table 1. A summary of responses of various primate species to EBV

Primate species	Common name	Natural occurrence of EBV-reactive antibodies	Sponta-neous for-mation of lymphoid cell lines	Transfor-mation of lymphocytes in vitro by EBV	Tumori-genesis
Great apes					
Hylobates lar	White-handed gibbon	+	+	+	−
Old-world monkeys					
Macaca mulatta	Rhesus monkey	+	+	−	−
New-world monkeys					
Saguinus mystax	Moustached marmoset (tamarin)	−	−	+	−
Saguinus oedipus	Cotton-top marmoset	−	−	+	+
Saguinus myncollis	White-lipped marmoset	−	−	+	−
Callothrix jacchus	Common marmoset	−	−	+	−
Lagothrix lagotricha	Woolly monkey	−	−	+	−
Saimiri sciurea	Squirrel monkey	−	−	+	−
Aotus trivirgatus	Owl monkey	−	−	+	+

II. IMMUNOCOMPETENCE

Immunocompetence may influence susceptibility to lymphoma caused by EBV. For example, immunosuppressive drugs may enhance tumor formation, although the number of inoculated animals is too small to evaluate this variable in systematic fashion. Malignant lymphoma was induced in 4 of 11 cotton-top marmosets which received azothiaprine and prednisone and in 2 of 9 animals which did not receive such agents (Miller et al., 1977).

There seems to be some question whether the cotton-top marmoset is as immunocompetent as some other species of primates. In one comparative study, marmoset cells were less responsive to phytohemagglutinin and marmosets produced lower levels of antibody to salmonella antigens than did baboons, cebus, or squirrel monkeys (Harvey et al., 1974). It may be relevant that cotton-top marmosets are always chimeric twins. This feature of placental structure may make them tolerant to a broader range of antigens.

The ability of malaria infection to enhance tumorigenicity of EBV has been investigated (Leibold et al., 1976). Three squirrel monkeys already infected with plasmodium were given large numbers of autologous EBV-transformed cells. A rapidly progressive, fatal malignant lymphoproliferative disease was induced and the animals died within 8–10 days after inoculation. The disease was clearly due to widespread proliferation of the transplanted cells. However, five other squirrel monkeys infected with malaria did not develop tumors when they were given cell-free virus.

D. PATHOLOGY OF THE EXPERIMENTAL DISEASE

The location of the grossly visible tumors seems influenced by the site of inoculation. Gibbons given intratonsillar injections developed tonsillar enlargement several weeks later (Werner et al., 1972). One cotton-top marmoset inoculated in the masseter muscle was subsequently found to have lymphosarcoma in the submandibular region (Wolf et al., 1977). In those animals that develop lymphoma following intraperitoneal injection palpably enlarged abdominal nodes are detected 3–4 weeks after inoculation. If surgical exploration of the abdomen is performed at this time the mesentery has numerous large lymph nodes, 1–2 cm in size, which are matted together and in some instances adherent to the wall of the gut (Fig. 1). The spleen and liver usually appear normal, although tumors in those locations have also been found (Rabin et al., 1977). Since many wild marmosets are chronically infested with a nematode, *Prosthenorcis elegans,* which burrows into the wall of the small intestine, two pathologic lesions caused by this parasite may on gross inspection be confused with the experimental lymphoma. One is an abscess due to perforation of the gut. The other is a hard fibrous nodule within the intestinal wall in which the head and hooks of the worm are embedded. In neither of these two complications of parasitism is the mesentery so filled with enlarged rubbery nodes. Histologic examination makes the appropriate diagnosis.

The histologic characterization of the lymphoma has been hampered by the extensive necrosis found in involved lymph nodes. The necrosis is likely to be due to the rapid growth of the tumor. However, much unsatisfactory material for histologic examination has been obtained from moribund animals, which were killed or which died. The best material is from surgical biopsies performed on animals with abdominal masses.

In uninoculated marmosets or in those that remain normal after inoculation the lymph nodes are small, usually less than 5 mm, with well-defined germinal centers and interfollicular zones. The follicles contain few cells in mitosis. In an occasional animal, irregularity and enlargement of follicle size indicate mild focal hyperplasia which was not considered abnormal (Fig. 2).

Hyperplasia of a pronounced degree was a prominent finding in the lymph nodes of 3 in a series of 20 inoculated marmosets (Miller et al., 1977). This change varied from increase in size and irregularity of germinal centers to massive confluence of follicles with abundant mitotic activity (Fig. 3). In the germinal centers of hyperplastic nodes the predominant cells had large vesicular uncleaved nuclei. In this form of hyperplasia

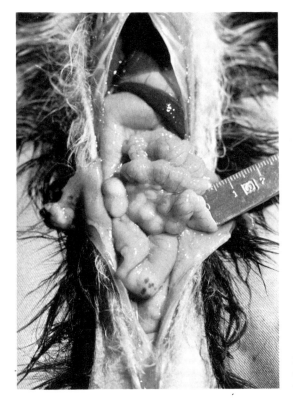

Fig. 1. Gross pathology of marmoset with a mesenteric lymphoma following inoculation with EBV

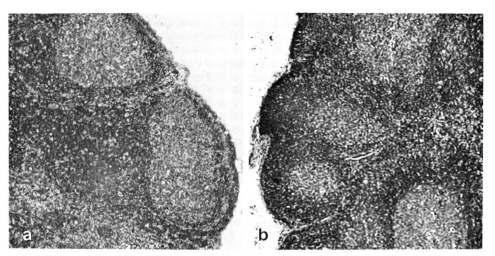

Fig. 2 a and **b.** Histology of normal marmoset lymph nodes (× 40)

Fig. 4 a–d. Histology of lymph nodes with malignant lymphoma. **a** A nodule involving the bowel wall (× 40). ▶ **b** Cords of tumor cells interspersed among zones of coagulation necrosis (× 40). **c** Lack of orientation of tumor cells (× 100). **d** Nuclei are irregular in size and shape, not cleaved or folded (× 250)

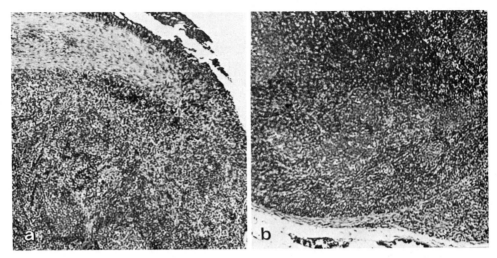

Fig. 3a and **b.** Hyperplastic marmoset lymph nodes. Note loss of normal follicular structures (× 40)

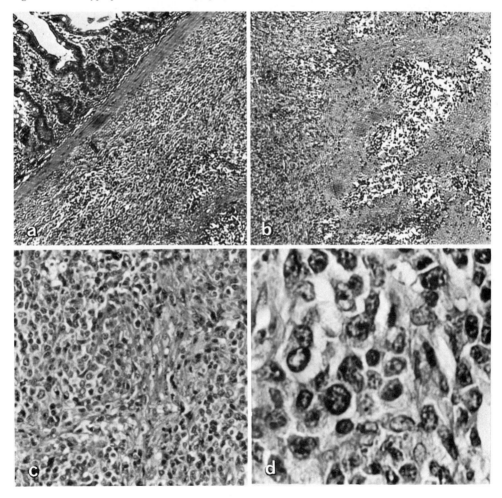

there was also an increase in number and crowding of lymphocytes in the interfollicular zones. Mitoses were present in the latter areas as well as numerous small foci of large reticular histiocytic cells giving rise to a "a starry sky" appearance (Fig. 4). Although such changes occasionally suggested the histologic appearance of malignancy, uniformity of cellular and nuclear size and shape, and some preservation of node architecture made such an interpretation unlikely.

Normal hyperplastic and malignant lymphoid nodules in the same animal were not uncommon. In the overtly malignant lymph nodes the component cells were arranged in irregular cords and masses which obliterated the basic lymph node architecture. Review of many sections suggested that the basis of the disruption of the normal landmarks of the node was enlargement and confluence of follicular structures.

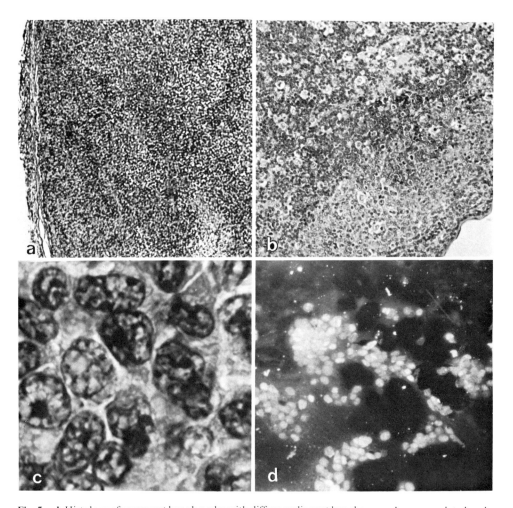

Fig. 5 a–d. Histology of marmoset lymph nodes with diffuse malignant lymphoma. **a** An encapsulated node in mesentery devoid of normal lymph node structure (× 40). **b** Areas of the node display a "starry sky" appearance (× 40). **c** Individual cells have large vesicular nuclei with prominent nucleoli (× 1000). **d** An impression smear of the node with EBV nuclear antigen

Necrosis and acute inflammatory changes of edema, hemorrhage, and accumulations of polymorphonuclear leukocytes were often observed in sections of tumor.

The tumor cells were arranged without polarization or organoid structure (Fig. 5). The majority were large and polygonal in shape with abundant cytoplasm. The nuclei were irregular in size and shape and always contained one or more nucleoli. Cleaved or folded nuclei were present among the tumor cells but were less common than uncleaved nuclei. On the basis of these cytologic features the tumors would fit either the large uncleaved follicular lymphoma or the immunoblastic sarcoma categories of human lymphomas (Lukes and Collins, 1975). The presence in some areas of the involved nodes of intense lymphoid hyperplasia with scattered "reactive" phagocytes simulates the histologic pattern of BL.

Focal collections of lymphoid cells and in some instances grossly visible tumor nodules have been seen in the liver, kidney, and lungs of some marmosets and the owl monkey with lymphoma (Shope et al., 1973; Epstein et al., 1973a). The spleen, although occasionally hemorrhagic, is not generally involved with tumor nor are the peripheral lymph nodes.

The experimental lymphomas are composed of two main types of cell which differ in many cytologic details evident at the ultrastructural level (Fig. 6). The nucleus of one has dense chromatin and nuclear pores are easily recognized. In the cytoplasm there are both free ribosomes and sparse rough endoplasmic reticulum. The surface of the cells is highly elaborated with microvilli and pseudopods. Neither Golgi apparatus nor lysosomes are prominent.

A second type of cell has distinctly different nuclear and cytoplasmic characteristics. The chromatin is dispersed and noncondensed and few nuclear pores are identified. The cytoplasm has few free ribosomes; instead there is massive elaboration of rough endoplasmic reticulum. The channels of the endoplasmic reticulum are swollen with a granular material. Microvilli are not a prominent feature of the latter cell.

Many features of the former cell type are preserved in lines cultivated from marmoset tumors. Cell lines from the owl monkey tumor are somewhat different. In particular, the cell surface is smooth. There is enough rough endoplasmic reticulum to suggest early activation toward the plasma cell series.

E. EBV GENOME IN THE EXPERIMENTAL TUMORS

EBV DNA has been demonstrated in the experimental lymphomas by the technique of DNA reassociation kinetics. Three lymphomas induced by B95-8 virus had an average of 8–30 genomes in every diploid cell (Miller et al., 1977). EBV DNA at a level of 3 genomes per cell was found in a lymph node with marked hyperplasia. The viral genome was not detected in normal lymph node or in a lymph node involved with an abscess following intestinal perforation. The lymphoma which resulted following inoculation of the Kaplan EBV strain appeared to contain 0.5 genomes per cell (Werner et al., 1975; Wolf et al., 1977), but since the tumor was extensively necrotic the number of EBV genomes in each viable tumor cell was likely to be higher.

There is no evidence that the tumor cells produce mature virus in the animal. Viral capsids have not been seen in a large number of cell profiles examined by electron

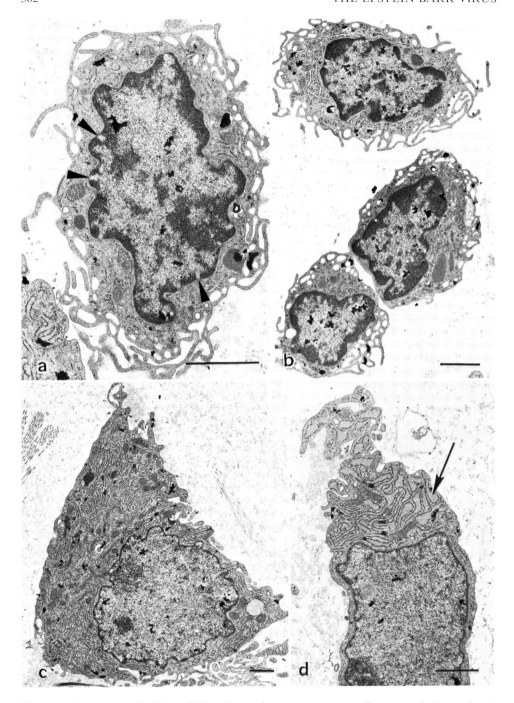

Fig. 6a–d. Ultrastructure of cells found in lymphoma of cotton-top marmoset. Two types of cells were found. The nucleus of the cell type shown in **(a)** and **(b)** has dense chromatin and nuclear pores are easily recognized *(arrowheads)*. There are both free ribosomes and sparse rough endoplasmic reticulum. The surface of the cells is highly elaborated with microvilli and pseudopods. Neither Golgi apparatus nor lysosomes are prominent. Cells are surrounded by a matrix of collagen.

microscopy. VCA has not been detected in tumor cell imprints stained by immunofluorescence. Therefore the measurement of the number of genome equivalents per tumor cell is not affected by the presence of cells which produce mature virus. It seems likely that the experimental tumors contain multiple latent genomes in every cell, as do BL tumors. The physical state of the genome in the experimental tumors has not yet been studied. It remains to be learned whether or not the genomes are integrated into cell DNA and whether episomal circular genomes are found in the marmoset tumor as they are in BL (Lindahl et al., 1976).

EBNA is found in nearly every nucleus of appropriately prepared imprints from tumors (Miller et al., 1977). In imprints made from lymph nodes with hyperplasia only a small proportion of the nuclei are positive. EBNA is probably a virus-coded protein and it is the single EBV genome product that is invariably expressed in human tumors (Klein, 1975). The presence of the EBV genome and the expression of EBNA in a majority of cells represent evidence that EBV caused the experimental tumor.

The tumor cells seem to harbor the entire EBV genome rather than only fragments of it. Thus, both owl monkey and marmoset cell lines have been obtained which release fully mature EB virions which are infectious as judged by transformation assays. The virions released from one such tumor cell line are also infectious for marmosets. One animal inoculated with virus recovered from a tumor developed "leukoviremia" and antibodies to EBV. That the animal did not proceed to lymphoma formation is evidence that there was no selection for a highly oncogenic virus variant.

There is little question that the virus shed by tumor lines is human EBV in its biologic, antigenic, and structural qualities. Thus, human sera with antibody to EBV neutralize the ability of this virus to transform lymphocytes in culture and antibody-negative human serum fails to do so.

Cell lines derived from both marmoset and owl monkey tumors contain multiple copies of EBV DNA per cell (Epstein et al., 1975; Miller et al., 1977). The amount of hybridization of viral cRNA with total cellular DNA corresponds to 50–200 genome equivalents per cell. Since as many as 5%–10% of cells in established marmoset lines produce virus, the number of genome equivalents per cell represents an average between producer and nonproducer cells.

Further fine molecular analysis of the DNA of EBV derived from experimental tumors will be required before it can be said with certainty that the genome found in the experimental tumors is identical to "feral" virus, which circulates naturally. Such future studies will undoubtedly include investigation of DNA homology and restriction enzyme patterns of the genomes of tumor-derived strains and of various virus isolates from man.

◀ **Fig. 6 a–d** *(continued)*. The cells in **(c)** and **(d)** have distinctly different nuclear and cytoplasmic characteristics. The chromatin is dispersed and noncondensed, and few nuclear pores are identified. The cytoplasm has few free ribosomes; instead there is massive elaboration of rough endoplasmic reticulum. The channels **c)** appear swollen with a granular material *(arrow)*. Microvilli formation is not as prominent as in cells shown in **(a)** and **(b)**. *Bars* represent 1 μm

F. EBV-SPECIFIC AND HETEROPHIL ANTIBODY RESPONSES OF
EXPERIMENTALLY INFECTED ANIMALS

Marmosets, gibbons, and owl monkeys have developed antibodies to a variety of EBV-associated antigens after inoculation. In gibbons, which do not develop tumors, antibody to VCA appears promptly, within 1–5 weeks after inoculation (Werner et al., 1972). In marmosets, the antibody response is delayed, often for 6–8 weeks, and some animals develop lymphoma and die before antibody is ever apparent. If marmosets which develop lymphoma survive their disease for a long period, their sera contain higher titers of antibody than inoculated animals without tumors (Miller et al., 1977). The first marmoset which we observed with lymphoma manifested a dramatic increase in anti-VCA between the 3rd and 6th month after inoculation.

Antibody to early antigen (EA) has also been found in marmoset sera. The anti-EA activity is directed against the diffuse component of the antigen. The highest titers were observed in sera of tumor-bearing animals. The pattern of antibody responses to VCA and EA resembl the serologic reactions observed in man (Henle et al., 1971). Monkeys with tumors had higher anti-VCA titers and more frequently developed anti-EA than did those with inapparent infection. One small group of marmosets, which died with malignant lymphoproliferative disease before antibodies appeared in their sera, is reminiscent of the boys with the X-linked immune deficiency disorder who did not develop antibodies to EBV and subsequently died of fatal IM (Bar et al., 1974).

A few marmoset sera have been analyzed for their content of neutralizing antibody to EBV. Preinoculation sera do not neutralize EBV. Sera taken after infection contain antibodies which neutralize several EBV strains. The titers are highest against the B95-8 strain with which the animals were inoculated (Miller et al., 1977).

One major difference between the antibody responses of marmosets and man to EBV is the general failure of the monkeys to demonstrate antibody to EBNA. Only one marmoset has developed a low level anti-EBNA titer (1:10). Another serologic difference is the failure of marmosets to develop antibodies to sheep erythrocytes analogous to the Paul-Bunnell heterophil antibodies. No heterophil responses were found in any of the marmosets in our series of inoculations, although injection of autologous EBV-transformed marmoset cells called forth a heterophil antibody in one of three animals studied by Falk et al. (1974). Squirrel monkeys seem to manifest this type of antibody regularly if they are hyperimmunized with autologous, transformed cells. However, squirrel monkeys do not elaborate the heterophil antibody if they are given cell-free EBV (Shope and Miller, 1973). These findings suggest that heterophil antigens may be present on EBV-transformed cells of some species and not others.

Cell-mediated immune responses of primates to EBV-induced changes in cellular membranes of infected cells have not yet been extensively investigated. That such responses do occur was demonstrated by showing that EBV-transformed marmoset cell lines stimulated the peripheral blood lymphocytes of a chimeric twin in a mixed-lymphocyte reaction (Falk et al., 1974).

The role that any immunologic reaction plays in limiting the infection in those marmosets that do not develop tumors can only be inferred. In one group of animals studied by Shope et al. (1975) "leukoviremia" developed in the 2 nd–4 th week after inoculation and terminated after the appearance of serum antibodies to VCA.

G. SPECIAL FEATURES OF TRANSFORMED MARMOSET CELLS

The incidence of malignant disease occurring in marmosets after inoculation of EBV is as high as 30%–40%. For a virus with low and geographically constrained oncogenicity in its natural host, man, this high rate of tumor induction raises questions about the special susceptibility of the experimental host. When the answers to such questions are known they will be complex and will undoubtedly involve many factors such as the nature of the immunologic response, possibly the route of administration, and the strain of virus as well. However, it is already clear that EBV-transformed cells originating from blood and lymphoid organs of certain new-world primates are different in a number of respects from comparable transformed cells of human origin.

I. VIRUS PRODUCTION

One marked difference lies in the frequency with which transformed cells are spontaneously activated to produce virus (Miller and Lipman, 1973). In most human cell lines obtained after transformation in vitro fewer than 1% of the cells are positive for VCA. This antigen is almost never seen in the lines originating from human umbilical cord blood. By contrast marmoset cell lines, whether derived from tumors or in vitro transformation, regularly display 5%–10% VCA-positive cells. Transformed marmoset and squirrel monkey cells also release more virus into the fluid phase of the culture. The increase in yield of EBV has been found for several strains of virus propagated in marmoset cells (Miller et al., 1976). That this increase in virus production is not due to a particular subpopulation of monkey cells which are completely permissive has been demonstrated by cloning studies (Miller and Lipman, 1973). All clones of transformed marmoset and squirrel monkey cell lines were similar to their parents and individual clones of each species produced extracellular virus in equivalent quantities.

The relatively high yield of extracellular virus from marmoset cells cannot be accounted for solely on the basis of an increase in the proportion of cells activated to produce virus. If this were the case one would expect only ten times more virus from marmoset than from human lines. However, since yields of virus from transformed marmoset cells are 1000 times the yield of virus from comparable transformed cells from adult humans, other factors must be involved as well. These factors may include more virions produced in each activated cell or more efficient processes of envelopment and release (Chap. 2).

A high rate of virus production by transformed cells may play a role in the high frequency of tumor formation by allowing spread of virus within the host. However, immunologically intact squirrel monkeys do not develop tumors following virus injection even though their cells transformed in vitro shed 10–100 times more virus than human cells.

II. SURFACE IG

Transformed marmoset cells still contain surface immunoglobulin and thus can clearly be identified as B lymphocytes (Deinhardt et al., 1975; Rabin et al., 1977). Cell lines obtained from several widely spread tumor nodules occurring in one animal were studied. There were many cells with μ and γ heavy chains and λ light chains, but there were no cells bearing κ light chains or α heavy chains. All the tumor cell lines from this animal also had a characteristic cytogenetic pattern; the median chromosome number was 45, and there was loss of a medium-size metacentric chromosome. These tumor cell lines also displayed a marker chromosome with an extra band in the centromeric region. These studies support the idea of monoclonality for a multiple, widely disseminated marmoset tumor (Rabin et al., 1977)

III. CYTOLOGY

The cytology of the EBV-transformed marmoset cell observed in culture is distinct from its human counterpart among lymphoblastoid lines. Marmoset transformants adhere to glass or plastic, though a portion of the cells is always loosely attached in clumps to the adherent ones and others float in the medium. This behavior of adherence by part of the culture is seen in cloned lines so that it is not due to heterogeneity among the cells. EBV-transformed marmoset and squirrel monkey lines have multinucleate giant cells that seem to be selective sites of virus production. Intranuclear inclusions and VCA are detected with greater frequency in multinucleate than in cells with single nuclei (Miller et al., 1972). Marmoset transformants growing in culture have extensively elaborated cellular membranes with pseudopods and microvilli, which are not seen on the surface of human lines.

IV. LYMPHOCYTE SURFACE MARKERS

Differences in the structure of the cell surface of transformed cells of one species could provide an explanation for a difference in oncogenicity. The lymphocyte surface markers on EBV-transformed marmoset cells were recently compared with those on comparable cell lines from humans or woolly monkeys (Robinson et al., 1977). The pattern of expression of receptors was different from one species to another. Human lines invariably expressed the receptor for C'. More than 90% of cells in human lines formed rosettes with sheep erythrocytes coated with antibody and fresh mouse serum as a source of complement (EAC rosettes). Transformants originating from woolly monkey blood are much like human lines in their morphologic appearance, in their low to absent virus production, and in their failure to adhere to glass. Such woolly monkey lines also form EAC rosettes though less than half the cells in any line are positive. In addition, more than half the cells in every woolly monkey line examined have a receptor for the Fc fragment of immunoglobulin as detected by rosette formation with erythrocytes coated with antibody. Fc receptors detected in this way are not usually found on human lymphoid cell lines obtained by in vitro transformation. Marmoset cell lines express neither the receptor for complement nor that for immunoglobulin.

The absence of classic B lymphocyte surface markers on transformed marmoset cells initially raised the possibility that in this species the lymphoblastoid lines originate from a cell other than a B lymphocyte. A monocyte, a non-B or non-T lymphocyte (thymus-dependent lymphocyte), or a stem cell were considered to be possible target cells. These possibilities now seem unlikely in view of results of experiments designed to determine the subpopulation of marmoset blood leukocytes which is susceptible to transformation (Robinson et al., 1977). If primary marmoset lymphocytes are first depleted of cells that bear the EAC receptor there is a marked decrease in the efficiency of transformation by EBV. The depletion of macrophages had no effect on the efficiency of transformation. Treatment of marmoset primary blood leukocytes by 5-bromodeoxyuridine and then a pulse of light, which kills cells in DNA synthesis, does not alter the transformation frequency either (Henderson et al., 1977). Thus, the cell in marmoset blood which is susceptible to transformation appears to be similar to that in human blood, namely a resting cell with the C′ receptor, i. e., a B lymphocyte.

One conclusion drawn from this series of experiments is that marmoset cells undergo an alteration in their normal differentiated B lymphocyte surface following transformation. This surface change which accompanies immortalization is not an invariable accompaniment of transformation in other species. Woolly monkey and human cells retain the surface markers found on normal B lymphocytes even though the cells have been transformed in their growth potential. The absence of the C′ receptor on marmoset cells by itself may not be the crucial event in the change to malignancy, but it may herald a more general change in the cell surface which accompanies oncogenic transformation.

The mechanism by which such surface changes occur is not known, but several hypotheses serve as the basis for further work. One hypothesis links the loss of the receptor for EAC to virus production by the transformants. There are several ways in which virus production might affect expression of the EAC receptor. The receptor may be blocked by virion envelope materials made by the cell and shed into the culture medium. Since the virus receptor and the EAC receptor are closely linked if not identical, virus envelope material would block the attachment of EAC rosettes. Another way to link virus production with the loss of the EAC receptor is to propose that viral glycoproteins are inserted in the membranes of all the cells in virus-producer lines. New glycoproteins alter the topology of the surface in some way so that binding of EAC is not possible. Alternatively virus production might select against cells with the EAC receptor. Such selection might operate by superinfection and lysis of cells with virus (or EAC) receptors or, more likely, by imposing a selective growth disadvantage in vitro on those cells with a virus receptor. The theory that relates virus production to loss of EAC receptors receives support from the observation that the single human BL line (P$_3$HR-1), which is also activated to release large amounts of mature virus, also lacks the ability to form rosettes with EAC.

The other major theory to account for the cell surface alteration of marmoset cells which have been transformed by EBV might be called the "dedifferentiation theory". This theory holds that transformed marmoset cells revert to a more primitive state than do human cells which have been transformed in culture. The marmoset cell may be more susceptible to "pleiotropic effects", which include changes in both growth and cell surface behavior. The fundamental difference in the surface of the transformed marmoset cell may not be the actual loss of receptors for complement but a physiologic change in the surface or in the cytoskeleton which prevents the receptors from functioning properly. For example, such receptors may not be able to move laterally in the membrane in order to form rosettes.

H. SIGNIFICANCE OF EXPERIMENTAL CARCINOGENICITY BY EBV

There can be little doubt that the ability to cause lymphoproliferative disease, some of which has the characteristics of overt malignancy, in certain species of primates is a biologic property of EBV. Several strains of virus can transform cells of nonhuman primates and cause lymphoma. Little seems lacking in the skein of proof that identifies EBV as the etiologic agent in the experimental tumors. Neutralization tests have been performed on a small scale in two laboratories (Shope, 1975; Wolf et al., 1977). When EBV is premixed with human antibody-positive serum, lymphoproliferative lesions, antibody formation, and "leukoviremia" do not occur. Human serum which is devoid of antibody to EBV fails to block infection. A variety of mock inocula which do not contain EBV do not induce tumors. These include BL biopsies, which do not contain mature virus, supernatant fluids from the nonproducer Raji cell line, and tissue culture medium. Such tumors do not develop spontaneously in the laboratory. When lymphomas did occur the animals were carefully monitored for infection with HVS, which is also capable of causing lymphomas in the same species. No antibodies to this agent were found. HVS could not be recovered from the tumors by cocultivation with permissive owl monkey kidney cells. Ultimately it was determined that EBV-induced lymphomas were of B cell origin and those caused by HVS were T cells. The biologic and biochemical evidence of the entire human EBV genome in the experimental tumors and their derivative cell lines is further proof that the tumors are caused by EBV.

These experiments strengthen the hypothesis that EBV causes lymphoproliferative disease, including malignant lymphoma, in man. As in man, a spectrum of responses occurs which varies from inapparent infection to malignant lymphoma. The incidence of the latter is by necessity higher in laboratory animals, which are selected on the basis of their susceptibility to cancer. The malignant disease produced experimentally shares many pathologic similarities with BL; these have been pointed out. Likewise there are parallels between natural and experimental infection in the pattern of serologic reactions. The virus-cell relationship, as far as it has been studied, is also identical. Tumor cells contain many copies of the genome. Transfer of tumor cells to the conditions of culture is associated with activation of the genome. The resultant cell lines have more EBV DNA, produce VCA, and release mature virions. The recent demonstration that cell lines from a multiple marmoset tumor are oligo-or monoclonal with respect to surface immunoglobulin and cytogenetic markers is an additional parallel with BL (Rabin et al., 1977).

There are also notable ways in which the experimental infection of primates differs from natural infection of man. The peculiar anatomic distribution of BL in the mandible has not been reproduced nor has involvement of the gonads; on the other hand, as with BL, so in the marmoset neither the spleen nor the peripheral lymph nodes are regularly affected. No atypical lymphocytes have been found in the peripheral blood of marmosets, the heterophil response is absent, and antibodies to EBNA were only detected at a very low level in one animal.

Perhaps the most important difference is the high incidence of malignant disease. It might be argued that tumor formation in the marmoset is an example of "crossed species virulence" and, as such, provides no evidence one way or the other about the potential oncogenic role of EBV in man. The phenomenon of a virus of low or moderate virulence in its natural host becoming highly lethal when it crosses species barriers is well known in virology. This possibility cannot be dismissed and will invariably cause confusion in the interpretation of the significance of any animal model of human disease. It is worth noting, however, that in other examples of crossed species virulence with the herpesviruses, the outcome is more severe and more invariable than in the case of EBV in marmosets. Every cotton-top marmoset infected with HVS develops malignant lymphoma. Nearly every human who contracts herpes simiae (B virus) infection incurs a severe encephalitis.

I.   FUTURE WORK WITH EBV IN PRIMATES

New-world monkeys are now in short supply as laboratory subjects. Their exportation has been stopped because many are endangered species. Small breeding colonies have been started, but their output does not promise to be sufficient for large scale in vivo experiments. Future projects involving these animals must therefore be selected carefully.

The EBV-transformed cotton-top marmoset cell is the most efficient system for generating extracellular EBV. Thus, lymphoid cells of this species will continue to serve as the source of different strains and genetic variants of EBV for comparative studies of structural and biologic properties. Another type of investigation which would not require killing the animal is analysis of factors influencing virus production and cell surface properties which differ so dramatically in transformants of different species.

Several areas of EBV research can be envisioned which will require some in vivo experimentation. The question of the oncogenic potential of naturally occurring EBV strains is not yet resolved. Most important is to learn whether wild-type EBV obtained directly from throat washing, with minimal further in vitro manipulation, is capable of inducing malignant lymphoma. The relative tumorigenic potency of EBV isolates from different geographic regions and from different pathologic states should be studied. A direct demonstration that EBV is capable of inducing epithelial tumors of the nasopharynx is still lacking. The virus strain recently recovered from a nasopharyngeal carcinoma biopsy passaged in nude mice is likely to be assayed for its capacity to induce a similar cancer in a primate (Trumper et al., 1977). The epidemiologic hypothesis linking BL with coinfection by EBV and malaria can be studied in a primate (Burkitt, 1969; Chap. 14). The influence of immunosuppressive regimens and transplants on the susceptibility to tumor formation and on reactivation of latent infection can also be best studied in an experimental animal.

From a practical viewpoint any vaccine regimen contemplated for use in man would best be tested for its protective effects against lymphoma in marmosets. The immunizing potential of various types of antigens, whether they be viral or cell membrane glycoproteins which induce neutralizing antibody, or nontransforming virus variants could first be evaluated in new-world monkeys (Chap. 19).

REFERENCES

Adams, A., Bjursell, G., Kaschka-Dierich, C., Lindahl, T.: Circular Epstein-Barr virus genomes of reduced size in a human lymphoid cell line of infectious mononucleosis origin. J. Virol. **22,** 373–380 (1977)

Andiman, W. A., Miller, G.: Properties of Epstein-Barr virus transformed woolly monkey lymphocytes. Proc. Soc. Exp. Biol. Med. **157,** 489–493 (1978)

Bar, R. S., Deler, C. J., Clausen, K. P., Hurtubise, P., Henle, W., Hewetson, J. F.: Fatal infectious mononucleosis in a family. N. Engl. J. Med. **290,** 363–367 (1974)

Blacklow, N. R., Watson, B. K., Miller, G., Jacobson, B. M.: Mononucleosis with heterophil antibodies and EB Virus infection. Acquisition by an elderly patient in hospital. Am. J. Med. **51,** 549–552 (1971)

Burkitt, D. P.: Etiology of Burkitt's lymphoma – an alternative hypothesis to a vectored virus. J. Natl. Cancer Inst. **42,** 19–28 (1969)

Deinhardt, F., Falk, L., Wolfe, L. G., Paciga, J., Johnson, D.: Response of marmosets to experimental infection with Epstein-Barr virus. In: Oncogenesis and herpesviruses II. de-Thé, G., Epstein, M. A., zur Hausen, H. (eds.), Part 2, pp. 161–168. Lyon: IARC 1975

Diamondopoulos, G. Ph., McLane, M. F.: Effect of host age, virus dose, and route of inoculation on tumor incidence, latency, and morphology in Syrian hamsters inoculated intravenously with oncogenic DNA simian virus 40. J. Natl. Cancer Inst. **55,** 479–482 (1975)

Epstein, M. A., Hunt, R. D., Rabin, H.: Pilot experiments with EB virus in owl monkeys *(Aotus trivirgatus)* I. Reticuloproliferative disease in an inoculated animal. Int. J. Cancer **12,** 309–318 (1973a)

Epstein, M. A., Rabin, H., Ball, G., Rickinson, A. B., Jarvis, J., Meléndez, L. V.: Pilot experiments with EB virus in owl monkeys *(Aotus trivirgatus)* II. EB virus in a cell line from an animal with reticuloproliferative disease. Int. J. Cancer **12,** 319–332 (1973b)

Epstein, M. A., zur Hausen, H., Ball, G., Rabin, H.: Pilot experiments with EB virus in owl monkeys *(Aotus trivirgatus)* III. Serological and biochemical findings in an animal with reticuloproliferative disease. Int. J. Cancer **15,** 17–22 (1975)

Falk, L., Wolfe, L., Deinhardt, F., Paciga, J., Dombos, L., Klein, G., Henle, W., Henle, G. Epstein-Barr virus: transformation of nonhuman primate lymphocytes *in vitro.* Int. J. Cancer **13,** 363–376 (1974)

Fialkow, P. J., Klein, G., Gartler, S. M., Clifford, P.: Clonal origin for individual Burkitt tumors. Lancet **1970 I,** 384–386

Frank, A., Andiman, W., Miller, G.: Epstein-Barr virus and non-human primates: natural and experimental infection. Adv. Cancer Res. **23,** 171–210 (1976)

Harvey, J. S. (Jr.), Felsburg, P. J., Heberling, R. L., Kniker, W. T., Kalter, S. S.: Immunological competence in non-human primates: differences observed in four species. Clin. Exp. Immunol. **16,** 267–278 (1974)

Henderson, E., Miller, G., Robinson, J., Heston, L.: Efficiency of transformation of lymphocytes by Epstein-Barr virus. Virology **76,** 152–163 (1977)

Henderson, E., Robinson, J., Frank, A., Miller, G.: Epstein-Barr virus: transformation of lymphocytes separated by size or exposed to bromodeoxyuridine and light. Virology **82,** 196–205 (1977)

Henle, G., Henle, W.: Immunofluorescence in cells derived from Burkitt's lymphoma. J. Bacteriol. **91,** 1248–1256 (1966)

Henle, W., Diehl, V., Kohn, G., zur Hausen, H., Henle, G.: Herpes-type virus and chromosome marker in normal leukocytes after growth with irradiated Burkitt cells. Science **157,** 1064–1065 (1967)

Henle, G., Henle, W., Zajac, B., Pearson, G., Waubke, R., Scriba, M.: Differential reactivity of human serums with early antigens induced by Epstein-Barr virus. Science **169,** 188–190 (1970)

Henle, G., Henle, W., Klein, G., Gunvén, P., Morrow, R. H., Ziegler, J. L.: Antibodies to early Epstein-Barr virus-induced antigens in Burkitt's lymphoma. J. Natl. Cancer Inst. **46,** 861–871 (1971)

Klein, G.: Studies on the Epstein-Barr virus genome and the EBV-determined nuclear antigen in human malignant disease. Cold Spring Harbor Symp. Quant. Biol. **39,** 783–790 (1975)

Leibold, W., Huldt, G., Flanagan, T. D., Andersson, M., Dalens, M., Wright, D. H., Voller, A., Klein, G.: Tumorigenicity of Epstein-Barr virus (EBV)-transformed lymphoid line cells in autologous squirrel monkeys. Int. J. Cancer **17,** 533–541 (1976)

Lindahl, T., Adams, A., Bjursell, G., Bornkamm, G. W., Kaschka-Dierich, C., Jehn, W.: Covalently closed circular duplex DNA of Epstein-Barr virus in a human lymphoid cell line. J. Mol. Biol. **102,** 511–530 (1976)

Lipman, M., Andrews, L., Niederman, J., Miller, G.: Direct visualization of enveloped herpes-like virus from throat washing with leukocyte transforming activity. J. Infect. Dis. **132,** 520–523 (1975)

Lukes, R. J., Collins, R. D.: New approaches to the classification of the lymphomata. Br. J. Cancer **31**, [Suppl. 2] 1–27 (1975)

Meléndez, L. V., Hunt, R. D., Daniel, M. D.: Herpesvirus saimiri II. Experimentally induced malignant lymphoma in primates. Lab. Anim. Care **19**, 378–386 (1969)

Menezes, J., Leibold, W., Klein, G.: Biological differences between Epstein-Barr virus strains with regard to lymphocyte transforming ability, superinfection and antigen induction. Exp. Cell Res. **92**, 478–484 (1975)

Miller, G., Shope, T., Lisco, H., Stitt, D., Lipman, M.: Epstein-Barr virus: transformation, cytopathic changes and viral antigens in squirrel monkey and marmoset leukocytes. Proc. Natl. Acad. Sci. USA **69**, 383–387 (1972)

Miller, G., Lipman, M.: Comparison of the yield of infectious virus from clones of human and simian lymphoblastoid lines transformed by Epstein-Barr virus. J. Exp. Med. **138**, 1398–1412 (1973)

Miller, G., Robinson, J., Heston, L., Lipman, M.: Differences between laboratory strains of Epstein-Barr virus based on immortalization, abortive infection and interference. Proc. Natl. Acad. Sci. USA **71**, 4006–4010 (1974)

Miller, G., Coope, D., Niederman, J., Pagano, J.: Biologic properties and viral surface antigens of Burkitt lymphoma and mononucleosis derived strains of Epstein-Barr virus released from transformed marmoset cells. J. Virol. **18**, 1071–1080 (1976)

Miller, G., Shope, T., Coope, D., Waters, L., Pagano, J., Bornkamm, G. W., Henle, W.: Lymphoma in cotton-top marmosets after inoculation with Epstein-Barr virus: tumor incidence, histologic spectrum, antibody responses, demonstration of viral DNA, and characterization of viruses. J. Exp. Med. **145**, 948–967 (1977)

Nilsson, K., Giovanella, B. C., Stehlin, J. S., Klein, G.: Tumorigenicity of human hematopoietic cell lines in athymic nude mice. Int. J. Cancer **19**, 337–344 (1977)

Nonoyama, M., Huang, C. H., Pagano, J. S., Klein, G., Singh, S.: DNA of Epstein-Barr virus detected in tissue of Burkitt's lymphoma and nasopharyngeal carcinoma. Proc. Natl. Acad. Sci. USA **70**, 3265–3268 (1973)

Pritchett, R. F., Hayward, S. D., Kieff, E. D.: DNA of Epstein-Barr virus. I. Comparative studies of the DNA of Epstein-Barr virus from HR-1 and B95-8 cells: size, structure and relatedness. J. Virol. **15**, 556–569 (1975)

Rabin, H., Neubauer, R. H., Hopkins, R. F., III, Levy, B. M.: Characterization of lymphoid cell lines established from multiple Epstein-Barr virus (EBV) induced lymphomas in a cotton-topped marmoset. Int. J. Cancer **20**, 44–50 (1977)

Reedman, B. M., Klein, G.: Cellular localization of an Epstein-Barr virus (EBV)-associated complement-fixing antigen in producer and non-producer lymphoblastoid cell lines. Int. J. Cancer **11**, 499–520 (1973)

Robinson, J. E., Andiman, W. A., Henderson, E., Miller, G.: Host-determined differences in expression of surface marker characteristics on human and simian lymphoblastoid cell lines transformed by Epstein-Barr virus. Proc. Natl. Acad. Sci. USA **74**, 749–753 (1977)

Shope, T. C., Miller, G.: Epstein-Barr virus: Heterophile responses in squirrel monkeys inoculated with virus-transformed autologous leukocytes. J. Exp. Med. **137**, 140–147 (1973)

Shope, T., Dechairo, D., Miller, G.: Malignant lymphoma in cottontop marmosets after inoculation with Epstein-Barr virus. Proc. Natl. Acad. Sci. USA **70**, 2487–2491 (1973)

Shope, T. C.: Prevention of Epstein-Barr virus (EBV)-induced infection in cotton-topped marmosets by human serum containing EBV neutralizing activity. In: Oncogenesis and herpes viruses II. de-Thé, G., Epstein, M. A., zur Hausen, H. (eds.), Part 2, pp. 153–159. Lyon: IARC 1975

Sugden, B., Summers, W. C., Klein, G.: Nucleic acid renaturation and restriction endonuclease cleavage analyses show that the DNA's of a transforming and a non-transforming strain of Epstein-Barr virus share approximately 90% of their nucleotide sequences. J. Virol. **18**, 765–775 (1976)

Sugden, B., Mark, W.: Clonal transformation of adult human leukocytes by Epstein-Barr virus. J. Virol. **23**, 503–508 (1977)

Sugden, B.: Comparison of Epstein-Barr viral DNA's in Burkitt lymphoma biopsy cells and in cells clonally transformed *in vitro*. Proc. Natl. Acad. Sci. USA **74**, 4651–4655 (1977)

Trumper, P. A., Epstein, M. A., Giovanella, B. C., Finerty, S.: Isolation of infectious EB virus from the epithelial tumour cells of nasopharyngeal carcinoma. Int. J. Cancer **20**, 655–662 (1977)

Werner, J., Henle, G., Pinto, C. A., Haff, R. F., Henle, W.: Establishment of continuous lymphoblast cultures from leukocytes of gibbons (Hylobates lar). Int. J. Cancer **10**, 557–567 (1972)

Werner, J., Pinto, C. A., Haff, R. F., Henle, W., Henle, G.: Response of gibbons to inoculation of Epstein-Barr virus. J. Infect. Dis. **126**, 678–681 (1972)

Werner, J., Wolf, H., Apodaca, J., zur Hausen, H.: Lymphoproliferative disease in a cotton-top marmoset after inoculation with infectious mononucleosis-derived Epstein-Barr virus. Int. J. Cancer **15**, 1000–1008 (1975)

Wolf, H., Werner, J., zur Hausen, H.: EBV DNA in nonlymphoid cells of nasopharyngeal carcinomas and in a malignant lymphoma obtained after inoculation of EBV into cotton-top marmosets. Cold Spring Harbor Symp. Quant. Biol. **39**, 791–796 (1977)

zur Hausen, H., Schulte-Holthausen, H., Klein, G., Henle, G., Henle, W., Clifford, P., Santesson, L.: EBV-DNA in biopsies of Burkitt tumors and anaplastic carcinomas of the nasopharynx. Nature **228**, 1056–1058 (1970)

17 Comparative Aspects: Oncogenic Animal Herpesviruses

F. Deinhardt and J. Deinhardt

Max von Pettenkofer-Institut, Ludwig-Maximilians-Universität, Pettenkofer Straße 9 a, D-8000 München 2 (FRG)

A. INTRODUCTION

A strong case can be made for including the oncogenic animal herpesviruses in a book on Epstein-Barr virus (EBV). Various proliferative diseases of animals are associated with RNA and DNA viruses and animal herpesviruses have been identified either as causative agents or as consistent associates of several, naturally occurring tumors. Close parallels can be drawn between some characteristics of these tumors and the expression of EBV infections in man. Exploration of the similarities (and disparities, too) of the malignancies seen in animals other than man, whether these diseases are induced experimentally or occur naturally, can cast light upon the human disease(s) caused by EBV. This chapter will review the animal oncogenic herpesviruses and the pathogenesis of the proliferative diseases they cause, in the hope that this somewhat different perspective will illuminate the role EBV plays in human disease.

Common to all herpesviruses is their mode of horizontal and not vertical transmission and a replicative cycle accompanied by stimulation of cellular meta-bolism in the early phase of infection. Cellular metabolism shuts down and cell death results if viral multiplication proceeds beyond a critical step in the replicative cycle. If, on the other hand, virus multiplication is blocked before that step, cell transformation may occur with maintenance of the entire or perhaps only part of the viral genome in the transformed cells and their progeny. Cells containing a viral genome in an integrated and/or extrachromosomal form can survive and multiply indefinitely, so long as the viral genome is not activated; activation of viral genomes may be temperature dependent, as in cells carrying Lucké's herpesvirus (LHV), may occur spontaneously, or may be induced chemically or by irradiation. In each instance, genome activation is followed by cell death even when virus activation does not proceed to the production of complete virus particles but is blocked again during a later stage of virus replication. The modes of latency of herpesviruses in the absence of cell transformation is still a matter of debate and will not be considered in detail, but transformation of cells by various herpesviruses is well documented and its possible mechanism and significance for certain tumors will be considered.

Before discussing individual herpesviruses it is necessary to consider some basic differences between the herpes and RNA tumor viruses, since a collaborative role between these viruses in the pathogenesis of certain tumors has been suggested. Both herpesviruses and RNA tumor viruses are widespread in the animal kingdom and it seems that each family or even species has its own representative of the two groups. The RNA tumor viruses or retraviruses (i. e., C-type leukemia, sarcoma and possibly nononcogenic endogenous viruses; B-type mammary tumor viruses of mice; and D-type or Mason Pfizer-like viruses of primates) can be transmitted vertically or horizontally and virus multiplication is compatible with normal survival or transfor-mation and rapid multiplication of infected cells. Synergism between herpes and RNA tumor viruses leading to cell transformation has been postulated, particularly for herpes simplex virus (HSV), EBV, and Marek's disease virus (MDV), but no final proof for such a mechanism exists in these systems. For a wider discussion the reader is referred to the published proceedings of Oncogenesis and Herpesviruses II (1975, edited by de-Thé et al.) and III (1978, edited by de-Thé et al.), Herpesvirus and Cervical Cancer (1973, edited by Wilbanks et al.), and Kaplan (1973). It was argued that infection of a cell by a herpesvirus under certain circumstances derepresses or activates an endogenous genome of a RNA tumor virus and that the activated RNA genome is actually responsible for the initiation and maintenance of cell transformation, but although activated RNA tumor viruses have been demonstrated in some cells transformed during an abortive herpesvirus infection, this finding has been inconsistent and it is unclear whether activation of the RNA genomes in these instances was accidental, without influence on cell transformation, or whether it played a causative role in the process. Interrelationships between MDV and avian C-type RNA viruses have been studied extensively and although some interaction and possibly a potentiating effect of C-type virus on the oncogenicity of MDV and/or of MDV on the expression of avian C-type viruses appears likely, MDV alone is without question capable of transforming cells and inducing typical neurolymphomatosis i. e., Marek's disease (Frankel et al., 1974, 1975; Witter et al., 1975a; Calnek and Payne, 1976). Similarly an activation of endogenous C-type viruses has been demonstrated during transformation of rodent cells by HSV, but it is unclear what (if any) role the activated C-type virus played in the transformation process (Munk et al., 1975). In this connection it should be pointed out once more that EBV free of detectable C-type viruses can transform human and nonhuman primate lymphocytes in vitro and induce lymphoproliferative diseases in nonhuman primates without any indication that activated C-type viruses play a role. Nor have C-type viruses been detected, despite extensive search, during transformation in vitro of T lymphocytes (thymus-dependent lymphocyte) or induction of lymphomas/leukemia in vivo in marmosets or owl monkeys with herpesvirus saimiri (HVS) or herpesvirus ateles (HVA).

Irrespective of the possibility that RNA viruses act synergistically it is clear that under certain circumstances infection of cells by herpesviruses induces cell transformation; the herpesviruses which have been associated with cell transformation in vitro or proliferative diseases in vivo are listed in Table 1. The association between cell transformation in vitro and/or tumor induction in vivo and herpesviruses is not restricted to mammals but has been observed in at least three animal classes. In addition, herpesviruses of at least three different virus taxa may cause cell proliferation, not only of lymphocytic cells but also of fibroblastic or epithelial cells. The herpesviruses in Table 1 are grouped according to the suggestions of the Herpes Virus Study Group of the International Committee for the Nomenclature of Viruses (Roizman, personal communication; Deinhardt and Wolf, 1978):

Alpha-herpesviruses (prototype: human HSV) generally have a wide host range, and although they are usually highly cytopathic, association with malignant diseases has been claimed.

Beta-herpesviruses (prototype: cytomegalovirus (CMV)) have a narrow host range and a slow replicative cycle and grow best in fibroblasts. CMV have been associated with naturally occurring, self-limited infectious mononucleosis(IM)-like diseases and Kaposi's sarcoma in man, with benign and malignant lymphoproliferative diseases after experimental infection of nonhuman primates, and with transformation of fibroblastic cells in vitro.

Gamma-herpesviruses (prototype: EBV) generally have a narrow host range (usually limited to the same order as the natural host), they multiply in and/or transform lymphocytic cells and some can also cause lytic infections in certain types of epithelial and fibroblastic cells. MDV, herpesvirus of turkeys (HVT), the EBV-like viruses of old-world and HVS and HVA of new-world monkeys belong to this group and all, with the exception of HVT, an attenuated strain of HVS, and some incompletely evaluated EBV-like viruses of old-world nonhuman primates, have been

Table 1. Potentially oncogenic herpesviruses

Virus	Natural host		Experimental host		Cell culture	
	Species	Disease	Species	Disease	Lytic infection	Trans-formation
Alpha-herpesviruses						
Herpes simplex virus types 1 and 2	Man	Lytic infection; (neoplasia)?	Many	Lytic infection	Yes	Yes (F)[a]
Equine herpesvirus 3	Equine	Lytic infection	Several species	Lytic infection	Yes	Yes (F)
Infectious bovine rhinotracheitis virus	Bovine	Lytic infection	Several species	Lytic infection	Yes	Yes (F)
Beta-herpesviruses						
Human cytomegalovirus	Man	Lytic infection; self-limited lymphopro-liferative disease (Kaposi's sarcoma)?	None		Yes	Yes (F)
Simian cytomegalovirus	Individual primate species	Lytic infection; proliferative disease not observed	Individual primate species	Lytic infection; self-limited lymphopro-liferative disease; lymphoma	Yes	?
Gamma-herpesviruses						
Marek's disease virus	Avian	Lytic infection in cells of feather follicles only; neurolympho-matosis	Restricted to avian species	Latent infection or lymphomatosis	Yes	Not known
Herpesvirus saimiri	*Saimiri sciureus*	None known	Several new-world monkeys	Lymphoma	Yes	(Yes) (LT)
Herpesvirus ateles	*Ateles* sp.	None known	Several new-world monkeys	Lymphoma	Yes	Yes (LT)
Epstein-Barr virus	Man	Infectious mononucleosis; Burkitt's lymphoma; (nasopharyngeal carcinoma)	*Saguinus* and *Aotus* sp.	Self-limited lymphopro-liferative disease; lymphoma	No[b]	Yes (LB)

[a] Cell type transformed: F, fibroblasts; LB, B lymphocytes; LT, T lymphocytes.
[b] With the exception of virus activation in occasional lymphoblastoid carrier cells.
[c] Only limited replication with some inconsistent results; see text.

Table 1 *(continued)*

Virus	Natural host		Experimental host		Cell culture	
	Species	Disease	Species	Disease	Lytic infection	Trans-formation
Unclassified Viruses						
Carp pox virus	Carp	Benign epithelioma	?	?	?	?
Lucké's herpesvirus	Frog	Kidney carcinoma; lytic infection at cold temperatures	?	?	(Yes)[c]	?
Herpesvirus sylvilagus	*Sylvilagus* sp.	Self-limited lympho-proliferation; lymphoma (?)	?	?	Yes	Not known
Guinea-pig herpesvirus	Guinea-pig	Lytic infection (leukemia)?	?	?	Yes	Yes (F)

shown to be associated with lymphoproliferative diseases and in the case of EBV, also with nasopharyngeal carcinoma (NPC).

Other currently unclassifiable herpesviruses (e. g., of fish and frogs) have not been studied as extensively as the mammalian and avian herpesviruses, but the association of frog LHV and kidney carcinomas is of particular interest in the context of this discussion.

A causative role between some herpesviruses and given tumors has been established with reasonable assurance in some instances, e. g., Lucké's renal carcinoma of frogs, Marek's disease (neurolymphomatosis) of chickens, Burkitt's lymphoma (BL) and NPC of man, the lymphoproliferative diseases caused by HVS and HVA in some nonhuman primate species, and the mostly self-limited lymphoproliferative disease of rabbits with herpesvirus sylvilagus. In other instances the role played by herpesviruses in tumor induction, as for example HSV in the pathogenesis of cervical carcinoma, remains almost speculative.

B. HERPESVIRUSES OF COLD-BLOODED ANIMALS

I. CARP POX VIRUS

Carp pox virus (CPV) is misnamed because it is a typical herpesvirus and the pathologic lesion with which it is associated, although commonly called "carp pox," is a benign epidermal tumor *(epithelioma papillosum)*, which was described as early as the sixteenth century (Wolf, 1973). CPV can be demonstrated regularly in the epitheliomas of carp *(Cyprinus carpio)*. Virus morphology and replication seem to be similar to other herpesviruses and, as with all other herpesviruses, cells harboring mature or immature herpes virions show signs of cell degeneration. As yet CPV has not been isolated or grown in cell cultures. The disease in carp is of little or no commercial importance, which may explain in part why few investigators have studied it.

II. LUCKÉ'S HERPESVIRUS

Already in 1934 Lucké postulated a virus etiology for the adenocarcinomas occurring in ~ 1%–9% of leopard frogs *(Rana pipiens)* (see Granoff, 1972, 1973 a, 1973 b; Rafferty, 1972; Mizell, 1975; Sharma, 1976). He observed acidophilic intranuclear inclusion bodies, similar to those induced by herpesviruses, in the tumor cells of hibernating frogs or frogs held at 4°–9 °C (Lucké, 1934) and successfully transmitted the tumors by cell-free extracts (Lucké, 1938, 1952). Herpesvirus particles were first demonstrated in tumor cells with electron microscopy by Fawcett in 1956, but proof of the etiologic or causative relationship between LHV and renal adenocarcinomas of frogs was long in coming (Naegele et al., 1974). With the possible exception of the reports of Wong and Tweedell of 1974, 1975, it has not yet been possible to grow LHV consistently in cell cultures to obtain purified cloned virus. Tweedell and Wong (1974) described the propagation of LHV in a pronephrotic cell line derived from stage 25 *Rana pipiens* embryos; the cultures also contained an adenovirus, at least in the early passages, and tumor induction by extracts of infected cells of the third virus passage (shown by electron microscopy to contain only herpesvirus particles) was reported in only one experiment. As yet this cell culture system has not yielded a reliable method for the propagation of LHV in vitro.

As a number of other viruses have also been isolated from these frog tumors in other experiments, tumor induction by herpesvirus purified by differential centrifugations of tumor extracts must be met with some reservation, as contamination of such preparations with other viruses cannot be excluded. Nevertheless, none of the other viruses (frog virus 4, a herpesvirus different from LHV; polyhedral cytoplasmic deoxyribovirus and a papova-like virus) have been shown to have any oncogenic potential (see Granoff, 1973 b). On the other hand, it has been established experimentally that inoculation of preparations containing LHV purified by rate zonal centrifugation induces tumors in frogs inoculated during the embryonic or larval stages when the kidney target cells for transformation are differentiating. Already differentiated kidney cells seem to be refractory to virus-induced transformation. In addition, the appearance of tumors depends on the development of the immunologic system of the frogs at the time of inoculation. A further proof of the causal relationship of LHV and renal tumors was provided by the demonstration of herpesvirus m-RNA in the virus-free "summer tumors" (Collard et al., 1973), the induction of virus in "summer tumors" by prolonged exposure to cold temperatures (4°–9 °C), and the demonstration of a LHV-induced cell surface antigen expressed on tumor cells irrespective of whether or not they contained complete virions, intracellular viral antigens, or only viral DNA in a repressed state (Naegele and Granoff, 1977). This membrane antigen must be an early gene product similar to the EBV-induced membrane antigen (MA) of BL cells and its expression must be compatible with the survival of the cells.

LHV is of particular interest in a discussion of herpesvirus-induced neoplasias since, except for CPV, it is the only animal herpesvirus having an established association with an epithelial tumor. It therefore parallels the interrelationships between EBV and NPC.

The dependence of LHV genome expression on temperature has been well studied, but the biochemical control mechanisms remain unknown. At an elementary level it can be said that at low temperatures (4°–9 °C) virus multiplication proceeds and infected cells are destroyed, whereas at higher temperatures (20°–25 °C) virus multiplication is arrested during an early step in the replicative cycle and transformation can occur and/or be maintained. However, in Tweedell and Wong's experiments LHV could be propagated in pronephric cell cultures kept at 25 °C, whereas tumor cells kept at 11.5 °C or higher in vitro by Breidenbach et al. (1971) showed no LHV replication even though LHV virions could be demonstrated in pieces of the same tumors kept at 7.5 °C. This system bears some similarities to the inhibition of virus multiplication of some temperature-sensitive mutants of a number of other viruses, but even this comparison brings us no closer to explaining the biochemical reactions responsible for LHV gene regulation.

C. HERPESVIRUSES OF WARM-BLOODED ANIMALS

I. MAREK'S DISEASE VIRUS

Until recently Marek's disease or neurolymphomatosis of chickens was important because of its world-wide effect on the supply of a relatively inexpensive source of protein; in the United States alone the disease cost 200 million dollars per annum. Marek's disease also has the distinction of being the first neoplastic disease to be controlled by a live nonpathogenic virus vaccine (see Biggs, 1973; Nazerian, 1973; Purchase, 1974, 1976; Nazerian et al., 1976; Payne et al., 1976), but of greatest interest to this discussion, in certain important respects Marek's disease is similar to BL of man.

Marek's disease was described first in Hungary at the beginning of this century (Marek, 1907). The disease became more prevalent in the late 1920s when for the first time it became a more frequent cause of death in commercial poultry. It continued to increase slowly throughout the 1930s, in part probably due to the concurrent development of high density, intensive systems of poultry farming. A more explosive increase developed in the 1950s with the appearance of a highly pathogenic form of disease which occurred in epizootic form and spread rapidly through all countries with developed poultry industries until control measures in the form of vaccines were developed.

Since a review of the entire literature on Marek's disease would exceed the objectives of this chapter, only a summary of current knowledge of the pathogenesis of Marek's disease follows and the disease is discussed in the context of its similarities and dissimilarities to EBV and other lymphotropic herpesviruses. Marek's disease consists of inflammatory and proliferative lesions, leading to swelling of peripheral nerves, with infiltration by proliferating lymphocytic cells, which can lead to demyelination and loss of axons. The infiltrating cells are not only those transformed by MDV but also inflammatory reactive elements. Similar lesions may occur in the brain and lymphomas may develop in all tissues, with or without a concurrent peripheral lymphocytosis. Degenerative changes are observed in the transitional, intermediate, and corneal layers of the germinative layer of the epithelium lining the feather follicles and these are the only lesions in which large amounts of MDV are produced.

Virus is disseminated through the shedding of MDV with cellular debris from the feather follicles; as the virus is relatively stable in this form (up to 6–8 weeks) transmission through chicken-pen dust is highly effective over considerable distances (Witter, 1972; Biggs, 1973; Nazerian, 1973).

MDV is recognized as a typical herpesvirus and as the causative agent of Marek's disease. The virus shares many structural, biochemical, and biologic similarities with other herpesviruses, particularly with EBV and the lymphotropic herpesviruses of new-world monkeys, HVS and HVA. Antigens cross-reacting between EBV and MDV have been reported by Naito et al., (1970), Ono et al. (1970), and Kato et al. (1972); between LHV, MDV, HSV, and CMV, by Kirkwood et al. (1972); between MDV, pseudorabiesvirus (PRV), and HSV, by Ross et al. (1972), Sharma et al. (1972a), and Nazerian (1973); between EBV, MDV, and bovine infectious rhinotracheitis virus (IBR), by Evans et al. (1972); between EBV and HVS, by Morgan (1977); and between CMV, HSV, and varicella-zoster virus by Krech and Jung (1971). In our laboratories no cross-reactivities between MDV, HVS, and EBV were found by neutralization and immunofluorescence (IF) tests (Deinhardt and Shramek, unpublished data). Since in the other published reports the apparent cross-reactivity was not associated with any of the defined virus structural or virus-induced proteins, the specificity of the observed reactions needs confirmation. Attempts to show common characteristics between the DNAs of these viruses failed (Wagner et al., 1970). Studies by molecular hybridization demonstrated partial DNA homologies between HSV, between EBV isolates from man and nonhuman primates (Falk et al., 1976a; Gerber et al., 1976), and between HVS and HVA (Fleckenstein et al., 1978), but no significant cross-hybridization could be demonstrated between HSV, EBV, HVS, HVA, MDV, or CMV (zur Hausen and Schulte-Holthausen, 1970; zur Hausen et al., 1970; Bachenheimer et al., 1972; Huang and Pagano, 1974; Roizman and Kieff, 1975; Fleckenstein et al., 1978). These findings do not necessarily contradict the reports of common antigens, but the relatedness between these groups of viruses as measured by cross-antigenicity or DNA homology is obviously not great and no common features which could be linked to the oncogenicity of these agents have been identified.

The question has been raised whether MDV alone is responsible for the lymphomas in Marek's disease or if the disease is caused by activation of an endogenous C-type RNA virus or through a concerted action of MDV and an avian C-type RNA virus. Early reports indicating that C-type RNA viruses were an essential part in the process of cell transformation or at least substantially enhanced the oncogenicity of MDV in cell cultures (Frankel and Groupé, 1971) or in vivo (Peters et al., 1973; Frankel et al., 1974, 1975) were not confirmed in later studies (Witter et al., 1975a; Calnek and Payne, 1976; Nazerian et al., 1976). Frankel et al. (1975) in a later study showed that chickens inoculated with MDV alone developed lymphomas without a demonstrable activation of C-type RNA viruses. Even so it cannot be denied that interaction between herpesviruses and C-type RNA viruses may take place and may to a certain extent influence the course of the disease, but at this time it would be erroneous to assign an essential role in herpesvirus oncogenesis to the ubiquitous C-type RNA viruses.

Infection with MDV under natural conditions occurs horizontally, very early in the life of the chicken (under commercial conditions within 1–3 weeks after hatching), mostly through inhalation or pecking of contaminated dust or litter. MDV multiplies regularly in the feather follicles but only very rarely and only in occasional cells of other normal or diseased tissues of infected chickens. MDV infects and transforms lymphocytic cells with T cell characteristics (Powell et al., 1975; Ross et al., 1977; Sharma et al., 1977), but in this case only an abortive infection results with transformation of the infected cells and maintenance of the viral genome over many cell generations, probably in a plasmid form like EBV, although true integration of at least part of the virus genome cannot be excluded (Nazerian et al., 1976). MDV-carrying tumor cells, like EBV-transformed cells, can be grown as permanent cell lines but with one major difference: MDV-transformed cells carry T cell markers, whereas the EBV-transformed cells have B cell (bone marrow-derived lymphocyte) characteristics. Virus expression varies in these cell lines and with time may be almost completely lost. In some but not all instances virus expression can be enhanced or induced by 5-iododeoxyuridine (IUDR) in lines that had lost virus genome expression, in a fashion similar to stimulation of EBV expression in cell lines derived from BL, normal individuals, or cell lines transformed in vitro (Dunn and Nazerian, 1977). Virus multiplication in these cells is inhibited early in the replicative cycle, before the major structural viral proteins are formed, since progression of viral multiplication to that stage is incompatible with cell survival, a situation very similar to that with EBV and the EBV-like or other lymphotrophic herpesviruses of primates. An early virus-associated nuclear antigen like EBV nuclear antigen (EBNA) has not been identified in MDV-transformed cells, but a probably nonstructural, MDV-induced membrane antigen similar to lymphocyte-detected membrane antigen (LYDMA) or early membrane antigen (EMA) present on EBV-transformed tumor cells (see Epstein and Achong, 1977) has been demonstrated. Marek's disease tumor-associated surface antigen (MATSA) does not stimulate the production of antibodies during the normal course of the disease (although chickens can react to this antigen with antibody formation during an intensive course of hyperimmunization) (Witter et al., 1975 b), but like LYDMA it triggers a cell-mediated immune response and probably plays a major role in the immunologic control of Marek's disease (Witter, 1976; Powell and Rowell, 1977; Ross, 1977).

Marek's disease has been controlled through the development of live attenuated virus vaccines (see Hilleman, 1972; Witter, 1976; Nazerian et al., 1976; Churchill, 1977) consisting either of (a) originally pathogenic strains of MDV attenuated through multiple passages in cell cultures, (b) naturally nonpathogenic field strains of MDV, or (c) the MDV-like HVT, which is nonpathogenic for chickens. Each of these vaccines has advantages, but HVT vaccines have been used most extensively and provide adequate protection for the commercial life of chickens. The mechanism of protection is not entirely clear; protection against challenge with MDV begins almost immediately after exposure to the vaccine virus and does not appear to be entirely dependent on antibody production. The vaccine virus establishes a generalized infection and HVT viremia usually persists for the life of the chicken. Viral interference may be a mechanism responsible for the immediate, at least partial protection against MDV challenge. Induction of MATSA-like antigens on the surface of some HVT-infected cells and induction of cell-mediated immunity rather than development of circulating antibodies may be the major factor of HVT-induced immunity. MATSA has been associated with the transformed state of lymphocytic cells and HVT is considered nononcogenic, but a few cells may be transformed by HVT. This may occur infrequently, without being enough to induce a clinically manifest neoplastic process, but frequently enough to stimulate immunity sufficient to reject even large numbers of transformed cells during subsequent infection with oncogenic MDV (Witter et al., 1975 a; Sharma and Coulson, 1977).

The possibility that MDV was dangerous for man became a concern when the dust from chicken pens was realized to be heavily contaminated and infectious, and the association of other herpesviruses such as EBV, HVS, and HVA with malignant lymphoproliferative diseases was established. The question of the possible suscepti- bility of man to MDV demanded urgent attention when the cultivation of MDV in human cells was reported, although the report was immediately shown to be erroneous due to contamination with HSV. Attempts in several laboratories to cultivate MDV in primate cells and other mammalian cells in vitro failed. Inoculation of MDV into marmoset monkeys (Sharma et al., 1972 b), which are highly susceptible to lymphoma induction with HVS or HVA and to an extent also with EBV, or into cynomolgus, rhesus and bonnet monkeys (Sharma et al., 1973), failed to induce any disease or detectable subclinical infection. In addition, surveys for antibodies among individuals heavily exposed to chicken dust of MDV-contaminated flocks were entirely negative.

Marek's disease is an avian disease caused by a herpesvirus similar to but not measurably genetically related to EBV. MDV cannot infect mammalian cells in vitro or in vivo and therefore does not pose a health hazard for mammals. The pathogenesis of the disease is similar to EBV, but the target cells are T and not B lymphocytes. There are now good prospects that Marek's disease will be completely eradicated through vaccination.

II. HERPESVIRUS SYLVILAGUS

Herpesvirus sylvilagus was isolated first by Hinze in 1968 from wild cottontail rabbits in Wisconsin, USA (Hinze 1968, 1969, 1971a, b; Hinze and Chipman, 1972). The first isolate was obtained from normal kidney cell cultures; later it was found that herpesvirus sylvilagus could also be isolated from blood cells. The virus proved to be different from herpesvirus III (herpesvirus cuniculi) and to be highly cell-associated (Ley and Burger, 1970). It was antigenically different from all known herpesviruses including HSV, EBV, HVS, HVA, PRV, and herpesvirus tamarinus and its host range was limited to cottontail rabbits. Inoculation of cottontail rabbits with herpesvirus sylvilagus generally caused a benign, self-limited lymphoproliferative disease, but disseminated lymphomas were seen in some animals. Virus could be isolated from proliferating cells by cultivation with rabbit kidney cells, but free virus was virtually absent in the inoculated animals and attempts to establish lymphoid cell lines from lymphoproliferating tissue or from the peripheral circulation have failed (Wegner and Hinze, 1974). Like LHV, EBV, HVS, and HVA, the virus is transmitted horizontally, not vertically, and excretion in saliva has been demonstrated (Spieker and Yuill, 1977a). Transmission by fleas or mosquitoes (Spieker and Yuill, 1976, 1977b) has not been found and the epidemiology of herpesvirus sylvilagus, other than its frequent occurrence in cottontail rabbits in Wisconsin, is largely unknown (Lewis and Hinze, 1976). The lymphoproliferative disease caused by this virus consists of accumulations of "immature lymphoid cells in various stages of development rather than a uniform population of lymphocytes arrested at one stage of maturation" (Hinze, 1971b), but, nevertheless, the massive cellular invasion with loss of normal structure in lymph nodes and kidneys justifies the classification of some of these lesions as truly neoplastic. As with MDV, EBV, HVS, and HVA infectious proliferating cells do not appear to contain virus structural antigens or complete virions in vivo, but virus activation takes place spontaneously when these cells are cocultivated with susceptible cottontail rabbit cells. It it not known whether herpesvirus sylvilagus infects B or T lymphocytes, if the disease is mono- or multiclonal, or where complete virus multiplication takes place in the animal. No explanation for the different reactivities of individual cottontail rabbits to inoculation with the same virus preparation (i. e., from a very mild, benign and limited lymphoproliferative response to a much more severe and truly malignant disease) has been found although this variability has been compared to the situation with EBV in man. The comparison seems unjustified as the response in rabbits appears to be a graded response to the initial infection, whereas the pathogenesis of IM, BL, or NPC is likely to be multifactorial.

III. GUINEA-PIG HERPESVIRUS

Guinea-pig herpesvirus (GPHV) was isolated originally by Hsiung and Kaplow (1969) from spontaneously degenerating kidney cell cultures of strain 2 guinea-pigs; during the following years further isolations were made from tissues such as buffy coat cells of leukemic and nonleukemic guinea-pigs (Hsiung and Kaplow, 1970; Hsiung et al., 1971b), from L_2C guinea-pig leukemia cells (Rhim, 1977), and occasionally also from strain 13, Hartley and Muta guinea-pigs (Bhatt et al., 1971; Hsiung et al., 1971b). The ultrastructure and morphogenesis of GPHV is typical for herpesviruses (Fong et al., 1973); the virus is highly cell-associated in vivo, existing mostly in a latent state, but it can be isolated readily by cocultivation. For example, leukemic lymphoblasts contain no detectable GPHV antigens in vivo, but antigens appear spontaneously in almost all cells within 48–72 h after explantation into cell cultures; death of the cells follows (Nayak, 1972). Only a few, if any, virus particles can be detected in such cultures, but GPHV can be isolated when such cells or other guinea-pig tissues are cocultivated with susceptible cell cultures. GPHV grows best in vitro in epithelioid cultures such as primary guinea-pig or rabbit kidney cells; some GPHV strains have been shown also to grow in Vero and mink lung cells, but other primary human, monkey, equine, hamster, and mouse cells have been reported to be resistant to infection with GPHV (Bhatt et al., 1971; Hsiung et al., 1971a; Rhim, 1977). The virus does not share antigens in common with human CMV, HSV, equine herpesviruses types 1 and 2, MDV, LHV, and EBV according to Hsiung et al. (1971a), but cross-reactions between GPHV and HSV in complement fixation (CF) have been reported by Rhim (1977).

GPHV is particularly interesting because it was isolated first only from strain 2 guinea-pigs, which are highly susceptible to the transplantable L_2C guinea-pig leukemia. In the light of findings with other herpesviruses such as LHV, MDV, EBV, and HVS the question of its possible relationship to this leukemia was raised. However, it was found that the L_2C leukemic cells also carried a RNA virus (Nadel et al., 1967; Opler, 1967), which although it could be induced in neoplastic and normal guinea-pig cells with 5-bromodeoxyuridine (BUDR) (Rhim et al., 1973, 1974; Hsiung, 1975) could not be grown in cell cultures. The characteristics of this virus put it into the class of endogenous murine B-type viruses; however, since it is serologically distinct from this group of viruses, with some unique morphologic characteristics, it may belong to an additional, as yet undefined group of retraviruses (Hsiung, 1975).

The relationship of either GPHV or guinea-pig retravirus alone or combined to L_2C leukemia is unresolved (Fong and Hsiung, 1977; Hsiung, 1977). Both viruses exist latently in leukemic and nonleukemic guinea-pigs and in animal strains that are susceptible or resistant to the L_2C leukemias. Inoculation of GPHV into guinea-pigs, mice, rabbits, hamsters, or rhesus monkeys did not induce disease (Bhatt et al., 1971; Lam and Hsiung, 1973a, b) and the mild and temporary lymphoid hyperplasia observed by Hsiung (1975) after infection of 1-day-old guinea-pigs with GPHV or a mixture of GPHV and guinea-pig retravirus was probably a response to an acute herpesvirus infection rather than an expression of neoplasia. The reported malignant transformation of hamster (Fong et al., 1973; Michalski et al., 1976) and rat embryo cells (Rhim, 1977) by GPHV in vitro adds to the large number of reports of transformation of rodent cells by various herpesviruses. This occurs not infrequently when infection takes place under partially nonpermissive conditions for virus multiplication. In this particular situation it is interesting that fully infectious GPHV can be used for infection under normally optimal temperatures for virus multiplication and that the block in virus multiplication leading to cell transformation must be entirely host-cell dependent. Although this is of considerable interest, it does not necessarily support the notion of a causal relationship between GPHV and guinea-pig leukemia.

IV. SHEEP PULMONARY ADENOMATOSIS

Sheep pulmonary adenomatosis (Jaagsiekte) is a contagious disease, which was thought to be caused by a herpesvirus isolated both in England and South Africa (Mackay, 1969 a, b; Smith and Mackay, 1969; Malmquist et al., 1972; de Villiers et al., 1975), but attempts to induce the disease with the isolated herpesvirus failed (Mackay and Nisbet, 1972). More recently a retravirus has been isolated from diseased lungs (Perk et al., 1974). In preliminary experiments published so far, pulmonary adenomatosis was induced in sheep inoculated with the retravirus and not in sheep inoculated with the herpesvirus, but much more extensive lesions developed in a higher percentage of animals when both agents were inoculated together (Martin et al., 1976). However, only a few animals were used in these studies and no final judgement can be made yet about the role one or both of these agents play in the pathogenesis of Jaagsiekte.

V. PRIMATE HERPESVIRUSES

1. Herpes Simplex Virus of Man

HSV has been associated by seroepidemiologic data with cervical carcinoma and DNA or mRNA sequences homologous to part of the HSV DNA have been reported in cervical carcinoma cells (Frenkel et al., 1972; Jones et al., 1978). However, the seroepidemiologic data are inconsistent, in some instances even contradictory, and the molecular hybridization data also need confirmation and clarification before human carcinoma cells can be believed regularly to carry all or part of the HSV genome. In addition, a number of nonstructural HSV-related antigens have been described in cervical carcinoma cells, but their specificity, either for cervical carcinoma or for HSV, has not been demonstrated consistently. In earlier seroepidemiologic studies neutralization tests were used, whereas in certain of the later studies antibodies to nonstructural antigens appearing early during the lytic cycle of infection were measured, but their specificity is somewhat doubtful. For this reason no detailed discussion of these systems will be given and the reader is referred to Nahmias (1972), Rapp (1974), Rapp and Buss (1974), Muñoz et al. (1975), Schneweis et al. (1975), Roizman and Kieff (1975).

However, none of the antigens described can be detected in all cervical carcinomas, or even in all cervical carcinomas of a given type or stage, and no consistent antibody patterns were demonstrated in double blind studies using sera of controls and carcinoma patients. Likewise the isolation of HSV from a cervical carcinoma reported by Aurelian (Aurelian et al., 1971; Aurelian, 1973) has not been repeated and probably represented a laboratory contamination. The "virus-specific, labile, nonvirion antigen in herpesvirus infected cells" (Tarro and Sabin, 1970, 1973; Sabin and Tarro, 1973; Sabin, 1974; Tarro, 1975) and the appearance of corresponding antibodies in cancer patients also belong in the group of irreproducible results and the fate of a number of HSV-associated antigens awaits final judgement (Hollinshead et al., 1972, 1973; Ibrahim et al., 1976). During the past few years complement-dependent cytotoxic antibodies against established cervical carcinoma cell lines and/or HSV-infected cells have been studied in carcinoma patients and controls and higher antibody titers have been reported for carcinoma patients. However, antibody titers against carcinoma cells or HSV-infected cells were often discordant and the specificity of the reactivities measured in these tests remains to be established (Thiry et al., 1974; Christenson, 1977).

Transformation of fibroblastic cells of rodents by HSV under experimental conditions in vitro has been demonstrated by a number of laboratories (Duff and Rapp, 1971a, b; Munyon et al., 1971; Rapp et al., 1973; Garfinkle and McAuslan, 1974; MacNab, 1974; Takahashi and Yamanishi, 1974; Boyd, 1975; Boyd and Orme, 1975; Boyd et al., 1975; Munk and Darai, 1975; Munk et al., 1975; Pope, 1975; Darai and Munk, 1976; Leiden et al, 1976; Darai et al., 1977; Donner et al., 1977; Gupta and Rapp, 1977; Schröder et al., 1977). Laboratory transformation of human cells has also been reported (Darai and Munk, 1973; Munk and Darai, 1973; Kucera and Gusdon, 1976; Marcon and Kucera, 1976). In these experiments transformation was achieved by infecting cells with partially inactivated virus or under only partially permissive conditions. The transformed rodent cells frequently, if not always, carried C-type RNA viruses (Flügel et al., 1977). It is undetermined whether transformation was caused solely by the herpesvirus, by cooperation between the herpesvirus and a C-type RNA virus, or solely by C-type RNA virus after activation by the herpesvirus infection. The transformed cells usually lost the expression of herpesvirus antigens on prolonged cultivation and it is unclear if survival of the entire or part of the herpesvirus genome was essential for maintaining the transformed condition of the cells. These systems are of great interest, but their relevance to carcinogenesis in vivo remains an open question and overinterpretation of these results, obtained in somewhat artificial systems, must be avoided.

2. Cytomegaloviruses

CMV are as widely distributed among animals of all classes as the alpha-herpesviruses. CMV causes silent or acute cytolytic infections, sometimes with a severe course in immunologically compromised patients. If infection occurs in utero it causes extensive embryopathies (fetal malformations) and distortion of normal development (see Wright, 1973). That an IM-like disease following transfusion of fresh blood in normal and particularly in debilitated or immunosuppressed patients could also be caused by CMV was first recognized by Klemola and Kääriäinen (1965) and studied subsequently by a number of laboratories (Nakao et al., 1967; Klemola et al., 1967, 1970; Rifkind, 1968; Foster and Jack, 1969; Evans, 1972; Fiala et al., 1975; Oill et al., 1977; Lerner and Sampliner, 1977). Oncogenic activity of CMV was considered for three reasons: CMV was isolated frequently from patients with malignant disease, particularly lymphomas; the lymphoproliferative nature of CMV-associated disease resembled IM; and other herpesviruses such as LHV, MDV, EBV, HVS, and HVA are associated with malignancy or with cell transformation in vitro (HSV). The isolation of CMV from patients with malignancies was probably due to activation of a latent CMV infection caused by a depression of the patients' immune system through their disease or chemotherapy. It is unlikely that CMV plays a causative role in the primary malignant disease. Even so inoculation of a CMV isolated from African green monkeys into *Cercopithecus aethiops, Macaca mulatta, M. speciosa, Papio hamadryas,* and *Saimiri sciureus* induced lymphoproliferative disease in all species inoculated except for the new-world species *S. sciureus*. The severity of the disease was related to the size of the inoculum and some animals died. Animals inoculated with 1×10^8 ID_{50} of CMV also developed a severe and uniform leukemoid reaction, described as follows: "In the bone marrow of all three infected monkeys a significant increase of the young forms of granulocytes and metamyelocytes was noticed together with relative decrease of mature neutrophiles . . . In the peripheral blood marked shift to the left of the leukocyte formula with an increase of abnormal rod-nuclear neutrophiles up to 23%–26% and leukocytosis were observed. On the third day of an acute phase of the disease single young forms of granulocytes (myelocytes and metamyelocytes) appeared in the blood," (Deichman et al., 1972 a, b; Deichman, personal communication). The experimentally induced disease had most of the characteristics of a self-limited IM-like disease and not those of a true lymphoma; the leukemoid reaction was comparable to those accompanying other infectious processes. The association of CMV with white blood cells in acute or persistent infections is unclear. Infection of buffy coat cells with CMV led to some virus production and possibly to prolonged survival of the cells but no lymphoblastoid cell lines carrying CMV have been established, with the exception that an EBV-transformed cell line may also carry CMV DNA (Joncas et al., 1975). Only already established lymphoblastoid cell lines with B cell characteristics but not T cell lines could be infected in one study by Huang and Pagano (1975). Another EBV-infected, nonproducer B lymphoblastoid cell line and peripheral buffy coat cells without differentiation between the various cell populations were infected in a more recent study by Jeor and Weisser (1977). A low-grade infection, which persisted for more than 10 days, was induced, but no permanent lymphoblastoid cell lines could be established from the infected buffy coat cells. The association of CMV in persistently infected patients with or without symptoms of CMV infection with mononuclear leukocytes has been repeatedly reported (Fiala et al., 1975; Joncas et al., 1975), but it is not known whether CMV is associated with one or more cell types and in which form the infection persists, i. e., a low-grade chronic infection or true latency.

Another approach for testing the oncogenic potential of CMV was evaluation of its transforming ability in vitro of other than lymphoid cells. Transformation of hamster embryo cells with ultraviolet(UV)-irradiated and partially inactivated CMV isolated from a human prostate gland was described by Rapp and his associates (Albrecht and Rapp, 1973; Nachtigal et al., 1974): the transformed cells carried virus-specific cytoplasmic and cell surface antigens (Albrecht and Rapp, 1973; Lausch et al., 1974; Rapp and Li, 1975), which could be detected by humoral and cell-mediated immune reactions (Murasko and Lausch, 1974, 1975, 1976; Lausch et al., 1975 a, b) and produced tumors in newborn hamsters (Albrecht and Rapp, 1973). Some of the CMV-specific antigens disappeared after prolonged cultivation in vitro or passage through animals and it has not been possible to re-isolate CMV from the transformed cells. The fate of the CMV genome in these cells is not entirely clear, i. e., it has not been shown whether the entire or only part of the viral genome is carried in the transformed cells or whether the genome, if present, is integrated or exists in a plasmid form.

Stimulation of cellular DNA synthesis by human CMV was shown by Jeor et al. (1974) and limited growth of human cells infected with CMV in agarose by Lang et al. (1974). Establishment of permanent human cell lines transformed by UV-irradiated CMV was described by Geder et al. (1976) and their oncogenic capacity was established in athymic mice (Geder et al., 1977). The transformed cells apparently share a cell surface antigen with the CMV-transformed hamster cells. A nuclear antigen has been observed which in an anticomplement IF test can be stained with some but not all human sera containing CMV antibodies (Geder and Rapp, 1977). This antigen is probably related to the early "6-h antigen" appearing in cells lytically infected with CMV and has been compared to EBNA. Both the nuclear and cell surface antigens are maintained during prolonged cultivation in vitro or passage through animals. It will be interesting to test human tumors for this antigen and sera from patients with malignancies for the corresponding antibodies.

In addition, CMV was isolated by Giraldo et al. (1972 a, b) from several African Kaposi's sarcomas. This group (1975) also showed that European patients, mostly with regressing Kaposi's sarcoma, had higher neutralizing antibodies against CMV than appropriately selected controls, but the correlation did not hold true for African patients, most of whom had progressing tumors. The virus was clearly identified as a CMV by Glaser et al. (1977), but the question of its role in the pathogenesis of Kaposi's sarcoma is completely open. Nevertheless, as Kaposi's tumors probably originate from reticuloendothelial tissues, sometimes in a fashion almost like an acute disease, and since it occurs preferentially in small areas in Africa like BL, a link with an oncogenic virus was discussed already in 1967 by Dayan and Lewis; further controlled studies of the possible interrelationships of this neoplasm and CMV deserve support.

3. Gamma-Herpesviruses of Primates

The group of gamma-herpesviruses should be discussed together because they share a number of biologic characteristics: all members of this group induce benign or malignant lymphoproliferative diseases, persist in lymphocytic cells of infected primates for life, and are transmitted horizontally by infectious virus produced in vivo at as yet unidentified sites. These viruses can be divided into two subgroups, those isolated from man and old-world monkeys and those isolated from new-world monkeys. The former consist of EBV-like herpesviruses isolated from chimpanzees (Gerber and Birch, 1967; Gerber et al., 1977; Landon et al., 1968), baboons (Deinhardt et al., 1976; Falk et al., 1976 a, 1977; Lapin, 1976; Gerber et al., 1977; Rabin et al., 1977a), and one orangutang (Rasheed et al., 1977). The second group consists of HVS (Meléndez et al., 1968, 1969 a, b; Falk et al., 1972 a, b; Deinhardt et al., 1973 a, b) and HVA (Meléndez et al., 1972; Deinhardt et al., 1973 b; Falk et al., 1974 a, c). All EBV-like viruses of old-world primates share common antigens and partial DNA base homology, as do HVS and HVA, but the two groups do not share any detectable antigens or DNA homology with each other. In addition, the EBV-like viruses infect and transform B cells, whereas HVS and HVA infect and transform T cells.

a) Herpesvirus Saimiri and Herpesvirus Ateles

HVS and HVA were first isolated from the new-world squirrel monkeys *(Saimiri sciureus)* and spider monkeys (*Ateles* sp.), respectively (see Deinhardt et al., 1974b; Wolfe and Deinhardt, 1978). The original isolations were made by chance when it was observed that kidney cell cultures derived from normal animals spontaneously degenerated with a cytopathic effect somewhat reminiscent of herpesvirus-infected cultures. It was shown subsequently that the cytopathic effect was indeed caused by herpesviruses and that these viruses were antigenically and biologically distinct from a previously isolated HSV-like agent of squirrel monkeys (Holmes et al., 1964; Melnick et al., 1964). The latter virus, plathyrrhine herpesvirus Type I (originally misnamed marmoset herpes virus or herpesvirus tamarinus, because it was isolated first from accidentally infected marmosets which had been housed together with squirrel monkeys after capture), was shown later to cause diseases in squirrel monkeys (the natural hosts) similar to the lesions caused by HSV in adult man; in marmosets and some other new-world primate species it almost always caused a fatal generalized infection similar to herpes neonatorum of man (Holmes et al., 1966). Understanding of the true nature of HVS and HVA evolved from a number of studies and can now be summarized as follows.

Morphology. Because lytic systems (see below) are available for HVS and HVA, the morphology of virus replication could be studied. HVS and HVA were identified as typical herpesviruses. Their relatively slow cycle of replication enabled investigators to distinguish clearly between cytoplasmic and nuclear phases of virus maturation (Morgan et al., 1970, 1973, 1976; Heine et al., 1971; Heine and Cottler-Fox, 1975; Friedmann et al., 1976; Banfield et al., 1977; Tralka et al., 1977). Intranuclear, unusual tubular and laminated structures as well as 40-nm rings were observed; the rings were seen also in a number of other herpesvirus infections (Tralka et al., 1977) and probably represent the inner capsid of a herpes virion (Roizman, 1972). The tubular and laminated structures have been described recently by Banfield et al. (1976, 1977) as lamella-particle complexes, similar to structures described in the cytoplasm of tumor cells in "hairy" cell leukemia, monoblastic leukemia, Waldenström's macroglobulinemia, chronic lymphatic leukemia, "lymphosarcoma cell leukemia," monkey renal proximal tubular cells, and a lymphoma of the northern pike. Structures consisting of "an elaborate system of paired membranes together with immature virus particles" were described already in the nuclei of chicken kidney cells infected with MDV by Epstein et al. (1968). Nuclear tubules were described in rabbit kidney cells infected with herpesvirus sylvilagus by Heine and Hinze (1972) and in a Lucké frog kidney carcinoma by McKinnell and Ellis (1972). Although, of course, the details of these structures differ somewhat in the various virus systems, they all may represent unusual forms of virus replication. Morgan et al. (1976) interpret these structures as "an aberrant assembly of virus components" and Banfield et al. (1977) state that the tubular lamella-particle complexes "may represent accumulation of virus structural proteins and nucleic acids" and that in HVS "the lamella may be composed of capsomeres, which on longitudinal or cross section would give a periodic striated structure; the sectioned capsomere of the herpesvirus saimiri virion has a periodicity and appearance identical to those of the sectioned lamella." Although these studies have furthered our understanding of the morphology of the replicative cycle of two oncogenic primate herpesviruses, virus structures have been detected neither in tumor tissues nor in circulating transformed lymphoblasts, as seems to be the rule with all gamma-herpesviruses, including EBV.

Nucleic Acids. The DNA of HVS and HVA has been characterized in a number of studies and was found to be similar, consisting of linear molecules of about 100×10^6 daltons (Laufs and Fleckenstein, 1973; Fleckenstein and Wolf, 1974; Fleckenstein and Bornkamm, 1975; Fleckenstein et al., 1975 a, b, 1976, 1977, 1978; Simonds et al., 1975; Bornkamm et al., 1976; Werner et al., 1977). Two populations of virions containing M genomes or H genomes were consistently isolated from various HVS stocks. The HVS M genome consisted of $\sim 28\%$ repetitive heavy (H)-DNA (70.6% guanine plus cytosine) and 72% unique light (L)-DNA (35.8% guanine plus cytosine) and had a density of 1.7045 g/ml in CsCl. The HVS H-DNA consisted of repeat units of 830,000 daltons arranged in a tandem configuration with a density of 1.7292 g/ml in CsCl. L-DNA had a constant length of 71.6×10^6 daltons and a density of 1.6951 g/ml in CsCl and was inserted between two pieces of repetitive H-DNA which were variable in length ($1-34 \times 10^6$ daltons), but the sum of the two H regions was almost constant ($30-35 \times 10^6$ daltons). The DNA of the M genome was infectious in cell culture and oncogenic in some species of marmosets (Fleckenstein et al., 1975b). The HVS H genome was not infectious and contained only repetitive H-DNA segments. Non integrated, episomal viral DNA in the form of covalently closed circular DNA molecules has been isolated from HVS-transformed nonproducer cells which could no longer be induced to produce complete infectious virus by various induction methods. These DNA molecules have a higher molecular weight (131.5×10^6 daltons) than the linear molecules isolated from various HVS virions. Partial denaturation mapping showed a uniform arrangement of H- and L-DNA sequences in all circles, containing two L-DNA regions (mol. wt. $54.0 \pm 1.8 \times 10^6$ daltons and $31.5 \pm 1.3 \times 10^6$ daltons) and two H-DNA regions (mol. wt. $25.6 \pm 1.9 \times 10^6$ daltons and $20.0 \pm 0.8 \times 10^6$ daltons) of constant length. The sequences of both L regions had the same orientation and the sequences of the shorter L-DNA piece appeared to be a subset of those of the longer pieces, containing totally only $\sim 75\%$ of the genetic information of the L-DNA isolated from HVS virions (Werner et al., 1977). The HVA genome is similar to the HVS genome, but some strain differences exist; the M genomes of strains 810 and 73, respectively, have a density of 1.7061 and 1.7064 g/ml in CsCl and consist of 74.2% and

73.6% of a unique light L-DNA (37.5% guanine plus cytosine with a density in CsCl of 1.6967 g/ml, mol. wt. 70×10^6 daltons) and of 25.8% and 26.4% of a highly repetitive heavy H-DNA (74.5% and 74.8% guanine plus cytosine with a density of 1.7330 and 1.7333 g/ml in CsCl). The HVA-H genome of both strains is composed of H-DNA subunits of about 0.93×10^6 daltons aranged in tandem.

About 35% of the L regions of HVA and HVS anneal with each other but with considerable mismatching (9% base sequence divergence), which leads to a reduction in the melting temperature of 13.5 °C. There is also only limited base sequence homologies (10%) between the H regions of HVS and HVA with at least 13% divergence of their base pairs.

Mismatching within the L regions of ∼ 2.4% was observed between two isolates of HVA (strains 810 and 73) with a reduction in melting point temperature of 3.4 °C. The H-DNA of the same two isolates showed a reduction of 5 °C of the melting temperature of heteroduplexes as compared with homoduplexes representing 3.3% mismatch (Fleckenstein et al., 1978). No base homology has been found between HVS or HVA DNA and EBV DNA. Digestion with endonucleases, especially with R. Sma I, provided an excellent tool for detailed and rapid characterization and allowed the differentiation by their cleavage pattern of at least three different strains of HVS and two strains of HVA (Fleckenstein and Mulder, personal communication).

Viral Proteins. The proteins of HVS and HVA have not been identified in detail, but several antigens have been recognized (Pearson et al., 1972, 1973; Klein et al., 1973; Rabin et al., 1973 b). An early antigen (EA), corresponding closely to the EA of EBV, is formed first in the nucleus and spreads later to the cytoplasm. It can be demonstrated in infected cells in two forms, punctate and trabecular, but an accurate analysis of these two forms has not been made and it is not known if the two forms are antigenically different. Formation of EA is not dependent on formation of new viral DNA; appearance of EA must be linked with inhibition of the host cell macromolecular synthesis because it is incompatible with cell survival, a relationship also seen in EBV. A late antigen (LA), similar to the VCA of EBV, is formed after new viral DNA is produced; antibodies to LA appear to be virus-neutralizing antibodies. Surface MA have been demonstrated on infected cells, but their exact nature needs to be established further. A nuclear antigen, similar to EBNA of EBV, has not been identified either in HVS- or HVA-transformed cells. However, nuclear antigens should be sought with indirect techniques that concentrate nuclear antigens by binding the antigens of a large number of cells to comparatively few indicator cells, as recently shown by Ohno et al. (1977a, b) for the EBV-like viruses of old-world nonhuman primates.

There is complete cross-reactivity between different isolates of HVS. Some minor antigenic differences may exist between HVA isolates from *Ateles geoffroyi* and *A. paniscus,* but this needs more detailed analysis. HVS and HVA cross-react only partially with each other and neither share detectable antigenic determinants with EBV or the other EBV-like viruses.

Propagation in vitro *of HVS and HVA:* In contrast to EBV, HVS, and HVA can be propagated in vitro in a number of fibroblastic or epithelioid cells of old-world and new-world primates, including man; both viruses undergo a complete lytic cycle of replication in culture (see Deinhardt et al., 1974 b). Both viruses grow best in cells of new-world primates, particularly owl monkey kidney cells and in some clones of Vero cells (derived originally from an African green monkey kidney). Multiplication in human cells, although reported by three laboratories, yields only very low virus titers and apparently pretreatment of the cell cultures with diethylaminoethyl-dextran is needed to enhance their susceptibility (Ablashi et al., 1971a; Meléndez et al., 1972; Falk et al., 1974 c).

On the other hand, infection and transformation in vitro of lymphocytic cells have been much more difficult to achieve with HVS and HVA than with EBV. It is possible to transform in vitro marmoset but not squirrel monkey lymphocytes with HVA (Falk et al., 1974 b) and probably with HVS (Wright and Deinhardt, unpublished data); transformation with HVA and probably also with HVS is enhanced when lymphocytes are stimulated before infection with low doses of mitogens. The transformed cells grow indefinitely, as lymphoblastoid cell lines (LCL); they are virus-producer or non-producer cells and have some T cell characteristics. Virus-carrying LCL can also be isolated from mononuclear cells from the peripheral circulation or from tumors of experimentally infected animals, and both types of LCL (cells transformed in vitro or in vivo) have the same characteristics. Tumor cells always lack virus expression in vivo, but after explantation some cells undergo spontaneous induction of virus genome expression during the first days of cultivation. LCL derived from tumor cell cultures (or through transformation in vitro) generally remain virus-positive for various lengths of time. Those individual cells of LCL which progress to formation of viral EA invariably die, EBNA-like nuclear antigen has not been identified, and the presence of cell surface MA will be discussed below. Spontaneous virus genome expression not infrequently ceases after prolonged cultivation over several months but continues to be inducible by IUDR or BUDR (Neubauer et al., 1974) in some but not all of such "nonproducer" LCL. It appears that those LCL which cannot be induced may have lost part of the viral genome. Neither the need for part of the HVS or HVA genome to be integrated into the host cell DNA for transformation to be induced or maintained, nor the possibility that existence as plasmid DNA is sufficient for transformation, has yet been established. Some evidence for the second possibility is provided by recent experiments by Werner et al. (1977) which showed in at least one noninducible, nonproducer cell line the presence of only circular extrachromosomal HVS DNA, which contained only ~ 75% of the total HVS L-DNA (see above).

A late virus-induced cell surface MA has been described by Pearson et al. (1972, 1973), Klein et al. (1973), Pearson and Davis (1976), and Prevost et al. (1976) in lytically infected cells. Current studies indicate that a LYDMA-like antigen (Svedmyr and Jondal, 1975; Klein et al., 1976) may be present on HVS- or HVA-transformed marmoset cells (Deinhardt, McGrath and Falk, unpublished data). In these experiments marmoset cells were transformed in vitro with EBV or HVA and were reacted in an autologous system against the lymphocytes of the same animal from which the lymphocytes for transformation had been obtained. Mixed lymphocyte cultures and lymphocytotoxicity tests were set up before and after reinoculation of the transformed nonproducer cells into the autologous animals. Initial results indicated that both EBV- or HVA-transformed cell lines carry a LYDMA-like antigen, but these preliminary data need confirmation. Of particular interest will be the testing for similarities or antigenic relationships between these cell surface MA of EBV and HVA.

The HVS- or HVA-induced LCL are classified as T cell-like because they do not exhibit surface-bound immunoglobulins (Ig), receptors for the Fc fragment of aggregated Ig, or the third component of complement (C'3). Most lines form rosettes with sheep or African green monkey erythrocytes (E rosettes) (Wallen et al., 1973;

Deinhardt et al., 1974b; Falk et al., 1974b; Wright et al., 1976, 1978) and react with specific anti-marmoset, T cell serum (Johnson, 1977; Wright et al., 1978). The ability of the transformed cells to form E rosettes was inconsistent and some LCL may lose this characteristic after prolonged cultivation. Treatment of LCL with neuraminidase usually enhanced E-rosette formation, but some LCL did not form E rosettes even after neuraminidase treatment under conditions previously established as optimal for other LCL. In addition, normal T cells as well as established LCL of *Callithrix jacchus* never formed E rosettes with the sheep erythrocytes commonly used for these tests but did form E rosettes with African green monkey erythrocytes (Wright et al., 1978). T cell markers were demonstrated with a specific anti-marmoset T cell serum by complement-dependent serum cytotoxicity and by IF tests (Johnson, 1977) in all HVS- or HVA-transformed LCL, including those which formed no E rosettes. These results should be compared to results of studies on the characteristics of EBV-transformed human and primate cells, which showed no T cell but some B cell characteristics (see below).

Infection in natural hosts: The natural hosts of HVS and HVA are squirrel monkeys *(Saimiri sciureus)* and spider monkeys *(Ateles* sp.) respectively. Seroepidemiologic studies of captured wild animals indicated that infection occurred early in life and antibodies probably persisted for the animals' lifetimes since almost all juvenile or adult captured wild animals had anti-LA and some also anti-EA antibodies (Falk et al., 1972b; Meléndez et al., 1972; Deinhardt et al., 1973a; Rabin et al., 1973b). In a large squirrel monkey colony, maintained for metabolic studies, it was shown that all adults had anti-LA antibodies and that babies were born with detectable levels of maternal antibodies which declined to nondetectable levels during the first 8–12 weeks of life. The first natural infections were detected by seroconversion at $\sim$ 6 months, and by 2–3 years of age all animals had developed antibodies. No disease was observed during natural seroconversion or after experimental infection of seronegative, 9–12 month-old squirrel monkeys with up to 10^5 plaque forming units (PFU) of HVS; these animals were observed closely with careful monitoring of hematologic values, but no abnormalities were observed even though inoculated animals became "viremic" at $\sim$ 17–24 days after inoculation, i.e., virus could be isolated from their circulating lymphocytes by cocultivation with susceptible cells, and they simultaneously developed antibodies to HVS-EA and HVS-LA. The antibody response to HVS-EA was generally lower than that to HVS-LA and it declined again after several months to a year, whereas antibodies to HVS-LA remained at fairly constant and higher levels. The circulating lymphocytes continued to yield virus over an observation period of more than a year and like naturally infected animals, these animals probably remain virus-positive for life. In summary, although antibodies have been demonstrated in these squirrel monkeys, their appearance and persistence in relation to natural infection needs further study. After natural infection virus could be recovered with an equally high incidence from the circulating lymphocytes of animals of all ages, an indication that "viremia" must persist for life once infection has occurred. Virus-yielding cells were identified as T cells (Wright et al., 1976) and it was shown that $\sim$ 1 in $0.5–1.0 \times 10^6$ circulating T cells yielded virus during cocultivation, although viral antigens were never detected in vivo in the lymphocytes, nor was it possible to establish LCL from seropositive squirrel monkeys. Excretion of virus from the oropharynx, in stool, or in urine during experimental infection has not been established accurately, because studies are greatly hampered by the unavailability of enough seronegative squirrel monkeys. However, it was shown that virus spreads from inoculated squirrel monkeys to uninoculated cagemate controls. HVS was isolated from a throat swab of such a control 163 days after inoculation of his cagemate (Falk et al., 1973 b). In another study with a group of ten females, captive for more than 1 year and shown to be HVS carriers, virus was isolated consistently from oropharyngeal secretions of nine of the animals for a period of over 5 months (Falk et al., 1973 a). Excreted virus was mostly cell-associated, but low levels of free virus could also be detected. Although no site of virus multiplication has been identified in the natural host (or in experimentally infected animals), it is probable that the virus is shed in the form of virus-carrying mononuclear cells from oropharyngeal lymphoid tissue and that virus is activated only in an occasional cell, thus explaining the small amount of cell-free virus found in oropharyngeal excretions. It is not known whether or not virus also multiplies in epithelial cells of the oropharynx as has been claimed recently for EBV (Lemon et al., 1977). Virus was never isolated from seronegative squirrel monkeys and so far no lymphomas which could be associated with certainty with HVS or HVA have been observed in squirrel or spider monkeys. This is hardly surprising since lymphomas appear to be rare in these species and the few that have been observed in squirrel monkeys have not been examined completely. If HVS and HVA do induce lymphomas in their natural hosts with a frequency similar to the induction by EBV of BL in man, insufficient squirrel and spider monkeys have been observed for too few years for many HVS- or HVA-induced lymphomas to have been seen.

In summary, HVS and HVA spread horizontally, they infect their natural hosts early in life without producing clinical disease, and infected animals become virus carriers for life. The virus infects lymphoid cells with T cell characteristics, without a measurable, complete cycle of virus replication in vivo. The site of virus multiplication in other cells is unknown although small amounts of cell-free virus are excreted in the oropharynx. Virus-carrying lymphocytes yield virus spontaneously when cocultivated in vitro with susceptible cells. The cells in which virus production is induced disintegrate, a situation identical to that in EBV, except that T and not B cells carry the virus and no fully permissive system for the propagation of EBV exists.

Infection of Experimental Hosts. Both HVS and HVA cause lymphomas and lymphoblastic leukemias in a number of new-world nonhuman primate species other than their natural hosts (see Deinhardt et al., 1974b; Rangan et al., 1977). "Natural" transmission has occurred occasionally when, for example, squirrel and owl monkeys (*Aotus* sp.) were kept in close contact immediately after capture or during transport from South America (Hunt et al., 1973; Rabin et al., 1975 a). Transmission of HVS to rabbits with induction of lymphoproliferative disease has been reported (Hunt et al., 1975), but attempts to transmit HVS to old-world nonhuman primates failed or were inconsistent. Similarly, occasional accidental inoculation of man has neither resulted in disease nor have antibodies to HVS been detected with certainty. Despite reports of limited, low-grade propagation of HVS in human fibroblastic cells, human lymphocytes seem to resist infection with HVS or HVA; however, the susceptibility of cells of old-world primates and man to infection in vitro with HVS and HVA needs further study.

Experimentally induced disease has been studied most extensively in some species of marmosets (Hunt et al., 1970, 1972; Wolfe et al., 1971) and owl monkeys (Hunt et al.,

1970; Ablashi et al., 1971b; Cicmanec et al., 1974). The disease induced in susceptible new-world nonhuman primates is lymphoma or lymphoblastic leukemia, which in most instances progresses rapidly and kills the animal within 20–150 days. Young animals of some species seem to be more susceptible than adults, whereas in other species no difference in susceptibility between newborn, juvenile, or adult animals was observed. Some species of marmosets (particularly *Saguinus* sp.) are particularly susceptible and as few as 10 PFU of HVS or HVA induces fatal lymphoproliferative disease in all inoculated animals. Some owl monkeys are more resistant and a chronic disease lasting for many months may ensue from which animals sometimes recover or may not get ill at all. Within days inoculated marmosets develop an infiltration of lymphoblastoid cells at the inoculation site which is histologically well developed by 5–7 days.Infiltration of local and systemic lymph nodes and almost all other organs with lymphoblastic cells follows rapidly over a period of a few weeks and death occurs from generalized lymphoma with or without peripheral lymphoblastic leukemia. The experimentally induced diseases are usually classified histologically as diffuse lymphomas of a poorly differentiated lymphocytic type, although stem cells sometimes predominate in HVS-induced lesions of cotton-topped marmosets *(Saguinus oedipus)* and small, well-differentiated lymphocytes predominate in HVS-induced lesions of white-lipped marmosets (*Saguinus fuscicollis* and *S. nigricollis*). Hematologic abnormalities are usually observed first in the peripheral circulation around 25 days after inoculation; the total white cell count rises from $\sim$ 6–15,000/mm^3 to $\sim$ 175,000/mm^3 with a steady increase in mononuclear lymphocytic cells with absolute lymphocyte counts from 6,500–117,000/mm^3 and the appearance of many immature or abnormal lymphoblasts. Cell-free virus has never been isolated from the oropharynx, stool, tissue extracts of normal or diseased organs, or blood plasma of inoculated animals or at death. Similarly, no viral antigens have been detected in circulating white cells, tumor cells, or normal tissues by IF and infection was never transmitted to noninoculated cagemate controls. However, when tumor cells were cultured in vitro, alone or together with cells susceptible to lytic infection by HVS or HVA, viral antigens appeared spontaneously in some cells as early as 48 h after explantation, with the subsequent production of complete infectious virus and death of the virus-producing cells. The progression of infection in inoculated animals could be followed by cocultivation with susceptible cells of cells obtained at various intervals post infection; during the entire course of the disease virus was isolated only from mononuclear cells with T cell characteristics. Isolations were made first 3 days post inoculation in cocultures of cells from the site of inoculation or regional lymph nodes, and after 14 days post inoculation also from circulating mononuclear cells. At 14 days post inoculation only 1 PFU of HVS was recovered from 10^5 circulating mononuclear cells; the number of cells yielding virus increased constantly during the following weeks and as few as ten cells were needed to recover one PFU of HVS during the week prior to death.

As described above, LCL can be established from abnormal circulating cells or tumor cells. Chromosomal analysis of tumor cells immediately after explant and during later cultivation showed that in contrast to BL, experimentally induced tumors were multiclonal. This could be shown because tumor cell lines consisted of cells with both male or female chromosomes (marmosets frequently twin and all heterosexual twins examined are hematopoietic chimeras, as proven by the presence of both sets of sex chromosomes in different hemopoietic cells of each twin) (Chu and Rabson, 1972; Marczynska et al., 1973; Rabin et al., 1973a).

Circulating HVS antibodies appear in experimentally infected marmosets, owl, and howler monkeys (Wolfe et al., 1971; Pearson et al., 1972, 1973; Klein et al., 1973; Rangan et al., 1977) much later than in similarly infected squirrel monkeys and often only after the animals had already become "viremic" (i. e., no free virus but virus could be isolated by cocultivation of circulating lymphocytes). Antibodies to HVS-LA usually became detectable 30–35 days after infection, but antibody production may be delayed in an occasional animal until shortly before death. Appearance of antibodies to HVS-EA lagged behind HVS-LA antibodies and sometimes reached only low titers or were undetectable. Antibodies both to HVS-LA and HVS-EA sometimes showed a pronounced decrease, with HVS-EA antibodies sometimes disappearing altogether, in parallel with a dramatic terminal increase in the white cell count and the relative number of lymphocytes. In animals with protracted disease (some owl monkeys) or Capuchin monkeys not developing lymphomas, antibodies to HVS-EA were detected over a prolonged period of time (Pearson et al., 1973, 1974; Rabin et al., 1975b). The persistent or even increasing titers of antibodies to HVS-EA were interpreted as a reflection of the presence of increasing numbers of virus genome-carrying cells and this accords with the ability to isolate virus at all times from circulating mononuclear cells. Antibodies to HVS-MA were evaluated by IF and by antibody-dependent lymphocytotoxicity (ADLC) (Prevost et al., 1976). ADLC, a particularly highly sensitive system, established that a close correlation exists between the increase of antibodies to HVS-MA, the progress of the disease, and the loss of responsiveness of T lymphocytes to mitogens (which is no paradox because Fc receptor-bearing cells and not T cells are responsible for the ADLC reaction). Antibodies to HVS-MA developed and remained at relatively low or moderate levels in animals not developing lymphoma or leukemia, but rose to high titers shortly before or simultaneously with the first signs of lymphoproliferation in those monkeys which developed malignant disease. Cell-mediated immune responses generally declined in experimentally infected animals as more and more normal T cells were replaced by immature abnormal lymphoblasts (Wallen et al., 1975a, b).

Vaccination Against HVS and HVA. Laufs (1974) and Laufs and Steinke (1975, 1976) vaccinated marmosets *(S. oedipus)* with heat- and formaldehyde-inactivated virus; the animals developed good neutralizing antibody titers after 4–6 inoculations, were resistant to challenge with small doses of live HVS (less than 500 LD$_{50}$) but succumbed through lymphoma development after challenge with higher doses. Another approach was the noninfectious vaccine suggested recently by Pearson and Scott (1977), who used preparations of antigen-positive, plasma membrane vesicles of lytically infected owl monkey kidney cells for immunization of marmosets. The vesicles were not infectious and inoculated animals developed good virus-neutralizing LA and MA but no EA antibodies; no data on the resistance of immunized animals to challenge with active virus have been reported yet. Schaffer et al. (1975) isolated an attenuated strain of HVS after serial passage of wild-type HVS in cell culture at 39 °C (HVS-39); this strain must have been a chance mutation because several subsequent attempts to isolate a similar strain from the same wild-type HVS by identical techniques failed. In susceptible marmosets the attenuated strain behaved like wild-type HVS in squirrel monkeys; marmosets infected with the attenuated strain developed antibodies against

HVS-LA and HVS-EA and became virus carriers, i. e., HVS could be isolated from circulating mononuclear cells by cocultivation techniques. HVS-39 seems to be a very stable mutant because over a prolonged period of time (> than 1 year) in virus-carrier animals, several passages in cell culture, and passage through marmosets, the virus has not acquired any pathogenicity. "Viremic" animals carrying HVS-39 in their lymphocytes with serum antibody titers to HVS-LA of 1:64–128, HVS-EA of 1:10–64, and a neutralizing titer of 1:32 nevertheless developed lymphomas and died when challenged with 770 PFU ($\geq 375 \, LD_{50}$) of wild-type HVS, although the disease course was significantly prolonged in comparison with the typical, shorter disease period in inoculated control marmosets. Two questions arise from these studies: (a) what mechanisms repress proliferation of virus-infected lymphocytes in marmosets inoculated with HVS-39 and (b) are these mechanisms similar to those regulating the interaction of HVS with lymphocytes in the natural hosts, squirrel monkeys? In contrast to marmosets infected with oncogenic HVS, infection of marmosets with HVS-39 resulted in a virus-cell interaction that did not lead to uncontrolled lymphoproliferation but to an apparently lifelong carrier state, comparable to the cell interaction occurring in squirrel monkeys after primary infection with wild HVS which also persists apparently for life. Although vaccination of man with live attenuated EBV vaccines may pose insurmountable problems (Chap. 19), comparative studies of oncogenic and attenuated HVS will provide valuable information about the pathogenesis of HVS-induced disease, the genetics of oncogenic and nononcogenic herpesviruses, and the nature of latent and malignant infections by these agents (Falk et al., 1976 b).

Treatment of HVS or HVA Infections. Attempts have been made to influence both the multiplication of HVS or HVA in vitro and induction of the disease in vivo. Although some retardation of virus multiplication was achieved with high doses of interferon in vitro, interferon did not substantially influence HVS- or HVA-induced disease in marmosets *(S. oedipus)* (Adamson et al., 1974; Laufs et al., 1974). Phosphonoacetic acid was shown by Ablashi et al. (1977) and Barahona et al. (1977) to have some inhibitory effect on HVS replication in cell cultures, but the effect was reversible and virus multiplication resumed when the drug was removed. Attempts at treating the malignant disease in vivo were reported by Adamson et al. (1974); cytosine arabinoside and adenine arabinoside induced a reduction in circulating transformed cells, somewhat similar to induction of remission through chemotherapy in leukemia in man, but nevertheless the animals died from recurrence of disease or other complications. Steroids, Oncovin, and cyclophosphamides had similar effects in preliminary studies. The lymphomatous diseases induced by the gamma-herperviruses in nonhuman primates, particularly the disease induced in marmosets and owl monkeys, should provide ideal systems for evaluation of future therapeutic agents.

b) EBV-Like Viruses of Nonhuman Primates

Antibodies to EBV in chimpanzees and other old-world nonhuman primates (baboons, cynomolgus, rhesus, and African green monkeys) were demonstrated first by Gerber and Birch in 1967, Gerber and Rosenblum (1968), and Goldman et al. (1968). Additional reports of the presence of EBV antibodies followed: in chimpanzees by

Landon and Malan (1971); in Taiwanese monkeys *(Macaca cyclopis)* by Chu et al. (1971); in four species of *Macaca* (rhesus, bonnet, cynomolgus, and Taiwanese monkeys) and *Cercopithecus* sp. (African green and talapoin monkeys) by Dunkel et al. (1972); in gorillas, chimpanzees, baboons, and rhesus monkeys by Kalter et al. (1973); and a number of others (discussed recently in detail by Frank et al., 1976). Initially it was unclear whether the antibodies found in nonhuman primates were due to infections contracted from man after capture, as had been shown to occur previously with other human viruses, or if the animals were infected naturally in the wild. Nor was it known if the viruses carried by the nonhuman primates were identical to human EBV or if they represented cross-reacting but distinct EBV-like agents. In 1968 Gerber and Rosenblum showed that rhesus monkeys bled 1–4 days after capture had antibodies to EBV and Levy et al. (1971) demonstrated EBV antibodies in chimpanzees bled immediately after capture in the wild. These studies clearly show that antibodies to EBV VCA and EA occur naturally in old-world nonhuman primates and it may be that all the old-world species are immune to EBV. On the other hand, EBV antibodies have not been identified in prosimians *(Lemur macaco, Galago crassicaudatus,* and *Nycticebus coucang)* or (with the exception of two studies) in new-world nonhuman primates (Hapalidae: *Saguinus mystax, S. oedipus, S. fuscicollis, S. nigricollis;* Cebidae: *Alouatta palliata, Ateles geoffroyi, Lagothrix lagotricha,* and *Saimiri sciureus)* – see Frank et al. (1976). An exception was reported by Gerber and Lorenz (1974), who detected CF antibodies reacting with crude EBV antigens (which could not however be demonstrated by IF) in *S. oedipus, S. fuscicollis,* and *S. mystax.* Recently some low titer antibodies against EBV VCA have been detected by IF in marmosets (*Saguinus* sp.), which had, however, been in captivity for a long time (Deinhardt et al., 1978). Whether new-world nonhuman primates have naturally acquired antibodies cross-reacting with EBV antigens must therefore be left open. If such antibodies can be detected in feral animals, it would indicate that the new-world nonhuman primates, like the primates of the Old World, harbor viruses antigenically related to EBV. However, such viruses have not been isolated from new-world primates despite many attempts, most of which succeeded only in detecting HVS- or HVA-like viruses. It seems more likely today that the antibodies observed in new-world primates, if proved to be specific, represent infections contracted from man after capture, since at least some new-world nonhuman primate species have been shown to be susceptible to experimental infection with human EBV (Chap. 16).

The actual presence of EBV-like herpesviruses in nonhuman primates was shown first by Landon et al. (1968), who established from uninfected normal chimpanzees permanent LCL with characteristics very similar to lines established from man. Herpesvirus-like particles were demonstrated by electron microscopy in occasional cells of these LCL and an antigenic relationship of these particles to EBV was established later. Comparisons of EBV VCA and EA with antigens detectable in the chimpanzee cell lines identified no difference between EBV and the EBV-like agent of chimpanzees and it was assumed that chimpanzees carried the same EBV as man. It was even conjectured that chimpanzees may serve as an animal reservoir for EBV and that arthropods may play a role in transmission between man and chimpanzee. The nature of the EBV-like virus of chimpanzees was clarified further only after the isolation of herpesvirus papio (HVP), another EBV-like virus isolated from baboons (Deinhardt et al., 1976, 1978; Falk et al., 1976a; Lapin, 1976; Gerber et al., 1977; Rabin et al., 1977a, b), restimulated interest in investigating the nature of the EBV-like nonhuman primate viruses, and the recognition of EBNA and development of molecular hybridization techniques allowed a further analysis. Gerber et al. (1976, 1977) reisolated EBV-like viruses from chimpanzee lymphocytes and also from the oropharynx of immunosuppressed chimpanzees. The LCL established from uninoculated normal chimpanzees had some B cell characteristics and the EBV-like agents, isolated from the oropharynx, infected and transformed B cells. VCA and EA of the chimpanzee agents were indistinguishable from those of EBV, but the chimpanzee EBNA, although cross-reacting with human EBNA, was antigenically clearly distinct. Hybridization between chimpanzee EBV DNA and human EBV DNA showed that chimpanzee EBV DNA contained sequences homologous only to 35%–45% of human EBV DNA.

The first baboon EBV-like virus (HVP) was isolated from lymphomatous baboons *(Papio hamadryas)* of a colony at the Institute of Experimental Pathology and Therapy, USSR Academy of Medical Sciences, Sukhumi. Over 30 cases of lymphoma and/or leukemia occurred there after the introduction into the colony of several baboons inoculated previously with human leukemic blood in 1967 (Lapin, 1974, 1976). Several LCL were established from lymphomatous baboons (Agrba et al., 1975) and these were shown to harbor the EBV-like virus, HVP. HVP was also isolated later from cocultures of peripheral lymphocytes of normal baboons of two colonies in the United States *(Papio hamadryas, P. anubis, P. papio, P. cynocephalus)* (Deinhardt et al., 1978).

Antibodies reacting with viral antigens in the HVP-carrying baboon LCL as well as with antigens of the EBV-carrying human LCL were demonstrated in a high percentage of animals of the Sukhumi colony, in a lymphoma-free colony near Sukhumi, and in normal baboons in the United States. The relationships of these viruses to human EBV is similar to the relationships between chimpanzee and human EBV; all three have apparently identical VCA and EA although the antigenic specificities of their EBNAs differ. At first EBNA-like antigens were not detected at all in HVP-infected cells but later, with the use of more sensitive techniques, HVP was shown to induce a nuclear antigen that partially cross-reacts with EBNA (Ohno et al., 1977a, b; Klein et al., 1978). However, its relationship to the chimpanzee EBV-induced nuclear antigen has not been determined.

HVP shares about 40% homology with human EBV by DNA-DNA hybridization; DNA-DNA hybridization between HVP and chimpanzee EBV has not been reported.

HVP transforms circulating lymphocytes of *Papio* sp., *Macaca mulatta, M. arctoides, Hylobates lar, Homo sapiens,* and *Saguinus* sp. in vitro (Falk et al., 1977; Rabin et al., 1977a) and in preliminary experiments HVP isolated from a lymphomatous baboon but not from a normal baboon induced lymphoproliferative disease in experimentally inoculated marmosets *(Saguinus* sp.) (Deinhardt et al., 1978). Adult and newborn animals were inoculated with the same virus preparations (live baboon cells producing HVP or autologous LCL transformed in vitro by HVP), but inoculated adults developed only a disease similar to an acute and often severe IM. Some animals died at the height of the illness. In the surviving animals the disease was self-limited and so far no late occurring relapses of lymphoproliferation have been observed. A precise histopathologic classification of the disease is difficult; the lesions were similar to a very strong reactive response, or to IM or immunoblastic lymphadenopathy, and in sections of some organs, to lymphoma. It is interesting that a response in newborn marmosets to inoculation of similar or even larger inocula of HVP than those used for adult animals has not been detected. This failure to react may parallel the difference in reaction of infants, older children, and adults to EBV. The complete lack of reaction to inoculation of HVP isolated from a healthy baboon may indicate that strain differences between various HVP isolates exist, similar to differences observed between various strains of EBV (Miller et al., 1975; Fresen et al., 1977; zur Hausen and Fresen, 1977). The lack of reactivity to the inoculation of the same or even greater numbers of lymphoblastoid cells carrying HVP isolated from a healthy baboon as compared to the response to inoculation of cells transformed by HVP isolated from a lymphomatous baboon also indicates that the lymphoproliferative disease is not merely a reactive response to inoculation of xenogenic cells but is more likely to be a virus-induced lymphoproliferation.

The lymphocytes transformed in vitro or in vivo by HVP have some B cell characteristics, but the extent of the expression of these markers was not uniform, different investigators reporting different results. The HVP- or EBV-transformed nonhuman primate cells did not form E rosettes nor did they react with specific anti-T cell serum and the extent of detectable, bound cell-surface immunoglobulins, $C'3$ or Fc receptors varied. Robinson et al. (1977, 1978) have discussed specific host-determined differences in expression of surface marker characteristics on human and simian LCL transformed by EBV; however, other studies indicate that a clear distinction between host species-regulated surface markers of EBV- or HVP-transformed LCL cannot be made. It has been shown that EBV or HVP also infect and transform B lymphocytes of nonhuman primates and these lymphocytes on prolonged cultivation may lose some of their B cell characteristics, as was shown to occur with EBV-transformed marmoset LCL by Rabin et al. (1977b) and Neubauer et al. (1978). They observed that these LCL formed rosettes with complement-coated erythrocytes after 2 months of cultivation but not after 15 months, whereas surface immunoglobulins and Fc receptors could be detected even after more than 16 months of cultivation. Similarly Fc receptors and at least low amounts of surface immunoglobulins have been demonstrated on EBV- or HVP-transformed LCL even after several years of culture (Deinhardt et al., 1974a; Falk et al., 1974b, 1977; Johnson, 1977). The differences in the results reported by Robinson et al. (1977, 1978) may be due to the different sensitivities of the test systems used.

The latest addition to this family of viruses is an EBV-like agent isolated from a LCL derived from an orangutang with spontaneous myelomonocytic leukemia (Rasheed et al., 1977). The orangutang LCL has no $C'3$ receptors, but 90%–100% of the cells have Fc receptors and surface-bound immunoglobulin. The VCA and EA of the orangutang EBV-like virus seem to be identical with human EBV; its EBNA-like antigen cross-reacts with both the chimpanzee and the human EBNA. The cell line has no detectable retraviruses and the orangutang EBV produced by this line transforms gibbon lymphocytes in vitro. DNA hybridization studies have not been reported and it is unclear whether the isolated virus has any causative relationship to malignant disease.

c) Other Viruses

A "rhesus leukocyte associated herpesvirus" was first described by Frank et al. (1973) and Bissell et al. (1973) and later named "herpesvirus macaca" by Graze and Royston (1975). Apparently the virus is common in wild as well as in laboratory rhesus monkeys; it is highly leukocyte-associated in vivo and has a narrow host range for growth in vitro. It induces lytic infection in vitro in human and rhesus fibroblastic cells and infects some human B cell but not T cell lines. The virus does not cross-react with known herpesviruses, including human and monkey CMV, EBV, HVS, and HVA. Squirrel monkeys can be infected experimentally; they seroconvert and become lifelong carriers. However, no disease or hematologic changes have been observed. The virus does not infect small laboratory animals or grow in embryonated hens' eggs. Although the virus has some similarities to EBV, its biologic significance is entirely unclear.

An outbreak of malignant lymphoma in the late 1960s and early 1970s in rhesus monkeys at the National Center for Primate Biology, University of California, resulted in the isolation of three herpesviruses from diseased animals (Stowell et al., 1971). Since materials from this outbreak were not available for study, the pathogenesis of the disease remains open. Apparently similar tumors were observed in three rhesus monkeys by Schneider (1975), who found them similar to human BL in histologic and electron-microscopic characteristics. Careful study of any further cases of this disease in rhesus monkeys is important, for it may provide a natural nonhuman primate model for EBV infection of man.

D. CONCLUSIONS

The recognition that EBV caused IM and was associated with BL and NPC of man revived general interest in the involvement of herpesviruses in cancers of other vertebrates. Today we recognize several herpesvirus groups, each of which is characterized by a distinct biologic behavior.

Two members of one of these herpesvirus groups, the LHV and the CPV, are related to epithelial cancers in their natural hosts (LHV with renal adenocarcinomas and CPV with benign epitheliomas). In their ability to transform epithelial cells in vivo these herpesviruses parallel the probable association of EBV with NPC. Unfortunately, drawing this parallel brings us no further to understanding why these viruses are predisposed to infecting tissues of epithelial origin or how they shift the fate of these cells, particularly as neither virus can be studied easily in lytic or transforming systems in vitro. LHV is of further interest because viral genome expression is temperature dependent but the relevance of this quality, biologically interesting as it is, to the expression of EBV in man is entirely speculative.

The relationships of the alpha- and beta-herpesviruses to proliferative disease, although far less than speculative, still rests on indirect evidence. Several alpha-herpesviruses, such as HSV 1 and 2, equine herpesvirus, and IBR grow in vitro to high titers in susceptible cell cultures and induce well-characterized lytic infections in their natural or experimental hosts. Under partially permissive conditions, i.e., infection with partially inactivated virus or culture incubation at supra- or suboptimal temperatures, these alpha-herpesviruses can transform cells in vitro so that they become able to cause tumors in syngeneic hosts. It remains unknown whether all or only part of the herpesvirus genome needs to persist in the cells to maintain transformation, or whether the herpesvirus acts like a physical or chemical carcinogen and induces cell transformation in a "hit-and-run" fashion without the need for a continued presence beyond the inducing event for the transformed cells to continue malignant proliferation. Understanding the underlying mechanism is hampered also by the fact that transformation is usually accompanied by an activation of endogenous retraviridae and a cocarcinogenic participation of herpesviruses and retraviruses must be considered. Much of the evidence for a causal relationship of HSV in inducing cervical and other carcinomas in man is indirect and apparently irrelevant to the situation with EBV. However, the knowledge of the molecular biology of this group of herpesviruses, and particularly of HSV, is far more advanced than for the other groups. Further definition of the events underlying complete and incomplete replicative cycles leading to lytic infection, latency, and (at least under experimental conditions) to transformation may become germane to the oncogenic role of EBV in man.

Far more relevant to the subject of this monograph are the beta- and gamma-herpesviruses. The beta-herpesviruses, i. e., human and simian CMV, occupy a position between the alpha- and gamma-herpesviruses: they cause lytic infection and latency in vivo and in vitro, transform fibroblastic cells in vitro under the same restrictive conditions required by alpha-herpesviruses to transform cells in vitro, and yet can become lymphocyte-associated and cause self-limited lymphoproliferative diseases similar to IM under natural conditions. After experimental infection of some species of nonhuman primates with high doses of virus they may even induce lymphomas. The importance of beta-herpesviruses lies in their apparently wide range of interactions with host cells or intact organisms, spanning from an interaction similar to lytic infections caused by HSV to lymphotropism and tumor induction similar to EBV or other members of the gamma-herpesvirus group. The recently intensified study of transformation by CMV promises further insights into the role of herpesviruses in lymphoproliferative disease. Gamma-herpesviruses have been recognized in birds, lagomorphs, and primates and the number of agents similar to EBV, HVS, or HVA identified during the past few years has risen remarkably. The gamma-herpesviruses have some striking characteristics: primary infection of the natural host leads to lymphoproliferation or, as in the case of HVS and HVA, to no detectable change at all. Virus multiplication cannot be detected in lymphocytic cells in vivo, in many cases the site(s) of virus multiplication being unknown. Reproduction of EBV in epithelial cells of tonsillar tissues in man has been reported, an observation requiring confirmation. This would explain the transmission of EBV by oral secretions, even though most of the virus in oropharyngeal secretions is cell-associated. Less is known about the multiplication of HVS or HVA in natural or experimental hosts: like EBV, HVS, and HVA are excreted and transmitted orally in the natural host, but excretion or transmission has not been shown in experimentally infected animals other than the natural host species. The gamma-herpesviruses have biologically similar early and late viral structural antigens; they probably all produce an early virus-induced nuclear antigen (although these have not yet been identified in HVS or HVA) and early and late cell surface membrane antigens. Appearance of the structural early antigens is incompatible with cell survival whereas the early nuclear antigens as well as some early cell surface membrane antigens are expressed in transformed cells and this production is obviously compatible with cell survival. Early structural antigens or later gene products have not been demonstrated in EBV-, MDV-, HVS-, or HVA- transformed cells in vivo, but spontaneous derepression occurs when cells are cultured in vitro. This is enigmatic because the mechanisms controlling apparently complete repression in vivo and spontaneous derepression in a few cells ($\sim$ 0.1%–10% of a population at any time) after explantation in vitro still await definition. Failure to detect virus expression in vivo in lymphocytic cells cannot depend solely on circulating antibodies or some other simple serum factor because cells cultured in the presence of antibodies to viral, structural, and virus-induced cell membrane antigens or in cell donor's own serum are not inhibited from spontaneous virus activation in vitro. On the other hand, virus activation in vivo may occur in occasional cells that are eliminated even before the stage of early structural or late cell membrane antigen formation; cell-mediated immune responses against even earlier cell membrane antigens may prevent the appearance of cells expressing EA or later gene products. However, this would require a highly efficient immune activity, operating against the surface antigens appearing on cells during initial stages of virus activation, perhaps at a time when these cells were more susceptible to immunologic attack. Nonproducer tumor cells lacking these particular antigens may be more stable and would therefore not be eliminated by this immune mechanism despite the fact that they carry other virus-induced cell surface membrane antigens. Studies of the immune response to HVS- or HVA-induced lymphomas, progressing rapidly or slowly, or studies of different species of marmosets inoculated with EBV or EBV-like viruses of old-world primates which develop a self-limited lymphoproliferative disease or overt lymphomas may help clarify the influence of the immune system on virus expression and tumor formation in vivo.

Association of retraviruses and gamma-herpesviruses has been reported: in some cases of BL retraviruses were detected. Extrapolation of this report to implicate such viruses in all BL and/or cell lines transformed by EBV would be unwise. No evidence for involvement of a retravirus has been found in nonhuman primates with EBV-induced lymphoproliferative disease or in nonhuman primate cells transformed by EBV in vitro. A retravirus was isolated from lymphomatous baboons of the Sukhumi colony; however, the causative role of the EBV-like herpesvirus (HVP) in the baboon lymphomatous disease is unclear. The retravirus does not transform cells in vitro and the Sukhumi isolate as well as other similar baboon endogenous retraviruses have not been shown to be oncogenic for baboons, other nonhuman primates, or other laboratory animals. On the other hand, HVP transforms B lymphocytes of several primate species in vitro and induces lymphoproliferative disease in at least two species of marmoset monkeys without detectable activation of retraviruses. This does not however establish that the lymphomatous disease in baboons is caused by HVP, since similar agents have been isolated from healthy baboons of several colonies. If undetected, dormant endogenous genomes of retraviruses were activated specifically in all cell transformations associated with herpesviruses, and if such genes would otherwise remain dormant, then it becomes a philosophical matter whether the oncogenic role is ascribed to the inducer, i.e., the herpesvirus, or to the induced gene. This question will not be settled until the precise molecular mechanism of cell transformation by herpesviruses has been determined.

Although the biologic activities of the EBV-like viruses of old-world nonhuman primates, of MDV and related viruses of the chicken, and of the HVS and HVA viruses of new-world nonhuman primates are similar in many aspects, there are also clear differences between the three groups. The EBV-like viruses transform B cells both in vivo and in vitro whereas MDV, HVS, and HVA infect and transform T cells. The disease induced by EBV in man is uniclonal whereas the disease induced experimentally by HVS and HVA is multiclonal. Natural distribution of EBV and EBV-like agents seems to be restricted to man and old-world nonhuman primates, although these viruses can transform cells of at least some new-world nonhuman primates in vitro and induce experimental lymphoproliferative diseases in vivo. The reverse situation, transformation of cells of old-world primates or induction of disease in old-world primates with HVS and HVA, has not been achieved regularly so their resistance or susceptibility remains unestablished. Relatedness between the members of the three virus groups can be demonstrated by analysis of antigens and DNA homology studies; extensive antigenic crossovers and considerable DNA homologies but no genetic relatedness have been demonstrated between the three groups. This does not contradict the genetic interrelationship of herpesviruses indicated by some of the studies on broadly cross-reacting herpesvirus-induced antigens, but the specificity of these antigens needs further definition. It is puzzling and of much interest to scholars of evolution that only B cell-tropic viruses are ubiquitous in old-world monkeys including man, whereas all similar viruses in new-world primates are T cell-tropic.

The regulatory mechanisms developing EBV infection into IM, BL, or NPC are unknown. Regulation may be host determined or may be due to the differences between EBV strains (Fresen et al., 1977; zur Hausen and Fresen, 1977). MDV, HVS, and HVA are more predictable in this respect, but although nononcogenic MDV and HVS strains exist we do not know what determines oncogenicity. HVS or HVA do not induce disease in their natural hosts but infection of some experimental hosts almost always leads to a fatal malignant lymphoproliferation. This difference in outcome has been argued to be due to a more efficient immunologic reaction against virus or virus-induced antigens in the natural hosts and a less efficient recognition and response to these antigens by the experimental hosts. Some experimental data support this view and biologically it makes good sense. Only some form of adaptation between host and virus could guarantee survival for both; this may have occurred by selection for genes which allow a rapid and effective immune response of the host. However, the difference between natural and experimental hosts in their response to infection may also be due to a different interaction of virus and host cell, which could result in a latent infection in cells of the natural hosts and in cell transformation of experimental hosts. This would not be an all-or-nothing effect since latent infection of cells must also occur in experimental hosts. In addition, some cell transformation, which is eliminated by the immune system, cannot be excluded in the natural hosts. Which of these mechansims, alone or in concert, controls the outcome of the infections of gamma-herpesviruses, cannot be decided yet, but the experimental systems provided by MDV, HVS, and HVA should help us to find out.

REFERENCES

Ablashi, D. V., Armstrong, G. R., Heine, U. Manaker, R. A.: Propagation of *herpesvirus saimiri* in human cells. J. Natl. Cancer Inst. **47**, 241–244 (1971 a)

Ablashi, D. V., Loeb, W. F., Valerio, M. G., Adamson, R. H., Armstrong, G. R., Bennett, D. G., Heine, U.: Malignant lymphoma with lymphocytic leukemia induced in owl monkeys by *herpesvirus saimiri*. J. Natl. Cancer Inst. **47**, 837–855 (1971 b)

Ablashi, D. V., Armstrong, G. R., Fellows, C., Easton, J., Pearson, G., Twardzik, D.: Evaluation of the effects of phosphonoacetic acid and 2-deoxy-d-glucose on *herpesvirus saimiri* and Epstein-Barr virus. In: Monograph of the 3rd International Symposium on Detection and Prevention of Cancer. Nieburgs, H. E. (ed.), Vol. **1**, pp. 245–262 (1977)

Adamson, R. H., Ablashi, D. V., Cicmanec J. L., Dalgard, D. W.: Chemotherapy of *herpesvirus saimiri* induced lymphoma-leukemia in the owl monkey. J. Med. Primatol. **3,** 68–72 (1974)

Agrba, V. A., Yakovleva, L. A., Lapin, B. A., Sangulija, I. A., Timanovskaya, V. V., Markaryan, D. S., Chuvirov, G. N., Salmanova, E. A.: The establishment of continous lymphoblastoid suspension cell cultures from hematopoietic organs of baboon *(papio hamadryas)* with malignant lymphoma. Exp. Pathol. **10,** 318–332 (1975)

Albrecht, T., Rapp, F.: Malignant transformation of hamster embryo fibroblasts following exposure to ultraviolet-irradiated human cytomegalovirus. Virology **55,** 53–61 (1973)

Aurelian, L.: Virions and antigens of herpes virus type 2 in cervical carcinoma. Cancer Res. **33,** 1539–1547 (1973)

Aurelian, L., Strandberg, J. D., Meléndez, L. V., Johnson, L. A.: Herpesvirus type 2 isolated from cervical tumor cells grown in tissue culture. Science **174,** 704–707 (1971)

Bachenheimer, S. L., Kieff, E. D., Lee, L. F., Roizman, B.: Comparative studies of DNAs of Marek's disease and herpes simplex viruses. In: Oncogenesis and herpesviruses. Biggs, P. M., de-Thé, G., Payne, L. N. (eds.), pp. 74–81. Lyon: IARC 1972

Banfield, W. G., Dawe, C. J., Lee, C. E., Sonstegard, R.: Cylindroid lamella-particle complexes in lymphoma cells of Northern Pike *(Esox lucius).* J. Natl. Cancer Inst. **57,** 415–420 (1976)

Banfield, W. G., Lee, C. W., Tralka, T. S., Rabson, A. S.: Lamella-particle complexes in nuclei of owl monkey kidney cells infected with *herpesvirus saimiri.* J. Natl. Cancer Inst. **58,** 1421–1425 (1977)

Barahona, H., Daniel, M. D., Bekesi, J. G., Fraser, C. E. O., King, N. W., Hunt, R. D., Ingalls, J. K., Jones, T. C.: *In vitro* suppression of *herpesvirus saimiri* replication by phosphonoacetic acid. Proc. Soc. Exp. Biol. **154,** 431–434 (1977)

Bhatt, P. N., Percy, D. H., Craft, J. L., Jonas, A. M.: Isolation and characterisation of a herpeslike (Hsiung-Kaplow) virus from guinea pigs. J. Infect. Dis. **123,** 178–189 (1971)

Biggs, P. M.: Marek's disease. In: The herpesviruses. Kaplan, A. S. (ed.), pp. 557–594. New York: Academic Press 1973

Bissell, J. A., Frank, A. L., Dunnick, N. R., Rowe, D. S., Conliffe, M. A., Parkman, P. D., Meyer, Jr., H. M.: Rhesus leukocyte-associated herpesvirus. II. Natural and experimental infection. J. Infect. Dis. **128,** 630–637 (1973)

Bornkamm, G. W., Delius, H., Fleckenstein, B., Werner, F.-J., Mulder, C.: Structure of *herpesvirus saimiri* genomes: Arrangement of heavy and light sequences in the M genome. J. Virol. **19,** 154–161 (1976)

Boyd, A. L.: Characterization of single-cell clonal lines derived from HSV-2-transformed mouse cells. Intervirology **6,** 156–167 (1975/76)

Boyd, A. L., Orme, T. W.: Transformation of mouse cells after infection with ultraviolet irradiation-inactivated herpes simplex virus type 2. Int. J. Cancer **16,** 526–538 (1975)

Boyd, A. L., Orme, T. W., Boone, C.: Transformation of mouse cells with herpes simplex virus type 2. In: Oncogenesis and herpesviruses II. de-Thé, G., Epstein, M. A., zur Hausen, H. (eds.), Part 1, pp. 429–435. Lyon: IARC 1975

Breidenbach, G. P., Skinner, M. S., Wallace, J. H., Mizell, M.: *In vitro* induction of a herpes-type virus in "summer-phase" Lucké tumor explants. J. Virol. **7,** 679–682 (1971)

Calnek, B. W., Payne, L. N.: Lack of correlation between Marek's disease tumor induction and expression of endogenous avian RNA tumor virus genome. Int. J. Cancer **17,** 235–244 (1976)

Christenson, B.: Complement-dependent cytotoxic antibodies in the course of cervical carcinoma. Int. J. Cancer **20,** 694–701 (1977)

Chu, E. W., Rabson, A. S.: Chimerism in lymphoid cell culture line derived from lymph node of marmoset infected with *herpesvirus saimiri.* J. Natl. Cancer Inst. **48,** 771–775 (1972)

Chu, C. T., Yang, C. S., Kawamura, A. (Jr.): Antibodies to Epstein-Barr virus in a Burkitt's lymphoma cell line in Taiwan monkeys *(Macaca cyclopis).* Appl. Environ. Microbiol. **21,** 539–540 (1971)

Churchill, A. E.: Herpes virus infections in chicken: control by vaccines. J. Antimicrob. Chemother. **3,** 15–19 (1977)

Cicmanec, J. L., Loeb, W. F., Valerio, M. G.: Lymphoma in owl monkeys *(Aotus trivirgatus)* inoculated with *herpesvirus saimiri:* clinical, hematological and pathologic findings. J. Med. Primatol. **3,** 8–17 (1974)

Collard, W., Thornton, H., Mizell, M., Green, M.: Virus-free adenocarcinoma of the frog (summer phase tumor) transcribes Lucké tumor herpesvirus-specific RNA. Science **181,** 448–449 (1973)

Darai, G., Munk, K.: Human embryonic lung cells abortively infected with herpes virus hominis type 2 show some properties of cell transformation. Nature (New Biol.) **241,** 268–269 (1973)

Darai, G., Munk, K.: Neoplastic transformation of rat embryo cells with herpes simplex virus. Int. J. Cancer **18,** 469–481 (1976)

Darai, G., Braun, R., Flügel, R. M., Munk, K.: Malignant transformation of rat embryo fibroblasts by herpes simplex virus types 1 and 2 at suboptimal temperature. Nature **265**, 744–746 (1977)

Dayan, A. D., Lewis, P. D.: Origin of Kaposi's sarcoma from the reticulo-endothelial system. Nature **213**, 889–890 (1967)

Deichman, G. I., Kashkina, L. M., Kokosha, L. V.: Isolation of cytomegalovirus of green monkeys from cultures of kidney tissues of clinically healthy monkeys. Vopr. Virusol. **17**, 309–312 (1972 a)

Deichman, G. I., Kashkina, L. M., Solov'eva, E. A.: Monkey disease, resembling infectious mononucleosis, induced by cytomegalovirus. Vestn. Akad. Med. Nauk. SSSR **27**, 24–29 (1972 b)

Deinhardt, F., Falk, L., Marczynska, B., Shramek, G., Wolfe, L.: *Herpesvirus saimiri:* A simian counterpart of Epstein-Barr virus of man? Bibl. Haematol. **39**, 416–427 (1973 a)

Deinhardt, F., Falk, L., Wolfe, L.: Simian herpesviruses. Cancer Res. **33**, 1424–1426 (1973 b)

Deinhardt, F., Falk, L., Wolfe, L.: Transformation of nonhuman primate lymphocytes by Epstein-Barr virus. Cancer Res. **34**, 1241–1244 (1974 a)

Deinhardt, F., Falk, L., Wolfe, L.: Simian herpesviruses and neoplasia. Adv. Cancer Res. **19**, 167–206 (1974 b)

Deinhardt, F., Falk, L. A., Nonoyama, M., Wolfe, L., Bergholz, C., Lapin, B., Yakovleva, L., Agrba, V., Henle, G., Henle, W.: Baboon lymphotropic herpesvirus related to Epstein-Barr virus (EBV); 3rd Herpesvirus Workshop. Cold Spring Harbor Laboratory 64 (1976) (Abs.)

Deinhardt, F., Wolf, H.: Similarities and differences between various herpesviruses: a review. In: Oncogenesis and herpesviruses III. de-Thé, G., Henle, W., Rapp, F. (eds.), pp. 169–176. Lyon: IARC 1978

Deinhardt, F., Falk, L., Wolfe, L. G., Schudel, A., Nonoyama, M., Lai, P., Lapin, B., Yakovleva, L.: Susceptibility of marmosets to Epstein-Barr virus-like baboon herpesviruses. Primates Med. **10**, 163–170 (1978)

de-Thé, G., Epstein, M. A., zur Hausen, H. (eds.): Oncogenesis and herpesviruses II. Lyon: IARC 1975

de-Thé, G., Henle, W., Rapp, F. (eds.): Oncogenesis and herpesviruses III. Lyon: IARC 1978

Donner, L., Dubbs, D. R., Kit, S.: Chromosomal site(s) of integration of herpes simplex virus type 2 thymidine kinase gene in biochemically transformed human cells. Int. J. Cancer **20**, 256–267 (1977)

Duff, R., Rapp, F.: Oncogenic transformation of hamster cells after exposure to herpes simplex virus type 2. Nature (New Biol.) **233**, 48–50 (1971 a)

Duff, R., Rapp, F.: Properties of hamster embryo fibroblasts transformed *in vitro* after exposure to ultraviolet-irradiated herpes simplex virus type 2. J.Virol. **8**, 469–477 (1971 b)

Dunkel, V. C., Pry, T. W., Henle, G., Henle, W.: Immunofluorescence tests for antibodies to Epstein-Barr virus with sera of lower primates. J. Natl. Cancer Inst. **49**, 435–440 (1972)

Dunn, K., Nazerian, K.: Induction of Marek's disease virus antigens by IdUrd in a chicken lymphoblastoid cell line. J. Gen. Virol. **34**, 413–419 (1977)

Epstein, M. A., Achong, B. G., Churchill, A. E., Biggs, P. M.: Structure and development of the herpes-type virus of Marek's disease. J. Natl. Cancer Inst. **41**, 805–820 (1968)

Epstein, M. A., Achong, B. G.: Recent progress in Epstein-Barr virus research. Ann. Rev. Microbiol. **31**, 421–445 (1977)

Evans, A. S.: Infectious mononucleosis and other mono-like syndromes. N. Engl. J. Med. **286**, 836–838 (1972)

Evans, D. L., Barnett, J. W., Bowen, J. M., Dmochowski, L.: Antigenic relationship between the herpesviruses of infectious bovine rhinotracheitis, Marek's disease, and Burkitt's lymphoma. J. Virol. **10**, 277–287 (1972)

Falk, L. A., Wolfe, L. G., Deinhardt, F.: Isolation of *herpesvirus saimiri* from blood of squirrel monkeys *(Saimiri sciureus)*. J. Natl. Cancer Inst. **48**, 1499–1505 (1972 a)

Falk, L., Wolfe, L., Deinhardt, F.: Epidemiology of *herpesvirus saimiri* infection in squirrel monkeys. In: Medical Primatology. Goldsmith, E. I., Moor-Jankowski, J. (eds.), pp. 151–158. Basel: Karger 1972 b

Falk, L. A., Nigida, S., Deinhardt, F., Cooper, R. W., Hernandez-Camacho J. I.: Oral excretion of *herpesvirus saimiri* in captive squirrel monkeys and incidence of infection in feral squirrel monkeys. J. Natl. Cancer Inst. **51**, 1987–1989 (1973 a)

Falk, L. A., Wolfe, L. G., Deinhardt, F.: Herpesvirus saimiri: Experimental infection of squirrel monkeys *(Saimiri sciureus)*. J. Natl. Cancer Inst. **51**, 165–170 (1973 b)

Falk, L. A., Nigida, S. M., Deinhardt, F., Wolfe, L. G., Cooper, R. W., Hernandez-Camacho, J. I.: *Herpesvirus ateles:* properties of an oncogenic herpesvirus isolated from circulating lymphocytes of spider monkeys *(Ateles* sp.). Int. J. Cancer **14**, 473–482 (1974 a)

Falk, L., Wolfe, L., Deinhardt, F., Paciga, J., Dombos, L., Klein, G., Henle, W., Henle, G.: Epstein-Barr virus: Transformation of non-human primate lymphocytes *in vitro*. Int. J. Cancer **13**, 363–376 (1974 b)

Falk, L., Wright, J., Wolfe, L., Deinhardt, F.: *Herpesvirus ateles:* transformation *in vitro* of marmoset splenic lymphocytes. Int. J. Cancer **14**, 244–251 (1974 c)

Falk, L., Deinhardt, F., Nonoyama, M., Wolfe, L. G., Bergholz, C.: Properties of a baboon lymphotropic herpesvirus related to Epstein-Barr virus. Int. J. Cancer **18**, 798–807 (1976 a)

Falk, L., Wright, J., Deinhardt, F., Wolfe, L., Schaffer, P., Benyesh-Melnick, M.: Experimental infection of squirrel and marmoset monkeys with attenuated *herpesvirus saimiri.* Cancer Res. **36**, 707–710 (1976 b)

Falk, L., Henle, G., Henle, W., Deinhardt, F., Schudel, A.: Transformation of lymphocytes by *herpesvirus papio.* Int. J. Cancer **20**, 219–226 (1977)

Fawcett, D. W.: Electron microscope observations of intracellular virus-like particles associated with the cells of the Lucké renal adenocarcinoma. J. Biophys. Biochem. Cytol. **2**, 725–742 (1956)

Fiala, M., Austin, T., Heiner, D. C., Imagawa, D. T., Guze, L. B., Payne, J. E.: Cytomegalovirus infection of polymorphonuclear and mononuclear leukocytes in immunosuppressed transplant patients, patients with CMV mononucleosis and a patient with leukaemia. In: Oncogenesis and herpesviruses II. de-Thé, G., Epstein, M. A., zur Hausen, H. (eds.), Part 2, pp. 109–112. Lyon: IRAC 1975

Fleckenstein, B., Wolf, H.: Purification and properties of *herpesvirus saimiri* DNA. Virology **58**, 55–64 (1974)

Fleckenstein, B., Bornkamm, G. W.: Structure and function of *herpesvirus saimiri* DNA. In: Oncogenesis and herpesviruses II. de-Thé, G., Epstein, M. A., zur Hausen, H. (eds.), Part 1, pp. 145–150. Lyon: IRAC 1975

Fleckenstein, B., Bornkamm, G. W., Ludwig, H.: Repetitive sequences in complete and defective genomes of *herpesvirus saimiri.* J. Virology **15**, 398–406 (1975 a)

Fleckenstein, B., Werner, J., Bornkamm, G. W., zur Hausen, H.: Induction of a malignant lymphoma by *herpesvirus saimiri* DNA. In: Epstein-Barr virus production, concentration and purification. IARC Internal Technical Rep. No. 75 003 159–164 (1975 b)

Fleckenstein, B., Bornkamm, G. W., Werner, F.-J.: The role of *herpesvirus saimiri* genomes in oncogenic transformation of primate cells. Bibl. Haematol. **43**, 308–312 (1976)

Fleckenstein, B., Muller, I., Werner, J.: The presence of *herpesvirus saimiri* genomes in virus transformed cells. Int. J. Cancer **19**, 546–554 (1977)

Fleckenstein, B., Bornkamm, G. W., Mulder, C., Werner, F.-J., Daniel, M. D., Falk, L. A., Delius, H.: *Herpesvirus ateles* DNA and its homology with *herpesvirus saimiri* nucleic acid. J. Virol. **25**, 361–373 (1978)

Fong, C. K. Y., Hsiung, G. D.: *In vitro* transformation of hamster embryo cells by a guinea pig herpes-like virus. Proc. Soc. Exp. Biol. Med. **144**, 974–979 (1973)

Fong, C. K. Y., Tenser, R. B., Hsiung, G. D., Gross, P. A.: Ultrastructural studies of the envelopment and release of guinea pig herpes-like virus in cultured cells. Virology **52**, 468–477 (1973)

Fong, C. K. Y., Hsiung, G. D.: Morphogenic studies of herpesvirus and oncornavirus from leukemic and normal guinea pigs. Fed. Proc. **36**, 2320–2327 (1977)

Foster, K. M., Jack, I.: A prospective study of the role of cytomegalovirus in post-transfusion mononucleosis. N. Engl. J. Med. **280**, 1311–1316 (1969)

Flügel, R. M., Darai, G., Braun, R., Munk, K.: Activation of an endogenous C-type RNA virus in rat embryo cells after transformation by herpes simplex virus types 1 and 2. J. Gen. Virol. **36**, 365–369 (1977)

Frank, A. L., Bissell, J. A., Rowe, D. S., Dunnick, N. R., Mayner, R. E., Hopps, H. E., Parkman, P. D., Meyer, H. M. (Jr.): Rhesus leukocyte-associated herpesvirus. I. Isolation and characterization of a new herpesvirus recovered from rhesus monkey leukocytes. J. Infect. Dis. **128**, 618–629 (1973)

Frank, A., Andiman, W. A., Miller, G.: Epstein-Barr virus and nonhuman primates: natural and experimental infection. Adv. Cancer Res. **23**, 171–201 (1976)

Frankel, J. W., Groupé, V.: Interactions between Marek's disease herpesvirus and avian leucosis virus in tissue culture. Nature (New Biol.) **234**, 125–126 (1971)

Frankel, J. W., Farrow, W. M., Prickett, C. O., Smith, M. E., Campbell, W. F., Groupé, V.: Responses of isolator-derived and conventional chickens to Marek's disease herpesvirus and avian leukosis virus. J. Natl. Cancer Inst. **52**, 1491–1497 (1974)

Frankel, J. W., Smith, M. E., Campbell, W. F., Mitchen, J. R., Groupé, V.: Experimental evidence for influence of type C viruses on Marek's disease virus associated oncogenesis. In: Oncogenesis and herpesvirus II. de-Thé, G., Epstein, M. A., zur Hausen, H. (eds.), Part. 2, pp. 17–25. Lyon: IARC 1975

Frenkel, N., Roizman, B., Cassai, E., Nahmias, A.: A herpes simplex 2 DNA fragment and its transcription in human cervical cancer tissue. Proc. Natl. Acad. Sci. USA **69**, 3784–3789 (1972)

Fresen, K.-O., Merkt, B., Bornkamm, G. W., zur Hausen, H.: Heterogeneity of Epstein-Barr virus originating from P$_3$HR-1 cells. I. Studies on EBNA induction. Int. J. Cancer **19**, 317–323 (1977)

Friedmann, A., Coward, J. E., Morgan, C.: Electron microscopic study of the development of *herpesvirus saimiri*. Virology **69**, 810–815 (1976)

Garfinkle, B., McAuslan, B. R.: Transformation of cultured mammalian cells by viable herpes simplex virus subtypes 1 and 2. Proc. Natl. Acad. Sci. USA **71**, 220–224 (1974)

Geder, L., Lausch, R., O'Neill, F., Rapp, F.: Oncogenic transformation of human embryo lung cells by human cytomegalovirus. Science **192**, 1134–1137 (1976)

Geder, L., Rapp, F.: Evidence for nuclear antigens in cytomegalovirus-transformed human cells. Nature **265**, 184–186 (1977)

Geder, L., Kreider, J., Rapp, F.: Human cells transformed *in vitro* by human cytomegalovirus: Tumorigenicity in athymic nude mice. J. Natl. Cancer Inst. **58**, 1003–1009 (1977)

Gerber, P., Birch, S. M.: Complement-fixing antibodies in sera of human and nonhuman primates to viral antigens derived from Burkitt's lymphoma cells. Proc. Natl. Acad. Sci. USA **58**, 478–484 (1967)

Gerber, P., Rosenblum, E. N.: The incidence of complement-fixing antibodies to herpes simplex and herpes-like viruses in man and rhesus monkeys. Proc. Soc. Exp. Biol. Med. **128**, 541–546 (1968)

Gerber, P., Lorenz, D.: Complement-fixing antibodies reactive with EBV in sera of marmosets and prosimians. Proc. Soc. Exp. Biol. **145**, 654–657 (1974)

Gerber, P., Pritchett, R. F., Kieff, E. D.: Antigens and DNA of a chimpanzee agent related to Epstein-Barr virus. J. Virol. **19**, 1090–1099 (1976)

Gerber, P., Kalter, S. S., Schidlovsky, G., Peterson, W. D., Daniel, M. D.: Biologic and antigenic characteristics of Epstein-Barr virus-related herpesviruses of chimpanzees and baboons. Int. J. Cancer **20**, 448–459 (1977)

Giraldo, G., Beth, E., Coeur, P., Vogel, C. L., Dhru, D. S.: Kaposi's Sarcoma: A new model in the search for viruses associated with human malignancies. J. Natl. Cancer Inst. **49**, 1495–1507 (1972a)

Giraldo, G., Beth, E., Haguenau, F.: Herpes-type virus particles in tissue culture of Kaposi's sarcoma from different geographic regions. J. Natl. Cancer Inst. **49**, 1509–1526 (1972b)

Giraldo, G., Beth, E., Kourilsky F. M., Henle, W., Henle, G., Miké V., Huraux, J. M., Andersen, H. K., Gharbi, M. R., Kyalwazi, S. K., Puissant, A.: Antibody patterns to herpesvirus in Kaposi's sarcoma: Serological association of European Kaposi's sarcoma with cytomegalovirus. Int. J. Cancer **15**, 839–848 (1975)

Glaser, R., Geder, L., Jeor, S. S., Michelson-Fiske, S., Haguenau, F.: Partial characterization of a herpes-type virus (K9V) derived from Kaposi's sarcoma. J. Natl. Cancer Inst. **59**, 55–60 (1977)

Goldman, M., Landon, J. C., Reisher, J.: Fluorescent antibody and gel diffusion reactions of human and chimpanzee sera with cells cultured from Burkitt tumors and normal chimpanzee blood. Cancer Res. **28**, 2489–2495 (1968)

Granoff, A.: Lucké Tumour-associated viruses, a review. In: Oncogenesis and herpesviruses. Biggs, P. M., de-Thé, G., Payne, L. N. (eds.), pp. 171–182. Lyon: IARC 1972

Granoff, A.: Herpesviruses and the Lucké tumor. Cancer Res. **33**, 1431–1433 (1973a)

Granoff, A.: The Lucké renal carcinoma of the frog. In: The Herpesviruses. Kaplan, A. S. (ed.), pp. 627–640. New York: Academic Press 1973b

Graze, P. R., Royston, I.: Infection of human and rhesus lymphoblastoid cells with *herpesvirus macaca*. Arch. Virol. **49**, 165–174 (1975)

Gupta, P., Rapp, F.: Identification of virion polypetides in hamster cells transformed by herpes simplex virus type 1. Proc. Natl. Acad. Sci. USA **74**, 372–374 (1977)

Heine, U., Ablashi, D. V., Armstrong, G. R.: Morphological studies on *herpesvirus saimiri* in subhuman and human cell cultures. Cancer Res. **31**, 1019–1029 (1971)

Heine, U., Hinze, H. C.: Morphological studies on *herpesvirus sylvilagus* in rabbit kidney cell cultures. Cancer Res. **32**, 1340–1350 (1972)

Heine, U., Cottler-Fox, M.: Electron microscopic observations on the composition of herpes-type virions. In: Oncogenesis and herpesviruses II. de-Thé, G., Epstein, M. A., zur Hausen, H. (eds.), Part 1, pp. 103–110. Lyon: IARC 1975

Hilleman, M. R.: Marek's disease vaccine: its implications in biology and medicine. Avian Dis. **16**, 191–199 (1972)

Hinze, H. C.: Isolation of a new herpesvirus from cottontail rabbits. Bacteriol. Proc. 147 (1968)

Hinze, H. C.: Rabbit lymphoma induced by a new herpesvirus. Bacteriol. Proc. 157 (1969)

Hinze, H. C.: New member of the herpesvirus group isolated from wild cottontail rabbits. Infect. Immun. **3**, 350–354 (1971a)

Hinze, H. C.: Induction of lymphoid hyerplasia and lymphoma-like disease in rabbits by *herpesvirus sylvilagus*. Int. J. Cancer **8**, 514–522 (1971b)

Hinze, H. C., Chipman, P. J.: Role of herpesvirus in malignant lymphoma in rabbits. Fed. Proc. **31,** 1639–1642 (1972)

Hollinshead, A., O'Bong, L., McKelway, W., Melnick, J. L., Rawls, W. E.: Reactivity between herpesvirus type 2 related soluble cervical tumor cell membrane antigens and matched cancer and control sera. Proc. Soc. Exp. Biol. Med. **141,** 688–693 (1972)

Hollinshead, A. C., O'Bong, L., Chrétien, P. B., Tarpley, J. L., Rawls, W. E., Adam, E.: Antibodies to herpesvirus nonvirion antigens in squamous carcinomas. Science **182,** 713–715 (1973)

Holmes, A. W., Caldwell, R. G., Dedmon, R. E., Deinhardt, F.: Isolation and characterization of a new herpes virus. J. Immunol. **92,** 602–610 (1964)

Holmes, A. W., Devine, J. A., Nowakowski, E., Deinhardt, F.: The epidemiology of a herpes virus infection of New World monkeys. J. Immunol. **90,** 668–671 (1966)

Hsiung, G. D.: Virological studies of guinea pig leukemia: an overview with reference to herpesvirus and oncornavirus. Fed. Proc. **36,** 2285–2289 (1977)

Hsiung, G. D., Kaplow, L. S.: Herpes-like virus isolated from spontaneously degenerated tissue culture derived from leukemia-susceptible guinea pigs. J. Virol. **3,** 355–357 (1969)

Hsiung, G. D., Kaplow, L. S.: The association of herpes-like virus and guinea pig leukemia. Bibl. Haematol. **36,** 578–583 (1970)

Hsiung, G. D., Fong, C. K. Y., Lamm, K. M.: Guinea pig leukocytes: *In vivo* and *in vitro* infection with a herpes-like virus. J. Immunol. **106,** 1686–1689 (1971 a)

Hsiung, G. D., Kaplow, L. S., Booss, J.: Herpesvirus infection of guinea pigs. I. Isolation, characterisation and pathogenicity. Am. J. Epidemiol. **93,** 298–307 (1971 b)

Hsiung, G. D.: Natural history of herpes and C-type virus infections and their possible relation to viral oncogenesis. An animal model. Prog. Med. Virol. **21,** 58–71 (1975)

Huang, E. S., Pagano, J. S.: Human cytomegalovirus. II. Lack of relatedness to DNA of herpes simplex I and II, Epstein-Barr virus, and nonhuman strains of cytomegalovirus. J. Virol. **13,** 642–645 (1974)

Huang, E. S., Pagano, J. S.: Replication of cytomegalovirus DNA in human lymphoblastoid cells. In: Oncogenesis and herpesviruses II. de-Thé, G., Epstein, M. A., zur Hausen, H. (eds.), Part 1, 475–482. Lyon: IARC 1975

Hunt, R. D., Meléndez, L. V., King, N. W., Gilmore, C. E., Daniel, M. D., Williamson, M. E., Jones, T. C.: Morphology of a disease with features of malignant lymphoma in marmosets and owl monkeys inoculated with *herpesvirus saimiri*. J. Natl. Cancer Inst. **44,** 447–465 (1970)

Hunt, R. D., Meléndez, L. V., Garcia, F. G., Trum, B. F.: Pathologic features of *herpesvirus ateles* lymphoma in cotton-topped marmosets *(Saguinus oedipus)*. J. Natl. Cancer Inst. **49,** 1631–1639 (1972)

Hunt, R. D., Garcia, F. G., Barahona, H. H., King, N. W., Fraser, C. E. O., Meléndez, L. V.: Spontaneous *herpesvirus saimiri* lymphoma in an owl monkey. J. Infect. Dis. **127,** 723–725 (1973)

Hunt, R. D., Daniel, M. D., Baggs, R. B., Blake, B. J., Silva, D., DuBose, D., Meléndez, L. V.: Clinicopathologic characterization of *herpesvirus saimiri* malignant lymphoma in New Zealand white rabbits. J. Natl. Cancer Inst. **54,** 1401–1412 (1975)

Ibrahim, A. N., Ray, M., Megaw, J., Brown, R., Nahmias, A. J.: Common antigens of herpes simplex virus 2, associated hamster tumors, and human cervical cancer. Proc. Soc. Exp. Biol. Med. **152,** 343–347 (1976)

Jeor, S. C. S., Albrecht, T. B., Funk, F. D., Rapp, F.: Stimulation of cellular DNA synthesis by human cytomegalovirus. J. Virol. **13,** 353–362 (1974)

Jeor, S. C. S., Weisser, A.: Persistence of cytomegalovirus in human lymphoblasts and peripheral leukocyte cultures. Infect. Immun. **15,** 402–409 (1977)

Johnson, D. R.: The lymphoid system of marmoset monkeys *(Saguinus* sp.) and effects of immunosuppression. Chicago, University of Illinois Graduate College: Ph. D. Thesis, 1977

Joncas, J. H., Menezes, J., Huang, E. S.: Persistence of CMV genome in lymphoid cells after congenital infection. Nature **258,** 432–433 (1975)

Jones, K. W., Fenoglio, C. M., Shevchuk-Chaban, M., Maitland, N. J., McDougall, J. K.: Detection of herpesvirus-2 mRNA in human cervical biopsies by *in situ* cytological hybridization. (In press) (1978)

Kalter, S. S., Heberling, R. L., Ratner, J. J.: EBV antibody in monkeys and apes. Bibl. Haematol. **39,** 871–875 (1973)

Kaplan, A. S. (ed.): The herpesviruses. New York: Academic Press 1973

Kato, S., Ono, K., Naito, M., Tanabe, S.: Immunological studies on Marek's disease virus and Epstein-Barr virus. In: Oncogenesis and herpesviruses. Biggs, P. M., de-Thé, G., Payne, L. N. (eds.), pp. 485–488. Lyon: IARC 1972

Kirkwood, J., Geering, G., Old, L. J.: Demonstration of group- and type-specific antigens of herpes viruses. In: Oncogenesis and herpesviruses. Biggs, P. M., de-Thé, G., Payne, L. N. (eds.), pp. 479–484. Lyon: IARC 1972

Klein, E., Klein, G., Levine, P. H.: Immunological control of human lymphoma: Discussion. Cancer Res. **36,** 724–727 (1976)

Klein, G., Pearson, G., Rabson, A., Ablashi, D. V., Falk, L., Wolfe, L., Deinhardt, F., Rabin, H.: Antibody reactions to *herpesvirus saimiri* (HVS)-induced early and late antigens (EA and LA) in HVS-infected squirrel, marmoset and owl monkeys. Int. J. Cancer **12,** 270–289 (1973)

Klein, G., Falk, L., Falk, K.: Antigen-inducing ability of *herpesvirus papio* in human and baboon lymphoma lines, compared to Epstein-Barr virus. Intervirol. **10,** 153–164 (1978)

Klemola, E., Kääriäinen, L.: Cytomegalovirus as a possible cause of a disease resembling infectious mononucleosis. Br. Med. J. **1965 II,** 1099–1102

Klemola, E., von Essen, R., Henle, G., Henle, W.: Infectious-mononucleosis-like disease with negative heterophil agglutination test. Clinical features in relation to Epstein-Barr virus and cytomegalovirus antibodies. J. Infect. Dis. **121,** 608–614 (1970)

Klemola, E., Kääriäinen, L., von Essen, R., Haltia, K., Koivuniemi, A., von Bonsdorff, C. H.: Further studies on cytomegalovirus mononucleosis in previously healthy individuals. Acta Med. Scand. **182,** 311–322 (1967)

Krech, U., Jung, M.: Antigenic relationship between human cytomegalovirus, herpes simplex, and varicellazoster virus studied by complement-fixation. Arch. Ges. Virusforsch. **33,** 288–295 (1971)

Kucera, L. S., Gusdon, J. P.: Transformation of human embryonic fibroblasts by photodynamically inactivated herpes simplex virus type 2 at supra-optimal temperature. J. Gen. Virol. **30,** 257–261 (1976)

Lam, K. M., Hsiung, G. D.: Guinea pig herpes-like virus infection. I. Antibody response and virus persistence in guinea pigs after experimental infection. Infect. Immun. **7,** 426–431, (1973 a)

Lam, K. M., Hsiung, G. D.: Guinea pig herpes-like virus infection. II. Antibody response and virus persistence in rabbits and mice. Infect. Immun. **7,** 432–437 (1973 b)

Landon, J. C., Ellis, L. B., Zeve, V. H. Fabrizio, D. P.: Herpes-type virus in cultured leukocytes from chimpanzees. J. Natl. Cancer Inst. **40,** 181–192 (1968)

Landon, J. C., Malan, L.: Seroepidemiologic studies of Epstein-Barr virus antibody in monkeys. J. Natl. Cancer Inst. **46,** 881–884 (1971)

Lang, D. J., Montagnier, L., Latarjet, R.: Growth in agarose of human cells infected with cytomegalovirus. J. Virol. **14,** 327–332 (1974)

Lapin, B. A.: The epidemiologic and genetic aspects of an outbreak of leukemia among hamadryas baboons of the Sukhumi monkey colony. Bibl. Haematol. **39,** 263–268 (1974)

Lapin, B. A.: Epidemiology of leukemia among baboons of Sukhumi monkey colony. Bibl. Haematol. **43,** 212–215 (1976)

Laufs, R.: Immunisation of marmoset monkeys with a killed oncogenic herpesvirus. Nature **249,** 571–572 (1974)

Laufs, R., Fleckenstein, B.: Purification of *herpesvirus saimiri* DNA. Bibl. Haematol. **39,** 457–461 (1973)

Laufs, R., Steinke, H., Jacobs, C., Hilfenhaus, J., Karges, H.: Influence of interferon on the replication of oncogenic herpesviruses in tissue cultures and in nonhuman primates. Med. Microbiol. Immunol. **160,** 285–294 (1974)

Laufs, R., Steinke, H.: Vaccination of non-human primates against malignant lymphoma. Nature **253,** 71–72 (1975)

Laufs, R., Steinke, H.: Vaccination of nonhuman primates with killed oncogenic herpesviruses. Cancer Res. **36,** 704–706 (1976)

Lausch, R. N., Murasko, D. M., Albrecht, T., Rapp, F.: Detection of specific surface antigens on cells transformed by cytomegalovirus with the techniques of mixed hemagglutination and I-labeled antiglobulin. Immunology **112,** 1680–1684 (1974)

Lausch, R. N., Jones, C., Christie, D., Hay, K. A., Rapp, F.: Spleen cell-mediated cytotoxicity of hamster cells transformed by herpes simplex virus: Evidence for virus-specific membrane antigen. J. Immunol. **114,** 459–465 (1975 a)

Lausch, R. N., Murasko, D. M., Jones, C., Hay, K. A.: Immunological studies with hamster cells transformed by cytomegalovirus and herpes simplex virus Type 1. In: Oncogenesis and herpesviruses II. de-Thé, G., Epstein, M. A., zur Hausen, H. (eds.), Part 1, pp. 315–321. Lyon: IARC 1975 b

Leiden, J. M., Buttyan, R., Spear, P. G.: Herpes simplex virus gene expression in transformed cells I. Regulation of the viral thymidine kinase gene in transformed L cells by products of superinfecting virus. J. Virol. **20,** 413–424 (1976)

Lemon, S. M., Hutt, L. M., Shaw, J. E., Li, J.-L. H., Pagano, J. S.: Replication of EBV in epithelial cells during infectious mononucleosis. Nature **268**, 268–270 (1977)

Lerner, P. I., Sampliner, J. E.: Transfusion-associated cytomegalovirus mononucleosis. Ann. Surg. **185**, 406–440 (1977)

Levy, J. A., Levy, S. B., Hirshaut, Y., Kafuko, G., Prince, A.: Presence of EBV antibodies in sera from wild chimpanzees. Nature **233**, 559–560 (1971)

Lewis, H. S., Hinze, H. C.: Epidemiology of *herpesvirus sylvilagus* infection in cottontail rabbits. J. Wildl. Dis. **12**, 482–485 (1976)

Ley, K. D., Burger, D.: Cell associated nature of cottontail rabbit herpesvirus *in vitro*. Appl. Environ. Microbiol. **19**, 549–550 (1970)

Lucké B.: A neoplastic disease of the kidney of the frog, *Rana pipiens*. Am. J. Cancer **20**, 352–379 (1934)

Lucké B.: Carcinoma in the leopard frog: its probable causation by a virus. J. Exp. Med. **68**, 457–468, (1938)

Lucké B.: Kidney carcinoma of the leopard frog: a virus tumor. Ann. N. Y. Acad. Sci. **54**, 1093–1109 (1952)

Mackay, J. M. K.: Tissue culture studies of sheep pulmonary adenomatosis (jaagsiekte). I. Direct cultures of affected lungs. J. Comp. Pathol. **79**, 141–146 (1969 a)

Mackay, J. M. K.: Tissue culture studies of sheep pulmonary adenomatosis (jaagsiekte). II. Transmission of cytopathic effects of normal cultures. J. Comp. Pathol. **79**, 147–154 (1969 b)

Mackay, J. M. K., Nisbet, D. I.: Pathogenicity tests in lambs with an ovine herpesvirus. In: Oncogenesis and herpesviruses. Biggs, P. M., de-Thé, G., Payne, L. N. (eds.), pp. 467–470. Lyon: IARC 1972

Macnab, J. C. M.: Transformation of rat embryo cells by temperature-sensitive mutants of herpes simplex virus. J. Gen. Virol. **24**, 143–153 (1974)

Malmquist, W. A., Kraus, H. H., Moulton, J. E., Wandera, J. G.: Morphologic study of virus-infected lung cell cultures from sheep pulmonary adenomatosis (jaagsiekte). Lab. Invest. **26**, 528–533 (1972)

Marcon, M. J., Kucera, L. S.: Consequences of herpes simplex virus type 2 and human cell interaction at supraoptimal temperatures. J. Virol. **20**, 54–62 (1976)

Marczynska, B., Falk, L., Wolfe, L., Deinhardt, F.: Transplantation and cytogenetic studies of *herpesvirus saimiri*-induced disease in marmoset monkeys. J. Natl. Cancer Inst. **50**, 331–337 (1973)

Marek, J.: Multiple Nervenentzündung (Polyneuritis) bei Hühnern. Deutsche Tierärztl. Wochenschr. **15**, 417–421 (1907)

Martin, W. B., Scott, F. M. M., Sharp, J. M., Angus, K. W.: Experimental production of sheep pulmonary adenomatosis (jaagsiekte). Nature **264**, 183–185 (1976)

McKinnell, R. G., Ellis, V. L.: Epidemiology of the frog renal tumour and the significance of tumour nuclear transplantation studies to viral aetiology of the tumour – a review. In: Oncogenesis and herpesviruses Biggs, P. M., de-Thé, G., Payne, L. N. (eds.), pp. 183–197. Lyon: IARC 1972

Meléndez, L. V., Daniel, M. D., Hunt, R. D., Garcia, F. G.: An apparently new herpesvirus from primary kidney cultures of the squirrel monkey *(Saimiri sciureus)*. Lab. Anim. Care **18**, 374–381 (1968)

Meléndez, L. V., Daniel, M. D., Garica, F. G., Fraser, C. E. O., Hunt, R. D., King, N. W.: *Herpes saimiri*. I. Further characterization studies of a new virus from the squirrel monkey. Lab. Anim. Care **19**, 372–397 (1969 a)

Meléndez, L. V., Hunt, R. D., Daniel, M. D., Garcia, F. G., Fraser, C. E. O.: *Herpes saimiri*. II. Experimentally induced malignant lymphoma in primates. Lab. Anim. Care **19**, 378–386 (1969 b)

Meléndez, L. V., Hunt, R. D., Daniel, M. D., Fraser, C. E. O., Barahona, H. H., King, N. W., Garcia, F. G.: *Herpesvirus saimiri* and *ateles* – their role in malignant lymphomas of monkeys. Fed. Proc. **31**, 1643–1650 (1972)

Melnick, J. L., Midulla, M., Wimberly, I., Barrera-Oro, J. G., Levy, B. M.: A new member of the herpesvirus group isolated from South American marmosets. J. Immunol. **92**, 596–601 (1964)

Michalski, F. J., Fong, C. K. Y., Hsiung, G. D., Schneider, R. D.: Induction of tumors by a guinea pig herpesvirus transformed hamster cell line. J. Natl. Cancer Inst. **56**, 1165–1170 (1976)

Miller, G., Robinson, J., Heston, L., Lipman, M.: Differences between laboratory strains of Epstein-Barr virus based on immortalization, abortive infection and interference. In: Oncogenesis and herpesviruses II. de-Thé, G., Epstein, M. A., zur Hausen, H. (eds.), Part 1, pp. 395–408. Lyon: IARC 1975

Mizell, M.: Tumor induction *in vivo*: major events leading to tumorigenesis in embryos inoculated with oncogenic herpesviruses. In: Oncogenesis and herpesviruses II. de-Thé, G., Epstein, M. A., zur Hausen, H. (eds.), Part 2, pp. 121–132. Lyon: IARC 1975

Morgan, D. G.: Observations on the antigenic relationships between Epstein-Barr virus and *herpesvirus saimiri*. J. Gen. Virol. **36**, 281–287 (1977)

Morgan, D. G., Epstein, M. A., Achong, B. G., Mélendez, L. V.: Morphological confirmation of the herpes nature of a carcinogenic virus of primates *(Herpes saimiri)*. Nature **228**, 170–172 (1970)

Morgan, D. G., Achong, B. G., Epstein, M. A.: Unusual intranuclear tubular structures associated with the maturation of *herpesvirus saimiri* in monkey kidney cell cultures. Br. J. Cancer **27**, 434–440 (1973)

Morgan, D. G., Achong, B. G., Epstein, M. A.: Morphological observations on the replication of *herpesvirus saimiri* in monkey kidney cell cultures. J. Gen. Virol. **32**, 461–470 (1976)

Munk, K., Darai, G.: Human embryonic lung cells transformed by herpes simplex virus. Cancer Res. **33**, 1535–1538 (1973)

Munk, K., Darai, G.: Transformation of embryonic rat fibroblasts by herpes simplex virus type 2. In: Oncogenesis and herpesviruses II. de-Thé, G., Epstein, M. A., zur Hausen, H. (eds.), Part 1, pp. 437–443. Lyon: IARC 1975

Munk, K., Darai, G., Deinhardt, F., Marczynska, B., Nonoyama, M., Silver, S.: Herpes simplex virus neoplastic transformation. Bibl. Haematol. **43**, 59–62 (1975)

Muñoz, N., de-Thé, G., Aristizabal, N., Yee, C., Rabson, A., Pearson, G.: Antibodies to herpesviruses in patients with cervical cancer and controls. In: Oncogenesis and herpesviruses II. de-Thé, G., Epstein, M. A., zur Hausen, H. (eds.), Part 2, pp. 45–51. Lyon: IARC 1975

Munyon, W., Kraiselburd, E., Davis, D., Mann, J.: Transfer of thymidine kinase to thymidine kinaseless L cells by infection with ultraviolet-irradiated herpes simplex virus. J. Virol. **7**, 813–820 (1971)

Murasko, D. M., Lausch, R. N.: Cellular immune response to virus-specific antigen in hamsters bearing isografts of cytomegalovirus-transformed cells. Int. J. Cancer **14**, 451–460 (1974)

Murasko, D. M., Lausch, R. N.: Spleen-cell cytotoxicity for cytomegelovirus-transformed cells. II. Inhibition by cytomegalovirus antiserum. Int. J. Cancer **16**, 24–32 (1975)

Murasko, D. M., Lausch, R. N.: Immunostimulation of cytomegalovirus-transformed cells and its inhibition by blocking sera. J. Natl. Cancer Inst. **56**, 1083–1085 (1976)

Nachtigal, M., Albrecht, T., Rapp, F.: Analysis of chromosomes of syrian hamster cells transformed with human cytomegalovirus. Intervirology **4**, 77–90 (1974)

Nadel, E., Banfield, W., Burstein, S., Tousimis, A. J.: Virus particles associated with strain 2 guinea pig leukemia (L₂C/N-B). J. Natl. Cancer Inst. **38**, 979–982 (1967)

Naegele, R. F., Granoff, A., Darlington, R. W.: The presence of the Lucké herpesvirus genome in induced tadpole tumors and its oncogenicity: Koch-Henle postulates fulfilled. Proc. Natl. Acad. Sci. USA **71**, 830–834 (1974)

Naegele, R. F., Granoff, A.: Viruses and renal carcinoma of *Rana pipiens*. XV. The presence of virus-associated membrane antigens(s) on Lucké tumor cells. Int. J. Cancer **19**, 414–418 (1977)

Nahmias, A. J.: Herpesvirus from fish to man – a search for pathobiologic unity. Pathobiol. Annu. **2**, 153–182 (1972)

Naito, M. K., Ono, S., Tanabe, T. R., Kato, S.: Detection in chicken and human sera of antibody against herpes-type virus from a chicken with Marek's disease and EB virus demonstrated by the indirect immunofluorescence test. Biken J. **12**, 205–212 (1970)

Nakao, T., Chiba, S., Ohsaki, M., Hanazono, H.: Cytomegalovirus mononucleosis. Lancet **1967 II**, 1153

Nayak, D. P.: Activation of guinea pig herpesvirus antigen in leukemic lymphoblasts of guinea pig. J. Virol. **10**, 933–936 (1972)

Nazerian, K.: Marek's disease: a neoplastic disease of chickens caused by a herpesvirus. Adv. Cancer Res. **17**, 279–317 (1973)

Nazerian, K., Lee, L. F., Sharma, J. M.: The role of herpesviruses in Marek's disease lymphoma of chickens. Prog. Med. Virol. **22**, 123–151 (1976)

Neubauer, R. H., Wallen, W. C., Rabin, H.: Stimulation of *herpesvirus saimiri* expression in the absence of evidence for type C virus activation in a marmoset lymphoid cell line. Virology **14**, 745–750 (1974)

Neubauer, R. H., Rabin, H., Hopkins, R. F., Levy, B. M.: Characteristics of cell lines established from Epstein-Barr virus induced marmoset tumors. In: Oncogenesis and herpesviruses III. de-Thé, G., Henle, W., Rapp, F. (eds.). Lyon: IARC (in press) 1978

Ohno, S., Luka, J., Lindahl, T., Klein, G.: Identification of a purified complement-fixing antigen as the Epstein-Barr virus-determined nuclear antigen (EBNA) by its binding to metaphase chromosomes. Proc. Natl. Acad. Sci. USA **74**, 1605–1609 (1977a)

Ohno, S., Luka, J., Falk, L., Klein, G.: Detection of a nuclear, EBNA-type antigen in apparently EBNA-negative *herpesvirus papio* (HVP)-transformed lymphoid lines by the acid-fixed nuclear binding technique. Int. J. Cancer **20**, 941–946 (1977b)

Oill, P. A., Fiala, M., Schofferman, J., Byfield, P. E., Guze, L. B.: Cytomegalovirus mononucleosis in a healthy adult: Assocation with hepatitis, secondary Epstein-Barr virus antibody response and immunosuppression. Am. J. Med. **62**, 413–417 (1977)

Ono, K., Tanabe, S., Naito, M., Doi, T., Kato, S.: Antigen common to a herpes-type virus from chickens with Marek's disease and EB virus from Burkitt's lymphoma cells. Biken J. **13**, 213–217 (1970)

Opler, S. R.: Observations on a new virus associated with guinea pig leukemia: preliminary note. J. Natl. Cancer Inst. **38**, 797–800 (1967)

Payne, L. N., Frazier, J. A., Powell, P. C.: Pathogenesis of Marek's disease. Int. Rev. Exp. Pathol. **16**, 59–154 (1976)

Pearson, G., Ablashi, D., Orr, T., Rabin, H., Armstrong, G.: Intracellular and membrane immunofluorescence investigations on cells infected with *herpesvirus saimiri*. J. Natl. Cancer Inst. **49**, 1417–1424 (1972)

Pearson, G. R., Orr, T., Rabin, H., Cicmanec, J., Ablashi, D., Armstrong, G.: Antibody patterns to *herpesvirus saimiri* (HVS)-induced antigens in owl monkeys infected with HVS. J. Natl. Cancer Inst. **51**, 1939–1943 (1973)

Pearson, G. R., Rabin, H., Wallen, W. C., Neubauer, R. H., Orr, T. W., Cicmanec, J. L.: Immunological and virological investigations on owl monkeys infected with *herpesvirus saimiri*. J. Med. Primatol. **3**, 54–67 (1974)

Pearson, G. R., Davis, S.: Immune response of monkeys to lymphotropic herpesvirus antigens. Cancer Res. **36**, 688–691 (1976)

Pearson, G. R., Scott, R. E.: Isolation of virus-free *herpesvirus saimiri* antigen-positive plasma membrane vesicles. Proc. Natl. Acad. Sci. USA **74**, 2546–2550 (1977)

Perk, K., Michalides, R., Spiegelman, S., Scholm, J.: Biochemical and morphologic evidence for the presence of an RNA tumor virus in pulmonary carcinoma of sheep (jaagsiekte). J. Natl. Cancer Inst. **53**, 131–135 (1974)

Peters, W. P., Kufe, D., Schlom, J., Frankel, J. W., Prickett, C. O., Groupé, V., Spiegelman, S.: Biological and biochemical evidence for an interaction between Marek's disease herpesvirus and avian leukosis virus *in vivo*. Proc. Natl. Acad. Sci. USA **70**, 3175–3178 (1973)

Pope, J. H.: Transformation *in vitro* by herpesviruses, a review. In: Oncogenesis and herpesviruses II. de-Thé, G., Epstein, M. A., zur Hausen, H. (eds.), Part 1, pp. 367–378. Lyon: IARC 1975

Powell, P. C., Payne, L. N., Frazier, J. A., Rennie, M.: T-lymphoblastoid cell lines from Marek's disease lymphomas. In: Oncogenesis and herperviruses II. de-Thé, G., Epstein, M. A., zur Hausen, H. (eds.), Part 2, pp. 89–99. Lyon: IARC 1975

Powell, P. C., Rowell, J. G.: Dissociation of antiviral and antitumor immunity in resistance to Marek's disease. J. Natl. Cancer Inst. **59**, 919–924 (1977)

Prevost, J.-M., Pearson, G. R., Wallen, W. C., Rabin, H., Qualtiere, L. F.: Antibody responses to membrane antigens in monkeys infected with *herpesvirus saimiri*. Int. J. Cancer **18**, 679–686 (1976)

Purchase, H. G.: Marek's disease virus and the herpesvirus of turkeys. Prog. Med. Virol. **18**, 178–197 (1974)

Purchase, H. G.: Prevention of Marek's disease: a review. Cancer Res. **36**, 696–700 (1976)

Rabin, H., Pearson, G., Chopra, H. C., Orr, T., Ablashi, D. V., Armstrong, G. R.: Characteristics of *herpesvirus saimiri*-induced lymphoma cells in tissue culture. In Vitro **9**, 65–72 (1973 a)

Rabin, H., Pearson, G., Klein, G., Ablashi, D. V., Wallen, W. C., Cicmanec, J. L.: *Herpesvirus saimiri* antigens and virus recovery from cultured cells and antibody levels and virus isolations from cultured cells and antibody levels and virus isolations from squirrel monkeys. Am. J. Phys. Anthropol. **38**, 491–497 (1973 b)

Rabin, H., Neubauer, R. H., Pearson, G. R., Cicmanec, J. L., Wallen, W. C., Loeb, W. F., Valerio, M. G.: Spontaneous lymphoma associated with *herpesvirus saimiri* in owl monkeys. J. Natl. Cancer Inst. **54**, 499–502 (1975 a)

Rabin, H., Pearson, G. R., Wallen, W. C., Neubauer, R. H., Cicmanec, J. L., Orr, T. W.: Infection of capuchin monkeys *(Cebus albifrons)* with *herpesvirus saimiri*. J. Natl. Cancer Inst. **54**, 673–677 (1957 b)

Rabin, H., Neubauer, R. H., Hopkins, R. F., Dzhikidze, E. K., Shevtsova, Z. V., Lapin, B. A.: Transforming activity and antigenicity of an Epstein-Barr-like virus from lymphoblastoid cell lines of baboons with lymphoid disease. Intervirology **8**, 240–249 (1977 a)

Rabin, H., Neubauer, R. H., Hopkins, R. F., Levy, B. M.: Characterization of lymphoid cell lines established from multiple Epstein-Barr virus (EBV)-induced lymphomas in a cotton-topped marmoset. Int. J. Cancer **20**, 44–50 (1977 b)

Rafferty, K. A.: Pathology of amphibian renal carcinoma, a review. In: Oncogenesis and herpesviruses. Biggs, P. M., de-Thé, G., Payne, L. N. (eds.), pp. 159–170. Lyon: IARC 1972

Rangan, S. R. S., Martin, L. N., Enright, F. M., Abee, C. R.: Herpesvirus *saimiri*-induced lymphoproliferative disease in howler monkeys. J. Natl. Cancer Inst. **59**, 165–171 (1977)

Rapp, F.: Herpesviruses and cancer. Adv. Cancer Res. **19**, 265–302 (1974)

Rapp, F., Li, L. J., Jerkofsky, M.: Transformation of mamalian cells by DNA-containing viruses following photodynamic inactivation. Virology **55**, 339–346 (1973)

Rapp, F., Buss, E. R.: Are viruses important in carcinogenesis? Am. J. Pathol. **77**, 85–100 (1974)

Rapp, F., Li, L. J.: Demonstration of the oncogenic potential of herpes simplex viruses and human cytomegalovirus. Cold Spring Harbor Symp. Quant. Biol. **39,** 747–763 (1975)

Rasheed, S., Rongey, R. W., Bruszweski, J., Nelson-Rees, W. A., Rabin, H., Neubauer, R. H., Esra, G., Gardner, M. B.: Establishment of a cell line with associated Epstein-Barr-like virus from a leukemic orangutan. Science **198,** 407–409 (1977)

Rhim, J. S.: Malignant transformation of rat embryo cells by a herpesvirus isolated from L_2C guinea pig leukemia. Virology **82,** 100–110 (1977)

Rhim, J. S., Duh, F. G., Cho, H. Y., Wuu, K. D., Vernon, M. L.: Activation by 5-bromo-2′-deoxyuridine of particles resembling guinea-pig leukemia virus from guinea-pig nonproducer cells. J. Natl. Cancer Inst. **51,** 1327–1331 (1973)

Rhim, J. S., Wuu, K. D., Ro, H. D., Vernon, M. L., Huebner, R. J.: Induction of guinea pig leukemia-like virus from cultured guinea pig cells. Proc. Soc. Exp. Biol. Med. **147,** 323–330 (1974)

Rifkind, D.: Cytomegalovirus mononucleosis. Ann. Intern. Med. **69,** 842–843 (1968)

Robinson, J. E., Andiman, W. A., Henderson, E., Miller, G.: Host-determined differences in expression of surface marker characteristics on human and simian lymphoblastoid cell lines transformed by Epstein-Barr virus. Proc. Natl. Acad. Sci. USA **74,** 749–753 (1977)

Robinson, J. E., Andiman, W. A., Henderson, E., Miller, G.: Differences in expression of surface marker characteristics on Epstein-Barr virus-transformed human and simian lymphoid cell lines. Primates Med. **10,** 149–155 (1978)

Roizman, B.: The herpesviruses, a biochemical definition of the group. Curr. Top. Microbiol. Immunol. **49,** 1–79 (1972)

Roizman, B., Kieff, E. D.: Herpes simplex and Epstein-Barr viruses in human cells and tissues: a study in contrasts. Cancer **2,** 241–322 (1975)

Ross, L. J. N.: Antiviral T cell-mediated immunity in Marek's disease. Nature **268,** 644–646 (1977)

Ross, L. J. N., Frazier, J. A., Biggs, P. M.: An antigen common to some avian and mammalian herpesviruses. In: Oncogenesis and herpesviruses. Biggs, P. M., de-Thé, G., Payne, L. N. (eds.), pp. 480–484. Lyon: IARC 1972

Ross, L. J. N., Powell, P. C., Walker, D. J., Rennie, M., Payne, L. N.: Expression of virus-specific, thymus-specific and tumour-specific antigens in lymphoblastoid cell lines derived from Marek's disease lymphomas. J. Gen. Virol. **35,** 219–235 (1977)

Sabin, A. B.: Herpes simplex-genitalis virus nonvirion antigens and their implication in certain human cancers: Unconfirmed. Proc. Natl. Acad. Sci. USA **71,** 3248–3252 (1974)

Sabin, A. B., Tarro, G.: Herpes simplex and herpes genitalis viruses in etiology of some human cancers. Proc. Natl. Acad. Sci. USA **70,** 3225–3229 (1973)

Schaffer, P. A., Falk, L. A., Deinhardt, F.: Brief Communication: Attenuation of *herpesvirus saimiri* for marmosets after successive passage in cell culture at 39° C. J. Natl. Cancer Inst. **55,** 1243–1246 (1975)

Schneider, P.: Malignant lymphoma resembling Burkitt's Tumour in rhesus monkeys: light- and electron microscopic studies. Beitr. Pathol. **155,** 285–296 (1975)

Schneweis, K. E., Haag, A., Lehmköster, A., Koenig, U.: Sero-immunological investigations in patients with cervical cancer: Higher rate of HSV-2 antibodies than in syphilis patients and evidence of IgM antibodies to an early HSV-2 antigen. In: Oncogenesis and herpesviruses II. de-Thé, G., Epstein, M. A., zur Hausen, H. (eds.), Part 2, pp. 53–57. Lyon: IARC 1975

Schröder, C. H., Kaerner, H. C., Munk, K., Darai, G.: Morphological transformation of rat embryonic fibroblasts by abortive herpes simplex virus infection: Increased transformation rate correlated to a defective viral genotype. Intervirology **8,** 164–171 (1977)

Sharma, J. M.: Marek's disease, Lucké's frog carcinoma and other animal oncogenic herpesviruses. Bibl. Haematol. **43,** 343–347 (1976)

Sharma, J. M., Coulson, B. D.: Cell-mediated cytotoxic response to cells bearing Marek's disease tumor-associated surface antigen in chickens infected with Marek's disease virus. J. Natl. Cancer Inst. **58,** 1647–1651 (1977)

Sharma, J. M., Burger, D., Kenzy, S. G.: Serological relationships among herpesviruses: Cross-reaction between Marek's disease virus and pseudorabies virus as detected by immunofluorescence. Infect. Immun. **5,** 406–411 (1972 a)

Sharma, J. M., Witter, R. L., Shramek, G., Wolfe, L. G., Burmester, B. R., Deinhardt, F.: Lack of pathogenicity of Marek's disease virus and herpesvirus of turkeys in marmoset monkeys. J. Natl. Cancer Inst. **49,** 1191–1197 (1972 b)

Sharma, J. M., Witter, R. L., Burmester, B. R., Landon, J. C.: Public health implications of Marek's disease virus and herpesvirus of turkeys. Studies on human and subhuman primates. J. Natl. Cancer Inst. **51,** 1123–1128 (1973)

Sharma, J. M., Nazerian, K., Witter, R. L.: Reduced incidence of Marek's disease gross lymphoma in T-cell-depleted chickens. J. Natl. Cancer Inst. **58**, 689–693 (1977)

Simonds, J. A., Robey, W. G., Graham, B. J., Oie, H., Vande Woude, G. F.: Purification of *herpesvirus saimiri* and properties of the viral DNA. Arch. Virol. **49**, 249–259 (1975)

Smith, W., MacKay, J. M. K.: Morphological observations on a virus associated with sheep pulmonary adenomatosis (jaagsiekte). J. Comp. Pathol. **79**, 421–424 (1969)

Spieker, J. O., Yuill, T. M.: *Herpesvirus sylvilagus* in cottontail rabbits. Antibody prevalence and flea burden relationships. J. Wildl. Dis. **12**, 310–314 (1976)

Spieker, J. O., Yuill, T. M.: *Herpesvirus sylvilagus* in cottontail rabbits: evidence of shedding but not trans placental transmission. J. Wildl. Dis. **13**, 85–89 (1977 a)

Spieker, J. O., Yuill, T. M.: *Herpesvirus sylvilagus* in cottontail rabbits: attempted laboratory transmission by 2 insect species. J. Wildl. Dis. **13**, 90–93 (1977 b)

Stowell, R. E., Smith, E. K., Espa, N. A. C., Nelson, V. G.: Outbreak of malignant lymphoma in rhesus monkeys. Lab. Invest. **25**, 476–479 (1971)

Svedmyr, E., Jondal, M.: Cytotoxic effector cells specific for B-cell lines transformed by Epstein-Barr virus are present with infectious mononucleosis. Proc. Natl. Acad. Sci. USA **72**, 1622–1626 (1975)

Takahashi, M., Yamanishi, K.: Transformation of hamster embryo and human embryo cells by temperature-sensitive mutants of herpes simplex virus type 2. Virology **61**, 306–311 (1974)

Tarro, G.: Analysis and description of procedures used in the study of the relationship of herpes simplex virus "non-virion" antigens to certain cancers. In: Oncogenesis and herpesviruses II. de-Thé, G., Epstein, M. A., zur Hausen, H. (eds.), Part 2, pp. 291–297. Lyon: IARC 1975

Tarro, G., Sabin, A. B.: Virus specific, labile, nonvirion antigen in herpesvirus-infected cells. Proc. Natl. Acad. Sci. **65**, 753–760 (1970)

Tarro, G., Sabin, A. B.: Nonvirion antigens produced by herpes simplex viruses 1 and 2. Proc. Natl. Acad. Sci. **70**, 1032–1036 (1973)

Thiry, L., Sprecher-Goldberger, S., Fassin, Y., Gould, I., Gompel, C., Pestiau, J., de Halleux, F.: Variations of cytotoxic antibodies to cells with herpes simplex virus antigens in women with progressing or regressing cancerous lesions of the cervix. Am. J. Epidemiol. **100**, 251–261 (1974)

Tralka, T. S., Costa, J., Rabson, A.: Electron microscopic study of *herpesvirus saimiri*. Virology **80**, 158–165 (1977)

Tweedell, K. S., Wong, W. Y.: Frog kidney tumors induced by herpesvirus cultured in pronephric cells. J. Natl. Cancer Inst. **52**, 621–624 (1974)

de Villiers, E. M., Els, H. J., Verwoerd, D. W.: Characteristics of an ovine herpesvirus associated with pulmonary adenomatosis (jaagsiekte) in sheep. South Afr. J. Med. Sci. **49**, 165–175 (1975)

Wagner, E. K., Roizman, B., Savage, T., Spear, P. G., Mizell, M., Durr, F. E., Sypowicz, D.: Characterization of the DNA of herpesviruses associated with Lucké adenocarcinoma of the frog and Burkitt lymphoma of man. Virology **42**, 257–261 (1970)

Wallen, W. C., Neubauer, R. H., Rabin, H., Cicmanec, J. L.: Nonimmune rosette formation by lymphoma and leukemia cells from *herpesvirus saimiri*-infected owl monkeys. J. Natl. Cancer Inst. **51**, 967–975 (1973)

Wallen, W. C., Neubauer, R. H., Rabin, H.: Evidence for suppressor cell activity associated with induction of *herpesvirus saimiri*-induced lymphoma. Clin. Exp. Immunol. **22**, 468–472 (1975 a)

Wallen, W. C., Rabin, H., Neubauer, R. H., Cicmanec, J. L.: Depression in lymphocyte response to general mitogens by owl monkeys infected with *herpesvirus saimiri*. J. Natl. Cancer Inst. **54**, 679–685 (1975 b)

Wegner, D. L., Hinze, H. C.: Virus-host-cell relationship of *herpesvirus sylvilagus* with cottontail rabbit leukocytes. Int. J. Cancer **14**, 567–575 (1974)

Werner, F.-J., Bornkamm, G. W., Fleckenstein, B.: Episomal viral DNA in a *herpesvirus saimiri*-transformed lymphoid cell line. J. Virol. **22**, 794–803 (1977)

Wilbanks, G. D., Deinhardt, F., Goodheart, C. R., Nahmias, A. J., Rawls, W. E.: Herpesvirus and cervical cancer. Cancer Res. **33**, 1345–1363 (1973)

Witter, R. L.: Epidemiology of Marek's disease. In: Oncogenesis and herpesviruses. Biggs, P. M., de-Thé, G. Payne, L. N. (eds.), pp. 111–122. Lyon: IARC 1972

Witter, R. L.: Natural mechanisms of controlling lymphotropic herpesvirus infection (Marek's disease) in the chicken. Cancer Res. **36**, 681–687 (1976)

Witter, R. L., Lee, L. F., Okazaki, W., Purchase, H. G., Burmester, B. R., Luginbuhl, R. E.: Oncogenesis by Marek's disease herpesvirus in chickens lacking expression of endogenous group specific chick helper factor Rous associated virus O and exogenous avian RNA tumor viruses. J. Natl. Cancer Inst. **55**, 215–218 (1975 a)

Witter, R. L., Stephens, E. A., Sharma, J. M., Nazerian, K.: Demonstration of a tumor-associated surface antigen in Marek's disease. J. Immunol. **115,** 177–183 (1975b)

Witter, R. L., Sharma, J. M., Offenbecker, L.: Turkey herpesvirus infection in chickens: Induction of lymphoproliferative lesions and characterization of vaccinal immunity against Marek's disease. Avian Dis. **20,** 676–692 (1976)

Wolf, K.: Herpesviruses of lower vertebrates. In: The herpesviruses. Kaplan, A. S. (ed.), pp. 495–520. New York: Academic Press 1973

Wolfe, L. G., Deinhardt, F.: Overview of viral oncology studies in *Saguinus* and *Callithrix* species. Primates Med. **10,** 96–118 (1978)

Wolfe, L. G., Falk, L. A., Deinhardt, F.: Oncogenicity of *herpesvirus saimiri* in marmoset monkeys. J. Natl. Cancer Inst. **47,** 1145–1162 (1971)

Wong, W. Y., Tweedell, K. S.: Two viruses from the Lucké tumor isolated in a frog pronephric cell line. Proc. Soc. Exp. Biol. Med. **145,** 1201–1206 (1974)

Wong, W. Y., Tweedell, K. S.: Viral carcinogenesis in a pronephric cell line: an ultrastructural study of rana-pipiens herpesviruses Lucké renal tumor. Am. J. Pathol. **80,** 143–152 (1975)

Wright, H. T.: Cytomegaloviruses. In: The herpesviruses. Kaplan, A. S. (ed.), pp. 354–388. New York: Academic Press 1973

Wright, J., Falk, L. A., Collins, D., Deinhardt, F.: Mononuclear cell fraction carrying *herpesvirus saimiri* in persistently infected squirrel monkeys. J. Natl. Cancer Inst. **57,** 959–962 (1976)

Wright, J., Falk, L. A., Wolfe, L. G., Deinhardt, F. W.: Lymphocyte populations of *Callithrix jacchus* marmosets. Cell. Immunol. **35,** 148–157 (1978)

zur Hausen, H., Schulte-Holthausen, H.: Presence of EB-virus nucleic acid homology in a "virus-free" line of Burkitt tumor cells. Nature **227,** 245–248 (1970)

zur Hausen, H., Schulte-Holthausen, H., Klein, G., Henle, W., Henle, G., Clifford, P., Santesson, L.: EBV DNA in biopsies of Burkitt tumors and anaplastic carcinomas of the nasopharynx. Nature **228,** 1056–1058, (1970)

zur Hausen, H., Fresen, K.-O.: Heterogeneity of Epstein-Barr virus II. Induction of early antigens (EA) by complementation. Virology **81,** 138–143 (1977)

18 Demographic Studies Implicating the Virus in the Causation of Burkitt's Lymphoma; Prospects for Nasopharyngeal Carcinoma

G. de-Thé[1]

International Agency for Research on Cancer (IARC) – W.H.O. – Lyon (France). On sabbatical leave to the Department of the Regius Professor of Medicine, University of Oxford (England)

[1] Present address: CNRS International Program on Human Tumors, Faculty of Medicine A. Carrel, Lyon and IRSC, Villejuif (France).

A. INTRODUCTION

The preceding chapters have described the basis and the strength of the association between the Epstein-Barr virus (EBV) and infectious mononucleosis (IM), Burkitt's lymphoma (BL), and nasopharyngeal carcinoma (NPC). They have shown how viral fingerprints can regularly be found in the tumor B lymphoblasts of BL and in the epithelial tumor cells of NPC, how humoral and cell-mediated immune responses to EBV antigens are greatly elevated in patients with BL or NPC, and how EBV has in vitro transforming activity for B lymphocytes (bone marrow-derived lymphocytes) of human and simian origin, as well as oncogenic potential in some new-world monkey species.

All these data favor the conclusion but do not *prove* that EBV is oncogenic in humans. Direct demonstration can only be obtained epidemiologically either by studying the sequence of events between infection and tumor development or by successful intervention against the virus (e. g., by a vaccine).

The epidemiologic approach is very rewarding if carried out in logical sequence. The first step would be to investigate the *natural history* of the viral infection and to compare it with that of the associated diseases. Can the epidemiologic characteristics of EBV infection explain those of BL and/or NPC? If successfully carried out, this step should lead to specific and testable hypotheses regarding the nature (noncausal, causal–direct or indirect) of the association between the virus and the development of the disease. The second step should consist of testing specific hypotheses, mainly through prospective studies. Very few prospective studies have, in fact, been carried out in cancer research but, as is described below, they represent a unique way of obtaining crucial information. These prospective studies naturally lead the way for intervention measures against the putative causative agent which can finally bring proof for a causal association and prevent the disease (the mission of epidemiology).

After comparing the epidemiologic characteristics of EBV infection with those of the associated tumors (BL and NPC), the results of the prospective BL study carried out in Uganda will be described and discussed in this chapter. We will examine the prospects for the epidemiologic approach in the field of NPC and then see how intervention might be undertaken to prevent EBV-associated diseases.

B. EPIDEMIOLOGIC CHARACTERISTICS OF EBV INFECTION AND OF THE ASSOCIATED TUMORS

Whereas the main epidemiologic characteristic of EBV is the variation in age at primary infection (depending on socioeconomic factors), that of BL is the critical role of geographic factors and that of NPC is the apparent role of genetic factors.

I. AGE AT EBV INFECTION DEPENDENT ON SOCIOECONOMIC (CULTURAL) FACTORS

The most important characteristic of EBV is its ubiquity: even the most remote and isolated tribes – such as in the Aleutian islands (Tischendorf et al., 1970), the

Amazonian plateau (Black et al., 1970), and the Melanesian islands (Lang et al. 1977) –
are infected by EBV (under these primitive conditions 100% of the population are
infected).

The second important characteristic was observed by Henle, who noted that the age
distribution of individuals with antibody to EB viral capsid antigen (VCA) varied with
hygienic and socioeconomic standards (Henle et al., 1969) (Fig. 1 of Chap. 4). He also
showed that in primitive societies EBV infection takes place earlier than in western
societies. In the latter there are significant differences in the age-specific prevalence
among socioeconomic classes. Hinuma et al. (1969) claimed that crowded conditions
led to early EBV infection.

The value of understanding the epidemiology of EBV infection was shown
when two technicians, who lacked antibody to the virus, seroconverted after developing acute IM (Henle et al., 1968; Chap. 13). The retrospective study carried out
on Yale medical students demonstrated that in fact only students lacking antibodies to EBV were candidates for IM (Niederman et al., 1968; Evans et al., 1968).
As will be discussed later, the prospective study on BL developed from the above
findings.

We conducted seroepidemiologic surveys on the prevalence of EBV infection in
populations suffering from different diseases associated with EBV – namely, Chinese
in Hong Kong and Singapore having a high incidence of NPC, Malays and Indo-
Pakistanis in Singapore having intermediate and low incidences of NPC, Ugandans in
the West Nile District of Uganda having a high BL incidence, and Caucasians in
France where IM is endemic. Representative samples of the general populations were
selected, visited, bled, and tested blind for EBV antibody serologic reactivity (see
details in International Agency for Research on Cancer (IARC) Annual Reports
1974–1976; de-Thé et al., 1975). Great care was taken to avoid any bias due to
differences in antigen batches, readings, etc. (Geser et al., 1974). Figure 1 shows the
prevalence and geometric mean titers (GMT) (of positive sera) of both VCA and early
antigen (EA) reactivities in three of these populations (Ugandan, Chinese Singaporeans, and Indian Singaporeans). It can be seen that in Uganda the prevalence of EBV
infection reaches 100% by the age of 3 years, whereas in Singapore the infection is
delayed in both ethnic groups (Chinese and Indo-Pakistani), who exhibited up to 20%
seronegative individuals in the 5–9 year-old age group. The number noted on the
curves refers to the number of sera tested in each age group. It can be seen that the
likelihood of finding seronegative children in Uganda after the age of 3 years is
practically nil. The curves on the *right* give the GMT of the positive sera in the different
age groups. The levels of the GMT reflect to a certain extent the mode of immune
response to primary EBV infection in the populations studied. The situation in
Uganda is striking: in the age group 1–2 years the GMT reaches a peak of 421, similar
to that observed in BL patients, whereas in Singapore it only averages 100. The
prevalence of antibodies to EA in the first 4 years of life in Uganda also confirms that
early infection takes place.

In Singapore and Hong Kong the population density is 1000 times higher than in
the West Nile District of Uganda, yet EBV infection takes place much later than in
tropical Africa! As the socioeconomic conditions in these areas are similar, one must
look for specific cultural habits favoring the transmission of the virus. The role of
saliva is believed to be critical. Viral infection could take place very early in life by
mouth-to-mouth "kiss feeding" between mother and baby. In equatorial Africa. 50%

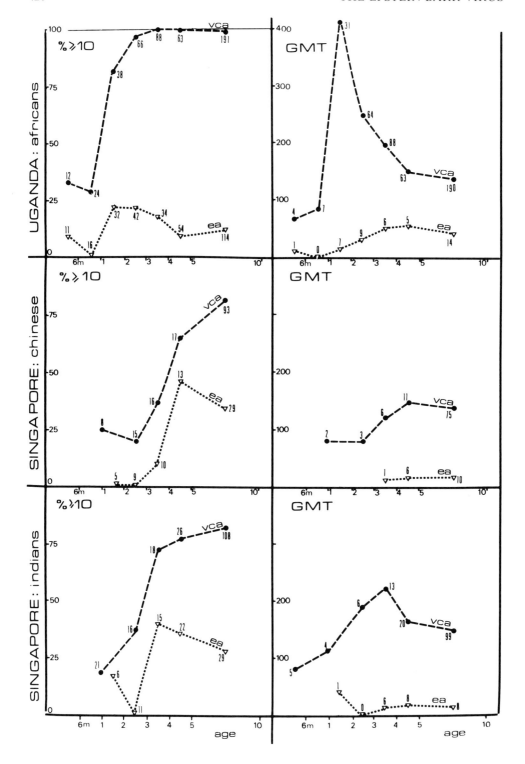

of the general population are shedding infectious EBV in the saliva compared to 10% in the United States (Gerber et al., 1976).

IM is caused by a relatively late primary EBV infection in adolescents of high social strata. In the early 1970s BL was thought to represent a "malignant" IM, resulting from an unusually late primary infection in tropical areas. BL, being a very rare condition, one could postulate that the few children who escaped primary infection before 4 or 5 years of age would represent the group at highest risk of developing BL. This formed the core of the discussions leading to the BL prospective study. However, later on, an alternative postulate seemed more likely – namely, that the children who suffered primary infection by EBV early in life might represent those at highest risk for BL (de-Thé, 1977). How early in life EBV infection can occur is debatable – prenatally, perinatally, or under maternal antibodies (i. e., 3–6 months after birth)? No data are yet available to confirm any of these possibilities, but collection of sera and saliva in newborns, with a 2-year follow-up, is in progress in Tanzania. The markers for such an early infection are not obvious, since the babies have maternal IgG. However, the presence of IgM antibodies specific for VCA and EA, of IgG to EA, and eventually of transforming EBV in the saliva of these babies could all be taken as indicating a primary infection by EBV. To obtain information on the mode of EBV transmission, saliva and milk are being collected from the mothers and will eventually be studied for the presence of transforming EBV.

The occurence of early EBV infection in tropical areas does not prove that it is related to BL development. Such proof would necessitate a long-term prospective study, which is not feasible at present. But there might be an alternative way to investigate this relationship. Deep social changes are taking place in equatorial Africa, particularly in Tanzania where cooperative ("ujamaa") villages were set up a few years ago. It would be of great value to follow the age-specific prevalence of EBV infection with the socioeconomic development of the country and to relate such changes to alterations in disease patterns. For example, improvements in maternal health and child care could be predicted to result in the disappearance of BL in equatorial Africa. If this were to occur, it would be reminiscent of the fall in the incidence of tuberculosis in industrialized countries accompanying the rising standard of living, which in fact preceded intervention by the medical profession (e. g., antibiotics and vaccines).

II. BURKITT'S LYMPHOMA DETERMINED BY CLIMATIC FACTORS

Since the epidemiology of BL has been well described in Chap. 14, the main point to be stressed here is that a number of epidemiologic characteristics of BL, such as the combined role of temperature, humidity, and altitude (Burkitt, 1962 a, b), space-time clustering well seen in the West Nile District of Uganda (Pike et al., 1967; Williams et al., 1978), and seasonal variation (Williams et al., 1974) cannot be explained by the characteristics of EBV infection described above. In contrast, the geographic

Fig. 1. Prevalence *(curves at left)* and geometric mean titers (GMT) of positive sera *(curves at right)* of antibodies to VCA and EA in representative samples of three populations: Ugandans (at high risk for BL), Chinese Singaporeans (at risk for NPC), and Indian Singaporeans (at no risk for BL or NPC). The numbers of sera for each point of the curves are noted. From de-Thé, G. (1977): Courtesy of the editor and publisher

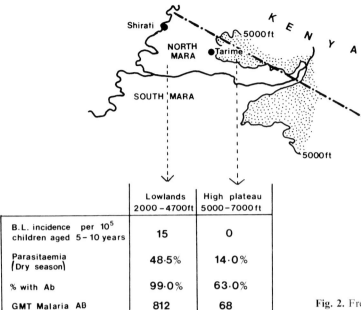

	Lowlands 2000–4700ft	High plateau 5000–7000ft
B.L. incidence per 10^5 children aged 5–10 years	15	0
Parasitaemia (Dry season)	48·5%	14·0%
% with Ab	99·0%	63·0%
GMT Malaria AB	812	68

AB = Antibodies to malaria ; GMT = Geometric mean titers

Fig. 2. Frequency of Burkitt's lymphoma and malaria in North Mara District, Tanzania

distribution of hyper- or holo-endemic malaria fits with that of BL (Dalldorf et al., 1964; Burkitt, 1970; O'Conor, 1970). Recent malaria surveys carried out by the IARC in the North Mara region of Tanzania have shown that both malaria parasite rates and GMT of antibodies to malaria differ markedly in the BL-free high plateaus and in the lowlands, where the incidence of BL is of the same order as that of the West Nile District of Uganda (Geser et al., in preparation; IARC Annual Reports 1976, 1977) (Fig. 2). Malaria could act either in facilitating a specific type of EBV infection by depressing the immune surveillance of the host or in increasing the size of the pool of target cells susceptible to a subsequent oncogenic event. Congenital malaria creates an extreme condition in which the placental barrier is obviously altered and congenital EBV infection could possibly result. Congenital overt malaria is very rare in African children (in contrast to Caucasian), but the finding of plasmodia in cord blood is not too rare an event (Draper, personal communication). On the other hand, heavy infection in newborns might create a condition in which a primary EBV infection results in a dramatic situation leading to a large pool of EBV-carrying cells (the size of this pool possibly being linked to the risk of later BL development).

III. NASOPHARYNGEAL CARCINOMA APPARENTLY DEPENDENT ON GENETIC AND CULTURAL FACTORS

The geographic distribution of NPC is uneven throughout the world, the incidence being very high in some populations of Chinese descent, intermediate in a number of countries around the Mediterranean and East Africa, and low in the rest of the world (Fig. 3). In Singapore the rate for NPC was found to be different in the different sublanguage groups, the Cantonese Chinese being at highest risk (the incidence in males being 30 per 100,000), intermediate in the Teochew (known in Hong Kong as Chiu Chau) (17 per 100,000), and somewhat lower in the Hokkien (originating from Fukien) (13 per 100,000) (Shanmugaratnam, 1973). Studies designed to look for specific differences in the cultural pattern of these various language groups have failed to date to uncover any risk factor related to NPC. However, immigrant Chinese in the United States appear to have a decreasing incidence, suggesting that environmental and cultural factors play a role (Buell, 1965, 1973; King and Haenszel, 1972; Fraumeni and Mason, 1974).

Intermediate incidence rates occur in northern and western Kenya, northern Uganda, and southern Sudan; also in a number of countries around the Mediterranean, such as Morocco, Algeria, Tunisia, Greece, and southern Italy, and amongst Israeli Jews born in Arab countries (de-Thé et al., 1976).

That genetic factors play a role in NPC development is suggested by the fact that many of the South East Asian populations, who have a high incidence of NPC, are also genetically related to the southern Chinese but have different cultural patterns. Furthermore, Ho (1967, 1972) has stressed the occurrence of familial clustering of NPC cases. Multicase families have also been described in intermediate incidence areas (Williams and de-Thé, 1974). One approach in investigating the role of genetic factors in NPC development has been to study blood genetic markers such as red cell antigens, red cell enzymes, and human leukocyte antigen (HL-A) profiles to determine whether NPC patients had specific characteristics. Simons and colleagues (1975) found an HL-A profile associated with high NPC risk in Cantonese Chinese consisting of A2-Bsin2 haplotype, the sin2 antigen being observed only in Mongolian populations. This haplotype was not observed in NPC patients from other parts of the world, but HL-A markers might differ with the genetic make-up of the race or ethnic group concerned. The existence of an NPC disease-susceptibility gene close to but outside the HL-A region of chromosome 6 has been postulated and may represent an immune-response gene.

C. THE IARC PROSPECTIVE STUDY OF BURKITT'S LYMPHOMA IN UGANDA AND THE CAUSATIVE ROLE OF THE VIRUS

The discovery of the role of the virus in the development of IM (thanks to retrospective studies) provided a model for BL. The question arose whether a prospective study on BL aimed at revealing the "pretumor" EBV profile was feasible. To answer such a question, an IARC conference was convened in Nairobi in December 1968 to consider prospects for conducting a longitudinal seroepidemiologic survey in a population with a high incidence of BL. At this conference specific hypotheses were formulated which could be tested in a 5-year prospective study involving 35,000 children aged 2–5 years. For an infection as ubiquitous as EBV, it was necessary to show that candidates for the disease were infected with, or reacted to, the virus in a way different from that of the general population: the difference being, for example, age at infection, degree of infection, or mode of response to infection. It was also possible that the serologic profile with respect to EBV observed in BL patients might have arisen *as a result* of the disease, since the tumor cells were of the type which harbors the virus.

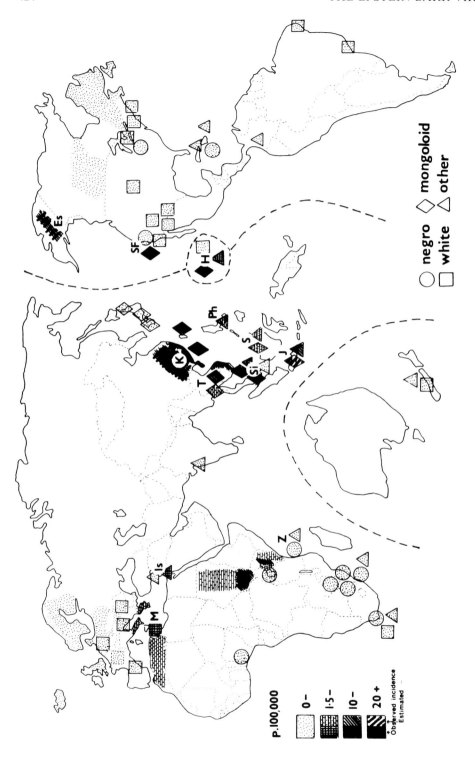

I. FOUR TESTABLE HYPOTHESES

Four testable hypotheses were therefore formulated (IARC, 1968; Geser and de-Thé, 1972).

Hypothesis 1 (the Null Hypothesis). There is *no causal* relationship between EBV and BL. The EBV serology profiles of children who later develop BL should not differ from those of age, sex, and locality matched controls. The high reactivities in BL patients after diagnosis would reflect a secondary reactivation of a passenger virus.

Hypothesis 2 (the IM Model). BL develops *shortly after a primary infection* (e. g., within 2 years) *with EBV*. Sera collected from patients before the incubation period would *lack* antibody to EBV.

Hypothesis 3. BL develops in children who have had a *long and heavy exposure to EBV*. The sera of "future" BL patients would exhibit high antibody titers long before the diagnosis of BL.

Hypothesis 4. EBV plays a causal role in BL, but the latent periods between infection and clinical onset are long and variable and the intervention of cofactors at critical times is also necessary. Prior to diagnosis the reactivity of the sera from BL patients might differ from that of controls, but in an unpredictable manner.

Two further workshops (in 1969 and 1970) were necessary to launch this large undertaking, designed primarily to test hypotheses 2 and 3. It was decided to implement it in the West Nile District of Uganda (Fig. 4), an area where the incidence of BL had been well documented for more than a decade.

Feasibility studies took place in 1969 to assess the cooperation of the population and the stability of EBV reactivities over an 18-month period (Kafuko et al., 1972). These studies also showed that $\sim 10\%$ of the population had titers lower than 1/10 and another 10%, greater than 1/160. Assuming that children in either of these groups (under hypotheses 2 and 3) might have at least a fivefold increase in risk of developing BL, then 30 cases of BL developing in the study cohort would be necessary to prove one of the hypotheses. It was estimated that a 5-year follow-up of around 35,000 children aged 4–8 years would yield 35 cases of BL.

◀ **Fig. 3.** Incidence of cancer of the nasopharynx. World distribution of NPC. One can recognize four levels of incidence:
1. The highest (20 per 10^5) is in the southern province of Kwang-tung in the People's Republic of China and in Cantonese immigrants in South East Asia (SEA).
2. The next highest (10–20 per 10^5) is in Cantonese immigrants outside SEA: e. g., in the United States (Hawaii and San Francisco).
3. There is intermediate incidence (1.5–9 per 10^5) around the Mediterranean and the Rift Valley in East Africa.
4. Low incidence (< 1.5) characterizes the rest of the world.
Geometric figures refer to Cancer Registries whereas *shaded areas* refer to estimated incidence from relative frequency data. (Map kindly prepared by Ms. Paula Cook from the Department of the Regius Professor of Medicine, University of Oxford, England.)
ES, Eskimos; *H*, Hawaii; *Is*, Israel; *J*, Java; *K*, Province of Kwang-tung in the People's Republic of China; *M*, Malta; *Ph*, Philippines; *S*, Sumatra; *SF*, San Francisco

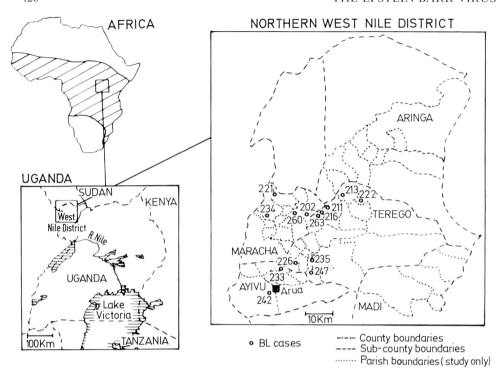

Fig. 4. Prospective study of BL in the West Nile District of Uganda. From de-Thé, G. et al. (1978 a):
Courtesy of the editor and publisher

II. IMPLEMENTATION OF THE STUDY

The prospective study was implemented in late 1971 when public meetings were held in
the localities where children were to be bled, in order to explain the purpose of the work
and gain the confidence of the population. A few days before the collection of blood in
each locality, house-to-house visits were made and all members of each household were
registered. Eligible children were thus identified and their parents asked to bring them,
2 or 3 days later, to a meeting point which was usually within 2–3 km of their homes.
Venous blood was collected whenever possible, but from very young children blood
was collected by finger prick. In order to look for malaria parasites, thick and thin
blood films were made at the same time. The blood samples were then placed in an
insulated box and centrifuged the following day at the field laboratory set up in Arua,
the capital of the district. The sera, stored in a deep freezer, were then shipped to
IARC, Lyon, for long-term storage in liquid nitrogen.

    Great care was taken to ensure that each serum sample could be easily located. A
number of checks were made by introducing small amounts of tritiated water at the
bleeding site into some of the blood samples and subsequently checking for tritium in
the stored sera. No major errors were detected.

    In the period February 1972 to September 1974, sera from 42,000 children aged 0–8
years were obtained. Systematic search for new cases of BL among the surveyed
children started early in 1973, with a "case detection" team regularly visiting all health
centers, dispensaries, and hospitals in the survey area. All suspected cases were sent to

Kuluva Hospital, where Dr. E. H. Williams examined the patients and took the following specimens: (1) a needle biopsy and touch smears for cytologic evaluation of the tumor; (2) a biopsy sent in part to the Department of Pathology at Makerere University in Kampala and in part to IARC in Lyon for evaluation by an international panel of pathologists (Dr. G. O'Conor, National Cancer Institute, Bethesda, and Prof. D. Wright, University of Southampton, U. K.); (3) a piece of tissue frozen for detection of EBV DNA by nucleic acid hybridization and for detection of EBV nuclear antigen (EBNA) by the indirect anti-complement immunofluorescence test; (4) a serum sample from the case together with serum samples from all members of his/her family; and (5) thick and thin blood films to be examined for malaria parasites.

Three types of control were used for comparison of EBV profiles with that of each new BL patient: (1) a neighbor of the same age and sex randomly selected in the field station from the list of those bled in the main survey, this control being revisited and bled again together with his/her family; (2) four control sera were selected from the serum bank at IARC, Lyon, taken from children of the same age, sex, and locality as the BL patient and bled in the main survey at about the same time; and (3) sera from a random sample of the surveyed population.

III. BUTKITT'S LYMPHOMA CANDIDATES HAVE HIGH VCA TITERS LONG BEFORE TUMOR DEVELOPMENT

Up to the end of November 1977, a total of 31 children with lymphomas were detected in the surveyed areas, 14 being bled previously, with time intervals ranging from 7 to 54 months between the main bleeding and clinical diagnosis. The "pre-BL" as well as the "post-BL" sera of the cases and of the various controls were tested simultaneously and blind in the IARC laboratory in Lyon (for VCA, EA, EBNA, and complement fixation) and in Dr. W. Henle's laboratory in Philadelphia (for VCA, EA, and EBNA). Whereas no significant differences were detected for EBNA and EA reactivities, higher VCA titers were observed in both laboratories in the pre-BL sera when compared to those of the matched controls (Fig. 5). The GMTs for BL patients were 425.5 and 176.7, respectively, in the two laboratories, whereas the GMTs for the controls were 125.8 and 52.7, respectively. Although the titers were higher in the IARC laboratory than in the Henle laboratory (due to differences in the cell line used and mode of reading), the ratios of the GMTs of patients and controls were $\sim$ 3.4–1 in both laboratories.

These differences were found to be significant in both laboratories (IARC: t, 3.00; p, 0.01; Henle: t, 2.65; p, 0.02 – two-sided Student's t test). A nonparametric test gave similar p values (0.008) when the probability was considered that 7 of the 14 pre-BL sera had VCA titers higher than any of their controls. The VCA titers of the pre-BL sera were also compared with the GMTs of representative samples of the general population in the surveyed areas. The titers of all but two of the patients were higher than the mean of the corresponding age group in the normal population (de-Thé et al., 1978 a).

The degree of increased risk of developing BL in children with VCA titers two or more dilutions above the mean of the normal population, standardized for age, sex, and locality, was 30 times that of the general population.

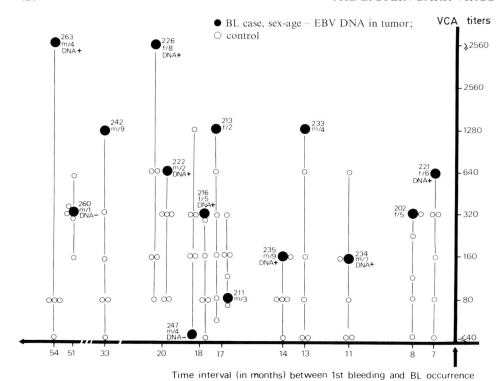

Fig. 5. EBV VCA antibody titers in sera collected from BL cases prior to tumor manifestation and from controls. By length of interval between bleeding and case detection. From de-Thé, G., et al. (1978a): Courtesy of the editor and publisher

IV. UNEXPECTED STABILITY OF VCA TITERS AT TUMOR ONSET

Figure 6 shows the evolution of VCA and EA titers from pre- to post-disease onset. A remarkable *stability* of VCA titers was observed over several years. This indicated that high VCA levels previously observed in BL patients were *present long before clinical onset of the disease*. Regarding the other EBV reactivities, only EA antibodies rose, in 8 of the 14 cases, subsequent to initial bleeding. Of these, 7 had antibodies directed against the restricted (R) component, the 5 long-term survivors all being in this category. No marked change was observed in the selected controls between initial bleeding and time of onset of the BL cases in the matched patients and no serologic differences were observed in pre- and post-sera from family members of cases and controls.

The pre- and post-BL sera as well as control sera were also tested for antibodies to herpes simplex virus (HSV), cytomegalovirus (CMV), and measles virus at the Center for Disease Control, Atlanta, Georgia, USA. No marked difference was observed in antibody level relative to cases and controls. Malaria parasite counts at the time of the main bleeding and onset of BL were investigated in cases and controls. No difference was observed between BL cases prior to diagnosis and controls, but at the time of disease onset BL patients had significantly less parasites than controls, possibly due to anti-malaria drugs being taken prior to presentation at hospital for BL diagnosis.

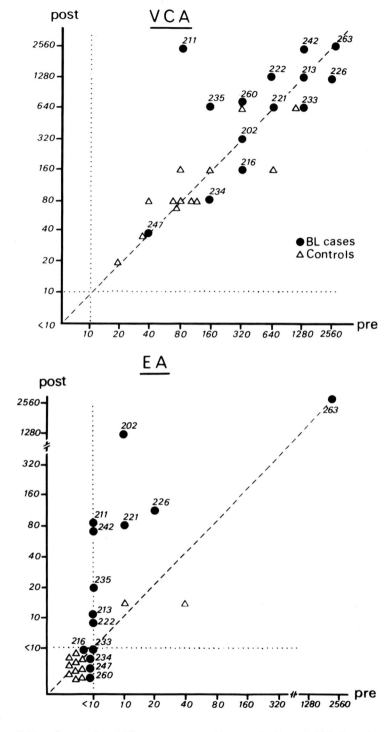

Fig. 6. EBV serologic reactivities of pre- and post-BL sera as compared to controls. From de-Thé, G., et al. (1978a): Courtesy of the editor and publisher

V. EPIDEMIOLOGIC EVIDENCE FOR EBV INVOLVEMENT IN CAUSATION OF BURKITT'S LYMPHOMA

The above data strongly support the third hypothesis mentioned earlier, i. e., that long and unusually heavy infection with the virus would lead to BL development, and discount the second hypothesis based on the IM model. Ten out of the 14 pre-BL sera had VCA titers as high as, or higher than, any of their controls. Of the remaining four patients, three had atypical characteristics: case 211, which presented with cervical lymph nodes, had a long history of 16 weeks before coming to the hospital and had EA antibody directed against the diffuse (D) component – all characteristics being atypical of BL. In two further cases (260 and 247) no viral DNA was detected: case 260 was diagnosed as "unclassified lymphoma"; while case 247 appeared to be an EBV-free lymphoma by all criteria (low serology before and after tumor onset and lack of viral markers in the tumor). The remaining case (234) had EBV markers in the tumor tissue, but its VCA titer preceding tumor development was average when compared to controls.

In the seven BL cases where tumor tissue showed EBV markers, all but one exhibited VCA titers higher than their matched controls prior to tumor onset. Although these data are insufficient to be conclusive, they strongly suggest that there are two types of lymphoma in tropical regions: EBV-associated and EBV-free. The EBV-associated lymphomas would have high VCA titers long before clinical onset and EBV markers in the tumor cells. The EBV-free lymphomas would have VCA titers similar to those of the general population prior to the disease and the tumor would have no detectable EBV markers. The EBV-free tumors form the great majority of childhood B lymphomas in temperate climates, while they are the exception in tropical areas: their etiology is unknown. The EBV-associated lymphomas would represent the disease described by Burkitt in tropical areas (Chap. 14).

VI. MEANING OF THE DISCREPANCY IN THE EBV REACTIVITIES ASSOCIATED WITH RISK OF BURKITT'S LYMPHOMA

The absence of an increase in EBV reactivities other than VCA in BL patients prior to disease onset creates some difficulties in interpreting the observed high VCA titers as evidence of a causal relationship between EBV and BL development. It should be recalled, however, that the various anti-EBV reactivities do not develop simultaneously after primary infection nor do they persist for equal periods afterward (de-Thé and Lenoir, 1977; Chap. 4). Soon after primary infection, IgM VCA antibodies develop, then IgG antibodies to VCA rise and remain stable, with only a moderate tendency to decline over the years. In contrast, antibodies to EA develop and decline rapidly, disappearing within months. In cases of EBV reactivation, they would reappear. Development of antibodies to EBNA is delayed when compared to that of EA and VCA, sometimes for several months to a year.

The level of antibody to VCA, because of its stability, appears to be the best marker of the *severity* of the primary infection, reflecting either the infective dose or the lack of a proper host control due, for example, to an infection occurring very early in life. As mentioned above, the author has proposed that very early infection by EBV might be the initiating event in the induction of BL (de-Thé, 1977). The present results of the prospective study are compatible with such a possibility. The oncogenic potential of both oncorna and oncodnaviruses is greatly enhanced when the virus is inoculated in newborn or very young animals (Gross, 1970).

VII. NEED FOR COFACTOR

As discussed above (Sect. B.II), malaria has repeatedly been suspected of playing a role in BL development by inducing immunologic disorders. The high EBV VCA titers might then be considered a consequence of a failure to control the viral infection due to severe malaria. However, if this were the case, the BL candidates would be expected to have elevated antibodies to other common infections such as CMV, HSV, and measles virus. This was not the case. The present results would suggest that EBV might act as an *initiator* of the malignancy, whereas other factors (such as heavy endemic malaria burden) would act as *promoters,* triggering the clinical onset.

VIII. CONCLUSION

The results to hand, taken in conjunction with the in vitro transforming ability of the virus for B lymphocytes and its oncogenic potential in new-world primates (Chap. 16), strongly support a *causal association* between EBV and BL. It would seem that the oncogenic potential of EBV in man is only expressed under unusual environmental conditions.

D. PROSPECTS FOR THE EPIDEMIOLOGIC APPROACH IN NASOPHARYNGEAL CARCINOMA

The association between the virus and NPC has been described in detail in Chap. 15, but proof of the causal nature of the association is still a matter for debate. The fact that the virus is naturally present in the oropharynx makes it possible that infection of NPC epithelial tumor cells is secondary to transformation of the epithelial cells into carcinoma. This view was raised recently by Henderson (1976, 1977), who found patients with various other tumors arising in the oropharyngeal area to have elevated titers to VCA and varying levels of antibodies in patients of various ethnic origins in Los Angeles.

To examine this point further, blind serologic tests were undertaken with standardized antigenic reagents on sera from NPC patients originating from high, intermediate, and low incidence areas, together with sera from patients with other ear, nose, and throat tumors as well as from normal individuals originating from the same geographic areas. Up to three fold differences were observed between the serologic reactivities of NPC patients of different ethnic origins, but the ratios of the GMTs of patients with NPC or other tumors were similar in the different areas – around 6 for VCA and EBNA and around 20 for EA (de-Thé et al., 1978b).

The regular presence of EBV DNA in the epithelial tumor cells of NPC originating from different geographic areas also supports the view that EBV plays an etiologic role in NPC development (Desgranges et al., 1975). However, as in the case of BL, a further step in understanding and establishing the role of EBV in NPC would be to determine the EBV profile preceding clinical onset of the tumor.

I. A PROSPECTIVE STUDY

A prospective study conducted in a high risk group, such as the Cantonese Chinese, could help to elucidate the following questions concerning the relationship between EBV and NPC:

1. Do candidates for NPC have an EBV profile different from that of the general population long before tumor development? If so, this would serve as a marker for identifying the cohort on which future etiologic studies could be carried out. Furthermore, if preventive measures, such as a vaccine, are to be developed, they should be applied as a priority to this highest risk group.
2. Are certain reactivities such as IgA or IgG antibodies to EA, either in the serum or the saliva, associated with *preclinical stages* of the disease? If this were the case, then early detection of the tumor in mass surveys in high incidence areas could be undertaken. This would lead to better control of the disease through early treatment.

From the methodologic point of view, a prospective study on NPC would be on a much smaller scale than that necessary for BL, due to the dramatic difference in incidence between the two tumors. In the 45–54 year age group, the incidence of NPC in Cantonese Chinese males is 98 per 100,000. Therefore, a follow-up of 5,000 male Cantonese Chinese (aged 45–54 years) should be sufficient to yield enough cases (around 25) over a period of 5 years to determine the EBV profile preceding tumor development.

The site for conducting such a prospective study would be a matter of feasibility. Singapore represents a very good site, because of the excellent cancer registry covering the whole island. The IARC is implementing a prospective study on liver carcinoma in Singapore which may also provide some pre-NPC sera. On the other hand, Dr. Ho in Hong Kong is following NPC family members prospectively and has already observed the presence of IgA specific for VCA in three sera which preceded the onset of the tumor by 9, 30, and 35 months, respectively (Ho et al., 1978). However, it must be borne in mind that 17% of the general population and 31% of NPC family members have serum IgA to VCA (Desgranges et al., unpublished). The area of choice for such a prospective study aimed at early treatment would be Kwang-tung Province of the People's Republic of China, where this tumor has its highest incidence.

II. CLINICALLY ORIENTED SEROLOGIC STUDIES

Apart from its importance for etiology, EBV serology may help the clinician in establishing the diagnosis of NPC in low incidence areas, in evaluating the prognosis of the tumor, and in monitoring treatment anywhere in the world. Clinically oriented studies are being implemented for assessing the respective values of serum and saliva IgA and IgG to EA and VCA, in this context, and there is little doubt that EBV serology should eventually become a routine biologic test in general ear, nose, and throat clinical oncology.

E. INTERVENTION AS THE FINAL STEP IN PROVING CAUSALITY

The ultimate aim of the epidemiologist is to *prevent the disease* by intervention against the causal factors. In addition, successful intervention can produce the ultimate evidence for causality, which may not otherwise be obtainable. In the case of EBV and human malignancies, intervention against cofactors such as malaria in BL is indeed easier to conceive than intervention against the virus, but discussion of the value and feasibility of an EBV vaccine represents an important topic.

I. INTERVENTION AGAINST MALARIA TO PREVENT BURKITT'S LYMPHOMA

As mentioned in Sect. B.II of this chapter, holo- or hyper-endemic malaria is associated with BL in equatorial Africa and the question as to whether an anti-malaria intervention would successfully decrease the incidence of BL can now be answered. The advantage of such an intervention is its public health appeal, providing that once established by a foreign organization in a population, malaria control is continued by the country concerned. The situation in the North Mara District of Tanzania (discussed above) provided a good opportunity for such a project, since BL cases had been monitored for approximately 10 years: the lowlands descending to shores of Lake Victoria (i. e., from 4,700 to 2,000 feet above sea level) have a BL incidence of the same order as that observed in the West Nile District of Uganda (15 per 100,000), whereas there were no registered cases on the high plateaus ranging from 5,000 to 7,000 feet above sea level.

In April 1977, an IARC/WHO/Tanzanian project was implemented whereby chloroquin tablets were distributed twice a month to all children aged 0–10 years in the North Mara District (around 70,000 children). Urine tests were carried out at random on these children to check their consumption of the drug. The control area was represented by the South Mara District, where there was no drug distribution by IARC but where BL case detection continues as in the North Mara. The value of this control area might, however, decrease with time, since in late 1977 the Tanzanian authorities initiated the distribution of chloroquin tablets in health centers throughout the whole area.

If the incidence of BL decreases dramatically in the immediate future (i. e., the next 2–3 years) in the study area but not in the control area, this will support the view that malaria acts as a promoter close to the time of development of BL and is responsible for the epidemiologic characteristics of the tumor. If congenital malaria represents a critical factor, possibly responsible for congenital EBV infection, or if malaria acts early in life (long before tumor development), one should not observe a decline in BL incidence before 6–8 years after the start of the study. During that period of time, socioeconomic changes will probably take place in socialist Tanzania and it might be difficult to interpret the results and to assess the respective roles of malaria intervention and of sociologic changes involving, primarily, maternal health and child care. If BL incidence does not change over a period of 7–10 years of active chloroquin distribution, then proof will be established that the vector and not malaria plays a key role in transmitting an oncogenic factor other than malaria.

II. INTERVENTION AGAINST THE VIRUS

When antiviral intervention is mentioned, vaccines come to mind as the most obvious means. In the common herpesvirus diseases, vaccines have been disappointing except for Marek's disease, a naturally occurring lymphoproliferative disease in chickens, for which immunization of 1-day-old chicks with either attenuated Marek's disease herpesvirus (MDV) or with a related apathogenic turkey herpesvirus has been very successful (Purchase, 1976). Furthermore, inoculation of soluble antigens extracted from MDV-infected cells was found to protect chicks against Marek's disease (Lesnick and Ross, 1975). These various vaccines are believed to act through cell-mediated immunity, humoral immunity being nonprotective (Nazerian, 1973; Chap. 17).

III. THE TIMING OF AN EBV VACCINE

Recently Epstein has proposed the development of an EBV vaccine as the only way to obtain final proof of the oncogenic potential of EBV in humans (Epstein, 1976 a, b). Three types of EBV vaccine could theoretically be envisaged. The first would be to use heat- or formaldehyde-killed EBV, in a way similar to that adopted by Laufs and Steinke in preventing herpesvirus saimiri (HVS)-induced tumors (Laufs and Steinke, 1976). The second possibility would be to use an apathogenic but interfering nonhuman herpesvirus. It should be borne in mind that, in the case of Marek's disease, this has proved to be the most effective way to prevent the disease. The third alternative would be to prepare membrane extracts of epithelial or lymphoid EBV-transformed cells, the latter being the technique suggested by Epstein. The successful utilization of membrane vesicle preparations of HVS-infected cells in preventing lymphomas induced by this virus in new-world nonhuman primates should form the experimental basis for developing similar research programs in the field of EBV (Chap. 19).

Epstein suggested that an eventual EBV vaccine for preventing EBV-induced malignancies, after being properly tested in nonhuman primate species, should be assayed for the prevention of IM in the Western world and, if this were successful, might then be applied to the prevention of BL. This is very appealing, but two difficulties could arise from the latter suggestion. The first difficulty is that high VCA antibody titers were shown in the BL prospective study (de-Thé et al., 1978 a; Sect. C) not to protect against tumor development but, instead, to represent an important risk factor. However, if the hypothesis is correct, namely that very early EBV infection is directly related to the risk of BL, then a vaccine given at birth might be effective. The second difficulty is the relative rarity of BL in Africa: one child per thousand develops BL and, although the grossness of the lesions could help to convince the public health authorities of the need to vaccinate against this rare disease, there will still be epidemiologic and ethical considerations to be overcome before implementing such a project (Higginson et al., 1971).

A vaccine in the field of NPC might be more readily acceptable. NPC is by far the most frequent ear, nose, and throat tumor in large parts of the world, representing the main cancer in males of Cantonese Chinese origin. A massive program of detection or, even better, of prevention by an eventual vaccine might be readily acceptable to the public health authorities of the countries concerned. However, a critical step before contemplating such an intervention is to determine whether certain antigenic preparations elicit a cell-mediated immune response in NPC patients and parallel the development of the disease.

The following priorities, therefore, arise: (a) to develop a nonhuman *primate model* for EBV-induced tumors in which the role of cell-mediated immunity in tumor induction by EBV could be evaluated and different types of vaccine tested (Chaps. 16 and 19); (b) to determine in humans the *pre-NPC tumor* events through a prospective seroepidemiologic study (discussed in Sect. D); and (c) to try and intervene in individuals at highest risk for NPC development. The ethical problems associated with vaccine trials could be more easily surmounted and accepted by such individuals.

F. CONCLUSIONS

The development of a cancer is a multifactorial event and the question for the epidemiologist is not to determine whether EBV is the sole cause of BL and/or NPC, but to determine if the virus is involved in any way in the causation of the diseases and if intervention against EBV is feasible. If BL can be prevented by an anti-malarial intervention, this would be very satisfying for the epidemiologist. The experimental researcher, on the other hand, wants to know if the virus is a necessary, even if not sole, factor. Secondly, he would like to know how the virus acts at the cellular level to transform cells into a premalignant or malignant state. Finally, his curiosity will lead him to intervention. The conquest of both BL and NPC will probably come by integrating further the epidemiologic approach and laboratory studies in multidisciplinary and collaborative ventures.

REFERENCES

Black, F. L., Woodall, J. P., Evans, A. S., Liebhaber, H., Henle, G.: Prevalence of antibody against viruses in Tiriyo, an isolated Amazon tribe. Am. J. Epidemiol. **91**, 430–438 (1970)

Burkitt, D.: A children's cancer dependent on climatic factors. Nature, **194**, 232–234 (1962a)

Burkitt, D.: A "tumour safari" in East and Central Africa. Br. J. Cancer **16**, 379–386 (1962b)

Burkitt, D. P.: An alternative hypothesis to a vectored virus. In: Burkitt's lymphoma. Burkitt, D. P., Wright, D. H., (eds.), pp. 210–215. Edinburgh, London: Livingstone 1970.

Buell, P.: Nasopharyngeal cancer in Chinese of California. Br. J. Cancer **19**, 459–470 (1965)

Buell, P., Race and place in the etiology of nasopharyngeal cancer: a study based on California death certificates. Int. J. Cancer **11**, 268–272 (1973)

Dalldorf, G., Linsell, C. A., Barnhart, F. E., Martyn, R.: An epidemiologic approach to the lymphomas of African children and Burkitt's sarcoma of the jaws. Persp. Biol. Med. **7**, 435–449 (1964)

de-Thé, G., Day, N. E., Geser, A., Lavoué, M. F., Ho, J. H.C., Simons, M. J., Sohier, R., Tukei, P., Vonka, V., Zavadova, H.: Seroepidemiology of the Epstein-Barr virus: preliminary analysis of an international study – a review. In: Oncogensis and herpesviruses II. de-Thé, G., Epstein, M. A., zur Hausen, H. (eds.), Part 2, pp. 3–16. Lyon: IARC 1975

de-Thé, G., Ho, J. H. C., Muir, C.: Nasopharyngeal carcinoma. In: Viral infections of humans. Evans, A. S. (ed.), pp. 539–563. New York: Plenum 1976

de-Thé, G.: Is Burkitt's lymphoma related to perinatal infection by Epstein-Barr virus? Lancet **1977 I**, 335–338

de-Thé, G., Geser, A., Day, N. E., Tukei, P. M., Williams, E. H., Beri, D. P., Smith, P. G., Dean, A. G., Bornkamm, G. W., Feorino, P. and Henle, W.: Epidemiological evidence for causal relationship between Epstein-Barr virus and Burkitt's lymphoma from Ugandan prospective study. Nature **274**, 756–761 (1978a) de-Thé, G., Lavoué, M. F., Muenz, L.: Differences in EBV antibody titres of patients with nasopharyngeal carcinoma originating from high, intermediate and low incidence areas. In: Proceedings of an International Symposium on Etiology and Control of Nasopharyngeal Carcinoma. Lyon: IARC (in press) (1978 b)

Desgranges, C., Wolf, H., de-Thé, G., Shanmugaratnam, K., Ellouz, R., Cammoun, N., Klein, G., zur Hausen, H.: Nasopharyngeal carcinoma X. Presence of Epstein-Barr genomes in epithelial cells of tumours from high and medium risk areas. Int. J. Cancer **16**, 7–15 (1975)

Epstein, M. A.: Implications for a vaccine for the prevention of Epstein-Barr virus infection: ethical and logistic considerations. Cancer Res. **36**, 711–714 (1976 a)

Epstein, M. A.: Epstein-Barr virus – is it time to develop a vaccine program? J. Natl. Cancer Inst. **56**, 697–700 (1976 b)

Evans, A. S., Niederman, J. C., McCollum, R. W.: Seroepidemiologic studies of infectious mononucleosis with EB virus. N. Engl. J. Med. **279**, 1121–1127 (1968)

Fraumeni, J. F. (Jr.), Mason, T. J.: Cancer mortality among Chinese Americans, 1950–69. J. Natl. Cancer Inst. **52**, 659–665 (1974)

Gerber, P., Nkrumah, F. K., Pritchett, R., Kieff, E.: Comparative studies of Epstein-Barr virus strains from Ghana and the United States. Int. J. Cancer **17**, 71–81 (1976)

Geser, A., de-Thé, G.: Does the Epstein-Barr virus play an aetiological role in Burkitt's lymphoma? (The planning of a longitudinal sero-epidemiological survey in the West Nile district, Uganda). In: Oncogenesis and herpesviruses, Biggs, P. M., de-Thé, G., Payne, L. N. (eds.), pp. 372–375. Lyon: IARC 1972

Geser, A., Day, N. E., de-Thé, G., Chew, T. S., Freund, R. J., Kwan, H. C., Lavoué, M. F., Simkovic, D., Sohier, R.: The variability in immunofluorescent viral capsid antigen antibody testing in population surveys of Epstein-Barr virus infection. Bull. WHO **50**, 389–400 (1974)

Gross, L.: Oncogenic viruses. Oxford: Pergamon Press 1970

Henderson, B. E., Louie, E., Jing, J. S., Buell, P., Gardner, M. B.: Risk factors associated with nasopharyngeal carcinoma. N. Engl. J. Med. **295**, 1101–1106 (1976)

Henderson, B. E., Louie, E. W., Jing, J. S., Alena, B.: Epstein-Barr virus and nasopharyngeal carcinoma: is there an etiologic relationship? J. Natl. Cancer Inst. **59**, 1393–1395 (1977)

Henle, G., Henle, W., Diehl, V.: Relation of Burkitt tumor associated herpes-type virus to infectious mononucleosis. Proc. Nat. Acad. Sci. USA **59**, 94–101 (1968)

Henle, G., Henle, W., Clifford, P., Diehl, V., Kafuko, G. W., Kirya, B. G., Klein, G., Morrow, R. H., Munube, G. M. R., Pike, M. C., Tukei, P. M., Ziegler, J. L.: Antibodies to EB virus in Burkitt's lymphoma and control groups. J. Natl. Cancer Inst. **43**, 1147–1157 (1969)

Higginson, J., de-Thé, G., Geser, A., Day, N.: An epidemiological analysis of cancer vaccines. Int. J. Cancer **7**, 565–574 (1971)

Hinuma, Y., Ohta-Hatuno, R., Suto, T.: High incidence of Japanese infants with antibody to a herpes-type virus associated with cultured Burkitt lymphoma cells. Jap. J. Microbiol. **13**, 309–311 (1969)

Ho, J. H. C.: Nasopharyngeal carcinoma in Hong Kong. In: Cancer of the nasopharynx. Muir, C. S., Shanmugaratnam, K. (eds.), pp. 58–63. UICC Monograph Series, Vol. 1. Copenhagen: Munksgaard, 1967

Ho, J. H. C.: Nasopharyngeal carcinoma (NPC). Adv. Cancer Res. **16**, 57–92 (1972)

Ho, J. H. C., Kwan, H. C., Ng, M. H., de-Thé, G.: Serum IgA antibodies to Epstein-Barr virus capsid antigen preceding symptoms of nasopharyngeal carcinoma. Lancet **1978 I**, 436

International Agency for Research on Cancer: Annual Reports, 1974, 1975, 1976, 1977

International Agency for Research on Cancer: Technical Report. Proceedings of a Planning Conference for Epidemiological Studies on Burkitt's Lymphoma and Infectious Mononucleosis. Nairobi, 16–18 December 1968

Kafuko, G. W., Henderson, B. E., Kirya, B. G., Munube, G. M. R., Tukei, P. M., Day, N. E., Henle, G., Henle, W., Morrow, R. H., Pike, M. C., Smith, P. G., Williams, E. H.: Epstein-Barr virus antibody levels in children from the West Nile District of Uganda: report of a field study. Lancet **1972 I**, 706–709

King, H., Haenszel, K.: Cancer mortality among foreign and native-born Chinese in the United States. J. Chron. Dis. **26**, 623–646 (1972)

Lang, D. J., Garruto, R. M., Gajdusek, D. C.: Early acquisition of cytomegalovirus and Epstein-Barr virus antibody in several isolated Melanesian populations. Am. J. Epidemiol. **105**, 480–487 (1977)

Laufs, R., Steinke, H.: Vaccination of non-human primates with killed oncogenic herpesvirus. Cancer Res. **36**, 704–706 (1976)

Lesnick, F., Ross, L. J. N.: Immunization against Marek's disease using MDHV specific antigens free from infectious virus. Int. J. Cancer **16**, 153–163 (1975)

Nazerian, K.: Marek's disease: a neoplastic disease of chickens caused by a herpesvirus. Adv. Cancer Res. **17**, 279–315 (1973)

Niederman, J. C., McCollum, R. W., Henle, G., Henle, W.: Infectious mononucleosis. J. Am. Med. Assoc. **203**, 139–143 (1968)

O'Conor, G.T.: Persistent immunologic stimulation as a factor in oncogenesis with special reference to Burkitt's tumor. Am. J. Med. **48**, 279–285 (1970)

Pike, M. C., Williams, E. H., Wright, D. H.: Burkitt's tumour in the West Nile District of Uganda, 1961–5. Br. Med. J. **1967 II**, 395–399

Purchase, H. G.: Prevention of Marek's disease: a review. Cancer Res. **36**, 696–700 (1976)

Shanmugaratnam, K.: Cancer in Singapore, ethnic and dialect group variations in cancer incidence. Singapore Med. J. **14**, 68–81 (1973)

Simons, M. J., Day, N. E., Wee, G. B., Chan, S. H., Shanmugaratnam, K., de-Thé, G.: Immunogenetic aspects of nasopharyngeal carcinoma (NPC). III. HL-A type as a genetic marker of NPC predisposition to test the hypothesis that EBV is an aetiologic factor in NPC. In: Oncogenesis and herpesviruses II. de-Thé, G., Epstein, M. A., zur Hausen, H. (eds.), Part 2, pp. 249–258. Lyon: IARC 1975

Tischendorf, P., Shramek, G. J., Balagdas, R. C., Deinhardt, F., Knospe, W. H., Noble, G. R., Maynard, J. E.: Development and persistence of immunity to Epstein-Barr virus in man. J. Infect. Dis. **122**, 401–409 (1970)

Williams, E. H., de-Thé, G.: Familial aggregation in nasopharyngeal carcinoma. Lancet **1974 II**, 295

Williams, E. H., Day, N. E., Geser, A. G.: Seasonal variation in onset of Burkitt's lymphoma in the West Nile District of Uganda. Lancet **1974 II**, 19–22

Williams, E. H., Smith, P. G., Day, N. E., Geser, A., Ellice, J., Tukei, P.: Space-time clustering of Burkitt's lymphoma in the West Nile District of Uganda, 1960–1975. Br. J. Cancer **37**, 109–122 (1978)

19 Vaccine Control of EB Virus-Associated Tumors

M. A. Epstein

Department of Pathology, The Medical School, University of Bristol, University Walk, Bristol BS8 1TD (England)

A. INTRODUCTION

The great progress which has been made in the understanding of Epstein-Barr virus (EBV) during the 15 years since the agent was first discovered (Epstein et al., 1964) is abundantly clear from the foregoing chapters of this book. It is also clear that work on EBV is more than justified on the basis of the interest and wide biologic and molecular insights it provides.

However, there can be no doubt that one of the central goals of tumor virology must be the prevention of a human cancer by the vaccine control of an oncogenic virus. This was explicitly recognized by the U.S. National Cancer Institute when it farsightedly set up the Special Virus-Leukemia Program in 1964 and should be kept even more to the fore now that the Program has been drastically diminished.

In order to implement work on such a vaccine it is naturally necessary to seek for unusual viruses in human cancers and thereafter to establish whether at least one such tumor might have an associated virus as cause. Thus, from the finding of a tumor-associated virus, investigation of it must proceed to the point where its behavior and properties suggest that it should be suspected of an oncogenic role in man (Rauscher et al., 1966; Baker et al., 1966).

B. EBV AS THE CAUSE OF A HUMAN CANCER

Sufficient compelling evidence for regarding EBV as a candidate human tumor virus has existed for some years (Epstein and Achong, 1973; Klein, 1973; Henle and Henle, 1974) and even 5 years ago it was not unreasonable to consider the agent not only as the leading such candidate, but also as the only convincing one. Since that time support for this view has become even firmer, and from everything discussed in this book it is obvious that all possible circumstantial evidence which can justifiably be required has been provided. EBV must now be recognized as playing an oncogenic role, at least in endemic Burkitt's lymphoma (BL) (Epstein, 1978), as the following facts bear witness:

1. BL patients have high titer antiviral antibodies with a characteristic pattern varying specifically with disease events (Chaps. 4 and 14).
2. Every tumor cell carries the virus DNA with at least one molecule linearly integrated into the host cell genome giving expression of virus-coded neoantigens (Chaps. 6, 7, 8, and 14).
3. The virus transforms normal human cells in vitro into continuously growing lines (Chaps. 10 and 11).
4. The virus induces malignant tumors experimentally in subhuman primates (Chap. 16).
5. An unusual response to the virus carries a remarkable risk factor for BL development in endemic zones (Chap. 18).
6. Known oncogenic animal herpesviruses show many similarities in behavior (Chap. 17).

Cofactors and possible ways in which they may interact with EBV to give expression to its oncogenic capability have been discussed in Chap. 14.

But despite all this circumstantial evidence, ethical constraints make direct proof of an etiologic role for EBV in BL hard to obtain; as has been emphasized before, such final proof can only come in the human context when tumor incidence can be shown to decrease following prevention of EBV infection by an antiviral vaccine (Epstein, 1975, 1976).

C. A VACCINE TO PREVENT EBV INFECTION

I. TIMING AND RATIONALE

The point has obviously now been reached in studies on EBV where the accumulation of yet more circumstantial indirect evidence on its carcinogenicity in man is quite unlikely to give definitive answers and where only the more dynamic approach of a vaccine program can resolve any last remaining uncertainties.

But quite apart from the scientific interest of showing that at least one human cancer actually has a viral etiology, there are far more important practical reasons for implementing an EBV vaccine program in relation to endemic BL. For, an effective vaccine to EBV protecting against BL in a high incidence area would give definitive proof of a causative role for the virus in this tumor and would thus immensely strengthen the likelihood that EBV is likewise an etiologic agent in the other human tumor with which it is associated, nasopharyngeal carcinoma (NPC) (Chap. 15). Although even in the high incidence areas BL does not involve very large numbers (Burkitt, 1963) and such areas are relatively restricted and have many more pressing medical problems, NPC, in contrast, affects very large numbers of people. High incidence areas of NPC are racially determined (Chap. 15), with southern Chinese having the greatest number of tumors; among the southern Chinese NPC is the most common tumor of men and second commonest tumor of women (Shanmugaratnam, 1967), and the southern Chinese and related races form about one-third of the population of the world (Shanmugaratnam, 1971). In addition, areas with a significant moderately high incidence have been recognized in South East Asia, North Africa, and East Africa (Clifford, 1970; Cammoun et al., 1974). NPC therefore constitutes a major cancer problem in terms of world health and considerable effort and expense for control would be fully justified.

An EBV vaccine program would clearly need to be carried out in two main steps: (1) a small-scale pilot experiment to prove carcinogenicity in endemic BL in a high incidence area and (2) the more difficult long-term control not only of BL but, more importantly, of NPC with its great significance in terms of numbers. Although the second step presents many problems, the first, involving the EBV and BL system, has certain unusual advantages; since EBV causes infectious mononucleosis (IM) (Chap. 13) the efficacy of a vaccine could be given preliminary testing by investigating its ability to protect those in the 15–25 age group at risk from delayed natural primary EBV infection with its high likelihood of being accompanied by IM symptoms (Niederman et al., 1970; University Health Physicians et al., 1971). Indeed, this in itself might be considered a justified objective because rising standards of living in Western communities are constantly increasing the numbers of young people suffering from IM, a disease of affluence which not only causes troublesome disruption among such groups as students and apprentices, but which is also known to carry an increased risk of subsequent Hodgkin's disease (Muñoz et al., 1978). Furthermore, there are well-recognized areas of high endemicity of BL in Africa (Pike et al., 1967; Williams et al., 1978) where the effect on tumor incidence of an efficacious anti-EBV vaccine could be tested. Finally, since endemic African BL has its peak incidence around the age of 6 years (Burkitt, 1963), the effect on tumor development of a blanket vaccination program of all 0–1 year old children could be judged in 5–10 years, far more rapidly than would be possible with most human cancers, which occur mainly late in life.

II. METHODOLOGY

The difficulties in preparing and administering to human populations a safe and effective vaccine for any suspected human tumor virus are obvious, but recent work with EBV and some oncogenic animal herpesviruses indicates that much less may be involved than has sometimes been feared in the past.

Control of a naturally occurring, herpesvirus-induced malignant tumor by an antiviral vaccine was achieved 10 years ago when live, apathogenic herpesvirus vaccines were introduced to protect chickens against Marek's lymphomas (Churchill et al., 1969; Okazaki et al., 1970; Chap. 17). The applicability of a live virus vaccine to the human situation is doubtful in the extreme because it would be impossible to administer to man a suspected tumor-inducing virus however attenuated. Indeed, even a conventionally inactivated virus of this kind would raise strong objections for use as a human vaccine because of the problem of ensuring total inactivation while maintaining antigenicity. However, further progress with vaccines against oncogenic animal herpesviruses has indicated that such difficulties can be overcome. Thus, chickens have been significantly protected against lymphomas of Marek's disease by vaccines free of viral nucleic acid; success has been obtained both with a vaccine consisting only of soluble viral antigens extracted from Marek's virus-infected tissue culture cells by treatment with nonionic detergents (Lesnick and Ross, 1975) and with a vaccine of purified plasma membranes from such cells (Kaaden and Dietzschold, 1974).

Subhuman primates have also been protected against a herpesvirus-induced malignant lymphoma; heat and formaldehyde have been used to inactivate herpesvirus saimiri (HVS), which is carcinogenic in marmosets (Meléndez et al., 1969; Chap. 17), and with this inactivated vaccine such animals have been protected against challenge with up to 200 times the usual tumor-inducing dose of the virus (Laufs and Steinke, 1975).

More recently, a nucleic acid-free plasma membrane vaccine has been developed for HVS, has so far been shown to be highly antigenic (Pearson and Scott, 1977), and will doubtless now be used to protect subhuman primates against HVS-induced malignant tumors.

As for the technical problems involved in the preparation of nucleic acid-free herpesvirus vaccines, here too, much progress has been made. The methodology for preparing cell membranes from human lymphoid cells and for purifying antigens from the isolated membranes is firmly established (Sanderson and Batchelor, 1968; Sanderson et al., 1971; Strominger et al., 1974; Crumpton and Snary, 1974) and clearly suitable for EBV-carrying cultured lymphoid cells in which the virus-determined cell surface antigens are just those responsible for eliciting virus-neutralizing antibodies (Pearson et al., 1970, 1971; Gergely et al., 1971; De Schryver et al., 1974, 1976). Suitable continuous cell lines expressing EBV membrane antigens (MA) are available and can be grown on a large scale without difficulty or special cost; furthermore, newer and simpler methods for obtaining cell membranes carrying herpesvirus antigens have been introduced (Scott, 1976) and improvements are also taking place in techniques for the enhancement of antigenicity.

III. TESTING

1. Safety

Two main safety factors must be taken into account with any EBV MA vaccine for administration to man. First, the total exclusion of virus DNA is of fundamental importance and must be confirmed in all material to be inoculated. The growth of cultures in (^{3}H)-thymidine-containing medium before harvesting cell membranes provides a highly sensitive radioactive label capable of revealing minute quantities of DNA when appropriate enzymic digestion steps are included in the tests (Pearson and Scott, 1977) and the whole procedure is both simple and straightforward.

Second, and equally important, safety also demands that the vaccine does not engender immunopathologic complications. Although such a hazard seems unlikely if purified MA are used, the problem of enhancement must be considered. It might be that the use of a killed vaccine to immunize a population at risk for BL would be justified only if immunity were maintained by booster doses through much of life, since a fall in immunity might permit late EBV infection with the development of blocking factors capable of enhancing the growth of any malignantly transformed BL cells which might subsequently emerge. However, it could equally well be that a high secondary antibody response to infection might result from previous but lapsed vaccination, might directly limit the growth of transformed cells, and would therefore be directly beneficial. These questions require preliminary testing in the laboratory using the South American subhuman primates susceptible to experimental infection and tumor induction by EBV (Epstein et al., 1973a, b, 1975; Shope et al., 1973; Deinhardt et al., 1975; Rabin et al., 1976; Miller et al., 1977; Chap. 16).

2. Efficacy

Susceptible subhuman primates are also necessary for the essential in vivo laboratory testing of the protective ability of a membrane vaccine, both as regards immunogenicity and prevention of tumors in species phylogenetically related to man. However, strict international control of the most desirable South American species has brought the supply and movement of wild-caught animals almost to a halt and the setting up of large breeding colonies for EBV vaccine work is therefore now an urgent priority.

Once vaccine protection against EBV and tumor induction has been demonstrated satisfactorily in animals and safety problems have been resolved, the efficacy of the vaccine in preventing infection by the virus in man is the next step. This can be judged in the context of seronegative young people in Western countries at risk for primary infection in the age group in which this event is accompanied by a 50% or higher incidence of IM symptoms (Niederman et al., 1970; Chap. 13). Apart from the essential information such a pilot program would provide, preliminary use of a vaccine in developed countries would be a sensible starting point from which to mount a tumor prevention program in a high incidence area for BL which will necessarily involve populations in developing countries (Chap. 14).

D. THE VACCINE PREVENTION OF EBV-RELATED TUMORS

Assuming that the preparation of a membrane vaccine, the safety testing of such a vaccine, the authentication of its effectiveness in animals, and the prevention by it of IM in EBV-negative individuals at risk can all be achieved, the stage will have been reached when a trial would be required to show that prevention of EBV infection significantly reduces BL in a high incidence area. It has already been pointed out that EBV cannot alone be responsible for the induction of endemic BL which is clearly a multifactorial disease (Epstein, 1978; Chap. 14), but as a necessary oncogenic component in the etiology, prevention of infection must have a consequential effect on the incidence of the tumor, just as in the parallel situation with the herpesvirus of Marek's disease. Here the agent is widespread in chicken populations but exerts its oncogenic effect only in combination with individual, environmental, genetic, hormonal, age, and other factors (Payne, 1973); nevertheless, vaccine protection against virulent virus prevents the development of lymphomas (Jackson et al., 1974).

For a field trial on children where BL is highly endemic, it is doubtful whether a membrane vaccine could induce sufficiently longlasting immunity, and revaccination would be required to maintain protection from the earliest postnatal months to the peak tumor age around 6 years. However, it is perfectly possible successfully to carry through complicated programs involving large numbers even in remote and underde- veloped regions as the report on the 7-year West Nile District of Uganda Prospective Study amply testifies (de-Thé et al., 1978; Chap. 18). Relatively simple financial and logistic support was required and blanket vaccination of an appropriate postnatal cohort in an area such as the West Nile District would not prove any more complicated even with the necessary follow-up and booster doses. The relatively small West Nile District has a dense population with a sufficiently high BL incidence (Pike et al., 1967; Williams et al., 1978) for a drop resulting from the antecedent vaccinations to be recognizable, and other suitable regions with similar high tumor incidences are also known (International Agency for Research on Cancer, 1976).

A vaccine program such as this seems to be the only way in which direct definitive proof can be obtained of the oncogenicity of EBV in endemic BL, along with the cofactors which clearly play a part (Chap. 14). Such proof will immensely strengthen the likelihood that the virus is also causally related to NPC and will thereby provide strong reasons for attempting the vaccine prevention of this numerically important tumor as well. However, NPC is a cancer of later life (Chap. 15) and therefore poses considerable problems in the maintenance of immunity to EBV over many years.

E. DISCUSSION

In view of the late age peak of NPC the difficulties for the vaccine control of EBV to decrease tumor incidence should not be minimized, but since NPC is the commonest tumor among a substantial section of the world population, no effort should be spared if control seems possible.

Although the circumstantial evidence incriminating EBV as the cause of NPC is less complete than with BL, nevertheless the relationship of the virus to the tumor has recently been shown to be very similar. It has long been recognized that all patients with NPC have antibodies to the virus with elevated titers and a quite characteristic pattern of reactions (Chaps. 4 and 15). In addition, the epithelial tumor cells carry EBV DNA and express the EBV nuclear antigen (EBNA) (Chaps. 6, 7, and 15). Information on the virus-cell interactions in NPC has now increased the closeness of the parallel with BL.

EBV particles cannot be found in NPC biopsy samples taken directly from patients (Svoboda et al., 1967; Gazzolo et al., 1972), but epithelial cells of some NPCs have been shown to be fully capable of supporting complete replication of the virus after separation from the usual nonmalignant infiltrating cells (Shanmugaratnum, 1971) by passage through nude mice (Klein et al., 1974) followed by treatment in vitro with 5-bromodeoxyuridine (BUDR) (Trumper et al., 1976). More importantly, further work has demonstrated that some NPC cells will replicate fully infectious EBV merely by passage in the nude mice (Trumper et al., 1977), showing that the degree of repression of the replicative function of the virus genome is capable of considerable variation and thus that it is in this respect similar to the situation in BL cells.

Activation by BUDR of EBV replication in cultured cells of some NPCs is exactly comparable to that seen in those BL tumors, such as Raji, which likewise do not produce the virus in vitro (Epstein et al., 1966) unless treated with this chemical (Hampar et al., 1972; Gerber, 1972). The "spontaneous" production of EBV by the cells of other NPC tumors when transplanted into nude mice brings the situation yet further into line with that of BL, since this effect of nude mouse passage is in many ways analogous to the activation of virus production in a proportion of cells when some BL biopsies are simply placed in culture (Epstein et al., 1965); this parallelism between the state of EBV in NPC and BL is actually complete in that examples of both tumors can be found in which virus production in vitro seemingly cannot be induced at all (Klein and Dombos, 1973; Glaser et al., 1976).

Major strain differences between EBV from different sources have not been demonstrated (Chaps. 1, 6, and 8) and the isolates so far available from NPC are like others in being both fully transforming and capable of productive infections (Trumper et al., 1977). In any event, comparison with the Marek's disease vaccine system suggests that minor strain differences do not affect control of tumor induction (Payne, 1973; Jackson et al., 1974).

It is true that the environmental cofactor(s) clearly playing a part in NPC causation (Clifford, 1970; Henderson, 1974; Henderson et al., 1976) has not been identified, but a genetic factor has been put on a firm basis (Simons et al., 1974, 1975, 1976). If the situation in NPC with its multiple causative factors should be like other similar diseases, then control of EBV infection should affect tumor incidence in just the same way that removal of cigarette smoking from among the factors causing lung cancer decreases the number of tumors in a given population (Doll and Peto, 1976).

Solution in the long-term future of the questions and problems in vaccine control of EBV-induced human malignancies should clearly be one of the main objectives for EBV research now that so many pointers have already been discovered showing the ways in which this difficult but compelling task should be undertaken. Success with this goal would more than justifiy all the world-wide effort expended on EBV so far, as well as the further endeavors which will doubtless be required in the future.

REFERENCES

Baker, C. G., Carrese, L. M., Rauscher, F.: The special virus-leukemia program of the National Cancer Institute: scientific aspects and program logic. In: Some recent developments in comparative medicine. Fiennes, R. N. T.-W. – (ed.), pp. 259–278. London, New York: Academic Press 1966

Burkitt, D.: A lymphoma syndrome in tropical Africa. Int. Rev. Exp. Pathol. **2**, 67–138 (1963)

Cammoun, M., Hoerner, G. V., Mourali, N.: Tumors of the nasopharynx in Tunisia: an anatomic and clinical study based on 143 cases. Cancer **33**, 184–192 (1974)

Churchill, A. E., Payne, L. N., Chubb, R. C.: Immunization against Marek's disease using a live attenuated virus. Nature **221**, 744–747 (1969)

Clifford, P.: *A review:* on the epidemiology of nasopharyngeal carcinoma. Int. J. Cancer **5**, 287–309 (1970)

Crumpton, M. J., Snary, D.: Preparation and properties of lymphocyte plasma membrane. Contemp. Top. Mol. Immunol. **3**, 27–56 (1974)

Deinhardt, F., Falk, L., Wolfe, L. G., Paciga, J., Johnson, D.: Response of marmosets to experimental infection with Epstein-Barr virus. In: Oncogenesis and herpesviruses II. de-Thé, G., Epstein, M. A., zur Hausen, H. (eds.), Part 2, pp. 161–168. Lyon: IARC 1975

De Schryver, A., Klein, G., Hewetson, J., Rocchi, G., Henle, W., Henle, G., Moss, D. J., Pope, J. H.: Comparison of EBV neutralization tests based on abortive infection or transformation of lymphoid cells and their relation to membrane reactive antibodies (anti MA). Int. J. Cancer **13**, 353–362 (1974)

De Schryver, A., Rosén, A., Gunvén, P., Klein, G.: Comparison between two antibody populations in the EBV system: anti-MA *versus* neutralizing antibody activity. Int. J. Cancer **17**, 8–13 (1976)

de-Thé, G., Geser, A., Day, N. E., Tukei, P. M., Williams, E. H., Beri, D. P., Smith, P. G., Dean, A. G., Bornkamm, G. W., Feorino, P., Henle, W.: Epidemiological evidence for causal relationship between Epstein-Barr virus and Burkitt's lymphoma: results of the Ugandan prospective study. Nature **274**, 756–761 (1978)

Doll, R., Peto, R.: Mortality in relation to smoking: 20 years' observation on male British doctors. Br. Med. J. **1976 II**, 1525–1536

Epstein, M. A.: Towards an anti-viral vaccine for a human cancer. Nature **253**, 6 (1975)

Epstein, M. A.: Epstein-Barr virus; is it time to develop a vaccine program? J. Natl. Cancer Inst. **56**, 697–700 (1976)

Epstein, M. A.: Epstein-Barr virus as the cause of a human cancer. Nature **274**, 740 (1978)

Epstein, M. A., Achong, B. G.: The EB virus. Annu. Rev. Microbiol. **27**, 413–436 (1973)

Epstein, M. A., Achong, B. G., Barr, Y. M.: Virus particles in cultured lymphoblasts from Burkitt's lymphoma. Lancet **1964 I**, 702–703

Epstein, M. A., Achong, B. G., Barr, Y. M., Zajac, B., Henle, G., Henle, W.: Morphological and virological investigations on cultured Burkitt tumor lymphoblasts (strain Raji) J. Natl. Cancer Inst. **37**, 547–559 (1966)

Epstein, M. A., Henle, G., Achong, B. G., Barr, Y. M.: Morphological and biological studies on a virus in cultured lymphoblasts from Burkitt's lymphoma. J. Exp. Med. **121**, 761–770 (1965)

Epstein, M. A., Hunt, R. D., Rabin, H.: Pilot experiments with EB virus in owl monkeys *(Aotus trivirgatus)* I. Reticuloproliferative disease in an inoculated animal. Int. J. Cancer **12**, 309–318 (1973 a)

Epstein, M. A., Rabin, H., Ball, G., Rickinson, A. B., Jarvis, J., Meléndez, L. V.: Pilot experiments with EB virus in owl monkeys *(Aotus trivirgatus)* II. EB virus in a cell line from an animal with reticuloproliferative disease. Int. J. Cancer **12**, 319–332 (1973 b)

Epstein, M. A., zur Hausen, H., Ball, G., Rabin, H.: Pilot experiments with EB virus in owl monkeys *(Aotus trivirgatus)* III. Serological and biochemical findings in an animal with reticuloproliferative disease. Int. J. Cancer **15,** 17–22 (1975)

Gazzolo, L., de-Thé, G., Vuillaume, M., Ho, H. C.: Nasopharyngeal carcinoma. II. Ultrastructure of normal mucosa, tumor biopsies, and subsequent epithelial growth *in vitro.* J. Natl. Cancer Inst. **48,** 73–86 (1972)

Gerber, P.: Acitvation of Epstein-Barr virus by 5-bromodeoxyuridine in "virus-free" human cells. Proc. Natl. Acad. Sci. USA **69,** 83–85 (1972)

Gergely, L., Klein, G., Einberg, I.: Appearance of Epstein-Barr virus-associated antigens in infected Raji cells. Virology **45,** 10–21 (1971)

Glaser, R., de-Thé, G., Lenoir, G., Ho, J. H. C.: Superinfection of epithelial nasopharyngeal carcinoma cells with Epstein-Barr virus. Proc. Natl. Acad. Sci. USA **73,** 960–963 (1976)

Hampar, B., Derge, J. G., Martos, L. M., Walker, J. L.: Synthesis of Epstein-Barr virus after activation of the viral genome in a "virus-negative" human lymphoblastoid cell (Raji) made resistant to 5-bromodeoxyuridine. Proc. Natl. Acad. Sci. USA **69,** 78–82 (1972)

Henderson, B. E.: Nasopharyngeal carcinoma: present status of knowledge. Cancer Res. **34,** 1187–1188 (1974)

Henderson, B. E., Louie, E., Jing, J. S., Buell, P., Gardner, M. B.: Risk factors associated with nasopharyngeal carcinoma. N. Engl. J. Med. **295,** 1101–1106 (1976)

Henle, W., Henle, G.: Epstein-Barr virus and human malignancies. Cancer **34,** 1368–1374 (1974)

International Agency for Research on Cancer: Annual Report 69–70 (1976)

Jackson, C. A. W., Biggs, P. M., Bell, R. A., Lancaster, F. M., Milne, B. S.: A study of vaccination against Marek's disease with an attenuated Marek's disease virus. Avian Pathol. **3,** 123–144 (1974)

Kaaden, O. R., Dietzschold, B.: Alterations of the immunological specificity of plasma membranes of cells infected with Marek's disease and turkey herpes viruses. J. Gen. Virol. **25,** 1–10 (1974)

Klein, G.: The Epstein-Barr virus. In: The herpesviruses. Kaplan, A. (ed.), pp. 521–555. London, New York: Academic Press 1973

Klein, G., Dombos, L.: Relationship between the sensitivity of EBV-carrying lymphoblastoid lines to superinfection and the inducibility of the resident viral genome. Int. J. Cancer **11,** 327–337 (1973)

Klein, G., Giovanella, B. C., Lindahl, T., Fialkow, P. J., Singh, S., Stehlin, J. S.: Direct evidence for the presence of Epstein-Barr virus DNA and nuclear antigen in malignant epithelial cells from patients with poorly differentiated carcinoma of the nasopharynx. Proc. Natl. Acad. Sci. USA **71,** 4737–4741 (1974)

Laufs, R., Steinke, H.: Vaccination of non-human primates against malignant lymphoma. Nature **253,** 71–72 (1975)

Lesnick, F., Ross, L. J. N.: Immunization against Marek's disease using Marek's disease virus-specific antigens free from infectious virus. Int. J. Cancer **16,** 153–163 (1975)

Meléndez, L. V., Hunt, R. D., Daniel, M. D., Garcia, F. G., Fraser, C. E. O.: Herpesvirus saimiri. II. An experimentally induced primate disease resembling reticulum cell sarcoma. Lab. Anim. Care **19,** 378–386 (1969)

Miller, G., Shope, T., Coope, D., Waters, L., Pagano, J., Bornkamm, G. W., Henle, W.: Lymphoma in cotton-top marmosets after inoculation with Epstein-Barr virus: tumor incidence, histologic spectrum, antibody responses, demonstration of viral DNA, and characterization of viruses. J. Exp. Med. **145,** 948–967 (1977)

Muñoz, N., Davidson, R. J. L., Withoff, B., Ericsson, J. E., de-Thé, G.: Infectious mononucleosis and Hodgkin's disease. Int. J. Cancer **22,** 10–13 (1978)

Niederman, J. C., Evans, A. S., Subrahmanyan, L., McCollum, R. W.: Prevalence, incidence and persistence of EB virus antibody in young adults. N. Engl. J. Med. **282,** 361–365 (1970)

Okazaki, W., Purchase, H. G., Burmester, B. R.: Protection agaitns Marek's disease by vaccination with a herpesvirus of turkeys. Avian Dis. **14,** 413–429 (1970)

Payne, L. N.: Marek's disease: a possible model for herpesvirus-induced neoplasms in man. In: Proceedings of the 3rd International Symposium of the Princess Takamatsu Cancer Research Fund: Analytic and experimental epidemiology of cancer. Nakahara, W., Hirayama, T., Nishioka, K., Sugano, H. (eds.), pp. 235–257. Tokyo: University of Tokyo Press 1973

Pearson, G., Dewey, F., Klein, G., Henle, G., Henle, W.: Relation between neutralization of Epstein-Barr virus and antibodies to cell-membrane antigens induced by the virus. J. Natl. Cancer Inst. **45,** 989–995 (1970)

Pearson, G., Henle, G., Henle, W.: Production of antigens associated with Epstein-Barr virus in experimentally infected lymphoblastoid cell lines. J. Natl. Cancer Inst. **46,** 1243–1250 (1971)

Pearson, G. R., Scott, R. E.: Isolation of virus-free Herpesvirus saimiri antigen-positive plasma membrane vesicles. Proc. Natl. Acad. Sci. USA **74**, 2546–2550 (1977)

Pike, M. C., Williams, E. H., Wright, B.: Burkitt's tumour in the West Nile District of Uganda 1961–5. Br. Med. J. **1967 II**, 395–399

Rabin, H., Pearson, G. R., Wallen, W. C., Neubauer, R. H., Cicmanec, J. L., Levy, B.: Comparative studies with different strains of Epstein-Barr virus in owl monkeys and marmosets. In: Comparative leukemia research 1975. Clemmesen, J., Yohn, D. S. (eds.). Bibl. Haemat. **43**, 326–330 (1976)

Rauscher, F. J., Carrese, L. M., Baker, C. G.: Survey of viral oncology with particular reference to lymphomas. Cancer Res. **26**, 1176–1184 (1966)

Sanderson, A. R., Batchelor, J. R.: Transplantation antigens from human spleens. Nature **219**, 184–186 (1968)

Sanderson, A. R., Cresswell, P., Welsh, K. I.: Involvement of carbohydrate in the immunochemical determinant area of HL-A substances. Nature New Biol. **230**, 8–12 (1971)

Scott, R. E.: Plasma membrane vesiculation: a new technique for isolation of plasma membranes. Science **194**, 743–745 (1976)

Shanmugaratnam, K.: Nasopharyngeal carcinoma in Asia. In: Racial and geographical factors in tumour incidence. Shivas, A. A. (ed.), pp. 169–188. Edinburgh: University of Edinburgh Press 1967

Shanmugaratnam, K.: Studies on the etiology of nasopharyngeal carcinoma. Int. Rev. Exp. Pathol. **10**, 361–431 (1971)

Shope, T., Dechairo, D., Miller, G.: Malignant lymphoma in cottontop marmosets after inoculation with Epstein-Barr virus. Proc. Natl. Acad. Sci. USA **70**, 2487–2491 (1973)

Simons, M. J., Wee, G. B., Chan, S. H., Shanmugaratnam, K., Day, N. E., de-Thé, G.: Immunogenetic aspects of nasopharyngeal carcinoma (NPC) III. HL-A type as a genetic marker of NPC predisposition to test the hypothesis that Epstein-Barr virus is an etiological factor in NPC. In: Oncogenesis and herpesviruses II. de-Thé, G., Epstein, M. A., zur Hausen, H. (eds.), Part 2, pp. 249–258. Lyon: IARC 1975

Simons, M. J., Wee, G. B., Day, N. E., Morris, P. J., Shanmugaratnam, K., de-Thé, G. B.: Immunogenetic aspects of nasopharyngeal carcinoma: I. Differences in HL-A antigen profiles between patients and control groups. Int. J. Cancer **13**, 122–134 (1974)

Simons, M. J., Wee, G. B., Goh, E. H., Chan, S. H., Shanmugaratnam, K., Day, N. E., de-Thé, G.: Immunogenetic aspects of nasopharyngeal carcinoma. IV. Increased risk in Chinese of nasopharyngeal carcinoma associated with a Chinese-related HLA profile (A2, Singapore 2). J. Natl. Cancer Inst. **57**, 977–980 (1976)

Strominger, J. L., Cresswell, P., Grey, H., Humphreys, R. E., Mann, D., McCure, J., Parham, P., Robb, R., Sanderson, A. R., Springer, T. A., Terhorst, C., Turner, M. J.: The immunoglobulin-like structure of human histocompatability antigens. Transplant. Rev. **21**, 126–143 (1974)

Svoboda, D. J., Kirchner, F. R., Shanmugaratnam, K.: The fine structure of nasopharyngeal carcinomas. In: Cancer of the nasopharynx. Muir, C. S., Shanmugaratnam, K. (eds.), pp. 163–171. Copenhagen: Munksgaard 1967

Trumper, P. A., Epstein, M. A., Giovanella, B. C.: Activation *in vitro* by BUdR of a productive EB virus infection in the epithelial cells of nasopharyngeal carcinoma. Int. J. Cancer **17**, 578–587 (1976)

Trumper, P. A., Epstein, M. A., Giovanella, B. C., Finerty, S.: Isolation of infectious EB virus from the epithelial tumour cells of nasopharyngeal carcinoma. Int. J. Cancer **20**, 655–662 (1977)

University Health Physicians and PHLS Laboratories: Infectious mononucleosis and its relationship to EB virus antibody. Br. Med. J. **1971 IV**, 643–646

Williams, E. H., Smith, P. G., Day, N. E., Geser, A., Ellice, J., Tukei, P.: Space-time clustering of Burkitt's lymphoma in the West Nile District of Uganda: 1961–1975. Br. J. Cancer **37**, 109–122 (1978)

Subject Index

Cyclic AMP, Cell Growth, and the Immune Response

Proceedings of the Symposium held at Marco Island, Florida, January 8–10, 1973. Editor: W. Braun, L. M. Lichtenstein, C. W. Parker. 1974. 106 figures, 82 tables. XV, 416 pages
ISBN 3-540-06654-3
Distribution rights for Japan:
Maruzen Co. Ltd., Tokyo

Gram-Negative Bacterial Infections and Mode of Endotoxin Actions

Pathophysiological, Immunological, and Clinical Aspects. Editors: B. Urbaschek, R. Urbaschek, E. Neter
1975. 155 partly colored figures.
XIV, 524 pages
ISBN 3-211-81292-X

W. Haas, H. von Boehmer
Techniques for Separation and Selection of Antigen Specific Lymphocytes

1978. 2 figures, 8 tables. II, 120 pages
(Current Topics in Microbiology and Immunology, Vol. 84)
ISBN 3-540-09029-0

The Immune System

27. Colloquium der Gesellschaft für Biologische Chemie. 29. April – 1. Mai 1976 in Mosbach/Baden. Editors: F. Melchers, K. Rajewsky.
1976. 104 figures. XII, 299 pages
(Colloquium Mosbach 27)
ISBN 3-540-07976-9

C. A. Knight
Chemistry of Viruses

2nd edition 1975. 54 figures. X, 325 pages
(Springer Study Edition)
ISBN 3-540-06772-8

J. L. van Lancker
Molecules, Cells, and Disease

An Introduction to the Biology of Disease.
1977. 60 figures. XV, 311 pages. (Springer Study Edition)
ISBN 3-540-90242-2

Lymphocyte Hybridomas

Second Workshop on "Functional Properties of Tumors of T and B Lymphocytes". Sponsored by the National Cancer Institute (NIH). April 3–5 1978 Bethesda, Maryland USA. Editors: F. Melchers, M. Potter, N. Warner
1978. 64 figures, 85 tables. XXIV, 246 pages
(Current Topics in Microbiology and Immunology, Vol. 81)
ISBN 3-540-08810-5

Lymphocytes, Macrophages, and Cancer

Editors: G. Mathé, I. Florentin, M.-C. Simmler
1976. 53 figures. IX, 160 pages
(Recent Results in Cancer Research, Vol. 56)
ISBN 3-540-07902-5

Lymphocytic Choriomeningitis Virus and Other Arenaviruses

Symposium held at the Heinrich-Pette-Institut für experimentelle Virologie und Immunologie, Universität Hamburg, October 16–18, 1972. Editor: F. Lehmann-Grube. Scientific Organizers of the Symposium: J. Hotchin, F. Lehmann-Grube, C. A. Mims
1973. 110 figures. XIII, 339 pages
ISBN 3-540-06403-6

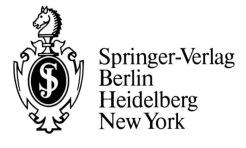

Springer-Verlag
Berlin
Heidelberg
New York

Virology Monographs/ Die Virusforschung in Einzeldarstellungen

Continuing/Fortführung von Handbook of Virus Research/ Handbuch der Virusforschung.
Editors: S. Gard, C. Hallauer, K. F. Meyer

Volume 1
H. A. Wenner,
A. M. Behbehani, L. Rosen
ECHO Viruses. Reoviruses
1968. 4 figures. IV, 107 pages
ISBN 3-211-80889-2

Volume 2
R. N. Hull, D. A. Tyrrell
**The Simian Viruses.
Rhinoviruses**
1968. 19 figures. IV, 124 pages
ISBN 3-211-80890-6

Volume 3
J. B. Hanshaw, W. Plowright, K. E. Weiss
**Cytomegaloviruses.
Rinderpest Virus. Lumpy
Skin Disease Virus**
1968. 26 figures.
IV, 131 pages
ISBN 3-211-80891-4

Volume 4
L. Hoyle
The Influenza Viruses
1968. 58 figures. IV, 375 pages
ISBN 3-211-80892-2

Volume 5
A. S. Kaplan
**Herpes Simplex and
Pseudorabies Viruses**
1969. 14 figures.
IV, 115 pages
ISBN 3-211-80932-5

Volume 6
J. Vilček
Interferon
1969. 4 figures. IV, 141 pages
ISBN 3-211-80933-3

Volume 7
B. E. Eddy, E. Norrby
**Polyoma Virus. Rubella
Virus**
1969. 22 figures. IV, 174 pages
ISBN 3-211-80934-1

Volume 8
J. Ponten
**Spontaneous and Virus
Induced Transformation in
Cell Culture**
1971. 35 figures. IV, 253 pages
ISBN 3-211-80991-0

Volume 9
W. R. Hess, P. G. Howell,
D. W. Verwoerd
**African Swine Fever Virus.
Bluetongue Virus**
1971. 5 figures. IV, 74 pages
ISBN 3-211-81006-4

Volume 10
F. Lehmann-Grube
**Lymphocytic Chorio-
meningitis Virus**
1971. 16 figures. V, 173 pages
ISBN 3-211-81017-X

Volume 11
M. J. G. Appel, J. H. Gillespie,
R. Siegert
**Canine Distemper Virus.
Marburg Virus.**
1972. 50 figures. III, 153 pages
ISBN 3-211-81059-5

Volume 12
D. Taylor-Robinson,
A. E. Caunt
Varicella Virus
1972. 10 figures. III, 88 pages
ISBN 3-211-81065-X

Volume 13
K. E. K. Rowson, B. W. J. Mahy
Lactic Dehydrogenase Virus
1975. 54 figures. IV, 121 pages
ISBN 3-211-81270-9

Volume 14
L. Philipson, U. Pettersson,
U. Lindberg
**Molecular Biology of Adeno-
viruses**
1975. 20 figures. III, 115 pages
ISBN 3-211-81284-9

Volume 15
G. Siegl
The Parvoviruses
1976. 1 figure, 10 tables.
III, 109 pages
ISBN 3-211-81355-1

Volume 16
R. W. Schlesinger
Dengue Viruses
With the collaboration of
S. Hotta
1977. 34 figures. III, 132 pages
ISBN 3-211-81406-X

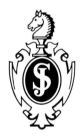

Springer-Verlag
Berlin
Heidelberg
New York